OXFORD MEDICAL PUBLICATIONS

Obstetrics and Gynaecology

Obstetrics and Gynaecology

A Critical Approach to the Clinical Problems

G. J. JARVIS

Consultant in Obstetrics and Gynaecology,
St James's University Hospital, Leeds
and
Senior Clinical Lecturer in Obstetrics and Gynaecology,
The University of Leeds

Oxford   New York   Tokyo
OXFORD UNIVERSITY PRESS
1994

Oxford University Press, Walton Street, Oxford OX2 6DP
Oxford New York Toronto
Delhi Bombay Calcutta Madras Karachi
Kuala Lumpur Singapore Hong Kong Tokyo
Nairobi Dar es Salaam Cape Town
Melbourne Auckland Madrid
and associated companies in
Berlin Ibadan

Oxford is a trade mark of Oxford University Press

Published in the United States
by Oxford University Press Inc., New York

A catalogue record for this book is available from the British Library

Library of Congress Cataloging-in-Publication Data
Jarvis, G. J. (Gerald Joseph)
Obstetrics and gynaecology : a critical approach to the clinical
problems / G. J. Jarvis.
(Oxford medical publications)
Includes bibliographical references and index.
1. Gynecology. 2. Generative organs, Female — Diseases.
3. Obstetrics. 4. Pregnancy — Complications. I. Title.
II. Series.
[DNLM: 1. Contraception. 2. Genital Diseases, Female. 3. Labor
Complications. 4. Menopause. 5. Pregnancy Complications. WQ 240J370]
RG101.J27   1991   618 — dc20   91–4298
ISBN 0–19–262058 4 (Hbk)

Typeset by Colset Private Ltd, Singapore.
Printed in Great Britain by
Bookcraft Ltd, Midsomer Norton

This book is dedicated to my wife, Liz, and my children, Thomas, Emma, and Sandy, without whose support it could not have been produced.

Preface

As medical science progresses, so medical practice evolves. Occasionally this progress is dramatic, as when a new investigative technique such as Doppler ultrasound, or a new surgical practice such as endometrial resection, is introduced. Generally, however, change arises by a multitude of smaller advances, each of which adds to our knowledge of a disease process, or influences the treatment that we give.

All doctors — both trainees and specialists — are expected to possess a detailed knowledge of the nature of the common disorders. In addition, however, they are expected to understand the scientific evidence upon which current practice should be based, and to keep abreast of recent research developments. There are innumerable areas of debate in clinical practice, yet in many cases these controversies can be largely resolved by overviewing and assessing the research data available, and applying the evidence to rational clinical practice.

This postgraduate text aims to provide such an overview, and thus hopes to encourage rational thinking and debate on topics of theoretical and clinical interest to doctors who practise obstetrics and gynaecology. Each chapter is introduced by an assessment of the relative importance of the condition under discussion to both the general population and the clinician. A detailed discussion of the subject follows which includes a synopsis of the research data upon which current practice should be based. The intention is that data should be presented in such a way that the reader may form his or her own opinion. Although my co-authors and I draw conclusions, enough information is given for the reader to assess the merit of these conclusions, and to challenge them if appropriate. Throughout the book, numerous areas where further research is indicated have been highlighted.

This book is written primarily by one author, but, where appropriate, chapters have been revised by acknowledged subject specialists. The single author approach allows for consistency of style and guards against repetition; it also enables the approach of the text to be that of a broad overview. The subject specialist input ensures that all areas are covered accurately, and that the latest research is included.

I would like to thank Jackie Maycock, Janet Thompson, and Sarah Craske for their secretarial help in producing this book and the staff of Oxford University Press for their faith and support.

Introduction to statistics

Since this book contains a significant amount of raw data upon which the conclusions which influence clinical practice are based, there is a need for a minimal number of statistical terms to be defined. The statistics used in this book are presented in such a way that the reader requires no specific knowledge of statistical methods, and statistical jargon is strenuously avoided.

The only two statistical terms regularly used in this book are 'statistically significant' and 'relative risk'. For an observation to be statistically significant, there must be a 95 per cent probability that it has not occurred by chance. A relative risk illustrates the observed result compared with the expected result. Thus, a relative risk of 1.0 means that the observed result occurred as often as the expected result, whilst a relative risk of 2.0 means that the observed result occurred twice as often as would have been expected, and a relative risk of 0.5 means that it occurred half as often as would have been expected.

Leeds   G.J.J.
March 1994

Contents

Co-authors

Professor F. Broughton Pipkin
Professor of Perinatal Physiology, The University of Nottingham.
24 Pre-eclampsia

Dr P. Crowley
Senior Lecturer, Department of Obstetrics and Gynaecology, Trinity College, Dublin.
26 Natural childbirth and intervention

Professor J. O. Drife
Professor of Obstetrics and Gynaecology, The University of Leeds.
2 The management of ectopic pregnancy

Dr M. Hamilton
Senior Lecturer in Obstetrics and Gynaecology, The University of Aberdeen.
4 The management of subfertility

Mr R. F. Lamont
Consultant in Obstetrics and Gynaecology, Northwick Park Hospital, Harrow.
22 The management of preterm labour

Mr G. Lane
Consultant Gynaecological Oncologist, St James's University Hospital, Leeds.
13 The management of carcinoma of the ovary

Professor R. J. Lilford
Professor of Obstetrics and Gynaecology, Chairman of the Institute of Epidemiology and Health Service Research, The University of Leeds.
16 Prenatal diagnosis

Dr D. T. Y. Liu
Senior Lecturer in Obstetrics and Gynaecology, The University of Nottingham.
15 Routine antenatal care

Mr D. Luesley

Senior Lecturer in Obstetrics and Gynaecology, The University of Birmingham.

11 The management of cervical intraepithelial neoplasia

12 The management of carcinoma of the cervix

Mr I. Z. MacKenzie

Clinical Reader in Obstetrics and Gynaecology, The University of Oxford.

25 The management of red cell alloimmunization

Mr M. J. A. Maresh

Consultant Obstetrician and Gynaecologist, St Mary's Hospital for Women and Children, Manchester.

23 Diabetes and pregnancy

Miss J. C. Montgomery

Consultant in Obstetrics and Gynaecology, Royal Sussex County Hospital, Brighton.

9 The management of menopause

Dr P. E. Munday

Consultant Genitourinary Physician, Watford General Hospital and St Mary's Hospital, London.

6 The management of gynaecological infections

Professor E. Newlands

Professor of Cancer Medicine, Charing Cross and Westminster Medical School, London.

3 The management of gestational trophoblastic disease

Professor P. M. S. O'Brien

Professor of Obstetrics and Gynaecology, The University of Keele.

8 The premenstrual syndrome

Mr J. M. Pearce

Consultant in Fetomaternal Medicine, St George's Hospital, London.

21 Specific infections during pregnancy

Mr J. A. D. Spencer

Senior Clinical Lecturer, Department of Obstetrics and Gynaecology, University College and Middlesex School of Medicine, University College, London.

18 The management of labour

Professor M. J. Whittle

Department of Fetal Medicine, Academic Department of Obstetrics and Gynaecology, The University of Birmingham.

17 The diagnosis and assessment of intrauterine growth retardation

1 The management of repeated miscarriage

The reported early loss rate among clinically recognizable pregnancies lies between 10 and 15 per cent overall, but rises to reach 13–26 per cent after one previous miscarriage, 17–29 per cent after two previous spontaneous miscarriages, and 25–46 per cent after three or more previous spontaneous miscarriages (Stirrat 1990). Malpas (1938) introduced the term 'habitual abortion' which is defined as three or more consecutive spontaneous miscarriages, on the assumption that there was a recurrent factor present in the 1 per cent of the population who had recurrent miscarriages which would limit the chance of this group ever having a live baby. It is important, when considering the statistics, to distinguish between primary recurrent spontaneous miscarriage (women who have never had a pregnancy which extended beyond 28 weeks) or secondary recurrent spontaneous miscarriage where even one pregnancy has extended beyond 28 weeks. Women who have had even one successful pregnancy at any stage are at a lower risk of subsequent repeated spontaneous miscarriage than are women who have not. Thus, a woman whose only previous pregnancy ended in a spontaneous miscarriage has a 16 per cent chance of a spontaneous miscarriage in a second pregnancy, whilst a woman whose first pregnancy resulted in a live birth has a 3 per cent chance of spontaneous miscarriage in the second pregnancy (Alberman 1988).

When counselling patients concerning the chance of repeated miscarriage, perhaps the statistics should be placed in a more positive fashion, thus, even after three unsuccessful pregnancies, the chance of a subsequent pregnancy being successful is at worst 54 per cent and at best 75 per cent, compared with 85 per cent for the whole population (Stirrat 1990).

The risks for spontaneous miscarriage should also be corrected for maternal age, since the incidence of spontaneous miscarriage is significantly raised in women over the age of 35 years. Poland et al. (1977) reported a prospective study of 638 women with a previous miscarriage and a spontaneous miscarriage rate of 22 per cent, not affected by gravidity. However, the risk of miscarriage was constant between maternal ages 20 and 34 years (23 per cent), but was only 13 per cent if the maternal age was less than 19, and was 48 per cent if the maternal age was between 35 and 39 (see Table 1.1). In a more recent study Cohen-Overbeek et al. (1990) reported that the spontaneous miscarriage rate between the 6th and 10th weeks of gestation rose from 1.9 per cent in women aged 36 years to 10.9 per cent for those aged 40 years or over. This increased spontaneous miscarriage rate in the older population is clearly of great

Table 1.1 Maternal age and abortion

Maternal age (years)	Pregnancies which aborted (%)
Overall (n = 638)	22
15–19	13
20–24	23
25–29	24
30–34	23
35–39	48

From Poland et al. (1977)

importance when counselling patients for invasive diagnostic procedures and is discussed in greater detail in Chapter 16 (Prenatal diagnosis).

All the above statistics are almost certainly a gross underestimate. Roberts and Lowe (1975) produced a mathematical model based on animal studies and the estimate of the number of periovulatory unprotected annual acts of the coitus in England and Wales. Although based on several assumptions, this model suggests that up to 78 per cent of conceptuses must abort, clearly mostly unrecognized. Edmonds et al. (1982) reported a prospective study in women trying to conceive. In 198 ovulatory cycles, 26 per cent resulted in a clinical pregnancy and 3 per cent in spontaneous miscarriage. However, there was chemical evidence of pregnancy in 60 per cent of the cycles, suggesting a particularly high level of unrecognized early pregnancy wastage. Other authors quote significant figures for unrecognized early pregnancy wastage although generally lower than the figures in the above study, Miller et al. (1980) quoting an unrecognized chemical pregnancy rate of 33 per cent and Wilcox et al. (1988) quoting 22 per cent. Having conceived and not aborted, patients with repeated previous miscarriage may have suboptimal subsequent pregnancy outcomes. Reginald et al. (1987) reported 118 pregnancies in 97 women with three or more spontaneous miscarriages and who reached the third trimester of pregnancy. Some 28 per cent delivered a preterm infant and 30 per cent delivered a baby whose birthweight was on or below the 10th centile for gestational age. There was a perinatal mortality rate of 161 per 1000. Parrazini et al. (1988) reported pregnancies in 158 couples who had had two or more previous spontaneous miscarriages without a previous term baby. The overall probability of delivering a live baby at term was only 64 per cent, and this fell to 46 per cent if there were four or more previous miscarriages. Similarly, such patients have a three-fold risk of bleeding at any stage during the pregnancy compared with the general obstetric population, a three-fold risk of delivering a baby with intrauterine growth retardation, a three-fold risk of a preterm delivery, and a 12-fold risk of perinatal death (Beard 1988).

There may, therefore, be a spectrum of pregnancy failure which extends from subfertility with unrecognized pregnancy loss, through recurrent miscarriage, and into perinatal loss. It is the management of those patients with recurrent miscarriage who are the subject of this chapter.

The prediction of spontaneous miscarriage

Some 25 per cent of all recognised pregnancies are complicated by bleeding but only 15 per cent miscarry, the other 10 per cent continuing (Everett *et al.* 1987). In those patients who are bleeding during early pregnancy and in those patients with a past history of miscarriage, a predictive test to distinguish between future spontaneous miscarriage and a continuing pregnancy would be of value both psychologically and economically. Biochemical tests have proved unsatisfactory for, although those patients in whom spontaneous miscarriage will occur have lower circulating levels of progesterone, oestradiol, and hCG than do patients in whom pregnancy will continue, there is too great a variation in the range of these tests to be prognostic. It may also be that the endocrine anomalies represent the effect of a poor pregnancy rather than a cause (Grudzinskas *et al.* 1988; Salem *et al.* 1984).

Ultrasonic examination of the uterus in early pregnancy has proved to be prognostic. Cashner *et al.* (1987) studied 489 patients with an ultrasonogram between the 8th and 12th weeks of pregnancy. The risk of spontaneous miscarriage occurring in women in whom a fetal heart was demonstrated was 2 per cent. Other authors have reported similar statistics in prospective studies (MacKenzie *et al.* 1988).

Ultrasound examination of early pregnancy failure in patients with a multiple conception has led to the observation of the 'vanishing twin'. Varma (1979) reported 1500 women with first trimester ultrasonic evidence of pregnancy, of whom 30 (2 per cent) showed multiple gestation sacs. Of these 30, only 15 delivered a twin pregnancy. Of the remaining 15, seven had a viable fetus in one sac and an empty second sac, (two of these seven subsequently miscarried and the other five delivered a singleton fetus), three patients had a first trimester missed abortion, and five had twin anembryonic sacs. Thus, of 30 patients with two gestation sacs, 50 per cent had a clinical multiple pregnancy, 33 per cent had a clinical abortion, and 17 per cent delivered a singleton.

The aetiology of repeated spontaneous miscarriage

Whilst a cause for repeated spontaneous miscarriage may not be found following investigation of patients with this complication, there have been claims for some degree of valid scientific evidence for the following associations with recurrent miscarriage:

(1) fetal chromosomal abnormality;

(2) parental chromosomal abnormality;

Table 1.2 Causes of repeated miscarriage and percentage of abnormalities

Cause	Tho (1979) (n = 100)*	Harger (1980) (n = 155)*	Stray-Pedersen (1984) (n = 195)*
Unknown	37	32	46
Parental chromosomes	12	15.4	3
Corpus luteal insufficiency	23	—	—
Uterine abnormality	15	27	19
Infection	—	48	15
Endocrine disorder	—	—	5
Cervical incompetence	—	—	13
Multifactorial	13	—	—

*n = no. of couples.

(3) uterine abnormality;

(4) progesterone deficiency;

(5) polycystic ovarian syndrome;

(6) intrauterine adhesions;

(7) cervical incompetence;

(8) immunological causes;

(9) collagen diseases;

(10) endocrine diseases;

(11) infections;

(12) psychological problems.

When investigating the parents with recurrent miscarriages, an abnormality may be found in up to 70 per cent of couples, and frequently more than one abnormality may be found. However, the finding of an abnormality does not necessarily mean that that is the cause of the problem, nor may it be treatable. The findings from several series in the literature are shown in Table 1.2, and it may be seen that more than one abnormality will be represented by a percentage of abnormalities greater than 100 per cent, whilst the relative incidence of some abnormalities may represent the 'special interest' of the authors. It should be noted that the only abnormalities found in all three series relate to parental chromosomes and uterine abnormality.

These abnormalities will now be discussed in detail.

Fetal chromosomal abnormality

Fetal chromosomal abnormality is a common finding in early spontaneous miscarriage. In one review of 400 spontaneous miscarriages an abnormal karyotype was reported in 21 per cent, of which the commonest types were trisomy, triploidy, and 45X (Kerr *et al*. 1966). Other authors have confirmed a similar incidence of chromosomal abnormalities in unselected spontaneous miscarriages as compared with an incidence of less than 0.5 per cent for abnormal chromosomes in the liveborn population (Carr 1967). Some authors have reported a higher statistic for the incidence of abnormal karyotypes in spontaneous miscarriages Thus, Hassold *et al*. (1980) karyotyped 1000 spontaneous miscarriages, of which 46 per cent were chromosomally abnormal, whilst Lauritsen (1976) found abnormal karyotypes in 55 per cent of 255 spontaneous miscarriages, the single most common abnormality being 45X.

It may be that spontaneous miscarriage represents a protective mechanism against the birth of some children with major chromosomal abnormalities.

Parents who have delivered a conceptus with a chromosomal abnormality may, in general, be reassured in situations other than trisomy. Boué *et al*. (1973) reported the subsequent pregnancy outcome in a 473 women with a previously karyotyped spontaneous miscarriage, of whom 60 per cent had a fetus with an abnormal karyotype. When the group with a previously abnormal karyotyped fetus was compared to the group with a previously normal karyotyped abortus, there were no differences in fecundity, incidence of congenital abnormalities in subsequent pregnancies, or incidence of subsequent spontaneous miscarriages.

Parental chromosomal abnormality

One or other of a couple who have had two previous consecutive spontaneous miscarriages are more likely to have a chromosomal abnormality (1.8 per cent) than the general population. If there have been three or more consecutive miscarriages, this abnormality rate rises to 2.3 per cent (Fitzsimmons *et al*. 1983). Tharapel *et al*. (1985) reviewed 79 published studies of approximately 8000 couples with two or more spontaneous miscarriages. The overall parental major chromosomal abnormality rate was 2.9 per cent per couple, and an abnormality was twice as likely to be found in the mother than the father. Some 50 per cent of the abnormalities were balanced translocations, and others included inversions and sex chromosome mosaicism.

As can be seen in Table 1.2 the finding of one or both partners with a major sex chromosomal abnormality in a series of patients with recurrent miscarriage is significant, and genetic counselling may be indicated in order to assess their chances of conceiving a subsequent baby with a normal karyotype.

Uterine abnormality

The commonest uterine abnormality to be found represents a failure of unification of the Mullerian system, resulting in a spectrum of abnormalities ranging from a subseptate uterus to a double uterus and cervix. The incidence of such abnormalities in the adult female population is approximately 2.3 per cent (range 1.1 to 3.5 per cent, Strassmann 1966) but may be identified in between

9.7 per cent and 17.4 per cent of all women with a history of habitual abortion (Harger *et al.* 1983; Stray-Pedersen and Stray-Pedersen 1984).

However, the finding of such an abnormality should not necessarily be taken to equate with its role as an aetiological factor in recurrent miscarriage (Stirrat 1990). A uterine abnormality, typically, is said to relate to the second trimester miscarriage of a live fetus rather than a first trimester loss (Carp *et al.* 1990). Although some authors do feel that an intrauterine anatomical abnormality may be of importance in disorders of implantation (Bennett 1987), other authors have concluded that there is no good evidence for a causal relationship between congenital uterine abnormality and first trimester miscarriage (Treffers 1990).

Fibroids are commonly found in association with subfertility (10–20 per cent), especially in older women, but are found in only 2 per cent of women with recurrent miscarriage. It is not clear just how often a submucous fibroid is the cause of miscarriage (Stray-Pedersen and Stray-Pedersen 1984; Treffers 1990).

Progesterone deficiency

Patients who are destined to miscarry will have a consistently lower pregnanediol excretion when compared with women who will continue their pregnancies, but it may be that this simply describes either a poor corpus luteum or poor placental development rather than an aetiological factor (Shearman and Garrett 1961).

Schweditsch *et al.* (1979) compared hormonal profiles in 18 women with ongoing pregnancies with six with a blighted ovum. In those with an ongoing pregnancy, β-hCG peaked at the 9th week and was consistently higher than in those patients with a blighted ovum. In ongoing pregnancies, serum pregnanediol declined between weeks five and eight, and then increased again from week eight onwards. Three of the six patients with the blighted ovum showed a normal pregnanediol profile, but three showed low pregnanediol excretions. Horta *et al.* (1977) reported a prospective study of progesterone profiles in 15 non-pregnant women of proven fertility and 15 women in early luteal phase of an ongoing pregnancy. The progesterone levels in the first seven days following ovulation were identical in both, but both the peak progesterone levels and the area of the progesterone profile were lower in 10 women with a past history of recurrent miscarriage.

Although progesterone deficiency and/or corpus luteum insufficiency have been implicated as a cause of recurrent miscarriage in some 35–60 per cent of cases, it is a difficult diagnosis to confirm, especially in a woman who is already pregnant (Carp *et al.* 1990; Lee 1987; Stirrat 1990).

Polycystic ovarian syndrome

Polycystic ovarian syndrome has been implicated as a possible cause of recurrent miscarriage. Evidence for the presence of polycystic ovarian syndrome (based on ultrasonic appearances and luteinizing hormone estimations) has been reported in 82 per cent of 56 women who had recurrent miscarriages compared with 18 per cent of parous controls, and 22 per cent of 'normal' women (Polson *et al.* 1988; Sagle *et al.* 1988).

The best and most recent evidence for the possibility of polycystic ovarian syndrome as an aetiological factor comes from Regan *et al.* (1990) who reported a prospective study based upon prepregnancy follicular phase luteinizing hormone concentrations in 193 women with regular spontaneous menstrual cycles. Of 147 women with normal LH concentrations, 88 per cent conceived but 12 per cent of these pregnancies miscarried. Of 46 women with raised LH concentrations, 67 per cent conceived but 65 per cent of these pregnancies miscarried.

In order to confirm this syndrome as an aetiological factor, further studies are indicated.

Intrauterine adhesions

Intrauterine adhesions or synechiae have been reported in women with recurrent miscarriage and it is thought that these adhesions may interfere with implantation (Bergquist *et al.* 1981). The diagnosis is generally made either by hysterosalpingography or by hysteroscopy. In a study of the world literature, 14 per cent of 2151 women with intrauterine adhesions presented with recurrent miscarriage, whilst 43 per cent of patients showed subfertility. In a population of patients with recurrent miscarriage, only 1 per cent had synechiae (Schenker and Margalioth 1982; Stray-Pedersen and Stray-Pedersen 1984).

Cervical incompetence

It is difficult to make an accurate assessment of the incidence of this condition since the diagnosis is generally made upon a classical history. Even the so-called 'objective tests', such as the resistance to the passage of a Hagar 8 dilator is itself subjective, whilst premenstrual hysterosalpingography may also be subject to reporter discretion (Edmonds 1988; Harger 1980). It is possible that the use of vaginal ultrasound assessment of the cervix during early pregnancy will allow for a more accurate assessment of this condition (Edmonds 1988; Stirrat 1990).

Some authors have implicated cervical incompetence as an aetiological factor in up to 13 per cent of women with recurrent miscarriages, whilst other estimates give up to 33 per cent of *all* miscarriages, especially those occurring during the second trimester (Harger *et al.* 1983; Stray-Pedersen and Stray-Pedersen 1984). There is also the suggestion that cervical incompetence should be considered as a possible cause of first trimester miscarriage even in the absence of a classical history (Edmonds 1988).

Immunological causes

The conceptus must demonstrate both paternal and maternal antigens, and there exists at least one mechanism whereby the conceptus is not rejected by the maternal tissues.

Most of the available information relates to the major histocompatibility antigens which were, initially, considered not to be expressed in trophoblast. However, it is now thought that this early work was technically inaccurate and that major (and minor) histocompatibility antigens may be detected in both the trophoblast and in the pre-implantation embryo (Billington 1988).

The sera of parous women contain antibodies with specific inhibitory activity against materno–fetal and materno–paternal allogenic reactions (so-called blocking antibody). It is argued that the maternal production of blocking antibodies after implantation prevents the immune rejection of the conceptus, and that a failure of this mechanism may be the cause of some first trimester miscarriages, especially in women who have never had a successful pregnancy (De Jong *et al.* 1990).

However, the evidence for this basic immunological theory is poor. The proponents of this theory would argue that couples with recurrent, consecutive spontaneous miscarriages are genetically more similar than those with successful pregnancies, and that this genetic similarity results in poor stimulation of blocking antibody (Beer *et al.* 1981; Mowbray *et al.* 1987). Other authors have not been able to identify a relationship between maternal cytotoxic alloantibody production and the subsequent protection from recurrent, spontaneous miscarriage (Sargent *et al.* 1988), whilst other workers have not been able to find evidence of increased recurrent, spontaneous miscarriages within religious sects characterized by intermarriage which should be associated with high levels of antigen sharing (Ober *et al.* 1985).

There has also been debate as to the nature of the antigens involved in the non-rejection of the conceptus, assuming that this theory is relevant in some patients. Initially it was considered that the major histocompatibility antigens, HLA-A,B,C, or D, were involved (Beer *et al.* 1981); however, it is now considered that these antigens are not the important, ones but that either HLA-G or the minor trophoblast–lymphocyte cross-reactive (TLX) antigens are involved (Ellis and McMichael 1939; McIntyre 1988). Other workers have suggested a different form of immunological cause for recurrent spontaneous abortion. Hill *et al.* (1992) have suggested that there is a cellular T lymphocyte produced in response to stimulation by sperm or trophoblast antigens which is found in some women with a history of recurrent spontaneous miscarriage (but not in women with a normal reproductive history) which is capable of toxicity against either embryo or trophoblast tissues.

There is no doubt that the complexities of the immunological non-rejection of the fetus have yet to be fully elucidated and even the relative importance of current observations is yet to be fully understood. In the meantime, it seems likely that at least some patients with recurrent spontaneous miscarriage have an immunological cause for their problems, and, in the absence of other detectable causes, are candidates for referral to a specialist centre for immunological evaluation either to receive direct help for themselves or to help in the accumulation of immunological information (Scott *et al.* 1987).

Collagen disorders

There are numerous series in the literature which associate an increased incidence of recurrent miscarriage with various collagen diseases, now termed autoimmune disorders. Of these, those associated with the lupus anticoagulant are probably the most important clinically.

Grigor *et al.* (1977) reported a series of 44 women with systemic lupus erythematosus (s.l.e.) sharing 137 pregnancies, 64 after the onset of the disease and 73 before the clinical onset. Only 32 live babies resulted from the 64 pregnancies, in which there was also a spontaneous miscarriage rate of 36 per cent and two stillbirths; this represented a perinatal mortality rate of 51 per 1000 total births. There was also suboptimal pregnancy performance in the 73 pregnancies before the clinical onset of disease, 18 pregnancies (25 per cent) terminating in a spontaneous miscarriage.

The lupus anticoagulant is an immunoglobulin which is associated to a varying degree with s.l.e. Although able to prolong coagulation times in the laboratory, it is associated with an increased risk of thrombotic episodes, both venous and arterial, together with an increased risk of repeated first trimester miscarriages, and second and third trimester intrauterine death (Lubbe *et al.* 1984). In another series of 81 pregnancies in women with lupus anticoagulant, there were 55 first trimester miscarriages (68 per cent), 16 *in utero* deaths (20 per cent), and only 10 live births (12 per cent) (Prentice *et al.* 1984). Numerous other series have confirmed this association between the presence of lupus anticoagulant and recurrent pregnancy loss (Branch *et al.* 1985; Lockshin *et al.* 1986; MacLean *et al.* 1994).

It is not clear how the presence of lupus anticoagulant results in pregnancy loss, but the favoured explanation relates to thrombosis in the placental vasculature. However, it is unlikely that this is the total explanation (Harris 1988).

Endocrine disorders

There is very little evidence to accept impaired glucose tolerance as a cause of repeated miscarriage. In a meta-analysis of over 50 published studies concerning diabetes and spontaneous miscarriage, Kalter (1987) concluded that diabetes is not a cause of miscarriage unless the prepregnancy diabetic control is particularly poor. This finding is confirmed by other authors (Miodovnik *et al.* 1986) and is discussed further in Chapter 23 (Diabetes in pregnancy).

Similarly, it is doubtful whether disorders of thyroid function are a cause of recurrent miscarriage (Stirrat 1990) even though some series have identified abnormalities of thyroid function in 2 per cent of couples with habitual miscarriages, possibly coincidentally (Stray-Pedersen and Stray-Pedersen 1984).

Infections

It is doubtful whether infection is a cause for recurrent miscarriage, the evidence being largely anecdotal and possibly relating to the enthusiasm with which the authors assess the patients microbiologically (Stirrat 1990). However, *Toxoplasma*, *Mycoplasma*, *Chlamydia*, and *Listeria* spp. have all been implicated in recurrent miscarriage.

Chlamydia sp. is found as frequently in patients with a history of recurrent miscarriage as it is in the normal sexually active population and cannot be considered to be a cause of recurrent miscarriage (Munday *et al*. 1984; Quinn *et al*. 1987; Sweet *et al*. 1987). Similarly, there is no convincing evidence to implicate *Listeria* sp. with recurrent miscarriage (Stray-Pedersen and Stray-Pedersen 1984).

Mycoplasma is no more common in couples with recurrent miscarriage than in those with successful pregnancies (Harger *et al*. 1983). At one time there was interest in the microorganism *Ureaplasma* which is closely related to *Mycoplasma* and was found in cultures taken from the cervix of 48 per cent of women with a history of recurrent miscarriage (Harger *et al*. 1983). Similarly, the organism was isolated from the endometrium in 28 per cent of women with recurrent miscarriages, but only from 10 per cent of normally fertile controls (Naessens *et al*. 1987). However, in a retrospective study of 4934 pregnant women, no differences were found in the gestational age of delivery between those women with positive cervical cultures for ureaplasma and those with negative cultures even though the organism was identified from 66 per cent of the entire population (Carey *et al*. 1991).

It seems unlikely that any of these organisms represent a cause of recurrent miscarriage.

Psychological problems

It is well recognized that couples with recurrent spontaneous miscarriage are under a great psychological strain. Although it is tempting to extrapolate that the high incidence of successful pregnancies associated with placebo seen in a few trials is evidence for a psychogenic aetiology in some cases of miscarriage, there is no real evidence to implicate psychological stress as a true aetiological factor.

From the above, it is clear that not all of the proposed aetiologies for recurrent miscarriage are equally valid. Similarly, as will be discussed below, they are not equally treatable. However, it is appropriate to investigate couples with recurrent miscarriage with a view to giving them an explanation for their problem and appropriate therapy where possible.

Examination of fetal material for chromosomes may enable a satisfactory explanation to be given, and couples with recurrent miscarriage should undergo chromosomal analysis with the appropriate genetic counselling when an abnormality is found. Uterine abnormalities should be looked for, although caution is required in attributing any abnormalities found to the underlying problem. Evidence for polycystic ovarian syndrome and autoimmune disease should also be sought. Evidence for progesterone deficiency and cervical incompetence may only really be obtained during a pregnancy, and intrauterine adhesions are relatively rare. Couples in whom the above series of investigations fail to demonstrate a cause may be referred for more detailed immunological assessment. It seems unlikely that a search for an endocrine disease or pelvic infection is of any value.

Treatment of recurrent early pregnancy loss

Only those conditions in which there is a possibility of specific treatment will be discussed. It is somewhat artificial to separate the aetiology of recurrent miscarriage from treatment, but the author felt that this would enable a clearer assessment of the literature to be obtained.

When the results of any treatment are considered, it should be borne in mind that a minimum of 54 per cent of patients would have a successful outcome without treatment and very few series in the literature have involved the use of placebo-controlled trials. These features make an accurate assessment of the results of treatment relatively difficult.

Uterine abnormality

The place of surgery in the treatment of uterine abnormality can only be gleaned from uncontrolled studies reported in the literature. The classical report by Strassmann (1966) reported a series of 263 metroplasties accumulated from various authors. Some 177 women conceived after this procedure, and pregnancy details are known for 170 of these women in 235 documented pregnancies. There were 32 spontaneous abortions or preterm pregnancies (14 per cent) and 203 term pregnancies (86 per cent). There is a more recent review of the literature (Treffers 1990), which looked at 11 series taken from the literature and involved 608 patients. Prior to metroplasty, the incidence of miscarriage ranged from 65 to 98 per cent of pregnancies, whereas after metro-plasty the incidence of miscarriage ranged from 12 to 26 per cent, suggesting the value of the procedure in selected patients. It is also possible to resect uterine septa using the hysteroscope. In one series involving 91 patients, 87 per cent of 63 post-operative pregnancies were successful compared with only 5 per cent of 240 pre-operative pregnancies (March and Israel 1987). More recent studies continue to produce such results (Fedele *et al.* 1993; Kirk *et al.* 1993).

The removal of fibroids, either by myomectomy or by hysteroscopy, should only be performed for a submucous fibroid (Treffers 1990). A literature review demonstrated that prior to myomectomy, 41 per cent of 1063 pregnancies ended in miscarriage, whereas after myometomy 19 per cent of 502 pregnancies miscarried (Buttram and Reiter 1981).

There is, therefore, good circumstantial evidence that metroplasty on patients with recurrent miscarriage may be successful, but the only way in which its exact place in the treatment of either early first trimester miscarriage due to disorders of implantation or later miscarriage can be assessed is by the use of randomized controlled trials.

Progesterone deficiency

There were numerous trials on the use of progesterone and recurrent abortion in the 1950s and 1960s which were either too small, or uncontrolled, or both.

There have been two recent meta-analyses of the effect of progesterone administration during pregnancy in an attempt to prevent miscarriage. Daya (1989) concluded a beneficial effect upon the risk of early pregnancy failure, whilst Goldstein et al. (1989) could find no such benefit. Goldstein et al. (1989) reported a meta-analysis of 15 randomized trials of progestogens, in which 9.5 per cent of 819 women taking a progestogen miscarried compared with 8.9 per cent of 841 controls. Daya (1989) reported a meta-analysis of three randomized trials, all included in the meta-analysis by Goldstein et al., but specifically selected to test progestogen therapy commenced in early pregnancy in women with repeated miscarriage. Daya reported that 22 per cent of 50 patients receiving progestogens miscarried compared with 47 per cent of 45 patients given placebo.

Polycystic ovarian syndrome

If polycystic ovarian syndrome is a cause of some recurrent miscarriages, then treatment of this syndrome should improve the results of pregnancy. Treatment may be achieved either by the use of clomiphene or by pituitary suppression followed by induction of ovulation.

Johnson and Pearce (1990) randomized 40 women with polycystic ovarian syndrome and primary recurrent spontaneous miscarriage to receive either clomiphene alone or buserelin for pituitary suppression followed by pure follicle-stimulating hormone (FSH). Spontaneous miscarriage occurred in 55 per cent of the 20 pregnancies in the women allocated to receive clomiphene but in only 10 per cent of the 20 following buserelin and FSH. However, since the buserelin–FSH treatment is expensive and time consuming, it is perhaps more appropriate to restrict it to those women who do not achieve a successful pregnancy following clomiphene.

Intrauterine adhesions

Intrauterine adhesions may be treated by either curettage, lysis with a hysteroscope, the insertion of an IUCD for up to two months, or the insertion of a

Foley catheter for seven days. The spontaneous abortion rate before treatment has been reported as 78 per cent and after treatment 20 per cent (Bergquist *et al.* 1981). Other authors have reported that, after treatment for synechiae, miscarriage occurred in 26 per cent of 245 pregnancies, or in 23 per cent of 298 pregnancies, compared with 40 per cent of 165 pregnancies prior to treatment (Schenker and Margalioth 1982; Treffers 1990).

Cervical incompetence

There are numerous reports about the value of cervical cerclage in uncontrolled trials, but the value of this technique in controlled trials is yet to be proven (Frieden *et al.* 1990).

The majority of the available information concerns the use of cervical cerclage on an elective basis in women with a past history suggestive of cervical incompetence. For instance, Harger (1980) reported that prior to the insertion of a McDonald suture in a group of 139 patients, only 19 per cent of pregnancies were successful, whereas after insertion the figure rose to 78 per cent. Similarly, after the insertion of a Shirodkar suture, the fetal survival rate rose from 20 per cent to 87 per cent. In a review of the world literature involving 33 series and almost 4000 patients, Treffers (1990) reported that the range for the delivery of surviving fetuses before insertion of the suture lay between 10 and 31 per cent but after insertion of the suture this figure rose to 60–100 per cent.

The randomized controlled MRC–RCOG trial (1988 and 1993) suggested some support for the use of cervical cerclage when obstetricians were 'uncertain' whether or not to recommend this treatment. In this trial, 13 per cent of 647 patients allocated to cervical cerclage delivered between 13th and 32nd weeks of pregnancy compared with 17 per cent of 645 patients who did not undergo a cerclage but cerclage was associated with a doubling of the risk of puerperal pyrexia (6 per cent compared with 3 per cent). The trial concluded that, on balance, cervical cerclage should be offered to women at high risk such as those with a history of three or more pregnancies ending before 37 weeks' gestation. Other randomized trials of cervical cerclage have failed to demonstrate any benefit in either the period of gestation at which delivery occurred, or in the survival rate following cervical cerclage compared with controls (Lazar *et al.* 1984).

There is some evidence that emergency insertion of a cervical suture may allow pregnancy to continue, although there are no randomized trials in this technique. Harger (1980) reported a fetal survival rate of 53 per cent after the insertion of an emergency McDonald suture and 68 per cent after the insertion of an emergency Shirodkar suture. Similarly, MacDougall and Siddle (1991) reported that 63 per cent of babies survived following the insertion of an emergency cervical suture in 19 women between the 16th and 28th weeks of gestation. It can only be assumed that both of these series represent a significant improvement over no treatment and it may not be ethical to perform a randomized controlled trial in this situation.

The observation that elective insertion would appear to be superior to emergency insertion, based upon the above statistics, may represent an over-treatment in the elective group.

There is some evidence from uncontrolled trials for the use of cervical cerclage in women with recurrent first trimester abortion. In a study of 37 patients who underwent first trimester cervical cerclage, 95 per cent delivered live babies (Edmonds 1988). The need to demonstrate that this is a statistically significant observation based upon a larger controlled study is clear.

Immunological causes

The hypothesis behind immunological treatment is that women without antipaternal antibodies may be stimulated into producing blocking antibody by receiving partner lymphocytes and this was supported by early anecdotal evidence (Taylor and Faulk 1981). However, there is some problem in accepting this hypothesis in that only 38 per cent of women who have had live births have detectable antipaternal antibody (Regan 1988).

In a randomized double-blind controlled trial of immunization, 27 women conceived having received their own leukocytes and 63 per cent aborted, whilst 22 women conceived following injection with their husband's leukocytes and 23 per cent aborted (Mowbray *et al.* 1985). These results were highly significant for the benefit of immunization with paternal cells compared with placebo immunization. There is a possibility of toxic reactions, including a 'flu-like malaise, swelling at the injection site, abdominal cramps, vomiting, and rigors. In subsequent reports, involving immunization of over 400 women, a success rate in the order of 80 per cent has been reported (Mowbray 1986, 1988). Other authors, but not in placebo controlled trials, have reported livebirth rates in the region of 89 per cent (McIntyre *et al.* 1986), but not all workers have demonstrated any benefit from this treatment (Beer 1986; De Jong *et al.* 1990). There is a need for larger, randomized, controlled trials on the use of immunotherapy in these patients since smaller trials have failed to show any benefit (Cauchi *et al.* 1991; Fraser *et al.* 1993; Ho *et al.* 1991).

There have been recent reports concerning other methods of immunization of women with a history of recurrent miscarriage. Following infusion with a placental trophoblast preparation, 76 per cent of 21 patients with recurrent miscarriage had a successful pregnancy (Johnson *et al.* 1988), whilst polyvalent immunoglobulin has been used in a series of 36 patients with recurrent miscarriage 81 per cent of whom reached the third trimester (Mueller-Eckhardt *et al.* 1991). Again, the need for larger, randomized, controlled trials is apparent.

Collagen diseases

In systemic lupus erythematosus, successful pregnancies have been reported following treatment with low-dose aspirin, systemic steroids, and heparin

(Lubbe *et al.* 1984; Regan 1991; Rosove *et al.* 1990). Such series have tended to involve small numbers of patients and be uncontrolled, such that a prospective randomized trials of therapy has yet to be reported (Harris 1988).

Psychological problems

The evidence for the benefit of psychological support in reducing the rate of recurrent spontaneous miscarriage is essentially anecdotal (Stack 1990). However, the benefits of 'tender loving care' have been assessed (Stray-Pedersen and Stray-Pedersen 1984, 1988). These authors reported 158 women with a history of recurrent miscarriage but without any detectable cause. Some 116 women received 'tender loving care' by which was meant psychological support with weekly medical and ultrasound examinations, with the avoidance of heavy work, travelling, and sexual intercourse until they had reached the mid-trimester of pregnancy. During the remainder of the pregnancy they received the usual style of antenatal care. Some 85 per cent of these women had successful pregnancies, whereas only 36 per cent of the other 42 women had a successful pregnancy. It is both important, and of interest, to discover which, if any, of these aspects of 'tender loving care' represents scientifically proven treatment for women with recurrent miscarriage.

Conclusions

Recurrent pregnancy failure is a difficult problem in that a cause may not always be found and the treatment may not always be available. Current methods of investigation will fail to identify a cause in almost 50 per cent of couples (Scott *et al.* 1987; Stray-Pedersen and Stray-Pedersen 1988). When treatment is available, the options have frequently not been assessed by means of randomized controlled trials and there is a great need for such studies in the management of patients with recurrent pregnancy loss.

The concept of a relationship between miscarriage and subfertility is not new, but since some causes of subfertility may also be causes of recurrent miscarriage, the treatment of these may result in an overall improvement in fecundity (Johnson and Pearce 1990).

Throughout this chapter, the author has observed the increasing trend towards the use of the word miscarriage rather than abortion (Chalmers 1992). As a generalization, women prefer a term other than abortion to be used since the overtones of induced or illegal abortion may contrast with the woman's disappointment at the unwanted loss of a pregnancy.

Acknowledgement

The author wishes to thank Professor G. M. Stirrat for his help and advice in the preparation of this chapter.

References

Alberman, E. (1988). The epidemiology of repeated abortion. In *Early pregnancy loss* (ed. R. W. Beard and F. Sharp), pp. 9–17. Springer–Verlag, London.

Beard, R. W. (1988). Clinical associations of recurrent miscarriage. In *Early pregnancy loss* (ed. R. W. Beard and F. Sharp), pp. 3–8. Springer–Verlag, London.

Beer, A. E. (1986). New horizons in the diagnosis, evaluation, and therapy of recurrent spontaneous abortion. *Clinics in Obstetrics and Gynecology* 13, 115–24.

Beer, A. E., Quebbeman, J. F., Ayers, J. W. T., and Haines, R. F. (1981). Major histocompatibility complex antigens and chronic habitual abortion. *American Journal of Obstetrics and Gynecology* 141, 987–9.

Bennett, M. J. (1987). Congenital abnormalities of the fundus. In *Spontaneous and recurrent abortion* (ed. M. J. Bennett and D. K. Edmonds), pp. 109–29. Blackwells, Oxford.

Bergquist, C. A., Rock, J. A., and Jones, H. W. (1981). Pregnancy failure following treatment of intra-uterine adhesions. *International Journal of Fertility* 26, 107–11.

Billington, W. D. (1988). Antigen expression by cells of the conceptus before, during, and after implantation. In *Early pregnancy loss* (ed. R. W. Beard and F. Sharp), pp. 205–12. Springer–Verlag, London.

Boué, J. G., Boué, A., Lazar, P., and Guguen, S. (1973). Outcome of pregnancy following spontaneous abortion with chromosomal anomalies. *American Journal of Obstetrics and Gynecology* 116, 806–12.

Branch, D. W., Scott, J. R., Kochenour, N. K., and Hershgolde, (1985). Obstetric complications associated with the lupus anticoagulant. *New England Journal of Medicine* 313, 1322–6.

Buttram, V. C. and Reiter, R. C. (1981). Uterine leiomyomata. *Fertility Sterility* 36, 433–45.

Carp, H. J. A., Toder, V., Mashiach, S., Nebel, L., and Serr, D. M. (1990). Recurrent Miscarriage. *Obstetric and Aynecdogical Survey* 45, 657–9.

Carr, D. H. (1967). Chromosome abnormalities as a cause of spontaneous abortion. *American Journal of Obstetrics and Gynecology* 97, 283–93.

Carey, J. C., Blackwelder, W. C., Nugent, R. P., Matterson, M. A., Rao, A. V., Eschenbuch, D. A., *et al.* (1991). Antepartum cultures for Ureaplasma urealyticum are not useful. *American Journal of Obstetrics and Aunecology* 164, 728–33.

Cashner, K. A., Christopher, C. R., and Dysert, G. A. (1987). Spontaneous fetal loss after demonstration of a live fetus. *Obstetrics and Gynecology* 70, 827–30.

Cauchi, M. N., Lim, D., Young, D. E., Kloss, M., and Pepperell, R. J. (1991). Treatment of recurrent aborters by immunization. *American Journal of Reproductive Immunology* 25, 16–17.

Chalmers, D. (1992). Terminology used in early pregnancy loss. *British Journal of Obstetrics and Gynaecology* 99, 357–8.

Cohen-Overbeek, T. E., Hop, W. C. T., Denouden, M., Pjipers, L., Jahoda, M. G. J., and Wladimiroff, J. W. (1990). Spontaneous abortion rate and advanced maternal age: consequences for prenatal diagnosis. *Lancet* ii, 27–9.

Daya, S. (1989). Efficacy of progesterone support for pregnancy in women with recurrent miscarriage. *British Journal of Obstetrics and Gynaecology* 96, 275–80.

De Jong, M. H. H., Bruinse, H. W., and Termijtelen, A. (1990). The immunology of normal pregnancy and recurrent abortion. In *Early pregnancy failure* (ed. H. J. Huisjes and T. Lind), pp. 27–38. Churchill Livingstone, Edinburgh.

Edmonds, D. K. (1988). Use of cervical cerclage in patients with recurrent first trimester abortion. In *Early pregnancy loss* (ed. R. W. Beard and F. Sharp), pp. 411–15. Springer–Verlag, London.

Edmonds, D. K., Lindsay, K. S., Miller, J. F., Williamson, E., and Wood, P. J. (1982). Early embryonic mortality in women. *Fertility Sterility* **38**, 447–52.

Ellis, S. A. and McMichael, A. J. (1989). Expression of unusual HLA class 1 on human extravillous trophoblast and a choriocarcinoma cell line. *Journal of Reproductive Immunology*, supp, 18–9.

Everett, C., Ashurst, H., and Chalmers, I. (1987). Repeated management of the threatened miscarriage by general practitioners in Wessex. *British Medical Journal* **295**, 583–6.

Fedele, L., Arcaini, L., Parazzini, F., Vercellini, P., and DiNola, G. (1993). Reproductive prognosis after hysteroscopic metroplasty. *Fertility Sterility* **59**, 768–72.

Fitzsimmons, J., Wapner, R. J., and Jackson, L. G. (1983). Repeated pregnancy loss. *American Journal of Medical Genetics* **16**, 7–13.

Fraser, E. J., Grimes, D. A., and Schultz, K. F. (1993). Immunization as treatment for recurrent spontaneous abortion. *Obstetrics and Gynecology* **82**, 854–9.

Frieden, F. J., Ordorican, S. A., Hoskins, I. A., and Young, B. K. (1990). The Shirodkar operation. *American Journal of Obstetrics and Gynecology* **163**, 830–3.

Goldstein, P., Berrier, J., Rosen, S., Sacks, H. S., and Chalmers, I. C. (1989). A meta-analysis of randomized controlled trials of progestogen agents in pregnancy. *British Journal of Obstetrics and Gynaecology* **96**, 267–74.

Grigor, R. R., Shervington, P. C., Hughes, G. R. V., and Hawkins, D. F. (1977). Outcome of pregnancy in systemic lupus erythematosus. *Proceedings of the Royal Society of Medicine* **70**, 99–100.

Grudzinskas, J. G., Stabile, I., and Campbell, S. (1988). Early pregnancy failure: biochemical and biophysical assessment. In *Early pregnancy loss* (ed. R. W. Beard and F. Sharp), pp. 183–90. Springer–Verlag, London.

Harger, J. H. (1980). Comparison of success and morbidity of cervical cerclage procedures. *Obstetrics and Gynecology* **56**, 543–8.

Harger, J. H., Archer, D. F., Marcheses, G., Muracca-Clems, M., and Garver, K. L. (1983). Aetiology of recurrent pregnancy losses and outcome of subsequent pregnancies. *Obstetrics and Gynecology* **62**, 574–81.

Harris, E. N. (1988). Clinical and immunological significance of anti-phospholipid antibodies. In *Early pregnancy loss* (ed. R. W. Beard and F. Sharp), pp. 43–60. Springer–Verlag, London.

Hassold, T., Chen, N., Funkhouser, J., Jones, T., Matsuura, J., *et al.* (1980). A cytogenic study of 1000 spontaneous abortions. *Annals of Human Genetics* **44**, 151–78.

Hill, J. A., Polgar, K., Harlow, B. L., and Anderson, D. J. (1992). Evidence of embryo- and-trophoblast-toxic cellular immune response in women with recurrent spontaneous abortion. *American Journal of Obstetrics and Gynecology* **166**, 1044–52.

Ho, H. N., Gill, T. J., Hsieh, H. J., Jiang, J. J., Lee, T. Y., and Hsieh, C. Y. (1991). Immunotherapy for recurrent spontaneous abortion. *American Journal of Reproductive Immunology* **25**, 10–15.

Horta, J. L. H., Fernandez, J. G., Leon, B. S., and Cortes-Gallegos, V. (1977). Direct evidence of luteal insufficiency in women with habitual abortion. *Obstetrics and Gynecology* **49**, 705–8.

Johnson, P. and Pearce, J. M. (1990). Recurrent spontaneous abortion and polycystic ovarian syndrome. *British Medical Journal* **300**, 154–6.

Johnson, P. M., Chia, K. V., Hart, C. A., Griffith, H. B., and Francis, W. J. A. (1988). Trophoblast membrane infusion for unexplained recurrent miscarriage. *British Journal of Obstetrics and Gynaecology* **96**, 342–7.

Kalter, H. (1987). Diabetes and spontaneous abortion. *American Journal of Obstetrics and Gynecology* **156**, 1243–53.

Kerr, M., Rashed, M. N., Christie, S., and Ross, A. (1966). Chromosome studies on spontaneous abortions. *American Journal of Obstetrics and Gynecology* **94**, 322–39.

Kirk, E. P., Chuang, C. J., Coulam, C. B., and Williams, T. J. (1993). Pregnancy after metroplasty for uterine anomalies. *Fertility Sterility* **59**, 1164–8.

Lauritsen, J. G. (1976). Aetiology of spontaneous abortion. *Acta Obstetrica et Gynaecologica Scandinavica*, Supp. 52, 1–29.

Lazar, P., Gueguen, S., Drewfus, J., Renorud, R., Pontonnier, G., and Papiernik, E. (1984). Multicentre controlled trial of cervical cerclage in women at moderate risk of preterm labour. *British Journal of Obstetrics and Gynaecology* **91**, 731–5.

Lee, C. S. (1987). Luteal phase defects. *Obstetric and Gynaecological Survey* **42**, 267–74.

Lockshin, C. J., Reece, E. A., Romero, R., and Hobbins, J. L. (1986). Antiphospholipid antibody and pregnancy wastage. *Lancet* **ii**, 742–3.

Lubbe, W. F., Butler, W. F., Palmer, S. J., and Liggins, G. C. (1984). Lupus anticoagulant in pregnancy. *British Journal of Obstetrics and Gynaecology* **91**, 357–63.

MacDougall, J. and Siddle, N. (1991). Emergency cervical cerclage. *British Journal of Obstetrics and Gynaecology* **98**, 1234–8.

McIntyre, J. A. (1988). In search of trophoblast–lymphocyte cross-reactiue (TLX) antigens. *American Journal of Reproductive Immunology and Microbiology* **17**, 100–10.

McIntyre, J. A., Faulk, W. P., Nichols-Johnson, V. R., and Taylor, C. J. (1986). Immunologic testing and immunotherapy in recurrent spontaneous abortion. *Obstetrics and Gynaecology* **67**, 169–75.

MacKenzie, W. E., Holmes, D. F., and Newton, J. R. (1988). Spontaneous abortion rate in ultrasonically viable pregnancies. *Obstetrics and Gynecology* **71**, 81–3.

MacLean, M. A., Cumming, G. P., McCall, F., Walker, I. D., and Walker, J. J. (1994). The prevalence of lupus anticoagulant and anticardiolipin antibodies in women with a history of first trimester miscarriages. *British Journal of Obstetrics and Gynaecology* **101**, 103–6.

Malpas, P. (1938). A study of abortion sequences. *Journal of Obstetrics and Gynaecology of the British Empire* **45**, 932–49.

March, C. M. and Israel, R. (1987). Hysteroscopic management of recurrent abortion caused by septate uterus. *American Journal of Obstetrics and Gynecology* **156**, 834–42.

Miller, J. F., Williamson, E., Glew, J., Gordon, Y. B., Grudzinskas, J. G., and Sykes, A. (1980). Fetal loss after implantation. *Lancet* **ii**, 554–6.

Miodovnik, M., Mimouni, F., Tsang, R. C., Ammar, E., Caplan, L., and Siddiqi, T. A. (1986). Glycaemic control and spontaneous abortion in insulin-dependent diabetic women. *Obstetrics and Gynecology* **63**, 666–9.

Mowbray, J. F. (1986). Effect of immunisation with paternal cells on recurrent spontaneous abortion. *Journal of Reproduction and Immunology*, Supp 9, 26.

Mowbray, J. F. (1988). Successes and failures of immunization for recurrent spontaneous abortion. In *Early pregnancy loss* (ed. R. W. Beard and F. Sharp), pp. 325–31. Springer–Verlag London.

Mowbray, J. F., Gibbings, C., Liddell, H., Reginald, P. W., Underwood, J. L., and Beard, R. W. (1985). Controlled trial of treatment of recurrent spontaneous abortion by immunization with paternal cells. *Lancet* **i**, 941–3.

Mowbray, J. F., Underwood, J. L., Michel, M., Thorbes, P. B., and Beard, R. W. (1987). Immunization with paternal lymphocytes in women with recurrent miscarriage. *Lancet* **ii**, 679–80.

MRC–RCOG Working Party (1988). Interim report of the MRC–RCOG multi-centre randomized trial of cervical cerclage. *British Journal of Obstetrics and Gynaecology* **95**, 437–45.

MRC–RCOG Working Party (1993). Final report of the MRC–RCOG multi-centre randomised trial of cervical cerclage. *British Journal of Obstetrics and Gynaecology* **100**, 516–23.

Mueller-Eckhardt, G., Heine, O, and Polten, B. (1991). Intravenous immunoglobulin to prevent recurrent spontaneous abortion. *Lancet* **337**, 424–5.

Munday, P. E., Porter, R., Falder, P. F., Carder, J. M., Holliman, R., Lewis, B. V., *et al.* (1984). Spontaneous abortion—an infectious aetiology? *British Journal of Obstetrics and Gynaecology* **91**, 1177–80.

Naessens, A., Foulon, W., Cammu, H., Goossens, A., and Lauwers, S. (1987). Epidemiology and pathogenesis of *Ureaplasma urealyticum* in spontaneous abortion and early preterm labour. *Acta Obstetrica at Gynaecologica Scandinavica* **66**, 513–16.

Ober, C. L., Hauck, W. W., Kostyu, D. D., O'Brien, E., Elias, S., Simpson, J. L., *et al.* (1985). Adverse effects of human leucocyte antigen-DR sharing on fertility. *Fertility Sterility* **44**, 227–32.

Parazzini, F., Acaia, B., Ricciardiello, O., Fedele, L., Liati, P., and Candiani, G. B. (1988). Short-term reproductive prognosis when no cause can be found for recurrent miscarriage. *British Journal of Obstetrics and Gynaecology* **95**, 654–8.

Poland, B. J., Miller, J. R., Jones, D. C., and Trimble, B. K. (1977). Reproductive counselling in patients who have had a spontaneous abortion. *American Journal of Obstetrics and Gynecology* **127**, 689–91.

Polson, D. W., Adams, J., Wadsworth, J., and Franks, S. (1988). Polycystic ovaries—a common finding in normal women. *Lancet* **i**, 870–2.

Prentice, R. L., Gatenby, L. A., Loblay, R. H., Shearman, R. P., Kronenberg, H., and Basten, A. (1984). Lupus anticoagulant in pregnancy. *Lancet* **ii**, 464.

Quinn, P. A., Petric, M., Barkin, M., Butany, J., Derzko, C., Gysler, N., *et al.* (1987). Prevalence of antibodies to *Chlamydia trachomatis* in spontaneous abortion and infertility. *American Journal of Obstetrics and Gynecology* **156**, 291–6.

Regan, L. (1988). A prospective study of spontaneous abortion. In *Early pregnancy loss* (ed. R. W. Beard and F. Sharp), pp. 23–37. Springer–Verlag. London.

Regan, L. (1991). Recurrent miscarriage. *British Medical Journal* **302**, 543–4.

Regan, L., Owen, E. J., and Jacobs, H. S. (1990). Hypersecretion of luteinizing hormone, infertility, and miscarriage. *Lancet* **336**, 1141–4.

Reginald, P. W., Beard, R. W., Chapple, J., Forbes, P. B., Liddell, H. S., Mowbray, J. F., *et al.* (1987). Outcome of pregnancies progressing beyond 28 weeks gestation in women with a history of recurrent miscarriage. *British Journal of Obstetrics and Gynaecology* **91**, 643–8.

Roberts, C. J. and Lowe, C. R. (1975). Where have all the conceptuses gone? *Lancet* **i**, 498–9.

Rosove, M. H., Tabsh, K., Wasserstrum, N., Howard, P., Hahn, B., and Kalunian, K. C. (1990). Heparin therapy for pregnant women with lupus anticoagulant. *Obstetrics and Gynecology* **75**, 630–4.

Sagle, M., Bishop, K., Ridley, N., Alexander, F. N., Michel, M., Bonney, R. C., *et al.* (1988). Recurrent early miscarriage and polycystic ovarian syndrome. *British Medical Journal* **297**, 1027–8.

Salem, H. T., Ghaneimah, S. A., Shaaban, M. M., and Chard, T. (1984). Prognostic value of biochemical tests in the assessment of fetal outcome in threatened abortion. *British Journal of Obstetrics and Gynaecology* **91**, 382–5.

Sargent, I. L., Wilkins, T., and Redman, C. W. G. (1988). Maternal immune responses to the fetus in early pregnancy and recurrent miscarriage. *Lancet* **ii**, 1099–104.

Schenker, J. G. and Margalioth, E. J. (1982). Intrauterine adhesions: an updated appraisal. *Fertility Sterility* **37**, 593–610.

Schweditsch, M. O., Dublin, N. H., Jones, G. S., and Wentz, A. C. (1979). Hormonal considerations in early normal pregnancy. *Fertility Sterility* **31**, 252–7.

Scott, J. R., Rote, N. S., and Branch, D. W. (1987). Immunologic aspects of recurrent abortion and fetal death. *Obstetrics and Gynecology* **70**, 645–56.

Shearman, R. P. and Garrett, W. J. (1963). Double-blind study of effect of 17-hydroxyprogesterone caproate on abortion rate. *British Medical Journal* **1**, 292–5.

Stack, J. M. (1990). Psychological aspects of early pregnancy loss. In *Early pregnancy failure* (ed. H. J. Huisjes and T. Lind), pp. 212–23. Churchill Livingstone, Edinburgh.

Stirrat, G. M. (1990). Recurrent miscarriage I and II. *Lancet* **336**, 673–5 and 724–33.

Strassmann, E. O. (1966). Fertility and unification of double uterus. *Fertility and Sterility* **17**, 165–76.

Stray-Pedersen, B. and Stray-Pedersen, S. (1984). Aetiological factors in habitual abortion. *American Journal of Obstetrics and Gynecology* **148**, 140–6.

Stray-Pedersen, B. and Stray-Pedersen, S. (1988). Recurrent abortion: the role of psychotherapy. In *Early pregnancy loss* (ed. R. W. Beard and F. Sharp), pp. 433–40. Springer–Verlag, London.

Sweet, R. L., Landers, D. V., Walker, C., and Schachter, J. (1987). *Chlamydia trachomatis* infection and pregnancy outcome. *American Journal of Obstetrics and Gynecology* **156**, 824–33.

Taylor, C. and Faulk, W. P. (1981). Prevention of recurrent abortion with leucocyte transfusion. *Lancet* **ii**, 68–70.

Tharapel, A. T., Tharapel, S. A., and Bannerman, R. M. (1985). Recurrent pregnancy losses and parental chromosomal abnormalities. *British Journal of Obstetrics and Gynaecology* **92**, 899–914.

Tho, P. T., Burd, J. R., and McDonough, P. V. (1979). Aetiology and subsequent reproductive performance in couples with recurrent abortion. *Fertility Sterility* **32**, 389–95.

Treffers, P. E. (1990). Uterine causes of early pregnancy failure. In *Early pregnancy failure* (ed. H. J. Huisjes and T. Lind), pp. 114–47. Churchill Livingstone, Edinburgh.

Varma, T. R. (1979). Ultrasound evidence of early pregnancy failure in patients with multiple conceptions. *British Journal of Obstetrics and Gynaecology* **86**, 290–2.

Wilcox, A. J., Weinberg, C. R., O'Connor, J. F., Baird, D. D., Schlatterer, J. P., Canfield, R. E., *et al.* (1988). Incidence of early loss of pregnancy. *New England Journal of Medicine* **319**, 189–94.

2 The management of ectopic pregnancy

The incidence of ectopic pregnancy varies throughout the world, and it is increasing. Douglas (1963) reported one ectopic pregnancy for every 28 live births in Jamaica, making tubal pregnancy the commonest gynaecological emergency. In Finland, in 1967, there were seven ectopic pregnancies per 1000 deliveries, whereas in 1983 there were 26 ectopic pregnancies per 1000 deliveries, this being 1 in 38 of total births (Makinen 1987). In Aberdeen, the incidence of ectopic pregnancy increased from 2.66 per 1000 births in 1950–1954 to 6.4 per 1000 births in 1980–1984 (Flett *et al*. 1988).

The incidence of ectopic pregnancy in the United States is also increasing, from 4.5 ectopics per 1000 pregnancies in 1970 to 9.4 per 1000 pregnancies in 1978, i.e. 1 in 106 pregnancies (Rubin *et al*. 1983). The current US incidence is 16.8 per 1000 live births (Centres for Disease Control 1990). The incidence of ectopic pregnancy throughout England and Wales has increased from 1 in 250 deliveries in 1970–1982 to 1 in 150 between 1982 and 1984. Although the incidence of ectopic pregnancy is increasing, in the UK its associated mortality rate is decreasing. In 1982–1984, there were 10 deaths directly due to ectopic pregnancy in the reported 138 'direct' maternal deaths (7.2 per cent), i.e. a mortality rate from ectopic pregnancy of 0.7 per 1000 ectopic pregnancies. Death occurred from either haemorrhage or anaesthesia (Department of Health 1989).

Bilateral simultaneous tubal pregnancy occurs in 1 in 200 000 live births (Edelstein and Morgan 1989).

The rest of this chapter will deal specifically with tubal pregnancy.

Why is tubal pregnancy increasing?

It has been claimed that the incidence of tubal pregnancy is not increasing but is merely being diagnosed with more certainty by laparoscopy. Although it is true that some tubal pregnancies may well resolve spontaneously, it is certain that the reported increase is, in fact, real.

There is no single convincing explanation for the increase in the incidence of tubal pregnancy; presumably this increase is multifactorial. The following are probably the major aetiological factors:

(1) pelvic inflammatory disease;

(2) intrauterine contraceptive devices;

(3) other methods of contraception;

(4) sterilization;

(5) tubal surgery;

(6) previous ectopic pregnancy;

(7) assisted reproduction.

Pelvic inflammatory disease

Chronic pelvic inflammatory disease, as evidenced by macroscopic damage to the tubes, has been reported as an aetiological factor in 6 per cent of ectopic pregnancies (Jones 1966). It is likely that the preceding infection was primarily pelvic and not related to appendicitis, for tubal pregnancy is no commoner in the right tube than in the left. When the tube containing a pregnancy is examined histologically, chronic pelvic inflammatory disease is found in 42 per cent of tubes (Breen 1970).

A history of pelvic inflammatory disease may be elicited. In a case-control study of 274 ectopic pregnancies compared with 548 controls, a history of pelvic inflammatory disease increased the relative risk of ectopic pregnancy to 3.3 (Marchbanks et al. 1988). The 'epidemic' of pelvic inflammatory disease in Finland is considered to be a major factor in that country's high incidence of tubal pregnancy (Makinen 1989). Immunological studies have also demonstrated an association between specific pelvic infections and ectopic pregnancy. Thus, Robertson et al. (1988) found that the serum of 76 per cent of 50 women with an ectopic pregnancy contained IgG antibodies to *Chlamydia* compared with 38 per cent of 550 age-matched controls with intrauterine pregnancies, whilst 32 per cent of the women with an ectopic pregnancy had gonococcal IgG antibodies compared with 4 per cent of controls. Most of the infections were subclinical.

Marjundar et al. (1983) reported histological evidence of salpingitis isthmica nodosa in 57 per cent of patients with a tubal pregnancy, and argued that the underlying aetiology of the salpingitis isthmica nodosa was previous tubal infection. The presumed mechanism relates either to a narrowing of the tubal lumen, or to an increased transit time within the tubes due to damage to ciliated epithelium.

Intrauterine contraceptive devices

Several studies have illustrated the importance of the current use of an IUCD as a risk factor in ectopic pregnancy (Makinen et al. 1989a; Marchbanks et al. 1988), current users having a relative risk of 11.9 compared with non-users. Vessey et al. (1974) reported 90 pregnancies in women with an IUCD *in situ*, of whom 8.9 per cent had a tubal pregnancy, whereas less than 1 per cent of failures of other methods of contraception were tubal pregnancies. The IUCD is an atypical method of contraception in that its primary effect is not to prevent fertilization but to prevent implantation. Hence, it would not be surprising that an IUCD was better protection against an intrauterine pregnancy than an extrauterine one.

Comparing the IUCD with other methods of contraception, women with an IUCD have an incidence of ectopic pregnancy only some 38 per cent that of women who use no contraception, but 204 times that of women who use oral contraception and 3.2 times that of women who have been sterilized (Franks *et al.* 1990). Ory *et al.* (1981) reported a case-control study of 615 women with an ectopic pregnancy compared to 3453 controls who were hospital in-patients, matched in age to those women with a tubal pregnancy and who were sexually active but were neither pregnant nor had recently been pregnant. They reported that:

1. Never users of IUCDs have the same risk of ectopic pregnancy as do past users.

2. All current contraceptive users, including IUCD users, were less likely to have an ectopic pregnancy than sexually active women who were not using contraception.

3. Longterm IUCD users (longer than two years) had an incidence of ectopic pregnancy which was 2.6 times that of short-term users (less than two years).

4. They were unable to find any difference in the risk of ectopic pregnancy between copper-containing IUCDs and plastic IUCDs.

5. IUCD users were three times more likely to have an ectopic pregnancy than any other users of contraception. The risk of an ectopic pregnancy with combined oral contraceptive therapy was the same as that using barrier methods.

6. The Progestasert IUCD was 1.3 times more likely to be associated with an ectopic pregnancy than any other IUCD.

It would seem, therefore, that the use of IUCDs cannot explain the increasing number of tubal pregnancies, although the association between tubal pregnancy and IUCD is greater than that with other contraceptive methods and is greater than that which might be expected from any association between an IUCD and chronic pelvic inflammatory disease.

The Progestasert device warrants special mention as this is the type of IUCD most likely to result in an ectopic pregnancy. Snowden analysed the data reported to the American FDA and the UK Committee on Safety of Medicines. These data suggested that the Lippes Loop reduced the rate of an ectopic pregnancy by 91–94 per cent, whereas a copper-containing device reduced the rate of an ectopic pregnancy by 96–97 per cent, but the Progestasert reduced the rate of an ectopic pregnancy only by between 56 and 71 per cent (Snowden 1977).

Table 2.1 Tubal pregnancy and contraception

Method	Number of tubal pregnancies per 1000 pregnancies
Combined oral contraceptive	0.005
Vasectomy	0.005
Condom	0.1
Diaphragm	0.15
Female sterilization	0.32
IUCD	1.0
None	2.6

From Franks *et al.* (1990)

Other methods of contraception

All methods of contraception have a failure rate, and a number of those failures will be tubal pregnancies. Franks *et al.* (1990) have estimated the number of ectopic pregnancies per 1000 pregnancy failures with different methods of contraception and this is shown in Table 2.1.

Between 4 per cent and 6 per cent of all pregnancies occurring in women using progestogen-only oral contraception are tubal (Smith *et al.* 1974; Tatum and Schmidt 1977). This represents a risk significantly greater than that from an IUCD, although Hawkins (1974) reported an incidence of only 1 per cent. When one considers that the mechanism of the contraceptive effect of progestogen-only pills is mainly on cervical mucus and endometrium, a poor protective effect against tubal pregnancy would be expected.

The risk of tubal pregnancy when medroxyprogesterone acetate is given intramuscularly for contraception is lower than that from the progestogen-only pill but greater than that from combined oral contraception. Post-coital contraception with oestrogen and a progestogen would also appear to carry an increased risk of tubal pregnancy, but the data are limited. Kubba and Guillebaud (1983) reported 17 pregnancies following the administration of post-coital contraception to 715 women. One pregnancy was tubal, suggesting a risk in the region of 58.8 per 1000 pregnancies.

Sterilization

The prevalence of sterilization as a method of contraception has increased greatly in the UK since the end of the 1960s. Although there is a substantial risk that any pregnancy following sterilization will be tubal, the statistics suggest that this is one of the major factors in the increase of tubal pregnancies, but by no means the only one. Thus, in Aberdeen between 1950 and 1954, no patient with a tubal pregnancy had had a previous sterilization procedure, whereas

Table 2.2 Pregnancy and sterilization

Technique	Number of tubal pregnancies per 1000 pregnancies
Open	200.0
Coagulation at laparoscopy	428.6
Coagulation plus transection	145.5
Falope ring application	60.0
'Clip' application	65.2

between 1980 and 1984 some 21 per cent of patients with an ectopic pregnancy had been previously sterilized.

Some 10 per cent of all patients who now present with a tubal pregnancy have had a previous sterilization (Davis 1986). It has been estimated that between 15 per cent and 76 per cent of all pregnancies following sterilization will be tubal (Davis 1986; Kjer and Knudsen 1989). It is generally considered that the tubotubal fistula or the tuboperitoneal fistula which allows conception to take place following sterilization must be narrow, and hence the relative disparity in size between a sperm and a fertilized ovum predisposes to the tubal pregnancy. However, Stock and Nelson (1984) argued that lumen size is not the only factor and proposed that the mechanism may be an alteration in the dynamics of the damaged portion of the tube within the fistula.

Different techniques of sterilization appear to carry different risks of tubal pregnancy should failure occur (Table 2.2). The greatest risk appears to follow tubal diathermy. The commonest methods of sterilization currently in use in the UK involve the application of either a ring or a clip to the fallopian tube and, should pregnancy follow either of these techniques, there is a 6 per cent risk that it will be tubal.

De Stefano *et al.* (1982) analysed the risk of tubal pregnancy following tubal sterilization, using age and method-specific cumulative risks. They demonstrated that the mean cumulative risk of tubal pregnancy per 1000 women who used any method of contraception was 15.6, whereas the specific risk after sterilization was 2.1, demonstrating that the *overall* risk to women of tubal pregnancy will fall following their sterilization.

Tubal surgery

Logic states that there ought to be an increased risk of tubal pregnancy following tubal surgery for infertility, partly because of the tubal damage which caused the infertility and partly because of surgical trauma, even by microsurgery. The overall incidence of tubal pregnancy in 653 patients from 14 series was reported by Winston (1981) as being 4.1 per cent of all patients but 24.8 per cent of all pregnancies. Marchbanks *et al.* (1988) reported that a history of tubal surgery was the second commonest risk factor for ectopic pregnancy, the commonest being current IUCD use.

Reversal of sterilization differs from other tubal surgery in that an operation has occurred but the fallopian tubes themselves are generally normal and the patient is usually of proven fertility. The risk of ectopic pregnancy after reversal of sterilization seems to be lower after microsurgical techniques than after macrosurgical ones. Winston (1981) reported 199 patients from 14 series who had undergone reversal of sterilization by macrosurgical technique. Some 46 per cent of all pregnancies were tubal. However, the same author reported 560 patients from 17 series who had undergone reversal of sterilization by a microsurgical technique—only 5.4 per cent of the pregnancies were tubal.

Previous ectopic pregnancy

Following a tubal pregnancy, the risk of a subsequent pregnancy being tubal is significantly increased. Hallatt (1975) reported a series of 1330 ectopic pregnancies in which 9.25 per cent were repeat tubal pregnacies.

Looking at the same problem in a different way, once a patient has had an ectopic pregnancy her chances of a repeat ectopic pregnancy in a subsequent pregnancy are increased. The level of this risk will depend to some degree upon the aetiology of the previous ectopic pregnancy and the treatment given, but most authors demonstrate that fertility is reduced. Timonen and Nieminen (1967) followed 743 patients after surgery for their first ectopic pregnancy. Of 50.2 per cent of patients who conceived, 28.8 per cent delivered a live baby, and 11.5 per cent had a repeat ectopic pregnancy. More recently, Makinen *et al.* (1989*b*) followed 110 women treated either radically or conservatively for tubal pregnancy. By the end of eight years, 65.6 per cent had delivered a live baby and 20 per cent had a subsequent ectopic pregnancy. The variation in these figures together with the technique used to treat the first ectopic pregnancy will be discussed later in this chapter.

Assisted reproduction

In vitro fertilization (IVF) and embryo transfer (ET) are associated with an increased risk of tubal pregnancy because of the high incidence of tubal damage in this group of patients. The first reported pregnancy after IVF and ET was tubal, and the risk of tubal pregnancy following IVF and ET appears to depend upon the indication for this procedure. Lancaster (1985) reported 13 tubal pregnancies in 201 clinical pregnancies following IVF, giving an incidence of ectopic pregnancy of 6.5 per cent.

The diagnosis of ectopic pregnancy

In 1853 Lawson Tait stated that the difficulty with ectopic pregnancy was in making the diagnosis. The classical triad of abdominal pain, abnormal uterine

Table 2.3 Diagnostic tests

Diagnostic aid	True +ve %	False +ve %	False −ve %
Urine pregnancy test	23–82	2–5	18–77
Serum β-hCG	80–100	25–33	0
Ultrasound	65–94	3–30	2–35
Culdoscopy	80–95	5–10	11–14
Laparoscopy	97	5	4

From Kim *et al.* (1987)

bleeding, and an adnexal mass occurs in only 30–40 per cent of patients, and a correct clinical diagnosis will be made in less than 50 per cent of all patients with an ectopic pregnancy at first presentation (Weckstein 1985). Other authors report a higher degree of clinical acumen; for instance, Hogston (1987) reported the correct diagnosis in 73 per cent of patients with tubal pregnancy. There are, therefore, a substantial number of patients with tubal pregnancy in whom a correct diagnosis is not made clinically. Clinical caution may also result in tubal pregnancy being overdiagnosed. Hogston also reported that in 32 per cent of patients who underwent laparoscopy because of 'suspected ectopic pregnancy' this diagnosis was wrong, in addition 20 per cent did not have any recognizable pelvic pathology at all.

Various diagnostic aids are, therefore, available in order to refute or confirm the diagnosis of suspected ectopic pregnancy; the relative merits of these aids were assessed by Kim *et al.* (1987) and they are compared in Table 2.3. The evidence which lies behind these statistics will now be discussed.

hCG measurement

A standard urinary pregnancy test is not a satisfactory diagnostic aid since it is neither particularly sensitive nor specific. In different series, a urine pregnancy test was positive in between 23 per cent and 82 per cent of women with an ectopic pregnancy (Kim *et al.* 1987; Tancer *et al.* 1981; Weckstein 1985).

The lack of sensitivity in the standard immunological pregnancy test may be overcome by β-hCG radioimmunoassay. Using monoclonal antibodies, serum β-hCG may be assayed in 20 minutes and may detect levels down to 2 IU per millilitre. The specificity and sensitivity of such a test will depend upon the 'cut-off' level for hCG used in the assay. Stenman *et al.* (1983) reported that all 22 women with an ectopic pregnancy had a positive test if the cut-off level was greater than 10 IU/ml. Similarly, all intrauterine pregnancies were positive at 10 IU/ml, but only 93 per cent at 25 IU/ml.

The value of this test in clinical practice has been reported by Goh *et al.* (1984) in a series of 30 patients with ectopic pregnancy. Three of these patients had been previously inadvertently discharged before a diagnosis of tubal pregnancy was made, yet on re-admission they all had demonstrable evidence of β-hCG. Goh *et al.* also reported one patient who had a false-negative and three with false-positive results. Stenman *et al.* (1983) also reported a false-positive incidence of 30 per cent for β-hCG detection in women attending with lower abdominal pain or bleeding who were not subsequently shown to be pregnant. No clinical diagnosis was made in these patients, and it may be that this does not represent a failure of the test but a failure of clinical diagnosis, in that some of these patients may have had an unrecognized complete abortion. Baber *et al.* (1988) demonstrated the value of combining clinical judgement with a rapid immunoassay test in the emergency department. Prior to the introduction of testing, 32 patients had a provisional diagnosis of ectopic pregnancy but only five (16 per cent) were surgically proven. During a similar period of time after the introduction of testing, there were only eight provisional diagnoses of ectopic pregnancy, seven (88 per cent) being surgically proven.

The use of serial measurements of β-hCG may have screening advantages. Kadar *et al.* (1981) reported two β-hCG titres 48 hours apart, in the presence of a continuing pregnancy, should have increased by at least 66 per cent. Some 85 per cent of those patients in whom this increase did not occur were subsequently shown to have either an ectopic pregnancy or a missed abortion. The predictive value of the rate of increase of β-hCG has been confirmed by other groups (Grudzinskas and Stabile 1993; Lindblom *et al.* 1989).

Ultrasound

The resolution of ultrasound machines limits their use in the positive diagnosis of ectopic pregnancy, but in practice the demonstration of an intrauterine pregnancy will exclude a coincidental ectopic pregnancy in all but 1 in 30 000 of pregnancies apart from those resulting from ovarian stimulation (Reece *et al.* 1983). The positive diagnostic finding of a live extrauterine fetal pole has been reported in 12 per cent of women with a proven ectopic pregnancy (Stabile *et al.* 1988), but in the absence of this sign there is no single other diagnostic ultrasound feature.

There may also be confusion with the findings of a 'pseudogestation sac' which has been reported in the uterus of 3 per cent of women with a tubal pregnancy. It is not possible by ultrasound to distinguish this from an early intrauterine pregnancy (Bateman *et al.* 1990). It presumably represents secretion of fluid by the decidua. The commonest other ultrasound finding is one of an 'adnexal swelling', or a mass in the Pouch of Douglas, which includes ectopic pregnancy in the differential diagnosis.

Transvaginal ultrasound is more sensitive than is abdominal ultrasound in the diagnosis of ectopic pregnancy (Burry *et al.* 1993; De Crespigny 1988). Kivikoski *et al.* (1990) compared the two techniques in 25 patients who were subsequently shown to have a tubal pregnancy at surgery. Transvaginal ultrasound predicted the diagnosis in 84 per cent of patients, whilst transabdominal ultrasound predicted the condition in only 68 per cent.

It may be that a combination of ultrasound and serum β-hCG will improve the diagnostic accuracy of either alone. Thus, an elevated serum β-hCG and empty uterus would support the diagnosis of an ectopic pregnancy in between 93 and 100 per cent of patients with this combination (Bateman *et al.* 1990; Weckstein 1985). It is possible that Doppler studies may become of diagnostic benefit in the future (Taylor and Meyer 1991).

Culdoscopy

Culdoscopy has been largely replaced by laparoscopy, which should diagnose all but the earliest tubal pregnancies. However Kim *et al.* (1987) reported a positive diagnosis on laparoscopy in only 112 of 122 patients (92 per cent), five patients having a 'failed laparoscopy' (4 per cent) and five being true diagnostic failures in that the tubes were reported as normal in the presence of a tubal pregnancy.

The treatment of tubal pregnancy

Not all tubal pregnancies are diagnosed and treated, since some tubal abortions undergo spontaneous resolution. Fernandez *et al.* (1988) reported 14 patients with an ampullary tubal pregnancy confirmed by laparoscopy, not actively bleeding, and in whom management was to be conservative. Four of these patients (29 per cent) ultimately required surgery because of pain or increasing hCG levels, but in nine patients (64 per cent) the tubal pregnancy resolved spontaneously. Six of these patients underwent a hystero–salpingogram three months later, and all six had patent tubes although one tube did look abnormal. Three of these patients ultimately conceived. Similarly Makinen *et al.* (1990) reported that 26 per cent of 102 patients with an ectopic pregnancy had successful spontaneous resolution when the clinical circumstances allowed conservative management with serum hCG monitoring. However, the majority of ectopic pregnancies will be treated by surgery.

The controversial aspects regarding surgical management relate to the choice of operative procedures. These are discussed and enumerated below:

(1) salpingectomy or salpingo–oophorectomy;

(2) salpingectomy or salpingotomy;

(3) laparoscopy or laparotomy.

Salpingectomy or salpingo–oophorectomy?

Jeffcoate advocated salpingo–oophorectomy, rather than salpingectomy, as a method of increasing the low fertility rates following an ectopic pregnancy in patients who wish to conceive. He suggested that the removal of the ovary together with the damaged tube in the presence of an apparently normal contralateral tube meant that ovulation would occur each month in the ovary adjacent to the remaining tube. No statistical evidence was offered (Jeffcoate 1955).

Schenker (1972) presented evidence which suggested that salpingo-oophorectomy did not improve fertility but did reduce the risk of a subsequent ectopic pregnancy, possibly by preventing transperitoneal migration of either an ovum or a blastocyst. He reported 257 women who underwent surgery for a tubal pregnancy and who wished to conceive. Of these, 205 women were treated by salpingectomy and 52 by salpingo–oophorectomy, but they were not randomly allocated. Of those treated by salpingectomy, 45.5 per cent became pregnant again, but 16.7 per cent of patients had an ectopic pregnancy in the remaining tube. Of those treated by a salpingo–oophorectomy, 40 per cent conceived again with two patients having a second ectopic pregnancy (5.7 per cent).

However, Franklin *et al.* (1973) reported a series of 492 women who had a previous tubal pregnancy and of whom 61 per cent had a subsequent pregnancy; 38 per cent of these women gave birth to a live baby, whilst 27 per cent had a second tubal pregnancy. There were no differences in conception rate, the rate of delivery of a live baby, or recurrent tubal pregnancy rate, whether these patients were treated by salpingectomy alone or salpingo–oophorectomy.

Although other small series do exist, there is no prospective randomly allocated trial of salpingectomy versus salpingo–oophorectomy in the management of tubal pregnancy. It is likely that the most important factor in the subsequent incidence of tubal pregnancy is not whether or not an ovary was conserved but the state of the remaining tube.

Salpingectomy or salpingotomy?

The earlier diagnosis of an unruptured tubal pregnancy, which is now possible with β-hCG measurement, ultrasound, and laparoscopy, gives the option of conservative surgery by salpingotomy, ampullary expression of the tubal pregnancy, or excision and re-anastomosis of an area of the tube (Maruri and Azziz 1993).

De Cherney and Kase (1979) reported 98 women with their first tubal pregnancy, of whom 50 were treated by either salpingectomy or salpingo-oophorectomy, whilst 48 were treated by salpingotomy with reconstruction of the tube. Table 2.4 shows that the incidence of a subsequent ectopic pregnancy was lower in those patients treated by radical surgery than in those in whom the tube was preserved. In a larger series, Timonen and Nieminen (1967) reported 743 patients, of whom 558 had undergone radical surgery and 185 conservative surgery. As can be seen from Table 2.4, the incidence of ectopic pregnancy was again greater in those patients in whom surgery had been conservative.

Linear salpingotomy may also be used in the presence of a ruptured tubal pregnancy, but meticulous debridement at the site of rupture prior to surgical repair is mandatory (Seifer *et al.* 1993; Thornton *et al.* 1991).

Table 2.4 Tubal pregnancy and surgery

Series	Pregnancies after radical surgery			Pregnancies after conservative surgery		
	No.	% Viable	% Ectopic	No.	% Viable	% Ectopic
De Cherney and Kase (1979)	50	42	12	48	39.6	18.6
Timonen and Nieminen (1967)	558	31.2	11.5	185	30.2	15.6

Fimbrial expression or 'milking' of an unruptured ectopic pregnancy out of a tube would seem to leave the patient at a greater risk of repeat ectopic pregnancy than do other conservative methods of surgery. Kadar (1988) pooled the data from several series and found that the ectopic pregnancy rate after 'milking' was 23 per cent compared with 17 per cent after salpingotomy.

When repeat ectopic pregnancy occurs, it is not always clear whether the conception has occurred in the repaired tube or in the contralateral tube. Oelsner et al. (1987) reported a retrospective analysis of 58 women undergoing conservative microsurgery for an ectopic pregnancy. Of 30 women who had two fallopian tubes remaining at the end of the procedure, 12 per cent had a subsequent ectopic pregnancy, whereas of 28 women who underwent microsurgery to their solitary tube, 38.5 per cent had a subsequent ectopic pregnancy, suggesting that the chance of subsequent tubal pregnancy is greater should the contralatral tube be absent. Moreover, an intrauterine pregnancy subsequently occurred in 58 per cent of patients who had both tubes and in only 46 per cent of those who had a solitary tube. Hallatt (1986) reported 200 women with an ectopic pregnancy treated by salpingotomy. Of these, 122 subsequently conceived and 24 of these pregnancies were tubal, 12 in the previously involved tube and 12 in the contralateral tube, suggesting that both tubes were at equal risk of subsequent ectopic pregnancy. Tuomivaara and Kauppila (1988) reported a five-year follow-up of 323 patients with a previous ectopic pregnancy and who wished to conceive in the future. Some 82 per cent did conceive, and, of these, 79 per cent had an intrauterine pregnancy which reached the third trimester, 13 per cent had another ectopic pregnancy, and 8 per cent a miscarriage. It made no difference whether the tube in which the ectopic pregnancy had been sited was removed or conserved. However, if the contralateral tube was damaged or absent ($n = 49$) 91 per cent were subfertile, whereas if the contralateral tube was 'normal' only 32 per cent were subfertile ($n = 262$).

It, therefore, seems that the major factor determining the risk of a subsequent ectopic pregnancy is the state of the contralateral tube, not the surgery performed (Ory et al. 1993; Silva et al. 1993). Since there may also be a small increase in the risk of subsequent ectopic pregnancy following conservative surgery compared with radical surgery, it may be that conservative management is appropriate only for the patient with either a contralateral blocked tube or absent tube. The only procedure which does seem to be associated with a pre-judiced future outcome is 'milking' of the tube in which an ectopic pregnancy was sited.

Laparoscopy or laparotomy?

The earlier detection of tubal pregnancy has also allowed the laparoscope to be used for treatment in the haemodynamically stable patient. This minimally invasive surgery carries the advantages of a shorter length of stay in hospital, a lesser need for analgesia, a more rapid return to full activity, and a low risk of adhesion formation (Meyer and De Cherney 1989). Other authors have reported similar small but successful series of tubal pregnancy treated by laparoscopic linear salpingotomy (Henderson 1989; Keckstein *et al.* 1990).

When conservative surgery is performed, it is important that the removal of trophoblastic tissue is complete since residual tissue is capable of prolifera-tion (Thornton *et al.* 1991). Residual tissue may be recognized by persis-tently elevated levels of β-hCG which should be assayed until it is no longer detectable. Kamrava *et al.* (1983) reported that hCG titres decreased and were then no longer detectable in 94 per cent of patients some 24 days after surgery.

The use of methotrexate

In view of the use of methotrexate in treating trophoblastic disease, there have been reports on the use of methotrexate as the sole treatment of tubal preg-nancy. Rodi *et al.* (1986) treated seven patients with systemic methotrexate and citrovorum rescue. All patients responded to treatment with a mean time of 31 days until the hCG levels became undetectable (range 5–50 days). Five patients underwent a hysterosalpingogram, with four demonstrating tubal patency, and one a unilateral occlusion on the side of the previous tubal pregnancy.

However, direct injection of methotrexate would seem preferable to systemic use of this potentially toxic agent. Pansky *et al.* (1989) injected 12.5 mg of methotrexate directly into 27 unruptured tubal pregnancies under laparoscopic control, without apparent side-effects. Some 89 per cent of patients showed resolution based on a falling serum hCG level with an average time of 12 days for the hCG to fall below 10 IU/ml, whilst 11 per cent of patients underwent a laparotomy because of increasing hCG levels. Ory (1991) reviewed 108 such managements reported in the literature. Successful resorption occurred in 94 per cent with a subsequent tubal patency rate of 70 per cent. This method of treatment may become increasingly popular in the haemodynamically stable patient with a small unruptured tubal pregnancy (Groutz *et al.* 1993; Pansky *et al.* 1993; Stovall and Ling 1993).

Conclusions

The incidence of tubal pregnancy appears to be rising throughout the world, and there is an increasing incidence of treatment by conservative means. With increasingly sensitive and specific methods of diagnosis, conservative surgery becomes a more realistic option. However, it is important that the methods of conservative surgery which are incorporated into clinical practice have been appropriately tested against radical surgery. The use of non-surgical methods of treatment, including observation and methotrexate, should become the subject of further study.

References

Baber, R. J., Bonifacio, M., and Saunders, D. M. (1988). The impact of an instant pregnancy test kit on the operations of a major hospital casualty department. *Australian and New Zealand Journal of Obstetrics and Gynaecology* 28, 134-6.

Bateman, B. G., Nunley, W. C., Kolp, L. A., Kitchin, J. D., and Felder, R. (1990). Vaginal sonography findings and hCG dynamics of early intrauterine and tubal pregnancies. *Obstetrics and Gynecology* 75, 421-7.

Breen, J. L. (1970). A 21 year survey of ectopic pregnancy. *American Journal of Obstetrics and Gynecology* 106, 1004-19.

Burry, K. A., Thurmond, A. S., Suby-Long, T. D., Patton, P. E., Rose, P. M., Jones, M. K., *et al.* (1993). Transvaginal ultrasound findings in ectopic pregnancy. *American Journal of Obstetrics and Gynecology* 168, 1796-802.

Centers for Disease Control (1990). Ectopic pregnancy. *Morbidity and Mortality Weekly Review* 39, 401-4.

Davis, M. R. (1986). Recurrent ectopic pregnancy after tubal surgery. *Obstetrics and Gynecology* 68, 445-55.

De Cherney, A. and Kase, N. (1979). Conservative surgical management of unruptured tubal pregnancy. *Obstetrics and Gynecology* 54, 451-5.

De Crespigpny, L. C. (1988). Demonstration of ectopic pregnancy by transvaginal ultrasound. *British Journal of Obstetrics and Gynaecology* 95, 1253-6.

De Stefano, J., Peterson, H. B., Layde, P. M., and Rubin, G. L. (1982). Risk of ectopic pregnancy following tubal sterilization. *Obstetrics and Gynecology* 60, 326-30.

Department of Health (1989). Report on confidential enquiry into maternal deaths in England and Wales 1982-84, pp. 41-6. Her Majesty's Stationery Office, London.

Douglas, C. P. (1963). Tubal ectopic pregnancy. *British Medical Journal* 2, 838-41.

Edelstein, N. C. and Morgan, M. A. (1989). Bilateral simultaneous tubal pregnancy. *Obstetric and Gynecologic Survey* 44, 250-2.

Fernandez, H., Rainhorn, J. D., Papiernik, E., Billett, D., and Frydman, A. R. (1988). Spontaneous resolution of ectopic pregnancy. *Obstetrics and Gynecology* 71, 171-4.

Flett, G. M., Urquhart, D. R., Fraser, C., Terry, P. B., and Flemming, J. C. (1988). Ectopic pregnancy in Aberdeen, 1950-85. *British Journal of Obstetrics and Gynaecology* 95, 740-6.

Franklin, E. W., Ziederman, A. N., and Laemmle, P. (1973). Tubal ectopic pregnancy. *American Journal of Obstetrics and Gynecology* 117, 220-5.

Franks, A. L., Beral, V., Cates, W., and Hogue, C. J. R. (1990). Contraception and ectopic pregnancy risk. *American Journal of Obstetrics and Gynecology* **163**, 1120–3.

Goh, B. N., Mountford, L., and MacKenzie, I. Z. (1984). A 1-hour hCG radio-immunoassay detection kit for the management of suspected ectopic pregnancy. *British Journal of Obstetrics and Gynaecology* **91**, 993–6.

Groutz, A., Luxman, D., Cohen, J. R., and David, M. P. (1993). Rising B-hCG titres following laparoscopic injection of Methotrexate into unruptured viable tubal pregnancies. *British Journal of Obstetrics and Gynaecology* **100**, 287–8.

Grudzinskas, J. G. and Stabile, I. (1993). Ectopic pregnancy, are biochemical tests at all helpful? *British Journal of Obstetrics and Gynaecology* **100**, 510–11.

Hallatt, J. G. (1975). Repeat ectopic pregnancy. *American Journal of Obstetrics and Gynecology* **122**, 520–4.

Hallatt, J. G. (1986). Tubal conservation and ectopic pregnancy. *American Journal of Obstetrics and Gynecology* **154**, 1216–21.

Hawkins, D. F. (1974). Progestogen-only contraception and tubal pregnancy. *British Medical Journal* **1**, 387.

Henderson, S. R. (1989). Ectopic tubal pregnancy treated by operative laparoscopy. *American Journal of Obstetrics and Gynecology* **160**, 1462–9.

Hogston, P. (1987). How should we diagnose ectopic pregnancy? *British Journal of Clinical Practice* **41**, 609–11.

Jeffcoate, T. N. A. (1955). Salpingectomy or salpingo–oophorectomy? *Journal of Obstetrics and Gynaecology of the British Commonwealth* **62**, 214–15.

Jones, D. H. (1966). Ectopic pregnancy. *British Journal of Clinical Practice* **20**, 377–83.

Kadar, N. (1988). Reproductive performance following conservative microsurgical management of tubal pregnancy. *British Journal of Obstetrics and Gynaecology* **95**, 538–9.

Kadar, N., De Vore, G., and Romero, R. (1981). Discriminatory hCG zone: its use in the sonographic evaluation for ectopic pregnancy. *Obstetrics and Gynecology* **58**, 156–61.

Kamrava, M. M., Taymor, M. L., Berger, M. J., Thompson, I. E., and Seidal, M. M. (1983). Disappearance of human chorionic gonadotrophin following removal of ectopic pregnancy. *Obstetrics and Gynecology* **62**, 486–8.

Keckstein, J., Hepp, S., Schneider, V., Sasse, V., and Steiner, R. (1990). The contact Nd: YAG laser; a new technique for conservation of the fallopian tube in unruptured ectopic pregnancy. *British Journal of Obstetrics and Gynaecology* **97**, 352–6.

Kim, D. S., Chung, S. R., Park, M. I., and Kim, Y. P. (1987). Comparative review of diagnostic accuracy. *Obstetrics and Gynecology* **70**, 547–54.

Kivikoski, A. I., Martin, C. M., and Smeltzer, J. S. (1990). Transabdominal and transvaginal ultrasonography in the diagnosis of ectopic pregnancy. *American Journal of Obstetrics and Gynecology* **163**, 123–8.

Kjer, J. J. and Knudsen, L. B. (1989). Ectopic pregnancy subsequent to laparoscopic sterilization. *American Journal of Obstetrics and Gynecology* **160**, 1202–4.

Kubba, A. A. and Guillebaud, J. (1983). Ectopic pregnancy after post-coital contraception. *British Medical Journal* **287**, 1343–4.

Lancaster, P. A. L. (1985). Obstetric outcome. *Clinics in Obstetrics and Gynaecology* **12**, 847–64.

Lindblom, B., Hahalam, M., and Sjoblom, P. (1989). Serial human chorionic gonadotrophin determinations by immunoassay for differentiation between intra-uterine and ectopic pregnancy. *American Journal of Obstetrics and Gynecology* **161**, 397–400.

Makinen, J. I. (1987). Ectopic pregnancy in Finland 1967–83: a massive increase. *British Medical Journal* **294**, 740–1.

Makinen, J. I. (1989). Increase of ectopic pregnancy in Finland. *Obstetrics and Gynaecology* **73**, 21–4.

Makinen, J. I., Erkkoloa, R. U., and Laippala, P. J. (1989*a*). Causes of the increase in the incidence of ectopic pregnancy. *American Journal of Obstetrics and Gynecology* **160**, 620–6.

Makinen, J. I., Salmi, T. A., Nikkanen, B. P. J., and Koskinen, E. Y. J. (1989*b*). Encouraging rates of fertility after ectopic pregnancy. *International Journal of Fertility* **34**, 46–51.

Makinen, J. I., Kivigarvi, A. K., and Irjala, K. M. A. (1990). Success of non-surgical management of ectopic pregnancy. *Lancet* **335**, 1099.

Marchbanks, P. A., Annegers, J. F., Coulam, C. B., Strathy, J. H., and Kurland, L. T. (1988). Risk factors for ectopic pregnancy. *Journal of the American Medical Association* **259**, 1823–7.

Marjunder, B., Henderson, P. H., and Semple, E. (1983). Salpingitis isthmica nodosa — high risk for tubal pregnancy. *Obstetrics and Gynecology* **62**, 73–8.

Maruri, F. and Azziz, R. (1993). Laparoscopic surgery for ectopic pregnancies. *Fertility Sterility* **59**, 487–98.

Meyer, W. R. and De Cherney, A. H. (1989). Laparoscopic treatment of ectopic pregnancy. *Ballière's Clinical Obstetrics and Gynaecology* **3**, 583–94.

Oelsner, G., Morad, J., Carp, H., Mashiach, S., and Serr, D. M. (1987). Reproductive performance following conservative microsurgery of tubal pregnancy. *British Journal of Obstetrics and Gynaecology* **94**, 1078–83.

Ory, H. W. and the Women's Health Group (1981). Ectopic pregnancy and IUCDs. *Obstetrics and Gynecology* **57**, 137–44.

Ory, S. J. (1991). Chemotherapy for ectopic pregnancy. *Obstetrics and Gynecologic Clinics of North America* **18**, 123–34.

Ory, S. J., O'Brien, P. S., Nnadi, E., Melton, L. J., and Hermann, R. (1993). Fertility after ectopic pregnancy. *Fertility Sterility* **60**, 137–9.

Pansky, M., Bukovsky, A., Golan, A., Langer, R., Schneider, D., Arieli, S., *et al.* (1989). Local methotrexate injection: a non-surgical treatment of ectopic pregnancy. *American Journal of Obstetrics and Gynecology* **161**, 393–6.

Pansky, M., Bukovsky, J., Golan, A., Langer, R., Weinraub, Z., Caspi, E., *et al.* (1993). Reproductive outcome after laparoscopic local Methotrexate injection for tubal pregnancy. *Fertility Sterility* **60**, 85–90.

Reece, E. A., Petrie, R. H., Sirmans, M. F., Finster, M., and Todd, W. D. (1983). Combined intrauterine and extrauterine gestation. *American Journal of Obstetrics and Gynecology* **146**, 323–30.

Robertson, J. N., Hodgeston, P., and Ward, M. E. (1988). Gonococcal and chlamydial antibodies in ectopic and intrauterine pregnancy. *British Journal of Obstetrics and Gynaecology* **95**, 711–16.

Rodi, I. A., Saver, M. V., Gorrill, M. J., Bustillo, M., Gunning, J. E., Marshall, J. R., *et al.* (1986). The medical treatment of unruptured ectopic pregnancy with methotrexate and citrovorum rescue. *Fertility Sterility* **46**, 811–13.

Rubin, G. L., Peterson, H. B., Dorfman, S. F., Layde, P. M., Maze, J. M., Ory, H. W., *et al.* (1983). Ectopic pregnancy in the United States: 1970 thro' 1978. *Journal of the American Medical Association* **249**, 1725–9.

Schenker, J. G. (1972). Surgery after tubal pregnancy. *Surgery Gynecology, and Obstetrics* **135**, 74–80.

Seifer, D. B., Gutmann, J. N., Grant, W. D., Kamps, C. A., and De Cherney, A. H.

(1993). Comparison of persistent ectopic pregnancy after laparoscopic salpingostomy and laparotomy for ectopic pregnancy. *Obstetrics and Gynecology* **81**, 378–82.

Smith, M., Vessey, M. P., Bounds, W., and Warren, J. (1974). Progesterone-only contraception and ectopic pregnancy. *British Medical Journal* **4**, 104–5.

Snowden, R. (1977). The Progestasert and ectopic pregnancy. *British Medical Journal* **2**, 1600–1.

Stabile, I., Campbell, S., and Grudzinskas, J. G. (1988). Can ultrasound really diagnose ectopic pregnancy? *British Journal of Obstetrics and Gynaecology* **95**, 1247–52.

Stenman, U., Alfthan, H., Myllynen, L., and Seppela, M. (1983). Ultrarapid and highly sensitive assay for chorionic gonadotrophin. *Lancet* **ii** 647–9.

Stock, R. J. and Nelson, K. J. (1984). Ectopic pregnancy subsequent to sterilization. *Fertility Sterility* **42**, 211–15.

Stovall, T. G. and Ling, F. W. (1993). Single dose Methotrexate. *American Journal of Obstetrics and Gynecology* **168**, 1759–65.

Tancer, M. L., Delke, I., and Veridiano, N. P. (1981). A 15-year experience with ectopic pregnancy. *Surgery, Gynecology, and Obstetrics* **152**, 179–82.

Tatum, H. J. and Schmidt, F. H. (1977). Contraceptive and sterilization practices and extrauterine pregnancy. *Fertility Sterility* **28**, 407–21.

Taylor, K. J. W. and Meyer, W. R. (1991). New techniques for the diagnosis of ectopic pregnancy. *Obstetric and Gynecologic Clinics of North America* **18**, 39–54.

Thornton, K. L., Diamond, M.P., and De (1991). Linear salpingotomy for ectopic pregnancy. *Obstetrics and Gynecologic Clinics of North America* **18**, 94–109.

Timonen, S. and Nieminen, U. (1967). Tubal pregnancy: choice of operative methods of treatment. *Acta Obstetrica et Gynaecologica Scandinavica* **46**, 327–39.

Tuomivaara, L. and Kauppila, A. (1988). Radical or conservative surgery for ectopic pregnancy? *Fertility Sterility* **50**, 580–9.

Vessey, M. P., Johnson, B., Doll, R., and Peto, R. (1974). Outcome of pregnancy in women using an IUCD. *Lancet* **i**, 495–9.

Weckstein, L. N. (1985). Current perspectives in ectopic pregnancy. *Obstetric and Gynecological Survey* **40**, 259–72.

Winston, R. M. L. (1981). Progress in tubal surgery. *Clinics in Obstetrics and Gynaecology* **8**, 654–79.

3 The management of gestational trophoblastic disease

The term 'gestational trophoblastic disease' covers a spectrum of diseases ranging from hydatidiform mole, the invasive mole or chorioadenoma destruens which is locally malignant but does not metastasize, and the truly malignant choriocarcinoma.

There is a wide variation in the incidence of hydatidiform mole worldwide, ranging from 1 in 85 deliveries in Indonesia, 1 in 120 in Taiwan, 1 in 500 in Japan, to approximately 1 in 1000 in the USA and the UK (Bagshawe *et al*. 1986; Bracken 1987; Currie 1991; Grimes 1984; Hayashi *et al*. 1982). The incidence of choriocarcinoma is always less than that for hydatidiform mole. Thus the incidence of choriocarcinoma is as high as 1 in 500 pregnancies in the Asian population with a range of incidences between 1 in 24 000 and 1 in 50 000 pregnancies in the US and the UK (Brinton *et al*. 1986; Grimes 1984).

Hydatidiform mole arises *de novo* as a form of abnormal pregnancy, whilst choriocarcinoma may arise either following an hydatidiform mole or following a previous pregnancy, either normal or abnormal. Thus, Bagshawe *et al*. (1971) reported a series of 191 choriocarcinomata, of which 63 per cent followed hydatidiform mole, 19 per cent followed live births, and 18 per cent followed either spontaneous miscarriages or stillbirths. When these relative incidences are analysed, the risk of choriocarcinoma is 5000 times more likely after a hydatidiform mole than after a normal pregnancy.

When a patient with a previous hydatidiform mole with apparently complete regression has a subsequent pregnancy, she is at risk of a recurrent hydatidiform mole. Bagshawe (1986) estimated the risk of a second mole as 1 in 76 with subsequent pregnancies, but if there have been two previous molar pregnancies the subsequent risk is 1 in 6.5. Other authors quote similar figures (Sand *et al*. 1984).

Factors in malignant change

Several risk factors have been reported which increase the likelihood of persistent trophoblastic disease resulting in the occurrence of an invasive mole, choriocarcinoma, or the need for chemotherapy. These are enumerated below. Parity appears not to be a significant factor in that the incidence of all

Table 3.1 Maternal age and relative risk of hydatidiform mole

Age (years)	Relative risk
< 15	6.0
15–19	1.5
20–24	1.1
25–29	1.0
30–34	1.1
35–39	1.6
40–44	3.0
45–49	26.3
> 50	411.0

trophoblastic tumours is, at most, 5 per cent higher in the first pregnancy than in any other pregnancies.

The major risk factors appear to be:

(1) maternal age;

(2) method of initial evacuation;

(3) ABO blood group;

(4) method of contraception after evacuation;

(5) complete or partial mole.

Maternal age is the most consistently reported risk factor in the aetiology of gestational trophoblastic disease (Table 3.1). The relationship between maternal age and the incidence of hydatidiform mole forms a J-shaped curve. The lowest incidence occurs in women aged between 20 and 34 years. Over the age of 40 years, there is a 3-fold increase of gestational trophoblastic disease and this rises to a 26-fold risk in women aged between 45 and 49 years, whilst the incidence in women over the age of 50 years is over 4000 times that of a woman aged between 25 and 29 years (Bagshawe *et al.* 1986; Baker 1991; Berkowitz *et al.* 1985; Currie 1991; Hayashi *et al.* 1982; La Vecchia *et al.* 1984). Paternal age is also a separate risk factor, but not as strong as maternal age. When controlled for paternal age, women married to men age 45 years or over had a relative risk of hydatidiform mole of 4.9 (La Vecchia *et al.* 1984). There is, therefore, a corresponding maternal age risk for choriocarcinoma, such that women over the age of 40 years have a 9-fold increase compared to women aged between 20 and 24 years (Brinton *et al.* 1986).

The initial method of evacuation of the hydatidiform mole may influence the need for chemotherapy, in that the lowest need for chemotherapy followed vacuum curettage and spontaneous evacuation, but there was an increased need after other methods (Bagshawe *et al.* 1986). However, this may not be a

Table 3.2 Effect of oral contraceptives within six months of evacuation of a hydatidiform mole

Total number of patients	8882
Total number receiving o.c.	1384 (16%)
Total number requiring chemotherapy	663 (7.5%)
Patients with normal hCG prior to o.c.	1049
Number requiring chemotherapy	5 (0.5%)
Patients with raised hCG prior to o.c.	335
Number requiring chemotherapy	103 (31%)

o.c., oral contraceptives

real risk factor; other methods might have been used in patients presenting with a larger volume of uterine contents, or, occasionally, in the older age group.

The influence of the ABO blood group system as a risk factor in the aetiology of trophoblastic neoplasia was reported by Bagshawe *et al.* in 1971, the risk of developing trophoblastic disease after any form of pregnancy being related to the ABO groups of both patient and husband. Thus a woman with blood group A married to a man with blood group O had the highest risk of developing trophoblastic disease, this risk being 10.4 times that of the lowest risk, that is a woman of blood group A married to a man of blood group A. However, other authors have failed to find any association between parental blood groups and the incidence of gestational trophoblastic disease (Curry *et al.* 1975; Messerli *et al.* 1985).

The early studies drew attention to the association between oral contraceptive use after evacuation of the mole and the need for subsequent chemotherapy. Thus, Stone and Bagshawe (1979) reported a series of 611 patients with hydatidiform moles. When oral contraception was used before the hCG levels became normal, 25 per cent of patients ultimately required cytotoxic therapy, whilst no patient required cytotoxic therapy when oral contraception was used after the hCG levels became normal. Some 9 per cent of patients who did not use oral contraception ultimately required cytotoxic therapy. A recent update on these figures (Bagshawe, unpublished), as shown in Table 3.2, has confirmed that the risk for subsequent chemotherapy is only increased in women who commence oral contraception before hCG levels become normal. Some 31 per cent of such women required subsequent chemotherapy. When oral contraceptives were delayed until hCG levels had become normal, only 0.5 per cent of women subsequently required chemotherapy.

Other studies have failed to show this conclusion but have generally comprised small numbers of patients (Berkovitz *et al.* 1981; Goldberg *et al.* 1987; Yuen and Burch 1983). In a prospective randomized trial, however, Curry *et al.* (1989) allocated 266 patients to receive either oral contraception or barrier methods of contraception after evacuation of a hydatidiform mole. Some

23 per cent of patients receiving oral contraceptives had evidence of postmolar trophoblastic disease as compared with 33 per cent who used barrier methods of contraception. Other studies have also suggested a lower incidence of postmolar trophoblastic disease following the use of oral contraception (Deicas *et al.* 1991).

The current advice to patients should remain that oral contraceptives should not be commenced until the hCG levels have returned to normal, and following this event there is no increased risk associated with the use of oral contraception. Until the hGG level return to normal, other methods of contraception should be used.

The relative risks for postmolar trophoblastic disease associated with complete and partial moles will be discussed towards the end of the following section.

Cytogenetics of trophoblastic tumours

Hydatidiform moles may be classed as either complete, that is trophoblastic tissue alone and no fetus, or incomplete, that is coexistence of trophoblastic tumour and fetus. The majority (72–74 per cent) of all hydatidiform moles are complete (Lawler *et al.* 1979; Stone and Bagshawe 1976).

All complete moles are diploid but the chromosomes are paternally derived, as reported by Kajii and Ohama based on banding studies of the moles and the 'parents' (1977). When the father's own two sets of chromosomes had different banding characteristics, the banding patterns of the mole's chromosomes were always identical with each other and with one of the paternal sets, suggesting that dispermy (fertilization with two sperms) was not the aetiological mechanism. They suggested that the aetiology was due to fertilization by a haploid sperm which, after meiosis, duplicated its chromosomes without cell division. This hypothesis is supported by the work of Yamashita *et al.* (1979). They reported that the HLA-types in complete moles were derived from the father. The moles were analysed for HLA-A and HLA-B specificities. Moles were not only homozygous for paternal HLA but even when the 'father' was heterozygous with HLA-A and -B, the mole was always homozygous for A or B, suggesting that the ovum was fertilized by a haploid sperm which had duplicated its own chromosomes after meiosis and without division. Subsequent work has also supported this view (Fisher and Newlands 1993; Grimes 1984; Jacobs *et al.* 1980; Lawler *et al.* 1991).

Partial moles are triploid, being either 69XXX or 69XXY. The source of the extra chromosomal set is paternal. The likeliest explanation for this is dispermy (Jacobs *et al.* 1982; Lawler *et al.* 1991; Ohama *et al.* 1986). Other chromosomal abnormalities have been described, including tetraploidy (Vassilakos *et al.* 1977).

Dyzygotic twinning may result in a normal fetus and a coexisting hydatidiform mole, albeit rarely (Khoo *et al.* 1986). Such a combination is associated with a poor obstetric performance, complicated by stillbirth (40 per cent), neonatal death (22 per cent), and survival of the coexisting fetus in only 38 per cent of cases (Vejerslev 1991).

The importance of the differentiation between complete and partial hydatidiform mole is of some relevance clinically. The malignant potential is greater for complete than for partial moles (Chen *et al.* 1994). Bagshawe *et al.* (1990) reported that only 1.2 per cent of 857 patients with a partial hydatidiform mole required chemotherapy, whereas 7.1 per cent of 5989 patients with a complete mole required chemotherapy. The risk of malignant change would, therefore, be considered to be minor (but not absent) should the molar pregnancy be triploid (Bagshawe *et al.* 1990; Deaton *et al.* 1989).

Why not histology?

A histological examination of a cohort of trophoblastic tumours would probably report choriocarcinoma in 3 per cent, chorioadenoma destruens in 1.25 per cent, tissue insufficient to make a diagnosis in 10 per cent, and hydatidiform mole in 85.75 per cent of cases. (Bagshawe 1963, Messerli *et al.* 1987).

However, there are two problems with the histological diagnosis. The first is that there is considerable inter- and intrapathologist variability in the diagnosis of gestational trophoblastic neoplasia. Messerli *et al.* (1987) reviewed histological specimens from 173 patients with gestational trophoblastic tumours. Of seven patients originally diagnosed as having choriocarcinoma, the first reviewing pathologist considered that this diagnosis was correct in only two of the seven, whilst the second reviewing pathologist considered the diagnosis was correct in three. Of the 162 cases of slides originally diagnosed as hydatidiform mole, one pathologist revised the diagnosis in two patients to choriocarcinoma, and the other pathologist agreed with those two but added a third case which the first pathologist did not consider to have gestational trophoblastic disease at all. Similarly, Javey *et al.* (1979) reviewed 256 patients who were considered to have hydatidiform mole. Twenty-two patients were not considered to have trophoblastic disease at all (8.6 per cent), and six were considered to have an invasive mole (2.3 per cent).

Secondly, and more importantly, there is poor correlation between the outcome and histology, with reports of metastases arising in patients with good histological evidence of a hydatidiform mole and other patients having clinical evidence of active disease, for example bleeding, metastases, or raised hCG levels, yet no tissue is obtainable on curettage (Genest *et al.* 1991).

Follow-up of trophoblastic tumours

In view of the fact that hydatidiform moles may progress to choriocarcinomata and in view of the fact that the histological diagnosis is not sufficiently 'hard', the need for biochemical follow-up of trophoblastic tumours is universally accepted. Trophoblastic cells produce a wide range of substances, but the usual marker is human chorionic gonadotrophin (hCG). Monitoring by means of pregnancy tests is not sufficiently sensitive since up to 30 per cent of choriocarcinomata do not produce sufficient hCG for a slide pregnancy test to become positive (700 IU per litre). Sensitive radioimmunoassays for hCG use antisera raised against the beta subunit of hCG in order to minimize cross-reactivity with LH.

Using this sensitive radioimmunoassay, the normal trend in patients who do not require subsequent chemotherapy is for a rapid initial fall in hCG production followed by a slower decay. Some 58 per cent of patients with a hydatidiform mole will still have evidence of hCG production by eight weeks, but the quantitative assay should continue to fall such that only a few patients still have detectable hCG production at 32 weeks (Bagshawe 1986).

The length of follow-up together with the advice to avoid pregnancy is of great clinical importance. Ideally, patients are advised to avoid pregnancy for six months after the hCG levels have returned to normal since the risk of choriocarcinoma beyond this time becomes negligible. The risk of any postmolar trophoblastic disease is only 1 in 286 once the hCG levels in urine have been undetectable for six months (Bagshawe *et al.* 1986).

The percentage of patients who receive cytotoxic therapy because of persistent trophoblastic disease varies between different series, ranging from 5.6 per cent (Stone and Bagshawe 1979) to 26 per cent (Morrow *et al.* 1977), because different criteria are used for selecting patients for treatment. There is clearly a balance between potential overtreatment and the risk of postmolar trophoblastic disease, and this balance is such that in current practice up to 10 per cent of patients with a hydatidiform mole in the UK will ultimately receive cytotoxic therapy, whereas 20 per cent of such patients in the US will receive cytotoxic therapy. Those patients who receive cytotoxic therapy will have either choriocarcinoma (arising in approximately 3 per cent of all patients with a hydatidiform mole) or persistent postmolar trophoblastic disease which may locally invade and perforate the uterus. In order to keep the proportion of patients requiring chemotherapy to a minimum, Bagshawe *et al.* (1973) produced criteria for treatment which are summarized below:

1. Serum hCG greater than 20 000 IU per litre at four to six weeks after evacuation.
2. Persistently raised levels of hCG some four to six months after evacuation.
3. Histological evidence of choriocarcinoma.
4. Evidence of brain, chest, hepatic, or gastrointestinal tract metastases.
5. Persistent or recurrent uterine haemorrhage in association with detectable hCG.
6. Rising hCG values.

The treatment of postmolar trophoblastic disease and choriocarcinoma

Without any treatment choriocarcinoma is invariably fatal. The original treatment was hysterectomy, and Ober *et al.* (1971) reported a survival rate of 19 per cent from an accumulated series of 436 patients. In his own unit, this survival rate could be increased to 52 per cent using a combination of surgery and chemotherapy with the early alkylating agents. With modern chemotherapy the overall survival rate is 96 per cent (Bagshawe *et al.* 1989).

Using the known prognostic criteria described earlier, together with a clinical assessment and sensitive hCG assays, patients may be divided into low-, medium-, and high-risk groups (Newlands *et al.* 1986; Smith *et al.* 1993).

Patients in the low-risk group are treated with methotrexate and folinic acid. Some 80 per cent achieve complete remission using this regime alone, with low toxicity (inflammation of the mucous membranes). However, 20 per cent of patients need to change treatment because of drug resistance and then join the medium-risk group (Bagshawe *et al.* 1989; Du Beschter *et al.* 1987).

The medium-risk group comprises patients with a higher incidence of resistance to methotrexate, and hence a combination of cytotoxic agents is used including methotrexate, 6-mercaptopurine, and folinic acid. More recently, etoposide has been added to this regime which has increased the incidence of complete remission, there have been no deaths in this group of patients since its introduction (Newlands *et al.* 1986). There is a variable incidence of reversible alopecia in this group and relapses are treated along with the high-risk patients.

The high-risk group consists of multiple drug therapy with or without salvage surgery, resulting in an overall survival of 85 per cent. The usual drug regime combines methotrexate, etoposide, cyclophosphamide, actinomycin-D, and vincristine (Mortakis and Braga 1990; Newlands *et al.* 1986, 1991). The long-term survival figures for patients treated with chemotherapy have been reported recently by Bagshawe *et al.* (1989).

Using the above regimes, the overall survival rate for patients with postmolar trophoblastic disease was 96 per cent, the only deaths being in the high-risk group (Bagshawe *et al.* 1989; Newlands *et al.* 1986, 1991). Mortality is due either to the extent of metastatic disease on presentation or the late development of drug resistance.

Prophylactic chemotherapy has been suggested by Goldstein (1971) who reported a series of 189 women with hydatidiform moles. One hundred and sixteen women acted as controls and were treated by evacuation only. Seventy-three women were treated by evacuation followed by methotrexate or actinomycin-D. Twenty per cent of the untreated patients showed evidence of persisting disease as did the prophylactic methotrexate group. Prophylaxis with low-dose actinomycin-D led to persistent disease in only 10 per cent of patients, whereas prophylaxis with high-dose actinomycin-D resulted in no patient having persisting disease. However, toxicity was not insignificant, and this included bone marrow depression, alopecia, and inflammatory changes of the mucous membranes. It would seem that prophylaxis using chemotherapy is inappropriate.

Although Hammond *et al.* (1980) demonstrated that hysterectomy at the commencement of cytotoxic therapy resulted in a marginal improvement in survival, surgery is not used as a first-line treatment, partly because of the efficacy of chemotherapy and partly because of the wish to preserve fertility. The indications for hysterectomy would now be severe uterine haemorrhage, perforation of the uterus by trophoblastic tissue, and, occasionally, when there is a drug resistant focus of disease within the uterus.

There is also an indication for hysterectomy in the presence of a placental site trophoblastic tumour. This rare tumour is composed mainly of cyto-trophoblast with very little syncytiotrophoblast. It tends to grow locally with a lower metastatic potential than does choriocarcinoma. The spread is mainly by local infiltration, management being different from other trophoblastic tumours in that these tumours are less chemosensitive and if localized to the uterus the treatment of choice is surgery, although occasional longterm remissions have been obtained with intensive chemotherapy (Dessau *et al.* 1990).

Twenty-five years ago the role of irradiation in the treatment of metastatic trophoblastic disease was reviewed by Brace (1968) in a series of 29 highly selected patients with disease resistant to chemotherapy. Only if the metastases were in the vagina did irradiation have a significant benefit. Some five out of 21 patients with cerebral metastases survived following irradiation and systemic chemotherapy. However, cerebral metastases would probably now be treated using intensive systemic treatment and intrathecal methotrexate.

Subsequent pregnancies

The risks of recurrence of trophoblastic disease in a subsequent pregnancy have already been discussed, and it is advisable that at least one hCG estimation is performed at approximately 12 weeks after delivery.

In a longterm study of 445 women treated with chemotherapy for gestational trophoblastic tumours, 90 per cent of those who wished for a pregnancy conceived and 86 per cent had at least one live birth; there was no excess of congenital malformations (Rustin *et al.* 1984).

Conclusions

Gestational trophoblastic diseases, therefore, represent a spectrum from the benign to the highly malignant choriocarcinoma. A variant of trophoblastic tumours is the placental site trophoblastic tumour which has only been recognized over the last decade. Whilst the latter tumour is generally treated by hysterectomy, very few other women should now require hysterectomy for gestational trophoblastic disease. Their management requires the integration of the information derived from serial hCG estimations, the clinical history and pattern of spread of the disease, and an understanding of the prognostic variables such that the patient has the maximum opportunity of obtaining complete remission with the minimum of toxicity. The major requirement for the future is a better understanding of the process of carcinogenesis of these tumours.

References

Bagshawe, K. D. (1963). Trophoblastic tumours-chemotherapy and development. *British Medical Journal* **2**, 1303–7.

Bagshawe, K. D. (1986). The U.K. registration scheme for hydatidiform mole, 1973–83. *British Journal of Obstetrics and Gynaecology* **93**, 529–31.

Bagshawe, K. D., Rawlins, G., Pyke, M. C., and Lawler, S. D. (1971). The ABO blood groups in trophoblastic neoplasia. *Lancet* **i**, 55 307.

Bagshawe, K. D., Wilson, H., Dublon, P., Smith, A., Baldwin, M., and Kardana, A. (1973). Follow-up after hydatidiform mole. *Journal of Obstetrics and Gynaecology of the British Commonwealth* **80**, 461–8.

Bagshawe, K. D., Dent. J., and Webb, J. (1986). Hydatidiform mole in England and Wales, 1973–83. *Lancet* **ii**, 673–7.

Bagshawe, K., Dent, J., Newlands, E. S., Begent, R. H. J., and Rustin, G. J. S. (1989). The role of low-dose methotrexate and folic acid in gestational trophoblastic tumours. *British Journal of Obstetrics and Gynaecology* **96**, 795–802.

Bagshawe, K. D., Lawler, S. D., Paradinas, F. J., Dent, J., Brown, P., and Boxer, G. M. (1990). Gestational trophoblastic tumours following initial diagnosis of partial hydatidiform mole. *Lancet* **i**, 1074–6.

Baker, V. V. (1991). The aetiology of epidemiology of gestational trophoblastic disease. In *Textbook of gynecologic oncology* (ed. G. Blackledge, J. Jordan, and H. Shingleton), pp. 437–43. W. B. Saunders, London.

Berkovitz, R. S., Goldstein, D. P., Marean, A. R., and Bernstein, M. (1981). Oral contraception and postmolar trophoblastic disease. *Obstetrics and Gynecology* **58**, 474–7.

Berkovitz, R. S., Cramer, D. W., Bernstein, M. R., Cassell, S., Driscoll, S. G., and Goldstein, D. P. (1985). Risk factors for complete molar pregnancy from a case control study. *American Journal of Obstetrics and Gynecology* **152**, 1016–20.

Brace, K. C. (1968). The role of irradiation in the treatment of metastatic trophoblastic disease. *Radiology* **91**, 540–53.

Bracken, M. B. (1987). Incidence and aetiology of hydatidiform mole. *British Journal of Obstetrics and Gynaecology* **94**, 1123–35.

Brinton, L. A., Bracken, E. N. M., and Connelly, R. R. (1986). Choriocarcinoma, incidence in the United States. *American Journal of Epidemiology* **123**, 1094.

Chen, R. J., Huang, S. C., Chow, S. N., Hsieh, C. Y., and Hsu, H. C. (1994). Persistent gestational trophoblastic tumour with partial hydatidiform mole. *British Journal of Obstetrics and Gynaecology* **101**, 330–4.

Currie, J. L. (1991). Gestational trophoblastic neoplasia. In *Textbook of gynecologic oncology* (ed. G. Blackledge, J. Jordan, and H. Shingleton), pp. 454–63. W. B. Saunders, London.

Curry, S. L., Hammond, C. B., Tyrey, I., Creasman, W. T., and Parker, R. T. (1975).

Hydatidiform mole, diagnosis, management, and follow-up. *Obstetrics and Gynecology* **45**, 1–12.

Curry, S. L., Schlaerth, J. B., Kohorn, E. I., Boyce, J. B., Gore, H., Twiggs, L. B., *et al.* (1989). Hormonal contraception and trophoblastic sequelae of the hydatidiform mole. *American Journal of Obstetrics and Gynecology* **160**, 805–11.

Deaton, J. L., Hoffman, J. S., Saal, H., Allred, C., and Koulos, J. P. (1989). Molar pregnancy co-existing with a normal fetus. *Gynecologic Oncology* **32**, 394–7.

Deicus, R. E., Millar, D. S., Rademher, A. W., and Lurain, J. R. (1991). The role of contraception and the development of post-molar gestational trophoblastic tumour. *Obstetrics and Gynecology* **78**, 221–6.

Dessau, R., Rustin, G. J. S., Dent, J., Paradinas, F. J., and Bagshawe, K. D. (1990). Surgery and chemotherapy in the management of placental site tumour. *Gynecologic Oncology* **39**, 56–9.

Du Beschter, B., Berkovitz, R. S., Goldstein, D. P., Cramer, D. W., and Bernstein, M. R. (1987). Metastatic gestational trophoblastic disease. *Obstetrics and Gynecology* **69**, 390–5.

Fisher, R. A. and Newlands, E. S. (1993). Rapid diagnosis and classification of hydatidiform moles by polymerase chain reaction. *American Journal of Obstetrics and Gynecology* **168**, 563–9.

Genest, D. R., Laborde, O., Berkovitz, R. S., Goldstein, D. R., Bernstein, M. R., and Lage, J. (1991). A clinico–pathological study of 153 cases of complete hydatidiform mole. *Obstetrics and Gynecology* **78**, 402–9.

Goldberg, G. L., Cloete, K., Bloch, B., Wiswedel, K., and Altaras, M. M. (1987). Medroxyprogesterone acetate in non-metastatic gestational trophoblastic disease. *British Journal of Obstetrics and Gynaecology* **94**, 22–5.

Goldstein, D. P. (1971). Prophylactic chemotherapy in patients with molar pregnancies. *Obstetrics and Gynecology* **38**, 817–22.

Grimes, D. A. (1984). Epidemiology of gestational trophoblastic disease. *American Journal of Obstetrics and Gynecology* **150**, 309–14.

Hammond, C. B., Weed, J. C., and Currie, J. L. (1980). The role of operation in the treatment of gestational trophoblastic disease. *American Journal of Obstetrics and Gynecology* **136**, 844–58.

Hayashi, K., Bracken, M., Freeman, D. H., and Hellenbrand, K. (1982). Hydatidiform mole in the U.S. *American Journal of Epidemiology* **115**, 67–77.

Jacobs, P. A., Wilson, C. M., Sprenkle, J. A., Rosenhelm, N. B., and Migeon, B. R. (1980). Mechanism of origin of complete hydatidiform mole. *Nature* **286**, 714–16.

Jacobs, P. A., Hunt, P. A., Matsuura, J. S., and Wilson, C. C. (1982). Complete and partial hydatidiform mole in Hawaii; cytogenetics, morphology and epidemiology. *British Journal of Obstetrics and Gynaecology* **89**, 258–66.

Javey, H., Behmard, S., and Langley, F. A. (1979). Discrepancies in the histological diagnosis of hydatidiform mole. *British Journal of Obstetrics and Gynaecology* **86**, 480–3.

Kajii, T. and Ohama, K. (1977). Androgenic origin of hydatidiform mole. *Nature* **268**, 633–4.

Khoo, S. K., Monks, P. L., and Davies, N. T. (1986). Hydatidiform mole co-existing with a live fetus. *Australian and New Zealand Journal of Obstetrics and Gynaecology* **26**, 129–32.

La Vecchia, C., Parazzini, F., DeCarli, A., Franceschi, S., Fasoli, M., Favalli, G., *et al.* (1984). Age of parents and risk of gestational trophoblastic disease. *Journal of the National Cancer Institute* **73**, 639–42.

Lawler, S. D., Pickthall, V. J., Fisher, R. A., Povey, S., WinEvans, M., and Szulman,

A. E. (1979). Genetic studies of complete and partial hydatidiform moles. *Lancet* **ii**, 580.

Lawler, S. D., Fisher, R. A., and Dent, J. (1991). A prospective genetic study of complete and partial hydatidiform mole. *American Journal of Obstetrics and Gynecology* **164**, 1270–7.

Messerli, M. L., Lilienfield, A. M., Parmley, T., Woodruff, J. D., and Rosenstein, N. B. (1985). Risk factors for gestational trophoblastic neoplasia. *American Journal of Obstetrics and Gynecology* **153**, 294–300.

Messerli, M. L., Parmley, T., Woodruff, J. D., Lilienfield, A. M., Bevilacqua, L., and Rosenstein, N. B. (1987). Inter- and intra-pathologist variability in the diagnosis of gestational trophoblastic neoplasia. *Obstetrics and Gynecology* **69**, 622–6.

Morrow, C. P., Kletzky, O. A., DiSaia, P. J., Townsend, D. E., Mishell, D. R., and Nakamura, R. M. (1977). Clinical and laboratory correlates of molar pregnancy and trophoblastic disease. *American Journal of Obstetrics and Gynecology* **128**, 424–30.

Mortakis, A. E. and Braga, C. A. (1990). Poor prognosis of metastatic gestational trophoblastic disease. *Obstetrics and Gynecology* **76**, 272–7.

Newlands, E. S., Bagshawe, K. D., Begent, R. H. J., Rustin, G. J. S., Holden, L., and Dent, J. (1986). Developments in chemotherapy for medium- and high-risk patients with gestational trophoblastic tumours. *British Journal of Obstetrics and Gynaecology* **93**, 63–9.

Newlands, E. S., Bagshawe, K. D., Begent, R. H. J., Rustin, G. J. S., and Holden, L. (1991). Results of the EMA/CO regimen in high-risk gestational trophoblastic tumours. *British Journal of Obstetrics and Gynaecology* **98**, 550–7.

Ober, W. B., Edgcomb, J. H., and Price, E. B. (1971). The pathology of choriocarcinoma. *Annals of the New York Academy of Science* **172**, 299–321.

Ohama, K., Ueda, K., Okamoto, E., Takenaka, M., and Fujiwara, A. (1986). Cytogenetics and clinicopathological studies of partial moles. *Obstetrics and Gynecology* **68**, 659–62.

Rustin, G. J. S., Booth, M., Dent, J., Solk, S., Rustin, F., and Bagshawe, K. D. (1984). Pregnancy after cytotoxic chemotherapy for gestational trophoblastic tumours. *British Medical Journal* **288**, 103–6.

Sand, P. K., Lurain, J. R., and Brewer, J. I. (1984). Repeat gestational trophoblastic disease. *Obstetrics and Gynecology* **63**, 140–4.

Smith, D. B., Newlands, E. S., and Bagshawe, K. D. (1993). Correlation between clinical staging and prognostic groups with gestational trophoblastic disease. *British Journal of Obstetrics and Gynaecology* **100**, 157–60.

Stone, M. and Bagshawe, K. D. (1976). Hydatidiform mole: two entities. *Lancet* **i**, 535–6.

Stone, M. and Bagshawe, K. D. (1979). An analysis of the influences of maternal age, gestational age, contraceptive method, and the primary mode of treatment of patients with hydatidiform mole on the incidence of subsequent chemotherpay. *British Journal of Obstetrics and Gynaecology* **86**, 782–92.

Vassilakos, P., Riotten, G., and Kajii, T. (1977). Hydatidiform mole: two entities. *American Journal of Obstetrics and Gynecology* **127**, 167–70.

Vejerslev, L. O. (1991). Clinical management and diagnostic possibilities in hydatidiform mole with co-existent fetus. *Obstetric and Gynecologic Survey* **46**, 577–88.

Yamashita, K., Ware, N., Araki, T., Ichinoe, K., and Makoto, K. (1979). Human lymphocyte antigen expression in hydatidiform mole. *American Journal of Obstetrics and Gynecology* **135**, 597–600.

Yuen, B. H. and Burch, P. (1983). Relationship of contraception to regression of beta-hCG. *American Journal of Obstetrics and Gynecology* **145**, 214–17.

4 The management of subfertility

It is generally stated that between 10 and 15 per cent of the adult population within reproductive age groups are subfertile. There is obviously no clear line where fertility ends and subfertility begins, but Southam (1960) reported the percentage cumulative pregnancy rates in 10 554 couples attempting to conceive. By the end of six months, 59 per cent of couples had conceived, by the end of 12 months 73 per cent, by the end of 24 months 84 per cent, but ultimately 10 per cent did not conceive. Hull *et al.* (1985) estimated that 1.2 couples per 1000 couples in the population attend a subfertility clinic in any one year, whilst Templeton *et al.* (1990) reported upon the prevalence of infertility in a cohort of 766 women aged 46–50 years of whom 79 per cent reported no difficulties in having children, 7 per cent chose not to conceive, and 14 per cent experienced subfertility, that is difficulty for more than two years in becoming pregnant. Of this 14 per cent, 9 per cent had primary infertility, of whom 60.3 per cent ultimately conceived, and 5 per cent had secondary infertility, of whom 57.5 per cent ultimately conceived. This left 6 per cent of those who wished to conceive with unresolved infertility. There was no difference in outcome between the 62 per cent of infertile couples who sought hospital care and the 38 per cent who did not! Other authors also draw attention to the observation that only a minority of childless couples seek medical help. Johnson *et al.* (1987) reported that only 20 per cent of the childless women aged 35 or over in their practice had ever consulted a doctor about their childlessness, and this may represent an incidence of voluntary childlessness together with a resignation to the state of subfertility (Johnson 1993; Johnson *et al.* 1987).

Female fertility may also decrease with increasing age. Menken *et al.* (1986) analysed the results of the United States National Fertility Study of 1965, and estimated that of wives aged 20–24 years, 3.6 per cent of couples were involuntarily infertile, of wives aged 30–34 years 14 per cent of couples were involuntarily infertile, and of wives aged 40–44, 25 per cent were involuntarily infertile. Schwartz and Mayaux (1982) analysed the cumulative success rates for AID in 2193 nulliparous women with azoospermic husbands. The cumulative success rates after 12 cycles are shown in Table 4.1. The effect of maternal age upon fertility has been well documented with regard to IVF. Using data taken from the Interim Licensing Authority Report (1991), Table 4.2 demonstrates that both the pregnancy rate per treatment cycle and the live birth rate per treatment cycle fall progressively beyond the age of 34 years. This probably relates to poor oocyte quality rather than implantation failure (Meldrum 1993; Navot *et al.* 1991).

Table 4.1 Age and fertility

Age of woman (years)	Cumulative pregnancy rate (%)
< 25	73.0
26–30	74.1
31–35	61.5
< 35	53.6

From Schwartz and Mayaux (1982)

Table 4.2 Age and fertility—IVF

Age of woman (years)	Pregnancy rate in each treatment cycle (%)	Livebirth rate per treatment cycle (%)
< 25	17.2	12.3
25–29	17.9	13.8
30–34	16.7	12.5
35–39	13.6	9.4
40–44	8.6	4.8
> 44	6.5	3.2

From Interim Licensing Authority Report (1991)

Table 4.3 Causes of infertility

Main cause	primary infertility (%) (n = 394)	Secondary infertility (%) (n = 239)
Male causes	26	21
Anovulation	21	16
Tubal causes	14	37
Endometriosis	13	8
Unexplained	26	18

From Randall and Templeton (1991)

The causes of infertility vary slightly from clinic to clinic and have been the subject of a recent review (Randall and Templeton 1991). This review, taken from a tertiary referral centre, demonstrated that 62 per cent of patients had primary and 38 per cent secondary infertility. The major causes of this infertility, following their investigations, are shown in Table 4.3. From this, it may be seen that male causes and unexplained infertility comprise over half of the causes of primary infertility, whereas tubal problems and male causes comprise over half of the causes of secondary infertility.

Although it is more important to describe the success rate for the treatment of individual causes of subfertility, it is of interest to note the success which may be achieved from a cohort of patients attending a subfertility clinic. The best prognosis appears to relate to secondary amenorrhoea which was not due to primary ovarian failure. Hull *et al*. (1979) reported that 93 per cent of such patients treated by either weight gain, clomiphene, bromocriptine or gonadotrophins conceived, 66 per cent within three cycles. The pregnancy rate for patients with tubal damage is, overall, significantly less, and pregnancy rates of up to 19 per cent are reported (Hull *et al*. 1985). These figures are significantly less than those quoted for the results of tubal surgery since these statistics will include all patients with tubal damage, not just those offered surgery. The lowest pregnancy rates appear to relate to severe sperm defects where pregnancy rates without AID of 0.3 per cent have been reported (Hull *et al*. 1985) but rising to 56 per cent with AID (Newton *et al*. 1974). The overall pregnancy rates for patients with unexplained infertility are in the region of 45–72 per cent (Hull *et al*. 1985; Newton *et al*. 1974). It has also been estimated that IVF could help up to 80 per cent of patients with tubal damage and 25 per cent of patients with unexplained infertility (Hull *et al*. 1985).

Patients who attend a subfertility clinic may also conceive without any specific treatment. Collins *et al*. (1983) reported that 38 per cent of all couples and 61 per cent of all pregnancies were 'treatment independent'.

The investigation of infertility

The basic investigation of the infertile couple may be grouped as:

(1) investigation of ovulation;

(2) investigation of tubal function;

(3) investigation of semen specimen;

(4) post-coital tests and antisperm antibodies.

The investigation of ovulation

It cannot be assumed that, simply because a women is menstruating regularly, she is ovulating. Some 20 per cent of women who are anovulatory have absolutely regular cycles, whilst 43 per cent have oligomenorrhoea, and 37 per cent have amemnorrhoea (Cox 1975).

A basal body temperature chart looking for a rise of approximately 0.3 °C in the luteal phase due to progesterone breakdown products is no longer considered to be an accurate method of assessment of ovulation. A monophasic temperature chart is found in 20 per cent of ovulatory cycles (Bauman 1981; Lenton *et al*. 1977*b*). Moreover, the day of ovulation is only predicted accurately in up to 34 per cent of patients based on a basal body temperature chart (Bauman 1981; Lenton *et al*. 1977*b*). Basal body temperature charts are thus insufficiently precise to give a meaningful indication of the day of ovulation (Templeton *et al*. 1982).

Endometrial biopsy was commonly used in order to determine ovulation. In

15 per cent of patients other pathology may be diagnosed by this technique, including submucous fibroids and pelvic tubercle. However, there is a wide range of histological appearance for any given progesterone level and vice versa, this is no longer the commonest method in use for the determination of ovulation. Intra-observer variation in endometrial dating is also known to occur (Li *et al.* 1989).

Mid-luteal serum progesterone levels are now widely used in the assessment of ovulatory cycles. There is no single luteal progesterone level which is totally characteristic of ovulation and pregnancies have been reported in cycles in which the mid-luteal progesterone level was as low as 12 nmol/l (Abdulla *et al.* 1983). Hull *et al.* (1982*a*) reported mid-luteal progesterone levels in 21 untreated single conceptual cycles all in excess of 28 nmol/l, and recommended that levels in excess of this should be taken as being highly suggestive of ovulation.

Serum or urinary oestrogen levels on radioimmunoassay during the proliferative phase may be used to predict ovulation, with a pre-ovulation peak approximately 37 hours before ovulation. Serial levels may also be used in the monitoring of follicular development but are not generally used in routine practice. A serum assay of both LH and FSH may be useful in patients who do not have a regular menstrual cycle as a ratio of LH to FSH of 3:1 may represent polycystic ovarian syndrome. Urinary LH dipstick kits are available and predict ovulation accurately (Barratt *et al.* 1989).

Hyperprolactinaemia will be found in 23 per cent of patients with secondary amenorrhoea and 8 per cent of patients with oligomenorrhoea. Some 2 per cent of patients with hyperprolactinaemia will have subnormal thyroid function. Prolactin levels, also measured by radioimmunoassay, may be elevated by stress and certain drugs, such as methyl-dopa and phenothiazines, but there is doubt as to the value of a prolactin measurement in the presence of a regular menstrual cycle. Some 96 per cent of women have a serum prolactin level of below 800 mU/l and hence this may be taken as representing the upper limit of normal (Glazener *et al.* 1987).

Ultrasound may be used to assess ovulation (Hackeloer *et al.* 1979) with a linear correlation between mean values of plasma oestradiol and follicular diameter in the five days prior to ovulation. The number of actively developing follicles may also be seen, and this is of particular use following hyperstimulation and IVF.

The investigation of tubal function

There are four methods for investigating tubal function; Rubin's test, hysterosalpingography (HSG), laparoscopy with dye test, and salpingoscopy. The Rubin's test (gas insufflation) is now rarely used because of its inaccuracy. Hysterosalpingography is also less accurate than laparoscopy with dye test. In one series of patients with bilateral tubal occlusion as seen on hysterosalpingography, 31 per cent had bilateral patent tubes and a further 19 per cent had unilateral patency on laparoscopy (Coltart 1970). Moreover, peritubular adhesions may be diagnosed with greater accuracy at laparoscopy than on hysterosalpingography (Leeton and Talbot 1973). Laparoscopy may also allow the diagnosis of endometriosis which is likely to have been missed on hysterosalpingography. Moreover, between 1–4 per cent of patients who undergo hysterosalpingography, even with aqueous media, will develop acute pelvic inflammatory disease (Moller *et al*. 1984; Pittaway *et al*. 1983). Although microorganisms may be cultured from the peritoneal cavity after laparoscopy and dye test, acute pelvic inflammatory disease in the presence of normal fallopian tubes is relatively unknown (Pyper *et al*. 1988).

Although it is too early to assess the procedure in clinical practice, salpingoscopy may be of value in obtaining additional information concerning tubal pathology, especially intraluminal adhesions or a circular stricture in patients with previous pelvic inflammatory disease (Brosens *et al*. 1987; Kerin *et al*. 1992). If the technique of salpingostomy does allow for a more accurate assessment of intratubular pathology, it may improve the success rate from tubal surgery (Reiss 1991). There is also good correlation between tubal damage as diagnosed by salpingoscopy and tubal damage as assessed histologically (Hershlag *et al*. 1991). It is likely that this technique will be of increasing importance in the assessment of patients prior to tubal surgery.

The investigation of a semen specimen

The commonest causes of male subfertility include primary spermatogenic failure, an obstructive lesion, disturbances of erection and ejaculation, and endocrine diseases (Jequier 1993).

Semen analysis is the commonest test for the assessment of male fertility; a sample of semen is produced by masturbation in order that the initial sperm-rich fraction of the ejaculate is included. A condom should not be used because many contain a spermicide. The sample should be transferred to a laboratory within two hours, avoiding excessive chilling or heating. The sample is generally analysed for volume, sperm density, sperm motility, and morphology. There are, however, great variations in these characteristics for the semen produced by any one man, leading to poor correlation between any given semenalysis result and the incidence of subsequent pregnancy. Zuckerman *et al*. (1977) compared the seminal analysis of 4000 men with proven fertility with the husbands in 1000 infertile couples. The only differences in the seminal analysis between the infertile and fertile group appeared to be an excess of sperm densities below 10×10^6/ml and below 25×10^6 sperms/ejaculate.

It becomes difficult to define a lower limit of normal in any aspect of semen analysis. It is likely that the results, based even on repeated semenalysis, should be considered as a spectrum, such that the chance of pregnancy will fall when there is a particularly low sperm count or a particularly low number of motile sperms but that so long as there are normally formed motile sperms in an ejaculate, the chance of pregnancy is not zero. Smith *et al*. (1977) assessed six semen samples from each man of 140 consecutive subfertile couples in whom

Table 4.4 Semen analysis

Sperm count	Pregnancy rate (%)	No. of motile sperm	Pregnancy rate (%)
$\times 10^6$ per ml			
< 5	42	< 5	37.5
5–60	50	5–60	60
> 60	70	> 60	78
$\times 10^6$ per ejaculate			
< 12.5	25	< 12.5	22.7
12.5–200	50	12.5–200	60
> 200	70	> 200	76.6

From Smith *et al.* (1977)

the overall subsequent pregnancy rate was 58 per cent. In general, sperm counts, whether number of sperm per millilitre or total number of sperm per ejaculate, broke down into three distinct groups when compared to subsequent pregnancy rates, as did sperm motility. These results are shown in Table 4.4. It can be seen that a pronounced reduction in either sperm count or sperm motility is required in order that the pregnancy rate should fall below the average for the population under study.

A varicocele is found in 10–20 per cent of otherwise normal males, in 30 per cent of males with subnormal semenalysis, but in up to 81 per cent of males with secondary infertility (Gorelick and Goldstein 1993; Vermeulen and Vandeweghe 1983, 1984). These authors reported a series of 82 men with varicoceles, 62 treated surgically and 20 untreated, but these groups were not randomly allocated. All patients had either oligozoospermia (less than 20 × 10^6/ml), asthenozoospermia (less than 40 per cent motility), or teratozoospermia (less than 30 per cent with ideal morphology). Within one year, 24 per cent of the patients treated by surgery achieved a pregnancy as compared to 40 per cent of those untreated. There was no significant increase in sperm density, motility, or normal morphology in the group treated surgically.

There are only minimal changes in semenalysis characteristics with increasing age. Schwartz *et al.* (1983) reported the semen characteristics in 833 fertile males between 21 and 50 years. There was no significant differences in count or volume. There was a small statistically significant decrease in motility with increasing age, from 70 per cent in men aged 20–25 to 65 per cent aged 46–50. There was also a small statistically significant increase in the incidence of abnormal forms, from 30 per cent in men aged 26–30 to 34 per cent in men aged 46–50. However, the greatest area of variation occurred not with age but with the length of pre-assessment abstinence, the best samples occurring after three days of abstinence.

Endocrine investigations in males are only really of help in the presence of severe oligospermia or azoospermia. De Kretser (1979) recommended measuring FSH, LH, and testosterone levels only in the presence of a sperm count of less than 5×10^6/ml, looking for either an androgen deficiency which may respond to androgen replacement or occasionally to gonadotrophins. Wu *et al.* (1981) observed that a single FSH level was just as valuable a discriminant between germ cell dysplasia (raised FSH) and tubular obstruction (normal FSH) as was testicular biopsy which is now rarely used.

The post-coital test and antisperm antibodies

The place of the post-coital test is controversial, partly because of doubt over the benefits of this procedure and partly because it is essential that the test is performed just before ovulation when cervical mucus production is at its peak, yet the majority of gynaecologists only hold a clinic once per week. The test is generally performed after two or three days abstinence and the examination may be carried out any time between 2–24 hours after intercourse, there being no good evidence that any narrower a range of examination times is beneficial. There is also debate as to the definition of a 'normal' post-coital test. In a review of the literature concerning the validity of the post-coital test (Griffiths and Grimes 1990) attention was drawn to the variation in definition which ranged from one sperm per high-power field (Jette and Glass 1972), through one sperm with forward penetration (Hull *et al.* 1982*b*), to five or more per high-power field (Collins *et al.* 1984). It is perhaps more useful to define the results as either fair (1–5 forward moving sperms per high-power field), good (6–20 forward moving sperms per high-power field), or excellent (greater than 20 forward moving sperms per high-power field) (Hull *et al.* 1982*b*).

In clinical practice, the post-coital test is more useful as a prognostic indicator of pregnancy rather than a specific investigation of subfertility (Hull *et al.* 1982*b*). He concluded 'until the alleged benefits of this test have been shown to merit its expense, inconvenience, and psychologic morbidity, the test should probably be used more selectively and interpreted with greater caution'. Some authors have shown that the length of time between presentation and conception was inversely proportional to the result of the post-coital test in couples with unexplained infertility (Hull *et al.* 1982*b*), whilst other workers have been unable to demonstrate any relationship between the outcome of the post-coital test and subsequent fertility (Eggert-Kruse *et al.* 1989).

There is evidence that abnormal immunological responses account for infertility in some couples, although the exact place of such investigations in current management has yet to be elucidated; in addition, differences in nomenclature have caused some confusion in the interpretation of available literature. However, Menge *et al.* (1982) analysed the serum of 698 infertile couples and found antisperm antibodies in 17 per cent of males, 22 per cent of females, and 31 per cent of at least one of each couple. The subsequent pregnancy rate where those males had antisperm antibodies was 7 per cent compared with 43 per cent in males without antibodies. The corresponding figures for females were 4 per cent and 46, respectively, and the corresponding pregnancy rates for couples were 13 per cent and 19 per cent, illustrating the adverse effect of antisperm antibodies upon fertility. Aitken *et al.* (1988) suggested a possible mode of action for these antibodies based on the examination of sperm and antibodies found in 8 per cent of men with infertility and up to 88 per cent of men after vasectomy. They postulated that the gamma-globulin fraction of such sera (from both groups) was capable of suppressing sperm–oocyte fusion *in vitro*.

Cellular immunity may also be implicated. Leukocytes from 14 infertile women were able to generate significantly greater inhibitory activity to sperm than did leukocytes from nine fertile women (McShane *et al.* 1985). The implications of such studies, and the appropriate treatments, remain unclear. The editor of *Obstetric and Gynaecologic Survey* (1989) stated 'this area seems loaded with disagreement and controversy'. Hopefully, such disagreement and controversy will become resolved and the appropriate treatment then given.

The treatment of subfertility

The following topics will be discussed:

(1) the induction of ovulation;

(2) the place of tubal surgery;

(3) the place of *in vitro* fertilization;

(4) artificial insemination.

The induction of ovulation

The prospect for patients with defects in ovulation will depend upon the nature of that defect, as discussed below. The prognosis is best for those patients with secondary amenorrhoea which was not due to primary ovarian failure, since their conception rates with treatment will equal those of normal women. Thus Hull *et al.* (1979) treated 59 such patients by either weight gain, clomiphene, bromocriptine, or gonadotrophins, and all patients ovulated, with 55 out of 59 (93 per cent) conceiving by the end of the study, 49 per cent within two cycles, and 66 per cent within three cycles.

The benefit of treating amenorrhoea related to weight loss by weight gain was demonstrated by Knuth *et al.* (1977). These authors considered that weight loss was the cause of secondary amenorrhoea in 23 per cent of patients, and when these women were encouraged to gain weight 58 per cent resumed an ovulatory cycle. It would appear that a significant percentage of body fat (26–28 per cent) is required in mature women in order that regular ovulatory cycles can occur (Frisch 1990).

Clomiphene

Clomiphene citrate is a non-steroidal agent acting mainly at the hypothalamic level where it competes for oestrogen receptor binding sites.

When the results from clomiphene therapy are assessed, it is important to distinguish between ovulation rates and pregnancy rates since all series show a significant discrepancy between these rates (Glasier 1990). The reasons for this discrepancy are multiple, but will include the criteria used for the diagnosis of ovulation and the observation that some patients being treated with clomiphene will have other undiagnosed factors involved in their subfertility. Whilst up to 90 per cent of patients who receive clomiphene will ovulate (Evans and Townsend 1976; Glasier 1990; Gysler *et al.* 1982; McGregor *et al.* 1968; Rust *et al.* 1974) the reported pregnancy rates have been variously quoted as being between 9 and 62 per cent, most studies reporting a conception rate of between 35 and 45 per cent (Evans and Townsend 1976; Glasier 1990; McGregor *et al.* 1968; Whitelaw 1970). These statistics are superior to those following placebo in which ovulation occurred in 40 per cent of patients and conception in 19 per cent (Evans and Townsend 1976).

The dose of clomiphene is important in that ovarian enlargement and hyperstimulation, much less common than with gonadotrophin therapy, is a dose-related complication, occurring in some degree in 7 per cent of women who receive 50 mg per day and in 9 per cent who receive 100 mg per day (McGregor *et al.* 1968). Of those women who will ovulate, 50 per cent will do so on a dose of 50 mg, but the dose may be increased by 50 mg increments to up to 200 mg per day in order for ovulation to occur (O'Herlihy *et al.* 1981). No patient requires treatment for more than five consecutive days in any one cycle.

If pregnancy is to occur, it tends to occur within the first few cycles. For example, in one series 52 per cent of the conceptions occurred during the first treatment cycle and 85 per cent of the conceptions occurred within the first three treatment cycles (Gysler *et al.* 1982). It, therefore, seems inappropriate to prescribe clomiphene in the longterm.

The day upon which clomiphene therapy should be instituted is also debated, but in a study of 414 clomiphene cycles in 87 patients, Wu and Winkel (1989) were unable to identify any differences in ovarian response or pregnancy outcome when clomiphene was initiated randomly upon the second, third, fourth, or fifth day of the menstrual cycle.

Over and above the incidence of ovarian enlargement, side-effects of clomiphene are not uncommon but rarely do they interfere with treatment. Approximately 10 per cent of women complain of hot flushes during treatment, whilst 1.6 per cent complain of visual disturbances (Glasier 1990). Multiple pregnancy should be considered to be a complication of treatment. The incidence of twins is generally reported in 6–8 per cent of all clomiphene pregnancies, whilst triplets occur in less than 0.5 per cent, both of those figures being greater than would be expected for the overall population (1.3 and 0.01 per cent, respectively) (Glasier 1990; Schenker *et al.* 1981).

There may be an increased incidence of first trimester spontaneous abortion following ovulation induction with clomiphene. The earlier series suggested that this was the case, the rate being variably quoted as between 16 and 26 per cent of conceptions (Adashi *et al.* 1979; McGregor *et al.* 1968). However, a recent meta-analysis of 3775 clomiphene-induced pregnancies showed that 16 per cent ended in miscarriage, a statistic similar to that expected from the overall population (Shoham *et al.* 1991). If an increased risk is present, it must be relatively small and may relate to the anti-oestrogenic effect of clomiphene (Scialli 1986).

There is no convincing evidence for an increase in the evidence of congenital abnormalities in pregnancies following ovulation induction with clomiphene (Mills *et al.* 1990). Shoham *et al.* (1991) analysed the published literature and found 40 major malformations in 3751 newborns following clomiphene induction, a rate of 10.7 per 1000, which is similar to the normal population.

Some patients taking clomiphene show evidence of follicular development but do not ovulate. In this situation, the addition of intramuscular hCG has been advocated with conception rates of up to 66 per cent (O'Herlihy *et al.* 1981). Although the theoretical risk of hyperstimulation and multiple pregnancy with this regime seems to be minimal (Ron-El *et al.* 1989) this regime is not superior to clomiphene alone in randomized trials (Quigley *et al.* 1984). This management has, therefore, failed to stand the test of time.

Bromocriptine

Bromocriptine is a dopamine agonist indicated in the treatment of hyperprolactinaemia, a condition found in 23 per cent of patients with secondary amenorrhoea and 8 per cent of patients with oligomenorrhoea. It is now generally accepted that empirical bromocriptine is not of benefit if the patient has a normal serum prolactin level, regardless of whether or not she is ovulating, nor is clomiphene of benefit in patients who have hyperprolactinaemia (Gorlitsky *et al.* 1978; Wright *et al.* 1979).

The use of bromocriptine in patients with a microprolactinoma or idiopathic disease results in between 85 and 95 per cent of patients ovulating and 70 and 80 per cent of all patients conceiving (Crosignani and Ferrari 1990; Pepperell *et al.* 1977). In order to minimize side-effects, therapy should be started with a low dose, 1.25 mg, taken with food, which is then gradually increased, usually to 7.5 mg, but occasionally up to 20 mg, depending upon prolactin levels (Crosignani and Ferrari 1990). These authors have reported that mild transient side-effects, such as nausea, headache, dizziness, and fatigue occurred in up to 69 per cent of patients receiving this treatment.

All the evidence currently available suggests that pregnancies which follow bromocriptine therapy are similar to the overall pregnancy population, with a spontaneous abortion rate of 11 per cent, a multiple pregnancy rate of 2 per cent, a fetal abnormality rate of 3 per cent, and no specific antenatal problems (Griffith 1978; Weil 1986).

Even in the presence of a macroadenoma and visual field defects, bromocriptine is probably preferable to surgery. Pituitary adenomata account for up to 10 per cent of all intracranial tumours, those of 10 mm or less in diameter are termed microadenomata and greater than 10 mm in diameter, macroadenomata. Corenblum and Taylor (1983) reported the use of bromocriptine

Table 4.5 Hyperprolactinaemia and pregnancy

	Untreated microadenoma	Untreated macroadenoma	Treated
Total no.	246	45	46
Increase in tumour size	15 (6.1%)	11 (24.4%)	2 (4.3%)
Visual disturbance and/or headache	4 (1.6%)	7 (15.6%)	2 (4.3%)

From Molitch (1985)

for between five and nine years in 75 women with hyperprolactinaemia, 10 with a normal sella, 49 thought to have a microadenoma, and 16 a macroadenoma. Menstruation recurred in 90 per cent of those patients with a normal sella, 98 per cent of those with a microadenoma, and 68.8 per cent of those with a macroadenoma. Of 46 patients who wished to conceive 80 per cent did so, and one-third of those patients with a macroadenoma in whom bromocriptine was discontinued showed clinical and radiological evidence of tumour growth which regressed when bromocriptine was reinstituted. In patients who have undergone surgical exploration of the sella turcica for a macroadenoma, 63 per cent still required bromocriptine at some stage postoperatively because of a continuation or recurrence of the hyperprolactinaemia (Thomson *et al.* 1985).

Since pregnancy is known to stimulate prolactin production, the risk of recurrence of the tumour, or the stimulation of tumour growth during pregnancy, has been specifically assessed. It would seem that this is only really a problem in patients who are untreated, whilst those patients who continue bromocriptine throughout pregnancy appear to be relatively free of these complications (Crosignani and Ferrari 1990). Molitch (1985) performed a meta-analysis based on 16 series of pregnant women with an untreated micro-adenoma, 11 series of pregnant women with an untreated macroadenoma, and eight series of previously treated women, regardless of the treatment modality used. As can be seen from Table 4.5, complications were significantly less in patients who had previously been treated. Although suprasella tumour growth is relatively unusual in treated patients, it may be excluded during pregnancy by repeated visual field evaluation (Crosignani and Ferrari 1990).

There are other dopamine agonists currently under assessment for the treatment of hyperprolactinaemia, of which cabergoline is currently the likeliest to be introduced into clinical practice, but these agents are not as yet available for routine patient treatment.

Cyclofenil

Cyclofenil is a weak anti-oestrogen, and, therefore, an alternative to clomiphene. Sato *et al.* (1969) treated 122 women with secondary amenorrhoea using dosages of 100–400 mg per day. Ovulation occurred in 43 per cent of patients and conception in 14 per cent, with just over half of the conceptions occurring during the first treatment cycle.

Tamoxifen

Tamoxifen is an anti-oestrogen, more powerful than clomiphene (Furr and Jordan 1984). Williamson and Ellis (1973) treated 32 anovulatory patients with either 20 mg daily for four days from the 2nd day of each cycle, if menstruating, or up to 80 mg if they remained amenorrhoeic. Ovulation occurred in 81 per cent of patients and pregnancy in 56 per cent either during treatment or in the first spontaneous cycle after treatment. There was no evidence of hyper-stimulation, excess multiple pregnancies, excess abortion, or fetal abnormality. Fukushima *et al.* (1982) treated 17 women with luteal phase insufficiency using 10 mg per day of tamoxifen for five days. The mean length of the luteal phase was elongated and pregnancy occurred in 24 per cent of patients.

Since clinicians have a greater experience of using clomiphene than tamoxifen, the latter tends only to be used if clomiphene has failed. There is some evidence that a combination of clomiphene and tamoxifen may be more effective than clomiphene alone (Suginami *et al.* 1993).

Gonadotrophin therapy

The basis of gonadotrophin therapy is the induction of follicular growth with human menopausal gonadotrophin (hMG) followed by the induction of ovulation with human chorionic gonadotrophin. A fixed regime may be used with preplanned doses of hMG, injections being administered on either day 1, 3, and 5, or days 1, 5, and 8 of the course of treatment, followed by an injection of hCG when follicular growth is ripe but not excessive. Alternatively, an individualized regime may be used whereby the number of injections of hMG and their dosages are based on follicular response, which is itself judged by either oestrogen excretion or ovarian ultrasound assessment, followed by a single injection of hCG. Individualized regimes tend to result in higher pregnancy rates and less hyperstimulation than do predetermined regimes (Lunenfeld and Insler 1974).

In a meta-analysis of 1286 patients undergoing 3002 treatment cycles, ovulation occurred in 75 per cent of patients and 64 per cent of cycles. Some 18 per cent of patients conceived, but 37 per cent of those pregnancies ended in an abortion. Some 25 per cent of pregnancies were multiple, whilst the fetal abnormality rate was 1.7 per cent and hyperstimulation occurred in 1.3 per cent of cycles (Thompson and Hansen 1970). A more recent review of the literature suggests that ovulation will occur in up to 90 per cent and pregnancy in up to 80 per cent of hypogonadotrophic patients using the above regimes (Bettendorf 1990). There is no hard evidence to suggest that the use of pure FSH therapy is superior to the use of hMG therapy (Bettendorf 1990).

The problem of hyperstimulation with gonadotrophins was reported by Mozes *et al.* (1965) who reported this complication in 7.6 per cent of cycles, with one death believed to be due to a pulmonary embolus and a cerebro-vascular accident, and a second patient who had a limb amputated due to arterial thromboembolism coexisting with massive venous thrombosis. It is now accepted that the risk of ovarian hyperstimulation may be minimized by the use of oestrogen concentration monitoring and follicular growth ultrasound monitoring. This should result in a decrease in the severity of hyperstimulation rather than a decrease in the incidence of all causes of hyperstimulation, mild, moderate, and severe (*Lancet*, 1991*b*; Smith and Cooke 1991). With such monitoring, Navot *et al.* (1988) reported that ovarian hyperstimulation occurred in 3 per cent of 1822 treatment cycles, especially in thin, young patients.

Provided the pituitary gland is responsive to gonadotrophin releasing hormone (GnRh), synthetic preparations of this agent given in a pulsatile fashion can mimic the normal pattern of secretion of gonadotrophins in the menstrual cycle (Leyendecker *et al.* 1980). High success rates in the treatment of anovulatory infertility have been reported, but women with polycystic ovaries are less responsive. In one such series (Homburg *et al.* 1989), ovulation occurred in 70 per cent of treatment cycles, pregnancy in 33 per cent of ovulation cycles, but miscarriage occurred in 28 per cent of the pregnancies.

Some patients fail to conceive after ovulation induction with the above approaches. In some cases this is due to premature luteinization where an LH surge occurs prior to adequate follicular development being achieved (Fleming and Coutts 1986). This tendency to premature luteinization, not uncommon in women with polycystic ovarian syndrome, can be overcome with the use of long-acting GnRH agonist therapy which suppresses endogenous release (down-regulation) followed by the use of an individualized HMG–hCG regime (Fleming *et al.* 1985). Down-regulation has also been used in patients who have a tendency to ovarian hyperstimulation with other regimes (Nilsson and Hamberger 1990).

There has also been some recent interest in the use of gonadotrophins to induce multifollicular development (superovulation) combined with intrauterine insemination of washed sperm in the management of couples with unexplained infertility (Chaffkin *et al.* 1991). Although the preliminary results of treatment are encouraging, the results of larger randomized studies must be awaited before the place for this treatment is established.

The cause of the high spontaneous abortion rate with gonadotrophin therapy, variably quoted as being between 12 and 31 per cent, is not clear, but likely explanations include premature ovulation, increased motility within the tube which caused the fertilized ovum to arrive at an ill-prepared uterus, and corpus luteum insufficiency. Shoham *et al.* (1991) reported a meta-analysis of 1340 gonadotrophin-induced pregnancies in which 18.8 per cent miscarried, a rate only slightly higher than that seen in the overall population. There may also be an increase in the incidence of fetal abnormality after gonadotrophin therapy. Shoham *et al.* (1991) reported that 1160 newborn infants had 25 major and 38 minor abnormalities, a total incidence of 54.3 per 100 which is higher than the usual ranges quoted for the population (3.1–22.5 per 1000 deliveries).

From the above, it is clear that the use of gonadotrophins in the induction of ovulation is an effective form of treatment but in view of the potentially high incidence of complications, especially hyperstimulation and multiple pregnancy, this treatment should be performed in subspecialist units.

Tubal surgery

The best results from tubal surgery cannot match the best results from the medical induction of ovulation, for inflammatory tubal disease may result in changes in tubal motility which are only partially reversible and alterations in the tubal nutritive function which is wholly irreversible. The assessment of results following tubal surgery is itself complicated by patient selection and, hence, results should only be quoted for any given operative procedure rather than tubal surgery generally; even then, bias in patient selection may have occurred. Lastly, the effect of intra-operative and post-operative measures may also modify the results and these will be discussed.

The reversal of a previous sterilization should be considered separately from other forms of tubal surgery because of the absence of previous pelvic inflammatory disease and the presence of a population of previous proven fertility. Winston (1980) reported a series of 126 reversals of sterilization resulting in 73 pregnancies (58 per cent); however, three pregnancies were tubal. The best results arose when the sterilization had been performed in the region of the isthmus (75 per cent pregnancy rate) and the worst relating to the ampulla (42 per cent). Rock *et al.* (1987) reported that 86 per cent of women who had undergone a previous Falope ring sterilization conceived following tubal reanastamosis, whilst only 67 per cent of women who had undergone a previous tubal diathermy conceived following tubal reanastamosis. This observation is one of the reasons why sterilization by application of a ring or clip is to be preferred to sterilization by diathermy.

Surgery performed for infertility involves either macroscopic or microscopic surgical techniques. The principles of microsurgery form a concept as much as a technique. The major principles have been enumerated by Winston (1980) and by Garcia and Mastroiann (1980); both involve the use of magnification over the range 2 × to 60 ×, minimal tissue handling and manipulation, the use of atraumatic instruments, such as glass rods to handle tissues, experience, tuition, the use of fine (for example 6–0) non-reactive suture material, attention to reperitonealization, keeping tissues moist with a warm saline irrigation, and precise haemostatis using bipolar microforceps coagulation.

There are numerous series in the literature which claim to show the advantage of microsurgery over macrosurgery in terms of higher incidences of pregnancy and to a lesser degree higher incidences of tubal patency, but virtually all series consist of a comparison of macrosurgery over one period of time with micro-surgery over a later period of time and, in the absence of any satisfactory controlled trial, it is possible that the results are as much related to surgical care as to the use of microsurgical techniques. Several series exist which claim to show the overall effect of microsurgical principles upon tubal surgery (Fayez and Suliman 1972; Frantzen and Scholosser 1982; Siegler and Kontopoulos 1979). The results from one of these series are illustrated in Table 4.6. During the period 1971–77, 99 macrosurgical tuboplasties were performed with a 77 per cent patency rate and a 36 per cent pregnancy rate. During the period 1977–9,

Table 4.6 Tubal surgery

Procedure	Macrosurgery			Microsurgery		
	No.	% Patent	No. Pregnant (%)	No.	% Patent	% Pregnant
Salpingolysis	24	100	63	8	100	75
Fimbrioplasty	16	88	39	6	84	50
Salpingostomy	32	77	25	16	80	38
Reanastamosis	20	66	40	27	88	59
Reimplantation	4	50	25	3	75	33
Combined procedures	3	42	0	2	67	0
Total	99	77	49	62	85	52

Data from Fayez and Suliman (1982)

62 microsurgical tuboplasties were performed with an 85 per cent patency rate and a 51 per cent pregnancy rate (Fayez and Suliman 1982). One area where these non-randomized series do seem to provide convincing evidence for the benefits of microsurgery concerns cornual blockage where the macrosurgical technique of reimplantation may be replaced by the microsurgical technique of reanastamosis. Diamond (1979) reported that following tubal reimplantation the patency rate was 57 per cent and the pregnancy rate 24 per cent, whereas after microsurgical reanastamosis, the rates were 82 per cent and 64 per cent, respectively.

The surgical treatment of hydrosalpinx by salpingostomy has been widely studied, partly because this is such a common situation when tubal damage has occurred. Non-randomized trials have suggested a significant improvement in outlook when microsurgical rather than macrosurgical salpingostomy is performed. Winston (1981) reported a meta-analysis of 14 series of macrosurgical salpingostomy in 653 patients and 10 series of microsurgical salpingostomy in a similar number of patients. Following macrosurgery, the term pregnancy rate was 9.5 per cent and the ectopic pregnancy rate 9 per cent. Following microsurgery, the rates were 19 per cent and 8 per cent, respectively. Similarly, Reiss (1991) quoted a meta-analysis of 16 series of microsurgical salpingostomy published since 1980 in which 1728 patients had a 26 per cent intrauterine and 8 per cent ectopic pregnancy rate. The largest single series of microsurgical salpingostomy, which was not included in the above series, reported that of 323 patients, the term pregnancy rate was 33 per cent and the ectopic pregnancy rate 10 per cent (Winston and Margara 1991). Other authors have quoted a similar conception rate (Singhal *et al.* 1991).

The above statistics for the results from microsurgical salpingostomy relate to all patients who were included in these series. This may be inappropriate since there is much evidence to suggest that the gross appearance of the hydrosalpinx will influence the outcome. These observations have allowed scoring systems to be devised in order that a better comparison of results may be possible (American Fertility Society 1988; Boer-Meisel *et al.* 1986). When such scoring systems are applied, it can be shown that the more severe is the damage, the lower is the intrauterine pregnancy rate. In one of the above series, the intrauterine pregnancy rate was 54 per cent in tubes of normal diameter, 30 per cent in tubes with moderate pre-operative distension, and 21 per cent in tubes with pre-operative severe dilatation (Singhal *et al.* 1991). In another series, term pregnancy occurred in 23 per cent of women with minimal tubal damage but in only 6 per cent of those with a tubo–ovarian mass (Winston and Margara 1991). The importance of such scoring systems will be discussed again when the relative merits of tubal surgery and IVF are assessed.

Repeat tubal surgery is generally unrewarding. Lauristen *et al.* (1982) reported a series of 71 patients undergoing their first tuboplasty in whom conception occurred in 59 per cent, whereas in 31 women undergoing a second tuboplasty by microsurgery, the conception rate was 16 per cent. Similarly, Thie *et al.* (1986) reported that of 161 patients undergoing primary microsurgical tuboplasty, 51 per cent conceived of whom 42 per cent had an intrauterine pregnancy and 9 per cent a tubal pregnancy, whereas of 21 women undergoing repeat microsurgical tuboplasty, only 18 per cent conceived, all intrauterine. Similarly, Winston and Margara (1991) reported that the 33 per cent pregnancy rate reported after a first attempt at microsurgical salpingostomy fell to 18 per cent in women undergoing a repeat procedure. Again, the implications of this observation will be discussed in the section which debates the merits of tubal surgery and IVF.

Additional procedures or techniques have been used during or after surgery in an attempt to produce improved results. These include the use of splints, surgical prostheses such as the Mulligan hood, drugs, and laparoscopy. It has now been demonstrated that there is no advantage from the use of splints for tubal surgery (Winston 1975). The use of Mulligan hoods at salpingostomy did improve tubal patency, from a pre-hood patency rate of 50 per cent to a post-hood patency rate of 70 per cent, but the need for a second surgical procedure and the advent of microsurgery have made these devices relatively redundant (Garcia and Mastroiann 1980).

Hydrotubation using a solution of hydrocortisone with or without an antibiotic was advocated by Grant and Robertson (1966) who argued that the hydrostatic pressure helped to expel mucus and tubal debris. In an uncontrolled trial, 108 patients who underwent post-operative hydrotubation had a pregnancy rate of 33 per cent, whereas 457 patients who did not had a pregnancy rate of 11.5 per cent. However, Winston (1980) was unable to find any benefit from hydrotubation, whilst Garcia and Mastroiann (1980) reported an incidence of post-operative pelvic inflammatory disease of 3 per cent following hydrotubation. In a randomized, controlled trial, the incidence of subsequent conception, tubal pregnancy, or live birth was similar whether or not post-operative hydrotubation was performed, hence the technique is no longer part of contemporary practice (Rock *et al.* 1987).

The potential benefit from dexamethasone or other anti-inflammatory agents in the reduction of post-operative adhesions is largely extrapolated from animal experimentation (Replogle *et al.* 1963). In the only randomized trial of steroids following surgery on human females, the use of steroids was of no benefit over placebo in the incidence of subsequent pregnancy (Larsson *et al.* 1985). Similarly, the use of intraperitoneal Dextran 70 is again largely extrapolated from animal experimentation rather than randomized trials in humans (Neuwirth and Khalaf 1975). The use of commercially available barriers to enhance the covering of deperitonealized areas following tubal surgery may also reduce adhesion formation (Li and Cooke 1994).

Laparoscopic tubal surgery has been advocated using either laparoscopic surgical instruments or laser (Donnez and Nisolle 1989; Fayez 1983) in the belief that these will reduce post-operative adhesion formation. In the absence of a randomized study, such conclusions may not be drawn (Reiss 1991). Other authors have reported a higher re-occlusion rate following laparoscopic tubal surgery (37 per cent) than after microsurgery (12 per cent) (Winston

and Margara 1991). Early laparoscopy, some 8–12 days after tubal reconstructive surgery, is advocated by some surgeons as the technique of choice
to reduce adhesion formation although the exact value is yet to be proven
(Jansen 1988).

From the above, it is clear that there have been numerous suggestions in
recent years aimed at improving the results following tubal reconstructive
surgery. However, in the absence of randomized trials it has become difficult
to convince all but the enthusiasts for these techniques that they provide benefits
for the patients.

The above series come from specialist centres and may represent the best
which can be achieved. Watson *et al.* (1990) reported the results of tubal surgery
performed in two non-specialist centres. Of 77 patients with a mean follow-up
of over three years, 12 per cent had term pregnancies. If bilateral distal tubal
occlusion alone was considered, only 5 per cent of patients had a pregnancy
which reached the third trimester. If adhesiolysis in the presence of patent tubes
was considered, only 21 per cent of patients had a pregnancy which reached
the third trimester. It may be that these poorer results are a reflection of
non-specialist centres or it may represent some degree of patient selection. These
results, however, raise the question whether tubal surgery should always be
performed in specialist units.

In vitro fertilization

In vitro fertilization has been used for tubal problems, unexplained infertility,
minimal endometriosis, and male fertility problems (Ord *et al.* 1993; Soliman
et al. 1993; Tucker *et al.* 1993). The current expectations from *in vitro* fertilization and embryo transfer have been reported by the American Fertility Society
(1991) and the Interim Licensing Authority (1991) and these statistics are shown
in Table 4.7. They allow for the expectation of a clinical pregnancy rate of 15.4
per cent per treatment cycle and a livebirth rate of 11.1–11.5 per cent per treatment cycle. The incidence of spontaneous abortion is in the region 18–23.3 per
cent, whilst the ectopic pregnancy rate is in the range 3.3–5.4 per cent. The
overall multiple pregnancy rate per treatment cycle is 24–26.8 per cent. The use
of freeze–thawed embryos does not have any significant effect upon these
results (Wood *et al.* 1984). The pregnancy rate following embryo transfer in a
natural cycle is 11.6 per cent but rises to 17 per cent in a stimulated cycle. The
effect of maternal age is very significant with a decreasing pregnancy rate
and livebirth rate beyond the age of 34 years, as shown in Table 4.2 (Interim
Licensing Authority 1991).

In patients with macroscopically normal fallopian tubes and without a past
history of tubal pregnancy, gamete intra-fallopian transfer (GIFT) may be
performed. The incidence of clinical pregnancy with this technique will depend
upon the number of ova transposed into the tube. Thus, with one or two ova,
there were no pregnancies but with three ova pregnancies occurred in 25 per
cent of cycles. There was no benefit from increasing the number of ova further

Table 4.7 IVF results

	Patients	Treatment cycles	Egg collections	Clinical pregnancies	Livebirths	Pregnancies per treatment cycle	Livebirths per treatment cycle
UK	8790	10 413	8930	1599	1157	15.4%	11.1%
USA	17 970	18 211	15 392	2811	2104	15.4%	11.5%

From American Fertility Society (1991); Interim Licensing Authority (1991)

(Molloy *et al.* 1986, 1987). Although some authors have suggested that GIFT will be associated with a higher pregnancy rate than will IVF and ET in patients with normal tubes (Yovich 1988), a randomized trial of IVF against GIFT showed no significant difference in the pregnancy rates and the management of patients with either unexplained or male infertility (Leeton *et al.* 1987).

Not only do stimulated cycles result in a greater pregnancy rate than do unstimulated, but the method of stimulation may also be of relevance. Rutherford *et al.* (1988), in an uncontrolled trial, reported better results using the synthetic LH–RH agonist buserelin with hMG, compared with clomiphene and hMG. Using buserelin, hyperstimulation occurred in 8 per cent of patients (resulting in cancellation of the treatment cycle) and an overall clinical pregnancy rate of 36 per cent in treatment cycles. Using clomiphene and hMG, there was a 31 per cent incidence of inadequate follicular development, no hyperstimulation, and a clinical pregnancy in 40 per cent of all treatment cycles. As the mean number of embryos obtained with buserelin was greater than that with clomiphene there was also a greater risk of multiple pregnancy, occurring in 33 per cent of the buserelin patients compared with 23 per cent of the clomiphene-treated patients.

The outcome of pregnancies associated with assisted conception was studied by the Medical Research Council (1990) who reported 1581 liveborn or stillborn children following IVF or GIFT. They confirmed an increased incidence of multiple pregnancy (23 per cent) and hence an increased incidence of preterm delivery (24 per cent). The incidence of major congenital abnormality was 2.2 per cent, a figure comparable to the normal population. The perinatal mortality rate was 11.7 per 1000 singleton births and 27.2 per 1000 for all births. Although international pooling of data to obtain larger series will be required to detect any small increase in morbidity or mortality, should there be such associated with assisted conception, these results would suggest that the technique does not result in a higher risk during pregnancy other than that expected from either multiple pregnancies or the underlying pathology which is causing the subfertility.

Tubal surgery or IVF?

The evidence presented in the previous sections opens a somewhat heated debate between the advocates of these treatment modalities (*Lancet* 1991*a*; Watson *et al.* 1990; Winston and Margara 1991). The advice which the clinician should give to the patients will depend upon many factors, not least of which is having both a microsurgical unit and an IVF unit to which one may refer. However, assuming that both are available, mild tubal distal occlusion should probably be treated microsurgically, whilst more severe disease, re-occlusion, or failure to conceive despite surgery should probably be treated by IVF (Reiss 1991). There will still remain a place for microsurgical techniques in the reversal of sterilization (Broadbent and Magos 1991). Other than the indications outlined above, 'it seems that salpingostomy is heading for obsolescence' (*Lancet* 1991*a*).

Table 4.8 IVF or AIH?

Problem	% Pregnancies per cycle	
	IVF	AIH
Male infertility (n = 86)	21	5
(if asthenospermia)	47	0
(if oligospermia)	11	9
Unexplained infertility (n = 68)	20	8
Cervical mucus hostility (n = 48)	38	3

From Hewitt *et al.* (1985)

Artificial insemination

The place of AID is well demonstrated, but frozen rather than fresh semen should now be used in order to allow adequate time for HIV testing to take place. Albrecht *et al.* (1982) reported a cumulative pregnancy rate of 85.1 per cent at the end of one year for 124 couples undergoing AID, with a pregnancy rate of 15 per cent for any single cycle. Mortimer and Richardson (1982) reported an alteration in the sex ratio of infants following AID. Following natural pregnancy, 51.5 per cent of babies are male; following AID with fresh semen this figure falls to 47.8 per cent; following AID with cryostored semen the percentage of male infants falls to 42.9 per cent, possibly due to cryodamage to Y chromosome.

Artificial insemination by husband has been advocated either for oligospermia or for cervical mucus hostility using high AIH (into the endocervical canal or uterine cavity) (Kerin *et al.* 1984; Nachtigall 1979). However, Glazener *et al.* (1987) reported a randomized, controlled study of 18 couples in whom infertility was thought to be due to low sperm density (less than 1×10^6 per ml), and in 28 couples in whom there was a negative post-coital test with a good sperm count (19 of these 28 men had antisperm antibodies in the semen). The trial alternated in six cycles of AIH with six cycles of normal intercourse. The cumulative conception rate following the six months of AIH was 4.7 per cent compared with 6.6 per cent following natural intercourse. There would appear to be very little evidence to support the use of AIH.

Moreover, IVF would appear to be superior to AIH in the treatment of male infertility, unexplained infertility, and cervical mucus hostility (Hewitt *et al.* 1985). The pregnancy rates per cycle for these conditions is shown in Table 4.8. The use of micromanipulative techniques may be of particular value in severe male factor infertility (Sakkas *et al.* 1992).

Endometriosis and infertility

Minimal endometriosis may be found in approximately 15 per cent of infertile women, whereas up to 40 per cent of patients with endometriosis are infertile (Bancroft *et al.* 1989). There are now four prospective randomized trials which suggest that there is no significant difference as regards fertility between treating minimal endometriosis actively, with placebo, or not at all. However, an indication for treating minimal endometriosis may be the prevention of worsening of the endometriosis rather than specifically improving the fertility.

Siebel *et al.* (1982) allocated 48 women with minimal endometriosis, and no other cause for their infertility, to either no treatment for one year, or danazol for six months, followed by no treatment for a further six months. Pregnancy occurred in 30 per cent of the patients in the danazol group and 50 per cent of those in the untreated group. Thomas and Cooke (1987) reported a randomized double-blind trial of either 12-months' treatment using the danazol-like drug, gestrinone, or placebo. The cumulative pregnancy rate at 12 months after treatment was 25 per cent in the gestinone arm and 24 per cent in the placebo arm. Following a second laparoscopy, the pregnancy rate in the presence of persisting disease was 30 per cent compared with 25 per cent in absent disease. Bayer *et al.* (1988) enlarged the trial performed by Siebel and reported a 12-month cumulative pregnancy rate of 57.4 per cent in the no-treatment group, whilst Telimaa (1988) allocated 49 patients to treatment with either danazol, medroxyprogesterone acetate, or placebo, each for six months, followed by a 30-month follow-up. The cumulative pregnancy rate in each group was 33 per cent, 42 per cent, and 46 per cent, respectively.

There would appear to be no direct benefit from the treatment of minimal endometriosis in the presence of otherwise unexplained infertility, although Thomas demonstrated that a minority of patients with minimal endometriosis, and who were not treated, had progression of their endometriosis which could ultimately affect fertility by tubal distortion.

Unexplained infertility

The incidence of unexplained infertility in the infertile population will depend to some degree upon the quality of the investigations performed, thus Haxton *et al.* (1987) reinvestigated 95 couples with apparently unexplained infertility and found abnormalities of sperm penetration in 22 and subnormal luteal progesterone profiles in 21. The suggested causes of unexplained infertility have included, over the years, a retroverted mobile uterus, abnormal oocyte development, luteinized unruptured follicles, fertilization abnormalities with a high occult abortion rate, luteal phase insufficiency, sperm antibodies, cervical mucus abnormalities (including cervical infection with mycoplasma and listeria), minimal endometriosis, and psychogenic factors.

Lenton *et al.* (1977*a*) followed 91 couples with unexplained infertility for up to 17 years, and, of these couples, 88 per cent had primary and 12 per cent secondary infertility. In the primary infertile couple the cumulative pregnancy rate at seven years was 36 per cent, a rate which would normally have been exceeded at three months in the fertile population, whereas in the secondary infertile patients the cumulative pregnancy rate at seven years was 79 per cent, also much lower than the normal population. Templeton and Penney (1982) estimated that unexplained infertility accounted for 24 per cent of the clinic population, and, using life-table analysis as a prognostic guide, estimated that only 66 per cent of patients with unexplained primary infertility will ever conceive, whilst only 79 per cent of those with secondary unexplained infertility will ever conceive.

The management of unexplained infertility must represent one of the major areas for advance in the future.

Conclusions

There have been major advances in the treatment of infertility, especially in the field of ovulation induction and *in vitro* fertilization. The concept of specialized units in Assisted Reproduction is now well accepted, yet there are only a limited number of treatments which have been subjected to controlled trials rather than cohort studies. Furthermore, the expectation of patients has altered, and many patients, probably quite appropriately, do not wish to encounter any significant delay in the investigation of their subfertility. Those patients with unexplained subfertility, even of short duration, are increasingly willing to try empirical *in vitro* fertilization, and it is perhaps in the area of unexplained infertility in which the next set of major advances will arise. Against this, there is recent anxiety (which may or may not be confirmed by future studies) because of a possible association between ovulation induction by ovarian stimulation and the subsequent development of malignant ovarian tumours (Harris *et al*. 1992; Spirtas *et al*. 1993; Willemsen *et al*. 1993). Moreover, the increased multiple births associated with the modern management of infertility have implications for obstetric and neonatal services (Levene *et al*. 1992).

References

Abdulla, U., Diver, M. J., Hipkin, L. J., and Davis, J. C. (1983). Plasma progesterone levels as an index of ovulation. *British Journal of Obstetrics and Gynaecology* **90**, 543–8.

Adashi, E. Y., Rock, J. A., Sapp, K. C., Martin, E. J., Wentz, A. C., and Jones, G. S. (1979). Gestational outcome of clomiphene-related conceptions. *Fertility Sterility* **31**, 620–6.

Aitken, R. J., Parslow, J. M., Hargreave, T. B., and Hendry, W. F. (1988). Influence of antisperm antibodies on sperm function. *British Journal of Urology* **62**, 367–73.

Albrecht, B. H., Cramer, D., and Schiff, I. (1982). Factors influencing the success of artificial insemination. *Fertility Sterility* **37**, 792–7.

American Fertility Society (1988). Classification of adnexal adhesions, distal tubal occlusions, occlusions secondary to tubal ligations, tubal pregnancies, anomalies, and intrauterine adhesions. *Fertility Sterility* **49**, 944–53.

American Fertility Society (1991). *In vitro* fertilization embryo transfer in the United States. *Fertility Sterility* **55**, 14–23.

Bancroft, K., Vaughan-Williams, C. A., and Elstein, M. (1989). Minimal–mild endometriosis and infertility. *British Journal of Obstetrics and Gynaecology* **96**, 445–60.

Barratt, C. L. R., Cooke, S., Shauhan, N., and Cooke, I. D. (1989). A prospective randomized controlled trial comparing urinary luteinizing hormone dipsticks and basal body temperature charts with timed donor insemination. *Fertility Sterility* **52**, 394–7.

Bauman, J. E. (1981). Basal body temperatures: unreliable method of ovulation detection. *Fertility Sterility* **36**, 729–33.

Bayer, S. R., Siebel, M. M., Saffan, D. S., Berger, M. J., and Taymor, M. L. (1988). Efficacy of danazol treatment for minimal endometriosis in infertile women. *Journal of Reproductive Medicine* **33**, 179–83.

Bettendorf, G. (1990). Pure follicle stimulating hormone. *Ballière's Clinical Obstetrics and Gynaecology* **4**, 519–34.

Boer-Meisel, M. E., Velde, E. R., Habbema, J. D. F., and Kardmaun, J. W. P. F. (1986). Predicting the pregnancy outcome in patients treated for hydrosalpinx. *Fertility Sterility* **45**, 23–9.

Broadbent, M. and Magos, A. L. (1991). I.V.F. or tubal surgery? *Lancet* **337**, 1291–2.

Brosens, I., Boeckx, W., Delattin, P., Puttemans, P., and Vasquez, G. (1987). Salpingoscopy: a new pre-operative diagnostic tool in tubal infertility. *British Journal of Obstetrics and Gynaecology* **94**, 768–73.

Chaffkin, L. M., Nulsen, J. C., Luciano, A. A., and Metzger, D. A. (1991). A comparative analysis of cycle fecundity rates. *Fertility Sterility* **55**, 252–7.

Collins, J. A., Wrixon, W., Janes, L. B., and Wilson, H. (1983). Treatment-dependent pregnancy among infertile couples. *New England Journal of Medicine* **309**, 1201–6.

Collins, J. A., Ying, S., Wilson, E. H., Wrixon, W., and Casper, R. F. (1984). The post-coital test as a predictor of pregnancy among 355 infertile couples. *Fertility Sterility* **41**, 703–8.

Coltart, T. M. (1970). Laparoscopy in the diagnosis of tubal pregnancy. *Journal of Obstetrics and Gynaecology of the British Commonwealth* **77**, 69–71.

Corenblum, B. and Taylor, P. J. (1983). Long-term follow-up of hyperprolactinaemic women treated with bromocriptine. *Fertility Sterility* **40**, 596–9.

Cox, L. W. (1975). Infertility: a comprehensive programme. *British Journal of Obstetrics and Gynaecology* **82**, 2–6.

Crosignani, P. G. and Ferrari, C. (1990). Dopaminergic treatments for hyperprolactinaemia. *Ballière's Clinical Obstetrics and Gynaecology* **4**, 441–55.

De Kretser, D. M. (1979). Endocrinology of male infertility. *British Medical Bulletin* **35**, 187–92.

Diamond, E. (1979). A comparison of gross and micro-surgical techniques for repair of cornual occlusion. *Fertility Sterility* **32**, 370–6.

Donnez, J. and Nisolle, M. (1989). Carbon dioxide laser laparoscopic surgery. *Ballière's Clinical Obstetrics and Gynaecology* **3**, 525–43.

Eggert-Kruse, W., Gerhard, I., Tilgen, W., and Runnebaum, B. (1989). Clinical significance of crossed *in vitro* sperm–cervical mucus penetration test in infertility investigations. *Fertility Sterility* **52**, 1032–40.

Evans, J. and Townsend, L. (1976). The induction of ovulation. *American Journal of Obstetrics and Gynecology* **125**, 321–7.

Fayez, J. A. (1983). An assessment of the role of operative laparoscopy in tuboplasty. *Fertility Sterility* **39**, 476-9.

Fayez, J. A. and Suliman, S. O. (1982). Infertility surgery of the oviduct. *Fertility Sterility* **37**, 73-8.

Fleming, R. and Coutts, J. R. T. (1986). Induction of multiple follicular growth in normal menstruating women with endogenous gonadotrophin suppression. *Fertility Sterility* **45**, 226-30.

Fleming, R., Haxton, M. J., Hamilton, M. P. R., McCune, G. S., Black, W. P., MacNaughton, M. C., *et al.* (1985). Successful treatment of infertile women with oligomenorrhoea using a combination of an LHRH agonist and exogenous gonadotrophins. *British Journal of obstetrics and Gynaecology* **92**, 369-73.

Frantzen, C. and Scholosser, H. W. (1982). Microsurgery and post-infectious tubal infertility. *Fertility Sterility* **38**, 397-402.

Frisch, R. E. (1990). Body fat, menarche, and ovulation. *Ballière's Clinical Obstetrics and Gynaecology* **4**, 419-39.

Fukushima, T., Tajima, C., Fukuma, K., and Maeyama, M. (1982). Tamoxifen in the treatment of infertility associated with luteal phase insufficiency. *Fertility Sterility* **37**, 755-61.

Furr, B. J. and Jordan, V. C. (1984). The pharmacologic and clinical uses of tamoxifen. *Pharmacology and Therapeutics* **25**, 127-205.

Garcia, C. R. and Mastroiann, L. (1980). Microsurgery for the treatment of adnexal disease. *Fertility Sterility* **34**, 413-24.

Glasier, A. F. (1990). Clomiphene citrate. *Ballière's Clinical Obstetrics and Gynaecology* **4**, 491-501.

Glazener, C. M. A., Kelly, M. J., and Hull, M. G. R. (1987). Prolactin measurement in the investigation of infertility in women with a normal menstrual cycle. *British Journal of Obstetrics and Gynaecology* **94**, 535-8.

Gorelick, J. F. and Goldstein, M. (1993). Loss of fertility in men with varicocoele. *Fertility Sterility* **59**, 613-19.

Gorlitsky, G. I., Kase, N. G., and Speroff, L. (1978). Ovulation and pregnancy rates with clomiphene citrate. *Obstetrics and Gynecology* **51**, 265-9.

Grant, A. and Robertson, S. (1966). Hydrotubation. *Medical Journal of Australia* **2**, 847-50.

Griffith, R. W. (1978). Outcome of pregnancy in mothers given bromocriptine. *British Journal of Clinical Pharmacology* **5**, 227-31.

Griffiths, C. S. and Grimes, D. A. (1990). The validity of the post-coital test. *American Journal of Obstetrics and Gynecology* **162**, 615-20.

Gysler, M., March, C. M., Mishell, D. R., Bailey, E. J. (1982). A decade's experience with an individual clomiphene treatment regime. *Fertility Sterility* **37**, 161-7.

Hackeloer, B. J., Fleming, R., Robinson, H. P., Adam, A. H., and Coutts, J. R. T. (1979). Correlation of ultrasonic and endocrine assessment of human follicular development. *American Journal of Obstetrics and Gynecology* **135**, 122-8.

Harris, R., Whittemore, A. S., Itnyre, J., and the Collaborative Ovarian Cancer Group (1992). Characteristics related to ovarian cancer risk. *American Journal of Epidemiology* **126**, 1204-11.

Haxton, M. J., Fleming, R., Hamilton, M. P. R., Yates, R. W., Black, W. P., and Coutts, J. R. T. (1987). Unexplained infertility results of secondary investigations in 95 couples. *British Journal of Obstetrics and Gynaecology* **94**, 539-42.

Hershlag, A., Seifer, D. B., Carcangio, M. L., Patton, D. L., Diamond, N. P., and De Cherney, A. H. (1991). Salpingoscopy: light microscope and electron microscopic correlations. *Obstetrics and Gynecology* **77**, 399-405.

Hewitt, J., Cohen, J., Krishnaswany, J., Fehilly, C. B., Steptoe, P. C., and Walters, D. E. (1985). Treatment of idiopathic infertility, cervical mucus hostility and male infertility: AIH or IVF? *Fertility Sterility* **44**, 350–5.

Homburg, R., Eshel, A., Armar, N. A., Tucker, M., Mason, P. W., Adams, J., *et al.* (1989). One hundred pregnancies after treatment with pulsatile LH RH to induce ovulation. *British Medical Journal* **298**, 809–12.

Hull, M. G. R., Savage, P., and Jacobs, H. S. (1979). Investigation and treatment of amenorrhoea resulting in normal fertility. *British Medical Journal* **1**, 1257–61.

Hull, M. G. R., Savage, P. E., Bromham, D. R., Ismail, A. A. A., and Morris, A. F. (1982*a*). The value of a single serum progesterone measurement. *Fertility Sterility* **37**, 355–60.

Hull, M. G. R., Savage, P. E., and Bromham, D. R. (1982*b*). Prognostic significance of the post-coital test. *British Journal of Obstetrics and Gynaecology* **89**, 299–305.

Hull, M. G. R., Glazener, C. M. R., Kelly, N. J., Conway, D. I., Foster, P. A., Hinton, R. A., *et al.* (1985). Population study of causes, treatment, and outcome of infertility. *British Medical Journal* **291**, 1693–7.

Interim Licensing Authority (1991). The sixth report of the Interim Licensing Authority for human *in vitro* fertilization and embryology, pp. 20–9. HMSO, London.

Jansen, R. P. S. (1988). Early laparoscopy after pelvic operations to prevent adhesions. *Fertility Sterility* **49**, 26–31.

Jequier, A. M. (1993). Male infertility. *British Journal of Obstetrics and Gynaecology* **100**, 612–14.

Jette, N. J. and Glass, R. H. (1972). The prognostic value of the post-coital test. *Fertility Sterility* **23**, 29–32.

Johnson, G. (1993). Childless women revisited. *British Medical Journal* **303**, 1116–17.

Johnson, G., Roberts, D., Brown, R., Cox, E., Evershed, Z., Goutham, P., *et al.* (1987). Infertility, or childless by choice? *British Medical Journal* **294**, 804–6.

Kerin, J. F. B., Kirby, C., Peek, J., Jeffrey, R., Warns, G. M., Mathews, C. D., *et al.* (1984). Improved conception rate after intrauterine insemination of washed spermatozoa for men with poor quality semen. *Lancet* **i**, 533–5.

Kerin, J. F., Williams, D. B., San Roman, G. A., Pearlstone, A. C., Giundfest, W. S., and Surrey, E. S. (1992). Falloposcopic classification and treatment of fallopian tube lumen disease. *Fertility Sterility* **57**, 731–41.

Knuth, U. A., Hull, M. G. R., and Jacobs, H. S. (1977). Amenorrhoea and weight loss. *British Journal of Obstetrics and Gynaecology* **84**, 801–7.

Lancet (1991*a*). I.V.F. or tubal surgery? *Lancet* **337**, 888–9.

Lancet (1991*b*). Ovarian hyperstimulation syndrome. *Lancet* **338**, 1111–12.

Larsson, B., Lalos, O., Marsk, L., Tronstad, S. E., Bygdeman, M., Pehrson, S., and Joelsson, I. (1985). Effect of intraperitoneal installation of 32% Dextran 70 on post-operative adhesion formation after tubal surgery. *Acta Obstetrica et Gynecologica Scandinavica* **64**, 438–41.

Lauritsen, J. G., Pagel, J. G., Vangsted, P., and Starrup, J. (1982). Results of repeat tuboplasties. *Fertility Sterility* **37**, 68–72.

Leeton, J. and Talbot, J. M. (1973). A comparative study of laparoscopy with hysterosalpingogram in 100 infertile patients. *Australia and New Zealand Journal of Obstetrics and Gynaecology* **13**, 169–71.

Leeton, J., Healy, D., Rogers, P., Yates, C., and Caro, C. (1987). A controlled study between the use of G.I.F.T. and I.V.F. and E.T. in the management of idiopathic male infertility. *Fertility Sterility* **48**, 605–7.

Lenton, E. A., Weston, G. A., and Cooke, I. D. (1977*a*). Long-term follow-up of the apparently normal couple with a complaint of infertility. *Fertility Sterility* **28**, 913–19.

Lenton, E. A., Weston, G. A., and Cooke, I. D. (1977*b*). Problems in using basal body temperature recordings in an infertility clinic. *British Medical Journal* 1, 803–5.

Levene, M. I., Wilde, J., and Steer, P. (1992). Higher multiple births and the modern management of infertility in Britain. *British Journal of Obstetrics and Gynaecology* 99, 603–13.

Leyendecker, G., Wid, T. I., and Hansmann, M. (1980). Pregnancies following chronic intermittant administration of Gn–RH by means of a portable pump. *Journal of Clinical Endocrinology and Metabolism* 51, 1214–16.

Li, T. C. and Cook, I. D. (1994). The value of an absorbable adhesion barrier in the prevention of adhesion reformation following microsurgical adhesiolysis. *British Journal of Obstetrics and Gynaecology* 101, 335–9.

Li, T. C., Dockery, P., Rogers, A. W., and Cooke, I. D. (1989). How precise is histologic dating of endometrium using the standard dating criteria? *Fertility Sterility* 51, 759–63.

Lunenfeld, B. and Insler, V. (1974). Classification of amenorrhoeic states. *Clinical Endocrinology* 3, 223–37.

MacGregor, A. H., Johnson, J. E., and Bunde, C. A. (1968). Further clinical experience with clomiphene. *Fertility Sterility* 19, 616–22.

McShane, P. M., Schiff, I., and Trentham, D. E. (1985). Cellular immunity to sperm in infertile women. *Journal of the American Medical Association* 253, 3555–8.

Medical Research Council (1990). Births in Great Britain resulting from assisted conception. *British Medical Journal* 300, 1229–33.

Meldrum, D. R. (1992). Female reproduction and ageing. *Fertility Sterility* 59, 1–5.

Menge, A. C., Medley, N. E., Mangione, C. M., and Dietrich, J. W. (1982). The incidence and influence of antisperm antibodies on infertile human couples. *Fertility Sterility* 38, 439–46.

Menken, J., Trussell, J., and Larssen, U. (1986). Age and infertility. *Science* 233, 1389–94.

Mills, J. L., Simpson, J. E., Rhodes, G. C., Graubard, B. I., Hoffman, H., Conley, M. R., *et al.* (1990). Risk of neural tube defects in relation to maternal fertility and fertility drug use. *Lancet* ii, 103–4.

Molitch, M. E. (1985). Pregnancy and the hyperprolactinaemic woman. *New England Journal of Medicine* 312, 1364–70.

Moller, B. R., Allen, J., Toft, B., Hansen, K. B., and Taylor-Robinson, D. (1984). Pelvic inflammatory disease after hysterosalpingography. *British Journal of Obstetrics and Gynaecology* 91, 1181–7.

Molloy, D., Speirs, A. L., Plessis, Y., Gellert, S., Bourne, H., and Johnston, W. I. H. (1986). The establishment of a successful programme of gamete intra-Fallopian transfer. *Australian and New Zealand Journal of Obstetrics and Gynaecology* 26, 206–9.

Molloy, D., Speirs, A., Plessis, Y., McBain, J., and Johnston, I. (1987). A laparoscopic approach to a program of GIFT. *Fertility Sterility* 47, 289–94.

Mortimer, D. and Richardson, D. W. (1982). Sex ratio of births resulting from artificial insemination. *British Journal of Obstetrics and Gynaecology* 89, 132–5.

Mozes, M., Bogokowsky, H., Antebi, E., Lunenfeld, B., Rabau, E., Serr, D. M., *et al.* (1965). Thrombo-embolic phenomena after ovarian stimulation with human gonadotrophins. *Lancet* ii, 1213–15.

Nachtigall, R. D. (1979). Artificial insemination with husband's sperm. *Fertility Sterility* 32, 141–7.

Navot, D., Relou, A., Birkenfield, A., Rabinowitz, R., Brzezinski, A., and Margalioth,

E. J. (1988). Risk factors and prognostic variables in the ovarian hyperstimulation syndrome. *American Journal of Obstetrics and Gynecology* **159**, 210–15.

Navot, D., Bergh, P. A., Williams, M. A., Garissi, G. J., Guzman, I., Sandler, B., et al. (1991). Poor oocyte quality rather than implantation failure as a cause of age-related decline in female fertility. *Lancet* **337**, 1375–7.

Neuwirth, R. S. and Khalaf, S. M. (1975). The effect of 32% Dextran 70 on peritoneal adhesion formation. *American Journal of Obstetrics and Gynecology* **121**, 420–2.

Nilsson, L. and Hamberger, L. (1990). Human gonadotrophins. *Ballière's Clinical Obstetrics and Gynaecology* **4**, 503–18.

Obstetric and Gynecologic Survey (1989). Assisted reproduction in the diagnosis and treatment of the male factor. *Obstetric and Gynecologic Survey* **44**, 19–20.

O'Herlihy, C., Pepperell, R. J., Brown, J. B., Smith, M. A., Sandri, L., and McBain, J. L. (1981). Incremental clomiphene therapy. *Obstetrics and Gynecology* **58**, 535–42.

Ord, T., Patrizio, P., Balmaceda, J. P., and Asch, R. H. (1993). Can severe male infertility be treated without micromanipulation? *Fertility Sterility* **60**, 110–15.

Pepperell, R. J., McBain, J. C., and Healy, D. L. (1977). Ovulation induction with bromocriptine in patients with hyperprolactinaemia. *Australian and New Zealand Journal of Obstetrics and Gynaecology* **17**, 181–91.

Pittaway, D. E., Winfield, A. C., Maxson, W., Daniell, J., Herbert, C., and Wentz, A. C. (1983). Prevention of acute pelvic inflammatory disease after hystero-salpingography. *American Journal of Obstetrics and Gynecology* **147**, 623–6.

Pyper, R. J. D., Ahmet, Z., and Houang, E. T. (1988). Bacteriological contamination during laparoscopy with dye injection. *British Journal of Obstetrics and Gynaecology* **95**, 367–71.

Quigley, M. M., Schmidt, C. L., Bauchamp, P. J., Pace-Owens, S., Berkowitz, A. S., and Wolf, D. P. (1984). Enhanced follicular recruitment in an *in vitro* fertilization program. *Fertility Sterility* **42**, 25–33.

Randall, J. M. and Templeton, A. A. (1991). Infertility: the experience of a tertiary referral centre. *Health Bulletin* **49**, 48–53.

Replogle, R. J., Johnson, R., and Gross, R. A. (1963). Prevention of post-operative intestinal adhesions with combined Promethazine and Dexamethasone. *Annals of Surgery* **163**, 580–8.

Reiss, H. (1991). The management of tubal infertility in the 1990s. *British Journal of Obstetrics and Gynaecology* **98**, 619–23.

Rock, J. A., Siegler, A. M., Boer-Meisel, M., Haney, A. F., Rosenwaks, Z., Pardo-Vargus, F., et al. (1988). The efficacy of post-operative hydrotubation. *Fertility Sterility* **42**, 373–6.

Rock, J. A., Zacur, H. A., Guzick, D. S., King, T. N., and Katz, E. (1987). Tubal anastamosis. *Fertility Sterility* **48**, 13–17.

Ron-El, R., Soffer, Y., Langer, R., Herman, A., Weintraub, Z., and Caspi, E. (1989). Low multiple pregnancy rate in combined clomiphene–human menopausal gonadotrophin treatment for ovulation induction or enhancement. *Human Reproduction* **4**, 495–500.

Rust, L. A., Israel, R., and Mishell, D. R. (1974). An individualised graduated therapeutic regime for clomiphene citrate. *American Journal of Obstetrics and Gynecology* **120**, 785–90.

Rutherford, A. J., Subak-Sharpe, R. J., Dawson, H. J., Margara, R. A., Franks, F., and Winston, R. M. L. (1988). Improvement of IVF after treatment with Buserelin. *British Medical Journal* **296**, 1765–8.

Sakkas, D., Lacham, O., Gianaroli, L., and Trounson, A. (1992). Subzonal sperm micromanipulation in cases of male factor infertility. *Fertility Sterility* **57**, 1279–88.

Sato, T., Ibuli, Y., Hirono, M., Igarashi, M., and Matsumotto, S. (1969). Induction of ovulation with Sexovid. *Fertility Sterility* **20**, 965-74.

Schenker, J. G., Yarokoni, S., and Granat, M. (1980). Multiple pregnancies following induction of ovulation. *Fertility Sterility* **35**, 265-9.

Schwartz, D. and Mayaux, M. J. (1982). Female fecundity as a function of age. *New England Journal of Medicine* **306**, 404-6.

Schwartz, D., Mayaux, M. J., Spira, A., Moscato, M. L., Jouannet, P., Czyglik, F., *et al.* (1983). Semen characteristics as a function of age. *Fertility Sterility* **39**, 530-5.

Scialli, A. R. (1986). The reproductive toxicity of ovulation induction. *Fertility Sterility* **45**, 315-23.

Shoham, Z., Zosmer, A., and Insler, V. (1991). Early miscarriage and fetal malformation after induction of ovulation, *in vitro* fertilization, and gamete intra-Fallopian transfer. *Fertility Sterility* **55**, 1-11.

Siebel, M. M., Berger, M. J., Weinstein, F. J., and Taymor, M. L. (1982). The effectiveness of danazol on subsequent fertility in minimal endometriosis. *Fertility Sterility* **38**, 534-7.

Siegler, A. M. and Kontopoulos, V. (1979). An analysis of macrosurgical and microsurgical techniques in the management of the tuboperitoneal factor in infertility *Fertility Sterility* **32**, 377-83.

Singhal, V., Li, T. C., and Cooke, I. D. (1991). An analysis of factors influencing the outcome of 232 consecutive tubal microsurgery cases. *British Journal of Obstetrics and Gynaecology* **88**, 628-36.

Smith, B. H. and Cooke, I. D. (1991). Ovarian hyperstimulation: actual and theoretical risks. *British Medical Journal* **302**, 127-8.

Smith, K. D., Rodriguez-Rigau, C. J., and Steinberger, E. (1977). Relationship between indices of seminal analysis and pregnancy rate in infertile couples. *Fertility Sterility* **28**, 1314-19.

Soliman, S., Daya, S., Colin, J., and Jarrell, J. (1993). A randomised trial of *in vitro* fertilisation versus conventional treatment for infertility. *Fertility Sterility* **59**, 1239-44.

Southam, A. L. (1960). What to do with the normal infertile couple. *Fertility Sterility* **11**, 543-9.

Spirtas, R., Kaufman, S. C., and Alexander, N. J. (1993). Fertility drugs and ovarian cancer—red alert or red herring? *Fertility Sterility* **59**, 291-3.

Suginami, H., Kitagawa, H., Nakahashi, N., Yano, K., and Masturbar, A. K. (1993). A Clomiphene citrate and Tamoxifen citrate combination therapy. *Fertility Sterility* **59**, 976-9.

Telimaa, S. (1988). Danazol and medroxyprogesterone acetate: inefficacious in the treatment of infertility and endometriosis. *Fertility Sterility* **50**, 872-5.

Templeton, A. A. and Penney, G. C. (1982). The incidence, characteristics, and prognosis of patients whose infertility is unexplained. *Fertility Sterility* **37**, 175-182.

Templeton, A. A., Penney, G. C., and Lees, M. M. (1982). Relation between the luteinizing hormone peak, the nadir of the basal body temperature, and the cervical mucus score. *British Journal of Obstetrics and Gynaecology* **89**, 985-94.

Templeton, A. A., Fraser, C., and Thompson, B. (1990). The epidemiology of infertility in Aberdeen. *British Medical Journal* **301**, 148-52.

Thie, J. L., Williams, T. J., and Coulan, C. B. (1986). Repeat tuboplasty compared with primary microsurgery for post-inflammatory tubal disease. *Fertility Sterility* **45**, 784-7.

Thomas, E. J. and Cooke, I. D. (1987). Successful treatment of asymptomatic endometriosis: does it benefit infertile women? *British Medical Journal* **294**, 1117-19.

Thompson, C. R. and Hansen, L. M. (1970). A summary of clinical experience in induction of ovulation and pregnancy. *Fertility Sterility* **25**, 844–53.

Thomson, J. A., Teasdale, G. M., Gordon, D., McCruden, D. C. C., and Davis, D. L. (1985). Treatment of presumed prolactinoma by transsphenoidal operation. *British Medical Journal* **291**, 1550–3.

Tucker, M. J., Wiker, S. R., Wright, G., Morton, P. C., and Toledo, A. A. (1993). Treatment of male infertility and ideopathic fertility failure with *in vitro* zonal insemination and direct egg injection. *American Journal of Obstetrics and Gynecology* **169**, 324–32.

Vermeulen, A. and Vandeweghe, M. (1984). Improved fertility after varicocele correction? *Fertility Sterility* **42**, 249–56.

Watson, A. J. S., Gupta, J. K., O'Donovan, P., Dalton, M. E., and Lilford, R. J. (1990). The results of tubal surgery in the treatment of infertility in two non-specialist hospitals. *British Journal of Obstetrics and Gynaecology* **97**, 561–8.

Weil, C. (1986). The safety of bromocriptine in hyperprolactinaemic women with infertility. *Current Medical Research and Opinion* **10**, 172–95.

Whitelaw, M. J. (1970). The significance of the high ovulation rate versus the low pregnancy rate with Clomid. *American Journal of Obstetrics and Gynecology* **107**, 865–77.

Willemsen, W., Kruitwagen, R., Bastiaans, B., Hanselaar, T., and Rolland, R. (1993). Ovarian stimulation and granulosa cell tumour. *Lancet* **341**, 986–8.

Williamson, J. D. and Ellis, J. D. (1973). The induction of ovulation with Tamoxifen. *Journal of Obstetrics and Gynaecology* **80**, 844–7.

Winston, R. M. L. (1975). Microsurgical reanastamosis of the rabbit oviduct. *British Journal of Obstetrics and Gynaecology* **82**, 513–22.

Winston, R. M. L. (1980). Microsurgery of the Fallopian tube. *Fertility Sterility* **34**, 521–30.

Winston, R. M. L. (1981). Is microsurgery necessary for salpingostomy? *Australian and New Zealand Journal of Obstetrics and Gynaecology* **21**, 143–52.

Winston, R. M. L. and Margara, R. A. (1991). Microsurgical salpingostomy is not an obsolete procedure. *British Journal of Obstetrics and Gynaecology* **98**, 637–42.

Wood, C., Downing, D., Trounsen, A., and Rogers, P. (1984). Clinical implications of developments in IVF. *British Medical Journal* **289**, 978–80.

Wright, C. S., Steele, S. J., and Jacobs, H. S. (1979). Value of bromocriptine in unexplained primary infertility. *British Medical Journal* **1**, 1037–9.

Wu, C. H. and Winkel, C. A. (1989). The effect of therapy inititiation day on clomiphene citrate treatment. *Fertility Sterility* **52**, 564–8.

Wu, F. C. W., Edmond, P., Raab, G., and Hunter, W. M. (1981). Endocrine assessment of subfertile couples. *Clinical Endocrinology* **14**, 493–507.

Yovich, J. L. (1988). The treatment of normospermic infertility by GIFT. *British Journal of Obstetrics and Gynaecology* **95**, 361–6.

Zuckerman, Z., Rodriguez-Rigau, C. J., Smith, K. E. D., and Steinbergher, G. (1977). Frequency distribution of sperm counts in fertile and infertile males. *Fertility Sterility* **28**, 1310–13.

5 Contraception

Contraception, in some form, is practised by over 80 per cent of the fertile population at any one time, but the technique of contraception employed varies both with time and with the age of the couples concerned. Before the introduction of oral contraception in the 1960s, barrier methods, withdrawal, and spermicides were the commonest methods in use. The oral contraceptive pill made a dramatic entrance and, by 1975, some 3.2 million of the 11 million fertile women in England and Wales were taking the pill, whilst 2.5 million males were using sheaths. By 1980, with an increased knowledge of the side-effects together with selective reporting by the media, oral contraceptive use fell by 15 per cent, whilst the use of sheaths increased by 32 per cent, and diaphragms or caps by 20 per cent. The oral contraceptive has increased again in popularity and approaches 3 million women users in England and Wales, and over 60 million oral contraceptive takers world-wide.

The method of contraception chosen by couples in the UK is illustrated in Table 5.1 (Office of Population, Census, and Surveys 1991). Whilst oral contraception is the commonest single method of contraception used, especially in women below the age of 35 years, sterilization of either the male or female partner is jointly the commonest method, especially in older couples. It should be noted that the percentages shown in Table 5.1 add up to more than 100 per cent since 4 per cent of couples use more than one method.

When counselling a couple about their future choice of contraception, it is now considered mandatory to include the failure rate, i.e. pregnancy rate, for any given method of contraception. A failure may be either a true failure of the method or a failure due to user error; the failure rates for different methods per 100 women-years, taken from the Oxford–Family Planning Association Study of over 17 000 women (Vessey *et al*. 1982*a*), are shown in Table 5.2. Failure may mean extrauterine pregnancy rather than intrauterine pregnancy and, even though this was discussed in Chapter 2 (Ectopic pregnancy), Table 2.1 is reproduced here as Table 5.3, after Tatum and Schmidt (1977).

There is increasing concern about the level of unplanned, and frequently unwanted, pregnancy in teenage girls (Royal College of Obstetricians and Gynaecologists, 1991). Since 1980, conception rates in England and Wales have remained static for women aged 35 and over, have increased in women aged 30–34, and have shown a decline in women aged 20–30, suggesting a planned delay in conception. However, conception rates have increased for women under 20 years, especially since 1983. As termination of pregnancy may represent, to some degree, the failure of contraception or of contraceptive advice, it is to be noted that the percentage of pregnancies terminated in England and Wales rose from 15 per cent in 1977 to 20 per cent in 1988. The percentage of

Table 5.1 Choice of contraception in UK*

Primary method used	All women (%)
Oral contraceptive	19
IUCD	7
Sheath	18
Cap/diaphragm	1
Withdrawal	5
Safe period	2
Spermicide	1
Female sterilization	14
Male sterilization	17
Previous hysterectomy	6
Trying to conceive	6
Pregnant	4
Others/none	4

*Office of Population, Census, and Surveys (1991)

Table 5.2 Contraceptive failure rates

Method	Failure rate per 100 women year	
	mean	range
Oral contraceptives $> 50 \mu g$	0.32	0.07–0.93
$\quad\quad\quad\quad\quad\quad\quad 50 \mu g$	0.16	0.12–0.21
$\quad\quad\quad\quad\quad\quad\quad < 50 \mu g$	0.27	0.17–0.41
Progestogen-only pill	1.2	0.7–1.8
Diaphragm	1.9	1.8–2.1
Sheath	3.6	3.3–3.9
Lippes loop	1.4	1.2–1.7
Copper IUCD	1.3	0.4–2.7
Rhythm	15.5	10.0–22.9
Withdrawal	6.7	4.9–8.9
Spermicides alone	11.9	8.3–16.4
Female sterilization	0.13	0.07–0.21
Male sterilization	0.02	0.004–0.06
DMPA	0.25	< 0.5

From Oxford—Family Planning Association Study (Vessey *et al.* 1982a)

Table 5.3 Contraceptive failure and tubal pregnancy

Method	No. of tubal pregnancies per 1000 pregnancies
Barrier	0
Combined oral contraceptives	0
Progestogen-only oral contraceptives	60.3
Medroxyprogesterone acetate	13.0
IUCD	29.7
Progestasert IUCD	163.0
Laparoscopic Falope rings	65.2

After Tatum and Schmidt (1977)

terminations varied by age group, with 36 per cent of pregnancies in women under the age of 20 years being terminated as compared with 55 per cent in women under 14 years. This represents an overall annual legal abortion rate of 14.2 per 1000 women of all ages but 20.9 per 1000 women for those under 20 years. Legal abortion rates for women under 20 years in other countries show a similar pattern, being 13.2 per 1000 in New Zealand, 15.2 in Canada, 19.5 in Australia, 21.5 in Sweden, but 45.7 in the USA (Royal College of Obstetricians and Gynaecologists 1991).

These trends and statistics have resulted in recommendations for better sex education in schools, an increased need for public education concerning the use of contraception and contraceptive services, and the provision and development of more effective and more acceptable contraceptive methods (Rimpela *et al.* 1993; Scally 1993).

The benefits and risks of oral contraception

Oral contraception is one of the most highly effective, yet reversible methods of contraception currently available. It is aesthetically acceptable and is the single most popular method of contraception for couples in the Western world. Although this chapter will devote much discussion to the possible risks from oral contraceptives, it must be stressed that oral contraception provides a 40 per cent reduction in the incidence and mortality of carcinoma of the ovary (please see Chapter 13 – (Ovarian cancer); Drife, 1989; Villard-Mackintosh *et al.* 1989). Women using oral contraception have a reduced incidence in surgery of 52 per cent for all functional ovarian cysts, of 31 per cent for cystadenomata, and of 17 per cent for benign cystic teratomata (Vessey *et al.* 1987). The use of oral contraception is also protective against endometrial cancer. Thus, the Centers for Disease Control (1983) compared 187 women with histologically proven endometrial cancer with 1320 controls with regard to their previous contraceptive practice. The use of combined oral contraception, at any stage, gave a relative risk for endometrial carcinoma of 0.5 when compared to 'never takers', with an enhanced protective effect for nulliparous women who had been previous combined oral contraceptive takers (relative risk 0.4). Similarly, Vessey *et al.* (1989) reported mortality statistics for the Oxford–FPA study in which a non-randomized cohort of 17 032 women were followed for a mean period of 16 years, representing 271 268 person-years. There were no deaths from carcinoma of the body of the uterus in the women in the oral contraceptive group, whilst two deaths occurred from this disease in the women in the IUCD group. Whilst such figures are small, they do suggest a significant protective effect from oral contraception upon this malignancy (Herbst and Berek 1993; Jick *et al.* 1993).

There is also some evidence that oral contraceptives protect against benign breast disease (Herbst and Berek 1993). Livolsi *et al.* (1979) reviewed 120 fibroadenomas in a case-controlled study, demonstrating a relative risk of 0.9 in oral contraceptive takers compared with non-takers. Since benign breast disease is a predisposing factor to malignant disease, this is an interesting finding.

Oral contraceptives and carcinoma of the cervix

The relative risks associated with contraceptives as a risk factor in the aetiology of cancer of the cervix will be discussed in Chapter 12. The Oxford–FPA study reported mortality rates in cohorts of women using different methods of contraception over a mean period of 16 years. The mortality rates from carcinoma of the cervix in all oral contraceptive users was 4.4 per 100 000 women-years compared with 0.9 per 100 000 women-years in the IUCD group. These mortality statistics were related to the length of oral contraceptive use. Thus, the mortality from carcinoma of the cervix was zero for less than 48 months' usage compared with 3.1 per 100 000 for 48–95 months' usage, and 7.4 per 100 000 for greater than 95 months' usage (Vessey *et al.* 1989). There would seem to be an excess risk of carcinoma of the cervix in women using longterm oral contraception (Herbst and Berek 1993).

Oral contraceptives and cancer of the breast

Approximately 6 per cent of British women and 9 per cent of American women develop carcinoma of the breast, especially ductal adenocarcinomata. Increased risk factors include an early age at menarche, late age at menopause, nulliparity, late age at first term pregnancy, a history of benign breast disease, and a family history of malignant breast disease. It is not surprising, therefore, that evidence of a connection between oral contraceptive use and breast cancer has been sought.

There are now numerous studies which assess the relative risk of carcinoma of the breast developing in the woman who is, or has been, a user of oral contraception, with conflicting results, and this is also true of the studies assessing the relationship between oral contraceptives and arterial disease, especially myocardial infarction. One possible explanation for the differing results would appear to be an in-built bias in the studies. This has been debated for carcinoma of the breast by Skegg (1988), and for arterial disease by Realini and Goldzieher (1985). The major causes of bias are listed below:

1. *Latent period*

If oral contraceptives are to induce disease or enhance the disease-producing effect of another agent, there will need to be a long enough latent period. For carcinoma of the breast, this may well be in excess of eight years, perhaps approaching 20 years. Any study, therefore, which does not allow a long enough assessment may not demonstrate an association, if association there be.

2. *Drug dosages*

The different dosages and potencies of the oestrogens and progestogens present in the pill may require some degree of substratification. Furthermore, the oestrogenic dosage of combined oral contraception has fallen steadily over the years.

3. *Errors of recall*

There may be errors of recall concerning whether or not oral contraception was ever taken, especially in the controls, and there may be even greater errors in recalling the type of oral contraceptive preparation taken.

4. *Selection of controls*

Most American studies use hospital-based controls, but these may not be a valid representation of the general population. Controls who are approached may refuse, or later drop out, and these will not be analysed. All other known aetiological factors must be included in a multivariate analysis. Control populations in different studies may not be comparable; for example Pike *et al.* (1981) found that 48 per cent of controls used oral contraceptives before their first pregnancy, whereas Vessey *et al.* (1982*b*) found only 23 per cent. This may not be relevant but, equally well, it may represent different control populations.

5. *Unknown variables*

Having accepted that the relative risks need to be adjusted for known variables such as age, parity, previous disease, socio-economic status, age at menarche, age at menopause, and smoking, there may be other factors which are less easy to assess, for example family history, and other factors which may be unknown.

There is *no* current evidence that carcinoma of the breast in women over the age of 45 years is increased by taking oral contraceptives (Centers for Disease Control 1983, 1986; McPherson *et al.* 1987; Miller *et al.* 1986; Murray *et al.* 1989; Paul *et al.* 1986; Stadel *et al.* 1985). It is likely that this observation is real, but it is theoretically possible that women over the age of 45 years have not yet had sufficient exposure to oral contraceptives and, should there be a latency period in the region of 20 years or longer, an effect may not be seen for another decade. However, current knowledge, suggests that there is no evidence for the development of breast cancer beyond the age of 45 years related to previous oral contraceptive usage.

The situation for oral contraceptive usage and carcinoma of the breast arising in women below the age of 45 years is not so optimistic and there may be an increased relative risk for the development of carcinoma of the breast. In a recent review of 27 major studies, there was an overall relative risk of 1.16 for the development of carcinoma of the breast in women who have used oral contraceptives and who are below the age of 45 years, compared with never-users. This increased relative risk rose to 1.2 in nulliparous women (compared with multiparous women) within this age group and further increased to a relative risk of 1.27 with greater than eight years' usage (Rushton and Jones 1992). The different relative risks for the development of carcinoma of the breast reported in 29 studies from the literature, relating to women below the age of 45 years and who have taken oral contraceptives, is shown in Table 5.4. The increased risk of 16 per cent reported for the development of breast cancer in younger women (Rushton and Jones 1992) is in keeping with the estimated increased risk of 15 per cent following oral contraceptive use suggested by the large World Health Organization Collaborative Study of Neoplasia and Steroid Contraceptive (1990), although this study found no association with duration of use (even allowing for a latency period of 20 years after cessation), the type of oestrogen used, or the type of progestogen used. There may however, be a dose-related effect, in that the relative risk for the development of breast carcinoma in younger women who used a 30 μg oestrogen preparation (1.04) compared with the relative risk associated with the use of a 50 μg oestrogen preparation (1.1) (United Kingdom National Study Group 1989).

There is no good evidence to suggest that the use of oral contraceptives, even longterm, contribute towards any increased risk of carcinoma of the breast in women with a family history of this disease. Thus, Murray *et al.* (1989) were unable to find any risk from oral contraceptive usage in 554 women with carcinoma of the breast and a first-degree family history compared with 280 controls without carcinoma of the breast. With our present state of knowledge, a family history of carcinoma of the breast should not itself be considered as a contraindication to oral contraceptive use.

Oral contraceptives and the cardiovascular system

The overview

Oral contraceptive use has been implicated in an increased risk of hypertension, coronary artery disease, and stroke, especially subarachnoid haemorrhage and intracerebral haemorrhage. The report of the Royal College of General Practitioners (1974) reported a follow-up of over 46 000 women, who included 23 611 takers and 22 766 controls. For oral contraceptive takers, the relative risk of acute myocardial infarction was 5.22, the relative risk of chronic ischaemic heart disease was 3.55, and the relative risk of subarachnoid haemorrhage was 3.77. The relative risk for other types of stroke was 1.22. When this data was analysed for mortality (RCGP 1977), there was an increased mortality of 40

Table 5.4 Risk of breast cancer in younger women and oral contraceptive use

Primary author	Year	Relative risk of breast cancer in users
Paffenbarger	1980	1.2
Pike	1981	2.2–3.5
RCGP	1981	0.7–1.7
Trapido	1981	0.8
Brinton	1982	0.8
Harris	1982	0.8
Vessey	1982	1.0
Pike	1983	1.0–3.5
Hennekens	1984	1.0
Rosenberg	1984	1.0
Stadel	1985	1.0
La Vecchia	1986	0.9
Lipnick	1986	0.9
Meirik	1986	1.0
Miller	1986	1.0
Paul	1986	2.2
Sattin	1986	1.0
McPherson	1987	1.3–5.4
Schlesselman	1987	0.9–10.3
Ravnihar	1988	1.1
RCGP	1988	0.8–5.8
Stadel	1988	1.0
Jick	1989	0.9
Miller	1989	2.0
UK National	1989	0.95–1.74
Vessey	1989	0.9
Schildkraut	1990	2.3
WHO	1990	1.15
Wingo	1991	1.4

per cent (relative risk 1.4) for pill-takers, 63.6 per 100 000 women-years compared to 46.0 per 100 000 women-years for non-takers. This mortality was almost exclusively due to death from circulatory disease, with an increased mortality from myocardial ischaemia of 10.4 per 100 000 women-years compared to 2.5 per 100 000 women-years in non-takers (relative risk 4.0), and a mortality from subarachnoid haemorrhage of 13.2 per 100 000 women-years for

Table 5.5 Oral contraceptive use and breast cancer

Relative risk for months of use	Type of oral contraceptive		
	$> 50 \, \mu g$	$< 50 \, \mu g$	progestogen-only
Never	1.0	1.0	1.0
1–48	1.08	0.99	1.33
41–96	1.52	1.44	0.73
97 +	2.63	0.89	0.59

From United Kingdom National Study Group (1989)

pill-takers compared with a risk of 2.8 per 100 000 women-years for non-takers (relative risk 4.7). The major duration of use, age of the patient, and smoking habits were also major factors. In another analysis of the 249 deaths in this study (RCGP 1981) the major synergistic effect of smoking and oral contraception was demonstrated. For all ages, the relative risk compared to non-user, non-smokers was 5.1 for oral contraceptive taking and smoking. The relative risk for oral contraceptive non-smokers was 3.2. If women aged 45 and over who took oral contraceptives smoked, the relative risk of dying became 18.0.

Vessey *et al.* (1977, 1981*a*, 1989), reported on the accummulated mortality from the Oxford–Family Planning Association Study. By 1989, with an average follow-up of 16 years and 152 597 women-years of observation on 9653 women taking oral contraceptives and 7379 women using IUCDs or diaphragms, a mortality analysis was possible involving 238 deaths. This is shown in Table 5.6. It should also be stated that the only death from liver tumour occurred in the IUCD–diaphragm group.

Porter *et al.* (1987), however, were not able to substantiate these results. In a comparison between 54 971 women-years of oral contraceptive usage compared with 245 567 women-years of non-usage in women belonging to a private health scheme in Boston, there was a mortality of 25 per 100 000 women-years in oral contraceptive users compared with 20 per 100 000 in non-users. However, no woman in the oral contraceptive group died from cardiovascular disease (14 other deaths), whereas 12 out of 64 deaths in the non-user group were due to cardiovascular disease. The size of the oral contraceptive group was almost certainly too small to allow satisfactory analysis.

It would, therefore, seem that there is some cause for concern relating to the use of oral contraceptives and the risk of cardiovascular disease. However, the next section will examine the size of this risk in greater detail and it will be seen that the risk with the newer oral contraceptive preparation is probably very small, especially when compared with other risk factors, especially smoking.

Hypertension

There is a small but real increased risk of hypertension in women taking oral contraceptives. The RCGP (1974) reported a relative risk of hypertension for

Table 5.6 Mortality and contraception

Mortality rate per 100 000 women years of observation	OC (n = 9653)	IUCD/diaphragm (n = 7379)	Relative risk for OC use
Total deaths	84.3	90.9	0.9
Ischaemic heart disease	9.2	2.8	3.3
Cerebrovascular accident	4.2	2.9	1.4
Cancer of breast	23.1	27.1	0.9
Cancer of cervix	4.4	0.9	4.9
Cancer of endometrium	0	1.4	—
Cancer of ovary	3.6	9.1	0.4
Other cancers	17.7	21.6	0.8

OC = oral contraception
From Oxford—Family Planning Association Study (Vessey *et al.* 1989)

pill-takers, when compared to controls, of 2.59, with a relative risk for ex-takers, compared to controls, of 0.99. The risk of hypertension, and the degree of that hypertension, have been well documented. Weir *et al.* (1974) reported a prospective controlled study in which there was no increase in mean diastolic or systolic blood pressure over a four-year period in 41 non-users, whilst in 73 women who were using oral contraceptives, there was a mean increase in diastolic blood pressure of 8.5 mmHg and a mean increase in systolic blood pressure of 14.2 mmHg. Some 4 per cent of users develop a blood pressure of greater than 140 mmHg systolic and 90 mmHg diastolic (Dalen and Hickler 1981).

There is little, if any, correlation between a past history of pregnancy-related hypertension and oral contraceptive-induced hypertension (Guillebaud 1989). Pritchard and Pritchard (1977) found no differences in the incidence of oral contraceptive-induced hypertension between 180 primiparous women with a history of pregnancy-related hypertension (including 26 women with eclampsia) and 200 nulligravid controls.

There is debate whether it is the oestrogen component or the progestogen component of oral contraception which is responsible for the development of hypertension. In the RCGP study (1974), there was no association between hypertension and oestrogen dosage, although there was a small association between hypertension and progestogen dosage. However, this study related to women receiving at least 50 μg of oestrogen. Some studies have found no significant change in the blood pressure of women using a 30 μg oestrogen oral contraceptive, but have found a significant increase in women using a 50 μg agent (Briggs and Briggs 1977). Other studies have shown that even 30 μg oestrogen contraceptives may result in an elevated blood pressure in susceptible women (Khaw and Peart 1982). This latter study also suggested a dose-response relationship between blood pressure and the progestogen content of oral contraceptives with the same oestrogen content, suggesting that both oestrogen and progestogen were aetiological factors in this effect. This is despite the observation that progestogen-only contraception is not associated with any elevation of blood pressure (Wilson *et al.* 1984).

These studies demonstrate the need for regular (six-monthly) blood pressure estimations. Once oral contraceptives are stopped, an elevated blood pressure will return to the pretreatment level within one month (Tsai *et al.* 1985).

Myocardial infarction

Some studies have suggested an association between the risk of myocardial infarction and oral contraceptive use (Table 5.6). Mann *et al.* (1975) compared 72 women who had experienced a myocardial infarction below the age of 45 years with 190 age-matched controls. Some 38.9 per cent of patients in the myocardial infarction group had used oral contraception at some stage compared with 21.2 per cent of the controls. Some 27.8 per cent of the patients in the myocardial infarction group had used oral contraception within a month of admission to hospital in comparison with 8.4 per cent of the controls. Slone *et al.* (1981) compared 556 women who had a myocardial infarction between the ages of 25 and 49 years with 2036 female hospital controls matched for age. The relative risk for current oral contraceptive use was 3.5.

However, the US Nurses' Health Study (Stampfer *et al.* 1988) could find no evidence of any increased risk from previous oral contraceptive usage, even longterm usage, in non-smokers for myocardial infarction, fatal or non-fatal. This study involved a total follow-up of 480 096 women-years in non-oral contraceptive users and 415 488 women-years in past oral contraceptive users. The follow-up on current oral contraceptive users was only 22 376 women-years and was considered too small to draw conclusions. There was, however, a significant excess of major coronary artery disease amongst smokers regardless of oral contraceptive usage. Similarly, when the RCGP study was updated (Croft and Hannaford 1989) to assess the risk factors present in 158 women with an acute myocardial infarction, the major risk was smoking (relative risk of 4.34 heavy smokers and 1.74 light smokers). Current oral contraceptive usage was only a risk factor in smokers, whereas previous oral contraceptive usage was neither a risk factor in smokers nor nonsmokers. Of the 18 women who died from myocardial infarction in the Oxford–FPA study, 17 were smokers and 15 were oral contraceptive users (Vessey *et al.* 1989).

It is clear from the above studies that smoking is a significantly greater risk factor for myocardial infarction in women than is oral contraceptive usage, although the two may be synergistic. Shapiro *et al.* (1979) demonstrated that a heavy smoker using oral contraceptives had a risk of myocardial infarction some 39 times that of a non-smoker non-oral contraceptive user, regardless of age (Table 5.7). Since oral contraceptive use, smoking, and age may combine to become significant risk factors for myocardial infarction, it is now generally accepted that women who smoke should not be prescribed oral contraceptives

Table 5.7 Age-adjusted relative risk of myocardial infarction

Cigarettes per day	No OC use	Recent OC use
None	1.0	4.5
1–24	3.4	3.7
$\geqslant 25$	7.0	39.0

OC = oral contraception
From Shapiro *et al.* (1979)

beyond the age of 35 years, unless they cease smoking (Loudon 1985). In women who do not smoke and who use a 30 or 35 μg preparation, the risk of myocardial infarction must be at most small and probably absent (Thorogood *et al.* 1991). Because of this, the upper age limit for the use of lower dose oral contraceptives by healthy non-smokers should be removed (*Drug and Therapeutics Bulletin* 1992; Szarewski and Guillebaud 1991).

Stroke

The evidence that oral contraceptive use is a risk factor in its own right for stroke is weak. The US Collaborative Group for the Study of Stroke in Young Women reported a case-controlled study in 1973. This involved 598 non-pregnant women, between the ages of 15 and 44 years, who were admitted to hospital with a cerebrovascular accident and compared with controls matched for age, sex, and race taken from both hospital and neighbourhood popula-tions. The overall relative risk for a CVA was 9.0 for oral contraceptive users, with the highest risk being 12.7 for white women undergoing a thrombotic CVA when compared with neighbourhood controls. Petiti and Windgred (1978) reported the Walnut Creek prospective study, where 17 939 women aged 18–54 were followed for an average of six and a half years, during which 11 of these women died from subarachnoid haemorrhage, four being current oral con-traceptive users, five being previous oral contraceptive users, and two being never-users. These 11 cases were compared with 3956 controls. This study demonstrated that the relative risk of death from subarachnoid haemorrhage was 1.6 for hypertensive women, 5.3 for previous oral contraceptive use, 5.7 for smokers, 6.5 for current oral contraceptive use, but 21.9 for both smoking and current oral contraceptive use, again demonstrating the synergistic effect of smoking and oral contraception. More recent studies confirm this view (Lidegaard 1993).

Not all studies have found this relationship. Inman (1979), however, was unable to find any adverse effect of oral contraception on the risk of subarachnoid haemorrhage. He compared 134 women, who were between the ages of 15 and 44 years, admitted with a subarachnoid haemorrhage with con-trols, and found that the only risk of oral contraception was that associated with hypertension. Thorogood *et al.* (1981) studied 446 women, between the ages of 15 and 44 years, who died from subarachnoid haemorrhage, in England

and Wales. When other known risk factors were excluded, 168 women remained and their oral contraceptive use was comparable with a control population. Vessey *et al.* (1984) found that the increased risk of death from subarachnoid haemorrhage was largely attributable to hypertension and smoking, the use of oral contraception in the absence of these other two factors being 'a weak factor'. The Nurses' Health Study (Stampfer *et al.* 1988) was also unable to find any difference in the incidence of stroke, fatal or non-fatal, between 62 718 non-users and 49 269 previous users of oral contraception. The authors considered that the current user group was too small to allow conclusions to be drawn.

Realini and Goldzieher (1985) analysed 14 case-controlled studies and 15 cohort studies designed to assess the relationship between oral contraceptive taking and stroke. The relative risk for oral contraceptive taking found in the studies ranged from 0.6 to 13.3, with 81.6 per cent of studies showing an increased relative risk for oral contraceptive ingestion in the region of 3.0. It would seem that CVA, either haemorrhagic or thrombotic, is increased in oral contraceptive users, especially should smoking or hypertension coexist.

The formulation of oral contraceptives

The formulation of oral contraceptives has been changed over the years in an attempt to reduce the risks of cardiovascular disease. It is accepted that there is an inverse relationship between the levels of circulating HDL-cholesterol and the incidence of cardiovascular disease mortality in both women and men (Jacobs *et al.* 1990). When controlled for age, smoking, and body mass, the inverse relationship between HDL levels and the risk of cardiovascular disease is greater than is the direct relationship between LDL levels and cardiovascular disease (Jacobs *et al.* 1990). The trend has been for a reduction in total steroid dosage and a modification of those steroids used. It is interesting to note that the first combined pill contained 150 μg ethinyloestradiol and 10 mg norethisterone (Szarewski and Guillebaud 1991).

That both the oestrogen and progestogen are risk factors in the development of ischaemic heart disease and cerebrovascular disease was demonstrated by the RCGP study (Kay 1982) in which the risk was greater in patients taking a 50 μg oestrogen pill than a 30 μg one and that for any given dosage of oestrogen, the risk increased when the dose of progestogen increased. However, the effects of oestrogens and progestogens upon the lipoprotein profile, as judged by the scientific literature, appears to be complex and at times contradictory. In 25 studies involving oral contraceptives containing 30 μg of ethinyloestradiol and 150 mg levonorgestrel, serum LDL was decreased in 12 and unchanged in 13 (Fotherby 1989*a*). This may be, in part, due to a complex metabolic effect and, in part, due to reporting of too few subjects. As a generalization however, oestrogens tend to increase serum triglyceride and HDL concentrations and decrease LDL concentrations, but this effect is modified by the progestogen (Fotherby 1989*a*). Thus, those progestogens derived from 19-nor-testosterone (for example norethisterone and levonorgestrel) may antagonize the benefits of oestrogen with an overall reduction in HDL and elevation in LDL, whereas those progestogens derived from progesterone (the pregnane progestogens, for example megestrol) have little or no effect upon lipoprotein levels. The so-called 'third generation' progestogens (for example desogestrel, gestodene, and norgestimate), although derived from 19-nor-testosterone, do not appear to have any significant antioestrogenic effect and, in combination with ethinyloestradiol, the effect on lipid metabolism is essentially neutral (Eyong and Elstein 1989; Gillmer 1989; Speroff and De Cherney 1993).

Godsland *et al.* (1990) studied the effects of nine different formulations of oral contraceptives upon lipoprotein levels. They found that compounds containing desogestrel gave the most favourable profiles, even compared with progestogen-only contraceptives and monophasic and triphasic agents. The best profiles were associated with a mean 14 per cent reduction in LDL concentrations and a mean 12 per cent increase in HDL concentrations. Although the changes in lipid metabolism with oral contraception, when they do occur, are small, it would seem prudent to use drug combinations which have either a neutral or a beneficial effect.

Looking to the future, it seems likely that lower doses of oestrogen may be associated with an even smaller risk of myocardial infarction (Thorogood and Vessey 1990). Hoppe *et al.* (1990) reviewed the evidence concerning changes in metabolism and the newer progestogens, and suggested that the minor changes which may now be measured were unlikely to be of longterm clinical significance.

Oral contraception and venous thrombosis

There is no doubt that a relationship between oral contraceptive usage and venous thrombosis exists. In 1968, Vessey and Doll analysed the predisposing factors for deep venous thrombosis and pulmonary embolus in 399 women aged between 16 and 40 years. Some 338 women had a known predisposing factor such as pregnancy, surgery, or coexisting disease, but 61 women had no known predisposing factors and these were compared with 122 hospital patient controls. There was no statistical difference between cases and controls for weight, smoking, family history, or thromboembolic disease. Some 45 per cent of the cases had used oral contraceptives during the month prior to admission compared with 9 per cent of controls, a relative risk for oral contraceptive use of 9.0. The authors estimated that the risk for thromboembolism in the population was 1 per 18 000 women per year, but this increased to 1 in 2000 for women taking oral contraception. The duration of oral contraceptive use was not significant. In 1969, the same authors analysed 84 patients, between the ages of 16 and 40 years, with deep venous thrombosis or pulmonary embolus and compared these to 168 controls. Oral contraceptives had been used in the previous month by 50 per cent of the patients but by only 14 per cent of controls. They also reported 19 women with cerebral thrombosis between the ages of 16 and 40 years. Some 58 per cent of this group had taken oral contraceptives

Table 5.8 Oestrogen and pulmonary embolus

Oestrogen dosage	Relative risk of fatal pulmonary embolus
50	1.0
70–80	1.2
100	1.6
150	2.4

From Inman *et al.* (1970)

within the previous month compared with 3.5 per cent of age-matched controls. For 17 cases of coronary thrombosis, some 12 per cent had used oral contraceptives within the previous month as compared with 21 per cent of age-matched controls.

Inman *et al.* (1970), giving evidence to the Committee on Safety of Drugs, reported upon 920 cases of thromboembolism in women taking oral contraceptives in the UK. They demonstrated that:

1. Sequential oral contraception was no more hazardous than combined oral contraception containing the same type and dosage of oestrogen.
2. The risk of fatal pulmonary embolus, non-fatal pulmonary embolus, but not deep venous thrombosis, was related to the dose of oestrogen, the risk increasing with the dose of oestrogen (Table 5.8).
3. The progestogen content was not a significant influence upon the risk of thromboembolic disease.

The Committee on Safety of Drugs of the UK, together with the Food and Drug Administration of the USA, advised that oral contraceptives containing greater than 50 μg of oestrogen should rarely be prescribed. There is little hard evidence which compares the risk of 30 μg of oestrogen oral contraceptives with 50 μg, but if the effect on clotting is dose-related, then the risk of thromboembolic disease should be less.

The changes in the coagulation system associated with oral contraceptives have been widely studied, and whilst the generally accepted trends are described below, these findings have not been demonstrated by all workers (Mammen 1982; Farag *et al.* 1988). There tends to be a decrease in concentration of the natural anticoagulant antithrombin III (Beller and Ebert 1985) and an increase in fibrinogen, prothrombin, and factors VII, IX, X, and XII, especially factor VII (Beller and Ebert 1985; Meade 1982). These authors have also found that the effects tend to be dose-related to the oestrogen content of the drug, whilst the progestogen content has either a neutral effect or may reduce the oestrogenic effect (Beller and Ebert 1985; Gillmer 1989).

Should oral contraceptives be stopped preoperatively?

The British National Formulary (1992) states that:

oestrogen-containing oral conraceptives should be discontinued (and adequate alternative contraceptive arrangements made) four weeks before major elective surgery and all surgery to the legs; they should normally be recommenced at the first menses occurring at least two weeks after the procedure.

Clearly, there is a balance between the risks of thromboembolic disease with surgery in patients taking oral contraceptives and the risks of unwanted pregnancy, even when other contraceptive advice is offered. There is no need to stop taking oral contraceptives for smaller procedures such as laparoscopy (Sue-Ling and Hughes 1988). These authors concluded that the use of prophylactic agents was not indicated in the absence of other risk factors unless prophylaxis would have been given even if the patient had not been taking oral contraceptives.

The view that women taking oral contraceptives and undergoing major abdominal surgery are at risk of thromboembolic disease is hotly debated. Sagar *et al.* (1976) reported upon the incidence of post-operative deep venous thrombosis, based on radioactive fibrinogen-uptake studies in 31 young women undergoing emergency abdominal surgery (largely appendicectomy). Evidence of deep venous thrombosis was found in six patients, none of whom had taken oral contraceptives within the month prior to surgery. Vessey *et al.* (1986) reported upon the incidence of post-operative thromboembolism in women in the Oxford–FPA study. In those women who were taking oral contraceptives during the month prior to surgery, 12 out of 1244 (0.96 per cent) had evidence of thromboembolic disease as compared with 22 out of 4359 (0.5 per cent) of women using an IUCD or diaphragm. This difference is not statistically significant, but does show a trend towards an increased thromboembolic risk. Current advice, therefore, remains contradictory with some authors suggesting that there is no need for women to stop oral contraception prior to major abdominal surgery (Sue-Ling and Hughes 1988), whilst other authors suggest that oral contraception should be stopped (Guillebaud 1985, 1988; Robinson *et al.* 1991). Until this debate is resolved, an individual clinician will need to evaluate his or her own policy, although a consensus of opinion would probably favour cessation of oral contraception. There is an increased risk of thromboembolic disease in women using oral contraception and undergoing leg surgery, and, therefore, oral contraceptives should be stopped in this situation (Sue-Ling and Hughes 1988).

Patients who have stopped taking oral contraceptives because of surgery may recommence oral contraception on the first day of the post-operative menses (Guillebaud 1985).

Oral contraceptives and liver disease

There is an increased incidence of gall-bladder and liver disease in women using oral contraceptives. The RCGP study (1974) demonstrated that the incidence of cholelithiasis was raised in users, with an overall relative risk of 1.37 when compared with non-users. The rate of reporting gallstones increased after two years of oral contraceptive usage, plateauing after five years with a relative risk of 3.0.

There is an increased incidence of benign liver tumours in patients using oral contraceptives. Edmondson *et al.* (1976) reported 42 women with hepatic adenomata compared with age-matched controls. The mean duration of oral contraceptive use in the cases was 73.4 months as compared with 36.2 months in controls, with a highly significant association between hepatomata and mestranol-containing oral contraceptives. Vana *et al.* (1977) reported 212 benign liver tumours in women, of which hepatocellular adenomata were the commonest and focal nodular hyperplasia the second commonest. The incidence of oral contraceptive use in both these two groups was 74 per cent. There may also be an increased incidence of malignant liver tumours in oral contraceptive users. Neuberger *et al.* (1986) reported 76 women with a hepatocellular carcinoma in a non-cirrhotic liver and compared them with 1300 controls. For a use of oral contraceptives of less than eight years there was no increased risk, but a relative risk of 4.4 if oral contraceptives had been used for longer than eight years. When these figures were adjusted to exclude serological evidence of previous hepatitis B virus, the relative risk after eight years became 7.2. Similarly, Forman *et al.* (1986) reported that the relative risk of hepatocellular carcinoma in oral contraceptive users was 3.8 for the series of 19 patients when compared with 147 controls, but that this risk was largely confined to women who had used oral contraceptives for longer than eight years, in which case it was 20.1. However, this figure may be inaccurate because of small numbers. There was no increased risk of cholangiocarcinoma.

Oral contraceptives and depression

It has been stated that there is an association between oral contraceptives and depression. Herzberg *et al.* (1971) assessed depression and loss of libido using psychological screening tests on 272 women before commencement of oral contraception. These women then commenced oral contraceptives (218 women) or had an IUCD inserted (54 women). There was no significant difference in depression and the use of either oral contraception or IUCDs, but 50 per cent of a small subgroup of women who either ceased or changed oral contraceptives during the trial were more likely to be depressed or become depressed whilst taking oral contraceptive treatment. Women choosing oral contraception were less likely to be depressed than were those choosing an IUCD. The mean depressive score fell on commencement of both oral contraception and IUCD use, perhaps related to the use of the reliable method of contraception. Both oral contraceptive and IUCD users showed an initial increase in libido with a further increase in the IUCD users, but the oral contraceptive group showed an early plateau which was only marginally higher than the pretreatment libido. The subgroup of women who ceased or changed oral contraception showed a small, but progressive, decrease in libido.

The RCGP report (1974) was unable to find any increase in endogenous psychotic depression in pill takers when compared to controls (relative risk 0.85). However, there was an increase in neurotic reactive depression (relative risk 1.3) but a significant increase in loss of libido (relative risk 4.54). The Oxford–FPA study found the incidence of suicide and para-suicide to be the same in both the oral contraceptive and the IUCD–diaphragm group (Vessey *et al.* 1989).

Adams *et al.* (1973) suggested that oestrogen caused a reduction in pyridoxine levels and that this pyridoxine deficiency resulted in inadequate 5-HT synthesis, a known aetiological factor for endogenous depression. They demonstrated the value of pyridoxine therapy in those women who did become depressed whilst taking oral contraception. In a group of 22 women who took oral contraceptives and suffered from depression, pyridoxine levels were measured and were shown to be low in 11 and normal in 11. In a double-blind, cross-over study, all 11 deficient patients became less depressed with pyridoxine therapy as did four with a placebo. Of the 11 patients who were not deficient, four became less depressed with pyridoxine and five with placebo. These results were statistically significant.

It would, therefore, seem likely that there is a small subgroup of women who may become depressed whilst taking oral contraceptives.

Oral contraception and drug interactions

The failure of combined oral contraception is not always due to patient non-compliance. It has been suggested that drug interactions may be an important factor.

The first drug thought to interfere with the efficacy of oral contraception was rifampicin, but other antibiotics have since been implicated, generally in the form of case reports, including ampicillin (Dossetor 1975) and tetracycline (Bacon and Shenfield 1980). More detailed reviews and prospective studies suggest that there is no significant risk of drug failure with ampicillin, tetracycline (even longterm) or co-trimoxazole (Back *et al.* 1982; Gillmer 1989; Murphy *et al.* 1991; Orme 1982). There is no reason to warn patients on oral contraception that antibiotics may reduce the efficacy. Such advice 'merely perpetuates inaccuracies' but is still recommended on medico-legal grounds! (Orme and Back 1991).

The situation with anticonvulsant therapy is more complex and pregnancy has been reported with most anti-epileptic agents, including phenytoin, carbamazepine, and ethosuximide, all of which induce hepatic microsomal enzymes and hence reduce the oestrogen effect (Gillmer 1989). Contraceptive efficacy may be maintained in such patients by increasing the oestrogen dosage, if necessary up to 100 μg daily, titrated against any breakthrough bleeding (Guillebaud 1989).

Oral contraception and pregnancy

There may be a temporary delay in the return of fertility in women who stop taking oral contraceptives in order to conceive. Pardthaisong and Gray (1981) surveyed 437 women who stopped taking the pill in order to conceive and found a mean delay of up to three months prior to conception as compared with that expected using cumulative life tables, although 94.3 per cent of women conceived within two years. Vessey *et al.* (1978) reported that women who ceased oral contraception had a short-term infertility when compared with other groups, but that no effect was detectable beyond 30 months in multiparae and 42 months in nulligravidae. There is no evidence to support the concept of 'post-pill amenorrhoea' being caused by oral contraception (Jacobs *et al.* 1977).

In women who conceive despite oral contraception, there is no evidence for either an increased incidence of miscarriage or for an increased incidence of fetal abnormality.

Harlap *et al.* (1980) could find no difference in the incidence of spontaneous abortion in 8412 women who ceased oral contraception prior to conception, even when it was stopped in the previous month, when compared with 23 711 women who used a different or no method of contraception prior to pregnancy. In those 781 women who continued to use the pill inadvertently during early pregnancy, when a multiple regression analysis for other factors was performed the risk of miscarriage was identical to that seen in the general population.

A study group of the World Health Organization could find no differences in the incidence of congenital abnormalities in the offspring of 22 953 women who used oral contraception prior to conception compared with 46 339 who did not (WHO Technical Report Series 1981). In an analysis of 1368 pregnancies where oral contraceptives were used during the conception cycle, this group further concluded that there was no increased risk of fetal anomaly, including chromosomal damage. A meta-analysis of 12 prospective studies on the risks of oral contraceptives during early pregnancy resulted in a relative risk of 0.99 for all malformations, suggesting that patients may be strongly reassured on this point (Bracken 1990). The WHO study group also reported that the perinatal mortality rates were consistently lower in pregnancies following oral contraceptive therapy, presumably due to the more favourable demographic and health characteristics of oral contraceptive users. This conclusion also applied following the cessation of oral contraceptives during early pregnancy.

Progestogens for contraception

Progestogens, used orally or intramuscularly, are discussed in this section, whilst some more recent methods of application are discussed under 'Newer methods of contraception'.

The progestogen-only pill is associated with a greater failure rate than is combined oral contraception (Table 5.2). The pregnancy rate appears to decrease with age, being 3.1 per 100 women-years in women aged 25–29, one per 100 in women over the age of 35, and 0.3 in those over 40 years of age (Vessey *et al.* 1985). Incorrect pill taking would appear to be a major factor in failure (Szarewski and Guillebaud 1991). This form of contraception would seem to be particularly indicated in women for whom oestrogen is less desirable; older smokers, and women with hypertension, diabetes, or during lactation. The commonest side-effect is disturbance of menstrual pattern. Fotherby (1989*b*) reported that 30 per cent of cycles were shorter than 24 days in women using progestogen-only contraception, 12 per cent were greater than 45 days, and some 15 per cent of women discontinued this method of contraception because of a disordered menstrual pattern. There have been no significant effects of progestogen-only contraception described upon carbohydrate metabolism (Blum *et al.* 1983), lipid metabolism (Radberg *et al.* 1982), or blood coagulation (Conrad *et al.* 1979).

Depomedroxyprogesterone acetate (DMPA or Depo-Provera) is a long-acting injectable contraceptive generally given in dosages of 150 mg once every 84–90 days, although greater dosages administered less frequently have been described (Fraser 1989). In major trials, the failure rates are less than 0.5 per 100 women-years (Fraser and Weisberg 1981) or even 0.25 per 100 women-years (Schwallie and Assenzo 1973). Menstrual irregularity is common and amenorrhoea becomes more likely with repeated use of DMPA. Thus, after one injection, 30 per cent of women have amenorrhoea, whilst after 12 months of use, 55 per cent of women have amenorrhoea (Schwallie and Assenzo 1973). Should bleeding become a clinical problem (4 per cent of patients), oestrogen (or rarely curettage) may be used (Fraser 1989). The median time from cessation of contraceptive efficacy to conception was 5.5 months in a group of 796 women, suggesting a minimal delay in the return of fertility (Pardthaisong *et al.* 1980) with 60 per cent of women conceiving within 12 months of discontinuation and 85 per cent within 24 months (Fraser 1989).

Controversy surrounded DMPA in the 1970s with reports that high-dose progestogens caused beagle bitches to develop benign and malignant breast lumps, but this evidence should not necessarily be extrapolated to humans. Until recently, clinical studies had not shown any association between DMPA and breast cancer in humans (Fraser 1989; Greenspan *et al.* 1980) or between DMPA and benign breast disease (Fraser and Weisberg 1981). Liang *et al.* (1983) followed 5000 women who received DMPA for between 4 and 14 years and found the relative risk to be 0.7 for breast cancer, 0.8 for ovarian cancer, and 1.2 for carcinoma of the body of the uterus. The recent WHO Collaborative Study (1991) demonstrated that there was no overall risk for breast cancer in women using DMPA for contraception other than during the first four years after commencing the agent (relative risk of 2.02). Thereafter, there was no increased risk in any woman, regardless of duration of use. This observation is difficult to explain, but is compatible with the stimulation of growth of an existing tumour rather than the initiation of tumour development.

The effect of DMPA on carbohydrate metabolism is negligible and because of its neutral pressor effect it is probably safer than the combined pill. Moreover, coagulation is not affected by DMPA. There is, however, some reduction of HDL and this factor needs to be considered when the risks for cardiovascular disease are also present in the user (Elder 1984).

DMPA would, therefore, appear to be a very effective method of contraception suitable for a specific group of patients.

Intrauterine contraceptive devices

The intrauterine contraceptive device is used by 7 per cent of couples (OPCS 1991). It is associated with a failure rate of 1.3–1.4 per 100 women-years (Vessey *et al.* 1982*a*), and with an ectopic pregnancy rate of 29.7 per 1000 pregnancies with non-medicated devices (Tatum and Schmidt 1977). This association is discussed further in Chapter 2 (Ectopic pregnancy).

The advice concerning the length of time for which an IUCD may remain *in situ* has changed over recent years. Most trials have shown that copper-containing IUCDs have either lower failure rates or similar failure rates to inert devices (Snowden 1981, World Health Organization 1987). Earlier studies suggested that this was only true for up to three years after insertion, but longer periods of follow-up have shown that the effective lifespan is in excess of the manufacturers' recommendations with failure rates no higher in the fourth, fifth, or even sixth year of use than in the first (range 0.1–1.5 pregnancies per 100 women-years) (Newton and Tacchi 1990; World Health Organization 1987). Some copper devices may even remain effective for up to 10 years (World Health Organization 1987).

It is now generally accepted that copper-containing IUCDs need not be changed more frequently than every five years and can be fitted into a woman over 40 years of age, the age-related reduced fecundity allowing the device to remain *in situ* until after the menopause (Newton and Tacchi 1990; Tacchi 1990). However, there is a risk of both pelvic inflammatory disease and actinomycosis associated with the use of IUCDs, and these risks are discussed below.

IUCDs and pelvic inflammatory disease

The association between IUCD use and pelvic inflammatory disease is well recognized, and following the recent litigation in the United States concerning

Table 5.9 Contraception and pelvic inflammatory disease

Type of contraception	Relative risk of pelvic inflammatory disease		
	Lee *et al.* (1983)	Kaufman *et al.* (1980)	Buchan *et al.* (1990)
None	1.0	1.0	1.0
Oral contraception	0.5	—	0.5
Barrier	0.6	—	0.6–1.2
All IUCDs	1.9	6.5	—
All IUCDs excluding Dalkon shield	1.6	—	—
Lippes loop	1.2	—	
Saf-T-Coil	1.3	9.2	3.3
Copper 7	1.9	3.8	
Progestasert	2.2	—	1.8
Dalkon shield	8.3	12.3	4.7
Sterilization	—	—	0.7

the Dalkon shield (now withdrawn), the rate of insertion of IUCDs in North America has dramatically decreased following the withdrawal of most IUCDs by manufacturers.

There are numerous studies which suggest an association between the use of an intrauterine contraceptive device and an increased incidence of pelvic inflammatory disease (Farley *et al.* 1992; Targum and Wright 1974; Westrom *et al.* 1976). Burkman and the The Women's Health Group (1981) compared 1447 patients with pelvic inflammatory disease with 3452 matched controls. The relative risk of pelvic inflammatory disease was 1.6 in the presence of an IUCD compared with a non-user. Similarly, Farley *et al.* (1992) reported that the overall rate of pelvic inflammatory disease in over 22 000 users was 1.6 cases per 1000 women-years of use.

The relative risk of pelvic inflammatory disease associated with different types of contraception is illustrated in Table 5.9. Compared with women who use no contraception, the relative risk of pelvic inflammatory disease in women using an IUCD ranged between 1.2 and 9.2, but rose to as high as 12.3 in women who used a Dalkon shield (Buchan *et al.* 1990; Kaufman *et al.* 1980; Lee *et al.* 1983; Vessey *et al.* 1981*b*).

The increased risk of pelvic inflammatory disease in patients using an IUCD compares with the decreased risk of pelvic inflammatory disease in patients using oral contraceptives. Thus, Senanayake and Kramer (1980) reported 18 studies from the literature, 16 of which showed a relative risk of between 0.3–0.9 for pelvic inflammatory disease in oral contraceptive takers compared with contraceptive non-users. Other studies have come to similar conclusions (Eschenbach *et al.* 1977; RCGP Study 1974; Rubin *et al.* 1982).

However, not all authors have found a protective effect from oral contraception. Washington *et al.* (1985) warned that the reduced incidence of pelvic inflammatory disease in oral contraceptive users did not apply to chlamydial infections. In a meta-analysis of 14 studies, they compared chlamydial pelvic inflammatory disease in 3255 oral contraceptive users with 3041 non-users. The relative risk of chlamydial pelvic inflammatory disease in users compared with non-users ranged from 1.0 to 3.9.

The protective effect of oral contraception against pelvic inflammatory disease may equate with the protective effect of barrier methods of contraception: Kelaghan *et al.* (1982) compared the contraceptive methods of 645 women admitted to hospital with pelvic inflammatory disease with a contraceptive method used by 2509 hospital controls without a history of pelvic inflammatory disease. The relative risk of pelvic inflammatory disease for women using barrier methods of contraception, when compared to those using no contraception, was 0.6.

The one problem with all these studies, however, is the paucity of data which corrects the relative risk of pelvic inflammatory disease, for any given method of contraception and for sexual behaviour. However, there is no doubt that there remains a statistically significant association between the use of an IUCD and pelvic inflammatory disease.

The two major risk factors which have been documented for pelvic inflammatory disease in IUCD users relate to the time of insertion and the presence of a tail.

The incidence of pelvic inflammatory disease is more than six times higher during the 20 days after insertion of an IUCD than during later times (Farley *et al.* 1992). This may relate to bacterial contamination of the endometrial cavity at the time of insertion, and there is some evidence that prophylactic antibiotics at the time of insertion will reduce the incidence of pelvic inflammatory disease and should, therefore, be considered (Sinei *et al.* 1990). There is also good evidence that the multifilament tail of an IUCD is a major factor in infection, whereas a monofilament-tailed IUCD or a tailless IUCD are not associated with infection (Skangalis *et al.* 1982, Sparks *et al.* 1981). Therefore, it seems inappropriate to insert IUCDs with a multifilament tail. There is also good evidence to suggest that a copper-containing IUCD is associated with a two-thirds reduction in the incidence of pelvic inflammatory disease compared with an inert device (Buchan *et al.* 1990; Kaufman *et al.* 1980). It would seem, therefore, that a copper-containing IUCD with a monofilament tail should be chosen.

The association between IUCDs and pelvic inflammatory disease may also result in subfertility. Daling *et al.* (1985) compared 159 nulligravid women with tubal infertility with a matched group of 159 controls who conceived their first child at the time when the infertile women started trying to conceive. The relative risk of primary infertility in 'ever-users' of IUCDs compared with 'never-users' was 2.6. The relative risk if the IUCD contained copper was 1.3, if the IUCD was a Lippes Loop or a Saf-T-Coil it was 3.2, and if a Dalkon shield was used it was 6.8. Other authors have reported similar findings (Cramer et al. 1985). It would seem that IUCD-related subfertility is largely primary infertility. There is no statistically increased risk of either secondary infertility, or of primary infertility in women who have had only one sexual partner (Cramer et al. 1985).

IUCDs and actinomycosis

There is also an association between IUCD use and colonization of the lower genital tract by the Gram-positive filamentous bacterium *Actinomyces*, especially *A. israelii*. The presence of an IUCD is said to enable the anaerobic spores to germinate; the colonies may be recognized macroscopically in pus as a yellow ('sulphur') granule, or be seen on cervical smears. Gupta (1982) reported 713 smears containing actinomycotic filaments, an incidence of 0.7 per cent in over 100 100 women, but present in 6.9 per cent of IUCD users.

Hager et al. (1979) reported a prospective controlled study of the relationship between actinomycosis and IUCD use. None of 50 patients without an IUCD had any evidence of actinomycotic infection, but four patients with an IUCD in situ (8 per cent) had evidence of actinomycosis on a smear, although all were asymptomatic. Petiti et al. (1983) reported the incidence of actinomycotic-like organisms on cervical smears as 0.13 per cent of 80 000 smears, but 97 per cent of the patients with evidence of this infection had an IUCD in situ. Duguid et al. (1980) reported that plastic IUCDs were more likely to predispose to actinomycotic colonization than were copper-containing devices. They reported evidence of actinomycotic-like structures on cervical smears in 31 per cent of 128 women with a plastic IUCD, 1.2 per cent of 165 women with a copper IUCD, and none of 300 women taking oral contraceptives.

Most workers have shown a relationship between the prevalence of actinomycosis and the duration of usage of the IUCD. Thus, Valicenti et al. (1982) were able to isolate actinomycotic organisms on a smear from 19 per cent of 26 women who had an IUCD in situ for only one year, from 29 per cent of 34 women who had an IUCD in situ for five years, and from 54 per cent of 13 women who had an IUCD in situ for ten years.

Although actinomycotic colonization may be noted, this does not necessarily equate with pelvic infection caused by actinomycosis. Duguid et al. (1982) reported 42 women with an IUCD in situ and actinomycotic organisms on a cervical smear. Some 45 per cent of the patients had pain, 45 per cent discharge, and 26 per cent abnormal bleeding. There was some overlap between the symptoms, but 18 per cent of the patients in this series were totally symptom-free. Valicenti et al. (1982) reported 112 women with actinomycotic organisms on a smear and who had an IUCD in situ. Some 72.8 per cent of these patients were completely symptom-free, the commonest symptom being described as vaginal discharge in 21.7 per cent. Only two patients (1.8 per cent) had any clinical evidence of pelvic inflammatory disease. Burkman et al. (1982) also reported on the association between actinomycosis and pelvic inflammatory disease in

IUCD users in a case-controlled study of 46 patients with acute pelvic inflammatory disease and 108 without. Evidence of actinomycotic organisms seen on a cervical smear was present in 17 per cent of those patients with pelvic inflammatory disease and in 5 per cent of the control group, the relative risk of hospitalization for pelvic inflammatory disease when actinomycotic organisms had been seen on the smear was 3.6 when compared with hospitalization without the presence of such organisms. Moreover, when infection did occur in the actinomycotic group, tubovarian abscess was a complication in 87.5 per cent compared with 28.9 per cent without actinomycosis.

Since only a minority of patients with actinomycotic organisms on a cervical smear will develop pelvic inflammatory disease, this is not an absolute indication for removal of the IUCD. However, this advice is generally given as a precaution. In the absence of clinical evidence of pelvic inflammatory disease, removal of the IUCD seems all that is required. Valicenti *et al.* (1982) removed the IUCD from 34 asymptomatic patients but with evidence of actinomycotic infestation, and in all instances there was no further evidence of actinomycotic-like organisms on cervical smears taken after the next menstrual period. Other authors have described a similar finding (Duguid *et al.* 1982). Should the patient wish, a new IUCD can be inserted at the time of removal of the infected device without a significant increased risk of reinfection (Mao and Guillebaud 1984). Should evidence of infection persist after removal of the IUCD, ampicillin may then be instituted (Bornstein 1987).

Emergency contraception

Emergency contraception is now the preferred term rather than post-coital contraception or 'morning-after' pill. The UK Attorney-General has ruled that emergency contraception is legal since it is administered before implantation has occurred. The techniques in use include combined oestrogen–progestogen, oestrogen alone, progestogens alone, and the insertion of an IUCD. When the efficacy of emergency contraception is considered, it should be remembered that the risk of pregnancy after one episode of unprotected intercourse is approximately 30 per cent at ovulation and between 2 and 10 per cent at other times (Drife 1993; Reader 1991).

Progestogen alone is the least effective of these methods; a single dose of 0.6 mg levonorgestrel given within 12 hours of coitus was associated with a pregnancy rate of 2.9 per cent in 205 patients (Yuzpe and Kubba 1989). Higher dosages may be used, but the incidence of side-effects such as nausea (20 per cent) or menstrual disturbance (21 per cent) may be increased. The association between ectopic pregnancy and emergency contraception is discussed in Chapter 2 (Ectopic pregnancy). This method is now only used when oestrogen or an IUCD are contraindicated.

The efficacy of oestrogen alone was demonstrated by Dixon *et al.* (1980) in 876 women with a single episode of intercourse, in whom there would have been

69 expected pregnancies based upon the day of the cycle at which intercourse took place. There were only 11 pregnancies, the most effective regime being ethinyl oestradiol, 5 mg per day for five days, commenced within 72 hours of unprotected intercourse. Some 70 per cent of patients experienced nausea and 33 per cent vomited. However, such regimes have been superseded by more effective methods.

Yuzpe and Lance (1977) reported 608 women receiving combined oestrogen and progestogen, in the form of 200 µg of ethinyl oestradiol and 2 mg of dl-norgestrel in two equally divided dosages 12 hours apart taken within 72 hours of unprotected intercourse. They had expected 12–20 pregnancies, but only one occurred. In a further study by Yuzpe *et al.* (1982) 692 women with an isolated episode of unprotected intercourse received the same regime within 72 hours. The estimate was for 31 pregnancies, but only 11 occurred, the estimated reduction in pregnancy being 65 per cent and the overall pregnancy rate for the entire group being 1.6 per cent. Some 29 per cent of patients vomited as a direct result of the treatment. Tully (1983) gave the same regime to 511 women, and reported an overall pregnancy rate of 2 per cent, but a rate of 5 per cent if the unprotected intercourse occurred at mid-cycle.

In a randomized trial of oestrogen alone against oestrogen–progestogen combined, the pregnancy rate in the oestrogen group ($n = 226$) was 0.9 per cent, whilst the pregnancy rate in the oestrogen–progestogen combined group ($n = 239$) was 0.4 per cent (van Santen and Haspels 1985). Vomiting occurred in 20.8 per cent of the oestrogen group and in 15.8 per cent of the combined group. Moreover, the oestrogen alone was taken for five days, whilst the combined treatment was taken for only one day. For these reasons, combined oestrogen–progestogen is the preferred method of emergency contraception, providing that treatment is commenced within 72 hours of coitus. Since there does not appear to be an increased risk of fetal abnormalities associated with the continued use of oral contraception in early pregnancy (p. 94), there is even less likely to be any excess risk of teratogenicity following emergency contraception.

An IUCD, inserted up to five days after unprotected intercourse, is probably the most effective form of emergency contraception available. The first reported failure occurred after over 1300 successful post-coital insertions (Kubba and Guillebaud 1985). It has the further advantage that, left in place, future contraception is provided and it may be especially indicated where oestrogen is contraindicated. However, it comes with the obvious disadvantages of insertion, including pain, especially in nulliparous patients (Yuzpe and Kubba 1989).

The two major options for emergency contraception will, therefore, be either a combination of oestrogen and progestogen, or the insertion of an IUCD (Webb *et al.* 1992).

Newer methods of contraception

Several new methods of contraception are under investigation and these include:

(1) subdermal implants of progestogen (Norplant);

(2) vaginal rings;

(3) progesterone antagonists;

(4) vaccines;

(5) male contraception;

(6) female condoms.

The World Health Organization conducted a study on subdermal implants of progestogen. The insertion of six capsules of levonorgestrel subdermally into the palmar aspect of the arm was associated with an annual pregnancy rate of 0.2–1.3 per cent, and a gross accummulative pregnancy rate of 2.6 per 1000 women-years (*Drug and Therapeutics Bulletin* 1994; WHO 1985).

The advantage of using a vaginal ring is the immediate reversal of contraception, the ring containing progestogen alone or oestrogen and progestogen combined. It is an effective method of contraception and is not associated with hypertension (Elkik and Elkik 1986).

The progesterone antagonist RU486 is a synthetic 19-norsteroid which competes with progesterone for receptor sites. Couzinet *et al.* (1986) reported that RU486 administered to 100 women resulted in abortion in 85 per cent of patients.

This drug is now licensed in the UK as mifepristone. When mifepristone in oral doses of 400–600 mg was followed 48 hours later by a vaginal prostaglandin pessary (Gemeprost 1 mg) complete abortion occurred in 95 per cent of 100 women who received these agents within 56 days of the previous period (Rodger and Baird 1987).

The UK Multicentre Trial (1990) reported 588 women seeking termination before the ninth week of pregnancy. They received 600 mg of oral mifepristone followed 48 hours later by 1 mg Gemeprost vaginally. Some 94 per cent of women had a complete abortion without the need for curettage and 81 per cent of the women remained in hospital for less than four hours. Side effects included severe pain (21 per cent), significant bleeding (9 per cent), vomiting (25 per cent), and diarrhoea (13 per cent). The French study of mifepristone followed by prostaglandin resulted in complete abortion in 96 per cent of 2041 women of whom 86 per cent expelled products of conception within the first 24 hours of insertion of the prostaglandin. In 1 per cent of women the pregnancy persisted and a further 3 per cent of women underwent evacuation of the uterus for either bleeding or retained products of conception or both. (Silvestre *et al.* 1990).

These studies suggest that mifepristone followed by prostaglandin represent a realistic alternative to early surgical termination of pregnancy (Henshaw *et al.* 1993; Norman *et al.* 1992; Thong and Baird 1992; World Health Organization Task Force 1993). This drug may also find use as a form of emergency contraception (Grimes and Cook 1992; Webb *et al.* 1992).

Mifepristone is teratogenic. Sirenomelia or caudal regression syndrome, characterized by fused lower limbs has been reported, but the true incidence of this or any other abnormality is yet to be described (Pons *et al.* 1991). Since the number of pregnancies which continue because mifepristone has failed and the woman has changed her mind will be very few, there is a need for the pooling of accurate data relating to the outcome of such pregnancies. Patients should be advised of the possible risk of teratogenicity until it is known whether this is a real possibility or not (Henrion 1989).

Although it may seem attractive to perform medical rather than surgical abortions, medical abortion may be more labour intensive and financial savings have yet to be demonstrated (Heard and Guillebaud 1992).

The use of a vaccine against hCG is also being studied by the WHO (Jones *et al.* 1988). Trials of the vaccine in non-human primates did not show any untoward effects, and resulted in corpus luteum regression, disruption of the peri-implantation embryo, and menstruation. The vaccine was also administered to 30 surgically-sterilized female volunteers who received two intramuscular injections six weeks apart. The potential contraceptive levels of anti-hCG appeared in all 30, and there were no important adverse effects, although several women suffered transient myalgia, pruritis, or a delayed erythema at the injection site. The efficacy of this vaccine as a contraceptive in humans is not yet known.

It seems unlikely that a male oral contraceptive will be in general use in the near future. Gonadotrophin releasing hormone analogues (GnRH) result in an adequate suppression of spermatogenesis accompanied by a loss of libido, whilst anti-androgens, such as cyproterone acetate, appear to be able to suppress spermatogenesis but they have impaired potency as a side-effect. The WHO (1990*b*) reported on the weekly injection of 200 mg of testosterone enanthate in 271 healthy fertile men. Within six months, 65 per cent became azoospermic and the treatment was discontinued as a failure in the other 45 per cent. After cessation of testosterone injections, the median time from azoospermia to recovery was 3.7 months. The need for weekly injections together with the limited success is unlikely to promote this as a method of contraception. There is increasing interest in the female condom (Femidom) which is a soft pliable polyurethane condom designed to line the vagina and hence may act as a barrier against sexually transmitted diseases as well as a contraceptive. However, it is not terribly easy to use and may have a failure rate of up to 15 per cent after 12 months of use (Bounds *et al.* 1992).

Conclusions

Contraceptive advice is a significant part of many gynaecological consultations and the whole area of family planning is emerging as a subspeciality in its own right. Newer methods of contraception await practical development, and what is appropriate for the Western world is not necessarily that which is appropriate for the Third World. It remains a valid observation that the woman who cannot, or does not wish to, use oral contraceptives is left with a suboptimal choice.

Acknowledgement

The author wishes to thank Mr A. Kubba for his help in the preparation of this chapter.

References

Adams, P. W., Winn, V., Rose, D. T., Seed, M., Folkard, J., and Strong, R. (1973). The effect of pyridoxine upon depression associated with oral contraception. *Lancet* i, 897–904.

Back, D. J., Breckenridge, M. A., MacIver, M., Orme, M., Rowe, P. H., Staiger, E., *et al.* (1982). The effects of ampicillin on oral contraceptive steroids in women. *British Journal of Clinical Pharmacology* 14, 43–8.

Bacon, J. F. and Shenfield, G. N. (1980). Pregnancy attributable to interaction between tetracycline and oral contraception. *British Medical Journal* 280, 293.

Beller, F. K. and Ebert, C. (1985). Effects of oral contraceptives on blood coagulation. *Obstetric and Gynecological Survey* 40, 425–36.

Blum, M., Rusecky, Y., and Gelernter, I. (1983). Glyco-haemoglobin levels in oral contraceptive uses. *European Journal of Obstetrics, Gynaecology, and Reproductive Biology* 15, 97–101.

Bornstein, J., Montgomery, L., and Kaufman, R. H. (1987). Actinomycosis documented by cervical smear and endometrial biopsy. *Acta Cytologica* 31, 955–7.

Bounds, W., Guillebaud, J., and Newman, G. B. (1992). Female condom – a clinical study of its use, effectiveness and patient acceptability. *British Journal of Family Planning* 18, 36–41.

Bracken, M. (1990). Oral contraception and congenital malformation in the offspring. *Obstetrics and Gynecology* 76, 552–7.

Briggs, M. and Briggs, M. (1977). Oestrogen content of oral contraceptives. *Lancet* ii, 1233.

Brinton, L. A., Hoover, R. N., Szklo, M., and Fraumeni, J. R. (1992). Oral contraceptives and breast cancer. *International Journal of Epidemiology* 11, 316–22.

British National Formulary (1992). Contraceptives. In *British national formulary*, p. 283. Published by British Medical Association and Royal Pharmaceutical Society of Great Britain London.

Buchan, H., Villard-Mackintosh, L., Vessey, M., Yeates, D., and McPherson, K. (1990). Epidemiology of pelvic inflammatory disease in parous women with special reference to IUCDs. *British Journal of Obstetrics and Gynaecology* 97, 780–8.

Burkman, R. T. and The Women's Health Group (1981). Association between intra-uterine contraceptive devices and pelvic inflammatory disease. *Obstetrics and Gynecology* **57**, 269–76.

Burkman, R., Schlesselman, S., McCaffrey, L., Gupta, P. K., and Spence, M. (1982). The relationship of genital tract actinomycetes and the development of pelvic inflammatory disease. *American Journal of Obstetrics and Gynecology* **143**, 585–9.

Centers for Disease Control, Cancer and Steroid Hormone Study (1983). Long-term oral contraceptive use and the risk of breast cancer. *Journal of the American Medical Association* **249**, 1591–5.

Centers for Disease Control, Cancer, and Steroid Hormone Group (1986). Oral con-traceptive use and the risk of breast cancer. *New England Journal of Medicine* **315**, 405–11.

Conrad, J., Samama, M., Horellou, M. H., Zorn, J. R., and Neau, C. (1979) Antithrombin III and oral contraception with progestogen-only preparations. *Lancet* **ii**, 471.

Couzinet, B., Le Strat, N., Ulmann, A., Baulieu, E. M. G., and Schaison, G. (1986). Termination of early pregnancy by the progesterone antagonist RU486. *New England Journal of Medicine* **315**, 1565–70.

Cramer, D. W., Schiff, I., Schoenbaum, S. C., Gibson, M., Belisle, S., Albrecht, B., *et al.* (1985). Tubal infertility and the IUCD. *New England Journal of Medicine* **312**, 941–7.

Croft, P. and Hannaford, P. C. (1989). Risk factors for acute myocardial infarction in women. *British Medical Journal* **298**, 165–8.

Dalen, J. E. and Hickler, R. B. (1981). Oral contraceptives and cardiovascular disease. *American Heart Journal* **101**, 626–39.

Daling, J. R., Weim, N. S., Metch, B. J., Chow, W. H., Soderscrom, R. M., Moore, D. E., *et al.* (1985). Primary tubal infertility in relation to use of an IUCD. *New England Journal of Medicine* **312**, 937–41.

Dixon, G. W., Schlesselman, J. J., Ory, J. W., and Blye, R.P. (1980). Ethinyl estradiol and conjugate estrogens as post-coital contraception. *Journal of the American Medical Association* **244**, 1336–9.

Dossetor, J. (1975). Drug interactions with oral contraceptives. *British Medical Journal* **4**, 467–8.

Drife, J. O. (1989). The benefits of combined oral contraceptives. *British Journal of Obstetrics and Gynaecology* **96**, 1255–8.

Drife, J. O. (1993). Deregulating emergency contraception. *British Medical Journal* **307**, 695–6.

Drug and Therapeutics Bulletin (1992). Starting oral contraceptives. *Drug and Therapeutics Bulletin* **11**, 41–4.

Drug and Therapeutics Bulletin (1994). Norplant — a contraceptive implant. *Drug and Therapeutics Bulletin* **32**, 17–19.

Duguid, H. L. D., Parratt, D., and Traynor, R. (1980). Actinomyces-like organisms in cervical smears from women using intra-uterine contraceptive devices. *British Medical Journal* **281**, 534–7.

Duguid, H. L. D., Parratt, D., Traynor, R., Duncan, I. D., Elias-Jones, J., and Duguid, R. (1982). Studies on uterine tract infections and the IUCD with special reference to actinomycetes. *British Journal of Obstetrics and Gynaecology* **89**, supp 4, 32–40.

Edmondson, H. A., Henderson, B., and Benton, B. (1976). Liver-cell adenomas asso-ciated with use of oral contraceptives. *New England Journal of Medicine* **294**, 470–2.

Elder, M. G. (1984). Injectable contraception. *Clinics in Obstetrics and Gynaecology* **11**, 723–41.

Elkik, F. and Elkik, E. (1986). Contraception in hypertensive women using a vaginal ring containing oestradiol and levonorgestrel. *Journal of Clinical Endocrinology and Metabolism* **63**, 29–35.

Eschenbach, D. E., Harnisch, J. P., and Holmes, K. K. (1977). Pathogenesis of acute pelvic inflammatory disease: role of contraception and at risk factors. *American Journal of Obstetrics and Gynecology* **128**, 838–50.

Eyong, E. and Elstein, M. (1989). Clinical update on a new progestogen – gestodene. *British Journal of Family Planning* **15**, 18–22.

Farag, A. M., Bottoms, S. F., Mammen, E. F., Hosni, M. A., Ali, A. A., and Moghissi, K. S. (1988). Oral contraceptives and the haemostatic system. *Obstetrics and Gynecology* **71**, 584–8.

Farley, T. M. M., Rosenberg, M. J., Rowe, P. J., Chen, J. F., and Meirik, O. (1992). Intra-uterine contraceptive devices and pelvic inflammatory disease. *Lancet* **339**, 785–8.

Forman, D., Vincent, J. T., and Doll, R. (1986). Cancer of the liver and oral contraception. *British Medical Journal* **297**, 1357–61.

Fotherby, K. (1989a). Oral contraceptives and lipids. *British Medical Journal* **298**, 1049–50.

Fotherby, K. (1989b). The progestogen-only pill. In *Contraception: science and practice* (ed. M. Filshie and J. Guillebaud), pp. 94–108. Butterworths, London.

Fraser, I. S. (1989). Systemic hormonal contraception by non-oral routes. In *Contraception: science and practice* (ed. M. Filshie and J. Guillebaud), pp. 109–25. Butterworths, London.

Fraser, I. S. and Weisberg, G. (1981). A comprehensive review of injectable contraception with special emphasis on depo medroxyprogesterone acetate. *Medical Journal of Australia*, (supp), **1**, 1–19.

Gillmer, M. D. G. (1989). Metabolic effects of combined oral contraceptives. In *Contraception: science and practice* (ed. M. Filshie and J. Guillebaud), pp. 11–38. Butterworths, London.

Godsland, I. F., Crook, D., Simpson, R., Proudler, T., Felton, C., Lees, B., *et al.* (1990). The effect of different formulations of oral contraceptive agents on lipid and carbohydrate metabolism. *New England Journal of Medicine* **323**, 1375–41.

Greenspan, A. R., Hatcher, R. A., and Moore, N. (1980). The association of depo medroxyprogesterone acetate and breast cancer. *Contraception* **21**, 563–8.

Grimes, G. A. and Cook, R. J. (1992). Mifepristone – an abortifacient to prevent abortion? *New England Journal of Medicine* **327**, 1088–9.

Guillebaud, J. (1985). Surgery and the pill. *British Medical Journal* **291**, 498–9.

Guillebaud, J. (1988). Should the pill be stopped pre-operatively? *British Medical Journal* **296**, 786–7.

Guillebaud, J. (1989). Practical prescribing of the combined oral contraceptive pill. In *Contraception: science and practice* (ed. M. Filshie and J. Guillebaud), pp. 69–93. Butterworths, London.

Gupta, P. K. (1982). Intra-uterine contraceptive devices. *Acta Cytologica* **26**, 571–613.

Hager, W. D., Douglas, B., Majmudar, B., Naib, Z. M., Williams, O. C., Ramsey, C., *et al.* (1979). Pelvic colonization with actinomyces in women using IUCDs. *American Journal of Obstetrics and Gynecology*, **135**, 680–4.

Harlap, S., Shiono, P. H., and Ramcharan, S. (1980). Spontaneous fetal losses in women using different contraceptives around the time of conception. *International Journal of Epidemiology* **9**, 49–56.

Harris, N. V., Weiss, N. S., Francis, A. M., and Polissar, L. (1982). Breast cancer in relation to patterns of oral contraceptive use. *American Journal of Epidemiology* **116**, 643–51.

Heard, M. and Guillebaud, J. (1992). Medical abortion. *British Medical Journal* **304**, 195–6.

Hennekens, C. H., Speizer, F. E., and Lipnick, R. J. (1984). A case-controlled study of oral contraceptive use and breast cancer. *Journal of the National Cancer Institute* **72**, 39–42.

Henrien, R. (1989). RU486 abortions. *Nature* **338**, 110.

Henshaw, R. C., Naji, S. A., Russell, I. T., and Templeton, A. A. (1993). Comparison of medical abortion with surgical vacuum aspiration. *British Medical Journal* **307**, 714–17.

Herbst, A. L. and Berek, J. S. (1993). Impact of contraceptives on gynecological cancers. *American Journal of Obstetrics and Gynecology* **168**, 1980–5.

Herzberg, B. M., Draper, K. C., Johnson, A. L., and Nichol, G. C. (1971). Oral contraceptives, depression, and libido. *British Medical Journal* **3**, 495–500.

Hoppe, G. (1990). Clinical relevance of oral contraceptive pill-induced plasma lipid changes. *American Journal of Obstetrics and Gynecology* **163**, 388–91.

Inman, W. H. (1979). Oral contraceptive and fatal subarachnoid haemorrhage. *British Medical Journal* **2**, 1468–70.

Inman, W. H., Westerholm, B., and Engelund, A. (1970). Thromboembolic disease and steroidal content of oral contraceptives. *British Medical Journal* **2**, 203–9.

Jacobs, D. R., Mebane, I. L., Bangdiwala, S. I., Criqui, M. H., and Tyroler, H. A. (1990). High density lipoprotein cholesterol as a predictor of cardiovascular disease mortality in men and women. *American Journal of Epidemiology* **131**, 32–47.

Jacobs, H. S., Kanuth, U. A., Hull, M. G. R., and Franks, S. (1977). Post-pill amenorrhoea—cause or coincidence? *British Medical Journal* **2**, 940–2.

Jick, S. S., Walker, A. M., Stergachis, A., and Jack, H. (1989). Oral contraceptives and breast cancer. *British Journal of Cancer* **59**, 618–21.

Jick, S. S., Walker, A. M., and Jick, H. (1993). Oral contraceptives and endometrial cancer. *Obstetrics and Gynecology* **82**, 931–5.

Jones, W. R., Bradley, J., Judd, S. J., Denholm, E. H., Ing, R. M. Y., Mueller, V. W., *et al.* (1988). Phase I clinical trial of a WHO birth control vaccine. *Lancet* **i**, 1295–8.

Kaufman, D. W., Shapiro, S., Rosenberg, L., Manson, R. R., Miettinen, O. D., Stolley, P., *et al.* (1980). Intra-uterine contraceptive device use and pelvic inflammatory disease. *American Journal of Obstetrics and Gynecology* **136**, 159–62.

Kay, C. R. (1982). Progestogens and arterial disease. *American Journal of Obstetrics and Gynecology* **142**, 762–5.

Kelaghan, J., Rubin, G. L., Ory, H. W., and Layde, P. M. (1982). Barrier methods of contraception and pelvic inflammatory disease. *Journal of the American Medical Association* **248**, 184–7.

Khaw, K. T. and Peart, W. S. (1982). Blood pressure and contraceptive use. *British Medical Journal* **285**, 403–7.

Kubba, A. A. and Guillebaud, J. (1985). Failure of post-coital contraception after insertion of an intrauterine device. *British Journal of Obstetrics and Gynaecology* **91**, 596–7.

La Vecchia, C., Decarli, A., and Fasoli, M. (1986). Oral contraceptives and cancers of the breast and of the female genital tract. *British Journal of Cancer* **54**, 311–17.

Lee, N. C., Rubin, G. C., Ory, H. W., and Burkman, R. T. (1983). Types of intrauterine contraceptive device and risk of pelvic inflammatory disease. *Obstetrics and Gynecology* **62**, 1–6.

Liang, A. P., Levenson, A. G., Layde, P. M., Shelton, J. D., Hatcher, R. A., Potts, M., *et al.* (1983). Risk of breast, uterine corpus, and ovarian carcinoma in women receiving medroxyprogesterone injections. *Journal of the American Medical Association* **249**, 2909–12.

Lidegaard, O. (1993). Oral contraception and risk of a cerebral thromboembolic attack. *British Medical Journal* **306**, 956–63.

Lipnick, R. J., Buring, J. E., and Hennekens, C. H. (1986). Oral contraceptives and breast cancer. *Journal of the American Medical Association* **255**, 58–61.

Livolsi, V. A., Stadel, B., Kelsey, J., and Holford, J. R. (1979). Fibroadenoma in oral contraceptive users. *Cancer* **44**, 1778–81.

Loudon, N. (1985). Oral contraception. In *Handbook of family planning* (ed. N. Loudon), p. 93. Churchill Livingstone, London.

McPherson, K., Vessey, M. P., Neila, A., Doll, R., Jones, L., and Roberts, M. (1987). Early oral contraceptive use and breast cancer. *British Journal of Cancer* **56**, 653–60.

Mammen, E. F. (1982). Oral contraceptives and blood coagulation. *American Journal of Obstetrics and Gynecology* **142**, 781–9.

Mann, J. I., Thorogood, M., Waters, S. E., and Pavell, C. (1975). Oral contraceptives and myocardial infarction in young women. *British Medical Journal* **3**, 631–2.

Mao, K. and Guillebaud, J. (1984). Influence of removal of intrauterine contraceptive devices on the colonization of the cervix by actinomyces-like organisms. *Contraception* **30**, 535–44.

Meade, T. W. (1982). Oral contraceptives, clotting factors, and thrombosis. *American Journal of Obstetrics and Gynecology* **142**, 758–61.

Mcirik, O., Lund, E., Adami, H. O., Bergstrom, R., Christoffersen, T., and Bergsjo, P. (1986). Oral contraceptive use and breast cancer in young women. *Lancet* **ii**, 650–3.

Miller, D. R., Rosenberg, L., Kaufman, D. W., Schottenfeld, A., Stolley, P. D., and Shapiro, S. (1986). Breast cancer in relation to early oral contraceptive use. *Obstetrics and Gynecology* **68**, 863–8.

Miller, D. R., Rosenberg, K., Kaufman, D. W., Stolley, P., Warshawer, M., and Shapiro, S. (1989). Breast cancer before aged 45 and oral contraceptive use. *American Journal of Epidemiology* **129**, 269–80.

Murphy, A. A., Zacur, H. A., Charach, E. P., and Burkman, R. J. (1991). The effect of tetracycline on levels of oral contraceptives. *American Journal of Obstetrics and Gynecology* **164**, 28–33.

Murray, P. P., Stadel, B. V., and Schlesselman, J. J. (1989). Oral contraceptive use in women with a family history of carcinoma of the breast. *Obstetrics and Gynecology* **73**, 977–83.

Neuberger, J., Forman, D., Doll, R., and Williams, R. (1986). Oral contraceptives and hepatocellular carcinoma. *British Medical Journal* **292**, 1355–7.

Newton, J. and Tacchi, D. (1990). Long-term use of copper intra-uterine devices. *Lancet* **335**, 1322–3.

Norman, J. E., Thong, K. J., Rodger, M. W., and Baird, D. T. (1992). Medical abortion in women of less than 56 days amenorrhoea. *British Journal of Obstetrics and Gynaecology* **99**, 601–6.

Office of Population Census and Surveys (1991). *General Household Survey, 1989*, pp. 185. Her Majesty's Stationery Office, London.

Orme, M. L. E. (1982). The clinical pharmacology of oral contraceptive steroids. *British Journal of Clinical Pharmacology* **14**, 31–42.

Orme, M. L. E. and Back, O. J. (1991). Unintended pregnancy and contraceptive use. *British Medical Journal* **302**, 789.

Paffenbarger, R. S., Kampert, J. B., and Chang, H. G. (1980). Characteristics that predict risk of breast cancer before and after the menopause. *American Journal of Epidemiology* **112**, 258–64.

Pardthaisong, T. and Gray, R. H. (1981). The return of fertility following discontinuation of oral contraceptives in Thailand. *Fertility Sterility* **35**, 532–4.

Pardthaisong, T., Gray, R. H., and McDaniel, E. B. (1980). Return of fertility following discontinuation of depo medroxyprogesterone and intra-uterine devices in Thailand. *Lancet* **i**, 509–11.

Paul, C., Skegg, D. C. G., Spears, G. F. S., and Kaldor, J. M. (1986). Oral contraceptives and breast cancer; a national study. *British Medical Journal* **293**, 723–6.

Petiti, D. B. and Windgred, J. (1978). Use of oral contraceptives, cigarette smoking and risk of subarachnoid haemorrhage. *Lancet* **ii**, 234–5.

Petiti, D. B., Tamamoto, D., and Morgenstern, N. (1983). Factors associated with actinomycosis-like organisms in Pap smear. *American Journal of Obstetrics and Gynecology* **145**, 338–41.

Pike, M. C., Henderson, B. E., Casagrande, J. T., Rosario, I., and Gray, G. E. (1981). Oral contraceptive use and early abortion as risk factors for breast cancer in young women. *British Journal of Cancer* **43**, 72–6.

Pike, M. C., Henderson, B. E., Krailo, M. B., Duke, A., and Roy, S. (1983). Breast cancer in young women and use of oral contraceptives. *Lancet* **ii**, 926–9.

Pons, J. C., Imbert, M. C., Elefont, E., Roux, C., Herschkorn, P., and Paperinik, E. (1991). Development after exposure to mifepristone in early pregnancy. *Lancet* **338**, 763.

Porter, J. B., Tick, H., and Walker, A. M. (1987). Mortality among oral contraceptive users. *Obstetrics and Gynecology* **70**, 29–32.

Pritchard, J. A. and Pritchard, S. A. (1977). Blood pressure response to oestrogen–progestin oral contraception after pregnancy-induced hypertension. *American Journal of Obstetrics and Gynecology* **129**, 733–9.

Radberg, T., Gustafson, A., Skryten, A., and Karlsson, K. (1982). Oral contraception in diabetic women. *Hormone and Metabolic Research* **14**, 61–5.

Ravnihar, S., Primic, Z. M., Kosmelj, K., and Stare, J. (1988). A case-controlled study of breast cancer in relation to oral contraceptive use in Slovenia. *Neoplasia* **35** 109–21.

Reader, F. C. (1991). Emergency contraception. *British Medical Journal* **302**, 801.

Realini, J. P. and Goldzieher, J. W. (1985). Oral contraceptives and cardiovascular disease. *American Journal of Obstetrics and Gynecology* **152**, 729–98.

Rimpelaah, M. K. and Kosunen, E. A. L. (1992). Use of oral contraceptives by adolescents in Finland. *British Medical Journal* **305**, 1053–7.

Robinson, G. E., Burren, T., Mackie, I. J., Bounds, W., Walshe, K., Faint, R., *et al.* (1991). Changes in haemostasis after stopping the combined contraceptive pill. *British Medical Journal* **302**, 269–71.

Rodger, M. W. and Baird, D. T. (1987). Induction of therapeutic abortion in early pregnancy with mifepristone in combination with prostaglandin pessaries. *Lancet* **ii**, 1415–18.

Rosenberg, L., Miller, D. R., Kaufman, D. W., Helmrich, S. P., Stolley, P. D., Schoffenfeld, D., *et al.* (1984). Breast cancer and oral contraceptive use. *American Journal of Epidemiology* **119**, 167–76.

Royal College of General Practitioners (1974). *Oral contraceptives and health*, pp. 43–50; 57–59. Pittman Medical, London.

Royal College of General Practitioners (1977). Mortality among oral contraceptive users. *Lancet* **ii**, 727–31.

Royal College of General Practitioners (1981). Further analyses of mortality in oral contraceptive users. *Lancet* **i**, 541–6.

Royal College of General Practitioners (1988). Breast cancer and the pill. *British Journal of Cancer* **58**, 676–80.

Royal College of Obstetricians and Gynaecologists (1991). *Report of the RCOG working party on unplanned pregnancy*, pp. 10–24. Chameleon Press, London.

Rubin, G. L., Ory, H. W., and Layde, P. M. (1982). Oral contraceptives and pelvic inflammatory disease. *American Journal of Obstetrics and Gynecology* **144**, 630–5.

Rushton, L. and Jones, D. R. (1992). Oral contraceptive use and breast cancer risk: a meta-analysis of variants with age at diagnosis, parity, and total duration of oral contraceptive use. *British Journal of Obstetrics and Gynaecology* **99**, 239–46.

Sagar, S., Stamatakis, J. D., Thomas, D. P., and Kakkar, B. V. (1976). Oral contraceptives, antithrombin III activity, and post-operative deep-vein thrombosis. *Lancet* **i**, 509–11.

Sattin, R. W., Rubin, G. L., Wingo, P. A., Webster, L. A. and Ory, H. W. (1986). Oral contraceptive use and the risk of breast cancer. *New England Journal of Medicine* **315**, 405–11.

Scally, G. (1993). Confidentiality, contraception, and young people. *British Medical Journal* **307**, 1157–8.

Schildkraut, J., Hulka, B. S., and Wilkinson, W. E. (1990). Oral contraception and breast cancer. *Obstetrics and Gynecology* **76**, 395–402.

Schlesselman, J. J., Stadel, B. V., Murray, P., Wingo, P. A., and Rubin, G. L. (1987). Consistency and plausibility in epidemiologic analysis. *Journal of Chronic Diseases* **40**, 1033–9.

Schwallie, P. C. and Assenzo, J. R. (1973). Contraceptive use—efficacy study utilizing medroxyprogesterone acetate. *Fertility Sterility* **24**, 331–9.

Senanayake, P. and Kramer, D. G. (1980). Contraception and the aetiology of pelvic inflammatory disease. *American Journal of Obstetrics and Gynecology* **138**, 852–60.

Shapiro, S., Slone, D., Rosenberg, L., Kaufman, D. W., Stolley, P. D., and Miettinen, O. S. (1979). Oral contraceptive use in relation to myocardial infarction. *Lancet* **i**, 943–6.

Silvestre, L., Dubois, C., Renault, M., Rezvani, Y., Baulieu, E. E., and Ullman, A. (1990). Voluntary interruption of pregnancy with mifepristone and a prostaglandin analogue. *New England Journal of Medicine* **322**, 645–8.

Sinei, S. K. A., Schulz. K. F., Lamptey, P. R., Grimes, D. A., Mati, J. K. G., Rosenthall, S. M., *et al.* (1990). Preventing IUCD-related pelvic infection. *British Journal of Obstetrics and Gynaecology* **97**, 412–19.

Skangalis, M., Mahoney, C. J., and O'Leary, W. M. (1982). Microbial presence in the uterine cavity as affected by varieties of intra-uterine contraceptive devices. *Fertility Sterility* **37**, 263–9.

Skegg, D. C. G. (1988). Potential for bias in case-controlled studies of oral contraceptives and breast cancer. *American Journal of Epidemiology* **127**, 205–12.

Slone, D., Shapiro, S., Kaufman, D. W., Rosenberg, I., Miettinen, O. S., and Stolley, P. D. (1981). Risk of myocardial infarction in relation to current and discontinued use of oral contraceptives. *New England Journal of Medicine* **305**, 420–4.

Snowden, R. (1981). Copper IUCDs and the pregnancy rate *British Journal of Family Planning* **6**, 104–8.

Sparks, R. A., Purrier, B. G. A., Watt, P. J., and Elstein, M. (1981). Bacteriological colonization of the uterine cavity. *British Medical Journal* **282**, 1189–91.

Speroff, L. and De Cherney, A. (1993). Evaluation of a new generation of oral contraceptives. *Obstetrics and Gynecology* **81**, 1034–47.

Stadel, B. V., Rubin, G. L., Webster, L. A., Schlesselman, J. J., and Wingo, P. A. (1985). Oral contraceptives and breast cancer in young women. *Lancet* **ii**, 970–3.

Stadel, B. V., Lai, S., Schlesselman, J. J., and Murray, P. (1988). Oral contraceptives and premenopausal breast cancer in nulliparous women. *Contraception* **38**, 287–99.

Stampfer, M. J., Willett, W. C., Colditz, G. A., Speizer, F. E., and Hennekens, C. H. (1988). A prospective study of past use of oral contraceptive agents and risk of cardiovascular disease. *New England Journal of Medicine* **319**, 1313–17.

Sue-Ling, H. and Hughes, L. E. (1988). Should the pill be stopped pre-operatively? *British Medical Journal* **296**, 447–8.

Szarewski, A. and Guillebaud, J. (1991). Contraception: current state of the art. *British Medical Journal* **302**, 1224–5.

Tacchi, D. (1990). Long-term use of copper intra-uterine devices. *Lancet* **336**, 182.

Targum, S. D. and Wright, N. H. (1974). Association of intra-uterine contraceptive device and pelvic inflammatory disease. *American Journal of Epidemiology* **100**, 262–77.

Tatum, H. J. and Schmidt, F. H. (1977). Contraception and sterilization practices and extra-uterine pregnancy. *Fertility Sterility* **28**, 407–21.

Thong, K. J. and Baird, D. T. (1992). Induction of abortion with Mifepristone and Misoprostol in early pregnancy. *British Journal of Obstetrics and Gynaecology* **99**, 1004–7.

Thorogood, M. and Vessey, M. P. (1990). An epidemiologic survey of cardiovascular disease in women taking oral contraceptives. *American Journal of Obstetrics and Gynecology* **163**, 274–8.

Thorogood, M., Adams, S. A., and Mann, J. I. (1981). Fatal subarachnoid haemorrhage in young women. *British Medical Journal* **283**, 762.

Thorogood, M., Mann, J., Murphy, M., and Vessey, M. (1991). Is oral contraceptive use still associated with an increased risk of fatal myocardial infarction? *British Journal of Obstetrics and Gynaecology* **98**, 1245–53.

Trapido, E. J. (1981). A prospective cohort study of oral contraceptives and breast cancer. *Journal of the National Cancer Institute* **67**, 1011–15.

Tsai, C. C., Williamson, H. O., Kirkland, B. H., Braun, J. O., and Lam, C. F. (1985). Low-dose oral contraceptives and blood pressure in women with a past history of elevated blood pressure. *American Journal of Obstetrics and Gynecology* **151**, 28–32.

Tully, B. (1983). Post-coital contraception – a study. *British Journal of Family Planning* **8**, 119–24.

United Kingdom Multicentre Trial (1990). The efficacy and tolerance of mifepristone and prostaglandin in first trimester termination of pregnancy. *British Journal of Obstetrics and Gynaecology* **97**, 480–6.

United Kingdom National Study Group (1989). Oral contraceptive use and breast cancer risk in young women. *Lancet* **i**, 973–82.

United Kingdom National Study Group (1990). Oral contraceptive use and breast cancer risk in young women. *Lancet* **i**, 1507–9.

US Collaborative Group for the Study of Stroke in Young Women (1973). Oral contraceptives and increased risk of cerebral ischaemia or thrombosis. *New England Journal of Medicine*, **288**, 871–8.

Valicenti, J. F., Pappas, A. A., Graber, C. D., Williamson, H. O., and Willis, N. F. (1982). Detection and prevalence of IUCD associated actinomycosis and related morbidity. *Journal of the American Medical Association* **247**, 1149–52.

van Santen, M. R. and Haspels, A. A. (1985). A comparison of high-dose oestrogens versus low-dose ethinyl oestradiol and norgestrel combination in postcoital interception. *Fertility Sterility* **43**, 206–13.

Vana, M., Murphy, G. P., Aronoff, B. L., and Baker, H. W. (1977). Primary liver tumours and oral contraceptives. *Journal of the American Medical Association* **238**, 2154–8.

Vessey, M. P. and Doll, R. (1968). Investigation of relationship between use of oral contraceptives and thromboembolic disease. *British Medical Journal* **2**, 199–205.

Vessey, M. P. and Doll, R. (1969). Investigation of relationship between use of oral contraceptives and thromboembolic disease. *British Medical Journal* **2**, 651–7.

Vessey, M. P., McPherson, K., and Johnson, B. (1977). Mortality amongst women participating in the Oxford–Family Planning Association centre study. *Lancet* **ii**, 731–3.

Vessey, M. P., Wright, N. H., McPherson, K., and Wiggins, P. (1978). Fertility after stopping different methods of contraception. *British Medical Journal* **1**, 265–7.

Vessey, M. P., McPherson, K., and Yeates, D. (1981*a*). Mortality and oral contraceptive users. *Lancet* **i**, 549–50.

Vessey, M. P., Yeates, D., Flavel, R., and McPherson, K. (1981*b*). Pelvic inflammatory disease and the IUCD: findings in a large cohort study. *British Medical Journal* **282**, 855–7.

Vessey, M. P., Lawless, M., and Yeates, D. (1982a). Efficacy of different contraceptive methods. *Lancet* **i**, 841–2.

Vessey, M. P., McPherson, K., Yeates, D., and Doll, R. (1982*b*). Oral contraceptive use and abortion before first term pregnancy in relation to breast cancer risk. *British Journal of Cancer* **45**, 327–31.

Vessey, M. P., Lawless, M., and Yeates, D. (1984). Oral contraception and stroke. *British Medical Journal* **289**, 530–1.

Vessey, M. P., Lawless, M., Yeates, D., and McPherson, K. (1985). Progestogen-only oral contraception. *British Journal of Family Planning* **10**, 117–21.

Vessey, M. P., Mant, D., Smith, A., and Yeates, D. (1986). Oral contraceptives and venous thromboembolism. *British Medical Journal* **292**, 526–9.

Vessey, M. P., Metcalfe, A., Wells, C., McPherson, K., Westhoff, C., and Yeates, D. (1987). Ovarian neoplasms, functional ovarian cysts, and oral contraceptives. *British Medical Journal* **294**, 1518–20.

Vessey, M. P., Villard-Mackintosh, L., McPherson, K., and Yeates, D. (1989). Mortality amongst oral contraceptive users: 20 year follow-up of women in cohort study. *British Medical Journal* **299**, 1487–91.

Villard-Mackintosh, L., Vessey, M. P., and Jones, L. (1989). The effects of oral contraceptives and parity on ovarian cancer trends in women under 55 years of age. *British Journal of Obstetrics and Gynaecology* **96**, 783–8.

Washington, A. E., Gove, S., Schachter, J., and Sweet, R. L. (1985). Oral contraception, chlamydial infection and pelvic inflammatory disease. *Journal of the American Medical Association* **253**, 2246–50.

Webb, A. M. C., Russell, J., and Elstein, M. (1992). Comparison of Yuzpe regimen — Danazol and Mifepristone in oral postcoital contraception. *British Medical Journal* **305**, 927–31.

Weir, R. H., Briggs, E., Mack, A., Naismith, L., Taylor, L., and Wilson, E. (1974). Blood pressure in women taking oral contraceptives. *British Medical Journal* **1**, 533–5.

Westrom, L., Bengtsson, I. P., and Mardh, P. A. (1976). The risk of pelvic inflammatory disease in women using IUCD as compared to non-users. *Lancet* **ii**, 221–4.

Wilson, E. S. B., Cruickshank, J., McMaster, M., and Weir, R. J. (1984). A prospective controlled trial of the effect on blood pressure of contraceptive preparations containing different types and dosages of progesterone. *British Journal of Obstetrics and Gynaecology* **91**, 1254–60.

Wingo, P. A., Lee, N. C., Ory, H. W., Beral, V., Peterson, H. B., and Rhodes, P.

(1991). Age-specific differences in the relationship between oral contraceptive use and breast cancer. *British Journal of Cancer* **78**, 161–7.

World Health Organization (1981). The effect of female sex hormones on fetal development and infant health. *World Health Organization Technical Report Series*, 657.

World Health Organization (1985). Facts about an implantable contraception. *Bulletin of the World Health Organization* **63**, 485–94.

World Health Organization (1987). Mechanism of action, safety, and efficacy of intrauterine devices. *World Health Organization Technical Report Series*, 753.

World Health Organization (1990*a*). The use of mifepristone for cervical preparation in the first trimester pregnancy termination by vacuum aspiration. *British Journal of Obstetrics and Gynaecology* **97**, 260–6.

World Health Organization (1990*b*). Contraceptive efficacy of testosterone-induced azoospermia in normal men. *Lancet* **336**, 955–9.

World Health Organization Collaborative Study of Neoplasia and Steroid Contraceptives (1990). Breast cancer and combined oral contraceptives. *British Journal of Cancer* **61**, 110–19.

World Health Organization Collaborative Study of Neoplasia and Steroid Contraceptives (1991). Breast cancer and depo-medroxyprogesterone acetate. *Lancet* **338**, 833–8.

World Health Organization Task Force (1993). Termination of pregnancy with reduced doses of Mifepristone. *British Medical Journal* **307**, 532–7.

Yuzpe, A. A. and Kubba, A. (1989). Post-coital contraception. In *Contraception: science and practice* (ed. M. Filshie and J. Guillebaud), pp. 126–43. Butterworths, London.

Yuzpe, A. A. and Lance, W. J. (1977). Ethinyl oestradiol and dl-norgestrel as a post-coital contraceptive. *Fertility Sterility* **28**, 932–6.

Yuzpe, A. A., Percival-Smith, R., and Rademaker, R. H. (1982). A multicentre clinical investigation employing ethinyl oestradiol and dl-norgestrel as a post-coital contraceptive agent. *Fertility Sterility* **37**, 508–13.

6 The management of gynaecological infections

This chapter is concerned with sexually transmitted diseases (STDs) and related genital infections, including vaginal candidiasis, and their complications. Pregnancy complications and other aspects of obstetric practice are discussed in Chapter 21 (Specific infections during pregnancy).

Epidemiology

Data on the incidence of STDs are collected in the United Kingdom from venereal disease clinics (now called departments of genitourinary medicine). It is believed that the majority of patients with classical venereal diseases, at least, are seen in these departments and trends are probably relatively accurate. Other STDs may be seen in other settings, (for example genital warts are seen by gynaecologists, urologists, dermatologists, and general practitioners) and reported changes in incidence may, therefore, be related to changes in referral patterns. In Table 6.1 trends can be seen in the incidence of some common STDs over the last 15 years.

STDs often occur together and the diagnosis of one STD should lead to a search for others. Thus a third of patients with gonorrhoea have a co-existing chlamydial infection (Oriel *et al.* 1974) and associated infections are common in patients with genital warts (Jenkins and Riley 1980). Pabst *et al.* (1992) found that 40 of 279 (14 per cent) patients attending a Baltimore STD clinic had more than one infection.

Gonorrhoea

Gonorrhoea is caused by a Gram-negative intracellular diplococcus, *Neisseria gonorrhoeae*. In practice non-sexual modes of transmission do not occur in adults and the presence of gonorrhoea has been regarded as prima facie evidence of adultery in matrimonial proceedings.

Epidemiology

In the last decade there has been a rapid decline in the number of cases, but this has been in part due to the dramatic decline in homosexually acquired disease, the ratio of male to female cases falling from 4:1 in 1962 to 1.7:1 in

Table 6.1 Changing incidence of infections seen in STD clinics in the UK*

Infection	No of cases in indicated year			
	1978	1983	1987	% Change
Syphilis	4866	3727	1538	− 68.4
Gonorrhoea	63 569	54 859	25 265	− 60.3
Non-specific infection	107 955	148 616	131 383	+ 21.7
Trichomoniasis	21 732	19 571	10 658	− 51.0
Candidiasis	42 524	62 199	59 768	+ 40.5
Herpes simplex	9036	17 908	16 699	+ 84.8
Genital warts	27 272	42 790	74 542	+ 173.3

*From Department of Health. Summary information from forms KC60 and SBH 60

1979 and to 1.3:1 in 1989 (Department of Health 1989). Disconcertingly, the most recent data suggest an upturn with increased numbers of cases reported from several parts of the world. The decline in incidence in Western countries in the last decade has not been mirrored in other parts of the world where the disease is still of major importance (Adler and Mindel 1988).

Gonorrhoea is a disease of young adults, and the largest rise in incidence since 1965 has been in girls under 20. The prevalence of infection depends on the population studied. In 1970, Driscoll *et al.* found gonorrhoea in 2.9 per cent of women attending a gynaecological clinic, whereas the infection was found in 17.6 per cent of women attending an STD clinic (Oriel *et al.* 1974). However, by 1989 (Department of Health), gonorrhoea accounted for only 3.4 per cent of diagnoses made at STD clinics in England and Wales.

Symptoms

Most men develop a purulent discharge and dysuria within two or three days of acquiring the infection and they then seek treatment. Approximately 10 per cent of men may be asymptomatic and are thus a reservoir of disease (Pariser, 1972). In contrast, women are commonly asymptomatic though the proportion of those with symptoms depends on the health care setting. In STD clinics, more than 80 per cent of women with gonorrhoea are the asymptomatic contacts of men attending with symptoms (Handsfield 1983). Some women may present with discharge or dysuria. The discharge may be purulent but the appearance is not sufficiently specific to allow a clinical diagnosis. In women, the endocervix, urethra, and rectum are the primary sites of infection, but the throat may also be infected following fellatio. Upper genital tract involvement occurs in about 10 per cent of cases (Rees and Annels 1969) and spread is most likely around the time of menstruation (Thin 1988). Instrumentation may also lead to gonococcal pelvic inflammatory disease (PID) following asymptomatic cervicitis (Bump and Fass 1985).

Complications

(1) skenitis;

(2) bartholinitis;

(3) pelvic inflammatory disease (PID);

(4) disseminated gonococcal infection (DGI);

(5) complication of pregnancy and the puerperium;

(6) adult conjunctivitis.

Skenitis and bartholinitis

Infection of Skene's glands and Bartholin's duct and gland are well recognized but are rare complications of gonorrhoea. The organism was isolated from 6 per cent of 63 women with a Bartholin's abscess (Bleker *et al.* 1990).

Pelvic inflammatory disease

The association between gonorrhoea and PID is discussed below.

Disseminated gonococcal infection

DGI is usually the result of a bacteraemia with a strain of *N. gonorrhoeae* which is very penicillin-sensitive. It complicates 1 per cent of cases of lower genital tract infection and is more common in women than men, and in the pregnant than the non-pregnant. The preceding infection is generally asymptomatic. It is characterized by joint pains, fever, pleomorphic skin lesions, and tenosynovitis. In some cases, infection of one large joint dominates the clinical picture; meningitis, endocarditis, and pericarditis are rare components of the syndrome. *N. gonorrhoeae* may be cultured from the blood in 20–30 per cent cases, from the joints in 50 per cent, and from the skin lesions rarely (*Lancet* 1984).

Complications of pregnancy and the puerperium

See Chapter 21 (Specific infections during pregnancy).

Adult conjunctivitis

Adult conjunctivitis is a rare complication and arises from direct spread of the organism from the genitals to the conjunctivae.

Diagnosis

Accurate diagnosis is dependent on correct swab-taking, appropriate transportation of specimens, use of selective media for culture, and the use of accurate confirmatory tests.

Since *N. gonorrhoeae* infects cervix, urethra, and rectum, swabs should be taken from these sites. A high vaginal swab will miss the infection in up to 30 per cent cases (Bhattacharya *et al.* 1973). A positive swab is most likely from the cervix (89 per cent), but an additional 6 per cent of cases have positive cultures only from the urethra and 4.8 per cent from the rectum (Barlow and Phillips 1978). Rectal infection is particularly common in women, and up to 40 per cent of infected women have the organism at this site (Barlow and Phillips 1978). A swab should also be taken from the pharynx if there is a history of oral contact. The diagnostic success is increased from 95 to 100 per cent by sampling more than one site and also by repeating the tests on up to three occasions (Thin 1988).

Direct plating of specimens at the patient's bedside is optimum but only possible in settings where gonococcal infection is sought regularly, for example in STD clinics. Alternatively, specimens should be sent to the laboratory in transport media such as Stuart's, Amies, or Transgrow. Gonococci are fastidious organisms and require culture on selective media, for example Thayer–Martin, to suppress the growth of contaminating bacteria. Colonies have a characteristic appearance, but colonial morphology is not sufficient to distinguish *N. gonorrhoeae* from other *Neisseria* spp. and another identification test(s) such as the oxidase, immunofluorescence, sugar fermentation, or coagglutination test is essential (Thin 1988).

When facilities for direct microscopy are available, examination of a Gram-stained smear of secretions will lead to a rapid presumptive diagnosis of gonorrhoea in 50 per cent of cases in women with a high degree of specificity (Ison 1990). New antigen detection tests have been developed, but they are currently insufficiently sensitive and specific to replace the combination of microscopy and culture. Furthermore, they cannot predict antibiotic sensitivity (Ison 1990).

Serological tests for gonorrhoea have been evaluated but are insufficiently sensitive or specific for the presence of current infection to be of any use to the practising clinician (Thin 1988).

Treatment

Penicillin was the mainstay of treatment for gonorrhoea from its introduction in the late 1940s until the mid-1970s, but the dose required to eradicate the organism has increased markedly. Intramuscular regimens have largely been replaced by orally active penicillins with the addition of probenecid (1 g) which delays the renal excretion of the drug. Single dose regimens are preferred to ensure compliance. Recommended regimens for penicillin-sensitive strains of *N. gonorrhoeae* include ampicillin 3.5 g plus probenecid 1 g in a single oral dose, or procaine penicillin 2.4 megaunits intramuscularly with 1 g of probenecid orally. These result in eradication of the organism in up to 98 per cent of cases (Thin 1988).

In 1976, there were two independent reports of strains of *N. gonorrhoeae* which were totally resistant to penicillin because they contained a beta-lactamase (penicillinase) producing plasmid which inactivated antibiotics with a beta-lactam ring structure (for example penicillins) (Arya *et al.* 1978). These strains (known as PPNG; penicillinase-producing *Neisseria gonorrhoeae*) spread rapidly from Africa and Asia, where they are now endemic (Sng *et al.* 1984), and it was only with strenuous efforts in the West that control was largely achieved by contact tracing (Arya *et al.* 1984). The prevalence in most Western countries is less than 5 per cent of strains isolated and these are mostly imported. Another problem which has developed is relative resistance to penicillin, which is chromosomally mediated (Ison *et al.* 1987). A number of tetracycline-resistant strains have also been described.

Treatment of PPNG and other resistant strains is with an injectable cephalosporin, for example cefotaxime 500 mg (Barlow and Phillips 1984), or spectinomycin 2 g (Barlow and Phillips 1978), or a quinolone derivative, for example ciprofloxacin 250 mg or 500 mg, orally (Ison *et al.* 1991).

Not all therapeutic regimens are active against oral and rectal infections (Collier *et al.* 1984).

In order to identify true treatment failure all isolates should be tested for their antibiotic sensitivity. Re-infection is common if a partner remains untreated and skilled contact tracing may be necessary to identify the source and secondary contacts (Talbot and Kinghorn 1985). The organism can be isolated from up to 66 per cent of the female contacts of men with gonorrhoea (Thin 1988). Follow-up tests are essential and all infected sites should be swabbed on at least two occasions. Since 30–60 per cent of women with gonorrhoea have a concurrent chlamydial infection, a diagnostic test for *C. trachomatis* is essential (Oriel *et al.* 1974). Trichomoniasis is also found commonly in association with gonorrhoea (Barlow and Phillips 1978).

Chlamydial infection

Chlamydia trachomatis is an obligate intracellular bacterium which causes genital and eye diseases. Other chlamydial species include *C. psittaci*, which causes ornithosis and psittacosis but which is also an important cause of fetal loss in commercial farming, and *C. pneumoniae*, a recently recognized cause of epidemic pneumonia in young adults. *C. trachomatis* has been classified into a number of serovars; A–C cause epidemic trachoma in tropical and subtropical countries, D–K cause oculogenital diseases in the West and probably also other parts of the world, and L1–L3 are responsible for lymphogranuloma venereum.

Epidemiology

C. trachomatis is transmitted sexually and is most commonly found in young adults. Worm and Petersen (1987) found the infection in 63 per cent of the partners of men with chlamydial urethritis. However, since the infection may be asymptomatic in both men and women, it may be found in couples who have been in a stable relationship for months or years. Unlike gonococcal infection, therefore, its presence does not indicate recent infidelity.

Table 6.2 Prevalence of chlamydial infection in various female populations

Population	Year	Prevalence (%)	Reference
STD Clinic, UK	1974	31	Hilton *et al.*
STD Clinic, UK	1978	20.4	Oriel *et al.*
STD Clinic, Sweden	1978	37	Paavonen *et al.*
STD Clinic, UK	1988	7.1	Shanmugaratnam *et al.*
STD Clinic, UK	1989	3.2	Sivakumar and Basu Roy
General practice, UK	1983	1.76	Fox
General practice, UK	1983	8	Southgate *et al.*
General practice, UK	1987	10.7	Longhurst *et al.*
Contraceptive Clinic, UK	1974	3	Hilton *et al.*
Contraceptive Clinic, UK	1987	3.4	Fish *et al.*
Gynae. clinic, Finland	1978	9	Paavonen *et al.*
Gynae. clinic, Sweden	1978	19.3	Ripa *et al.*
Gynae. clinic, UK	1983	5	Munday

In studies conducted in the late 1960s and early 1970s when diagnostic tests first became widely available, the organism was found in 20–25 per cent of women attending STD clinics. More recently, the prevalence of infection in these populations seems to be less than 10 per cent (Shanmugaratnam and Pattman 1989; Sivakumar and Basu Roy 1989). This may be a true decline in incidence but may also represent new cases occurring in a well-screened population, whereas the early studies detected all infections acquired over many years in a previously unscreened population.

The prevalence of infection in various populations is shown in Table 6.2. As can be seen, prevalence varies widely in different clinical and geographic settings, but there is no doubt that this is a very common and frequently under-diagnosed condition (Faro 1991). Data from various parts of the world now indicate that chlamydial infection is several times more common than gonorrhoea (Cates and Wasserheit 1991; Taylor-Robinson 1994).

Symptoms and signs

Like *N. gonorrhoeae*, *C. trachomatis* infects cervix, urethra, and rectum, but rarely, or if at all, the pharynx (Bowie *et al.* 1977). Although there may be symptoms of discharge or dysuria, these are often attributed to other causes. Asymptomatic infection is common and is found in up to two-thirds of chlamydia-positive women seen in STD clinics. In other settings, more women may present with symptoms (Sweet and Gibbs 1990). A mucopurulent cervicitis associated with hypertrophic ectopy is said to be characteristic of chlamydial cervicitis (Brunham *et al.* 1984), and although this condition is commonly found in women with chlamydial infection the appearance is not specific enough to obviate the need for a diagnostic test. Dunlop *et al.* (1989) described a characteristic colposcopic appearance with erythema and follicles but this lacks specificity. Furthermore, many women with chlamydial infection have a clinically normal cervix.

C. trachomatis is the commonest cause of non-gonococcal urethritis in men, presenting with discharge and dysuria which is less severe than in gonorrhoea. A considerable proportion of men, perhaps up to 50 per cent, are however asymptomatic.

Diagnosis of chlamydial infection

There are a number of different techniques, all of which have their limitations:

(1) tissue culture;

(2) direct immunofluorescence;

(3) ELISA;

(4) polymerase chain reaction (PCR) and the Dot–blot test;

(5) serology.

Tissue culture

This technique has many variants, perhaps the most popular of which is culture on cycloheximide-treated McCoy cells with Giemsa staining to identify characteristic inclusions (Ripa and Mardh 1977), regarded by many as the 'gold standard' (Taylor-Robinson and Thomas 1991). In experienced hands it is specific and sensitive but does require the expertise of a laboratory skilled in tissue culture techniques. Specimen handling is important, and if the specimen is not to be processed immediately, it should be kept in liquid nitrogen.

Direct immunofluorescence

This test is simple to perform and in experienced hands is very sensitive and specific (Thomas *et al.* 1984). It is, however, labour intensive and requires considerable experience to recognize the characteristic appearances of fluorescing chlamydial particles (elementary bodies). False-positives may thus occur. The test has not been properly evaluated for specimens from non-genital sites and should not be used in these situations. Some authorities believe that it may be even more sensitive than culture because it has the potential to detect a single elementary body (Taylor-Robinson and Thomas 1991). No special transport requirements are necessary; a swab is smeared over the well of a special slide and fixed with acetone. Slides may be stored indefinitely at +4 °C.

ELISA

This semi-automated test is now widely used in diagnostic laboratories. There are a number of kits of startlingly different sensitivities and specificities, and it would be wise for the clinician to know something of the characteristics of the test which his laboratory uses. The test cannot match direct immunofluorescence in sensitivity, but large numbers of specimens can be batched and tested together making it a more cost-effective test. Specificity is controversial but some kits contain a confirmation step which helps to improve specificity to acceptable levels (Moncada *et al.* 1990). The test should not be used in medico-legal work, for example in cases of suspected child abuse, as its accuracy would be challenged in court. Specimens should be collected into special media provided with the test kit, but no special precautions are required for transportation.

PCR and Dot-blot techniques

These are research tools which are not available commercially. PCR promises to be a very sensitive and rapid test (Palmer *et al.* 1991; Taylor-Robinson 1994; Witkin *et al.* 1993).

Serology

A microimmunofluorescence test for the detection of serum antibody to the various serovars (Wang and Grayston 1970) has been promoted by some as a useful diagnostic test for detecting chlamydial infection (Treharne *et al.* 1977). Unfortunately, in the majority of clinical situations this is not so (Schachter *et al.* 1979). Serum antibody is not invariably produced in superficial infections and when it is, it may persist for long periods. Furthermore, some tests fail to distinguish between antibody to *C. trachomatis* and *C. pneumoniae*. In pelvic inflammatory disease and Fitz-Hugh–Curtis syndrome very high titres of antibody, for example greater than 1 in 1024, may be suggestive of disease as may be the presence of IgM, but these tests should not be relied on. Recently, diagnostic tests for locally produced IgA have been developed as an alternative to culture and antigen detection techniques but they appear to lack sensitivity and specificity.

Serology should, therefore, be perceived as a useful epidemiological tool for looking at populations, and perhaps the association of distant infection with current disease (Sellors *et al.* 1988) but not as a diagnostic test in the individual case.

Complications

(1) bartholinitis;

(2) urethral syndrome;

(3) PID and its sequelae;

(4) pregnancy complications;

(5) adult eye disease;

(6) Reiter's syndrome;

(7) chlamydial eye disease;

(8) cervical intraepithelial neoplasia.

Bartholinitis

C. trachomatis is a rare cause of bartholinitis. Bleker *et al.* (1990), cultured the organism in 2 per cent of cases.

Urethral syndrome

This condition, also known as abacterial cystitis, produces symptoms indistinguishable from bacterial cystitis in the absence of a significant number of bacteria. Many causes have been proposed (Maskell *et al.* 1979) but it seems likely that chlamydial infection of the urethra accounts for some cases. Stamm *et al.* (1980) investigated university students with symptoms of cystitis and found that those who did not fulfil standard criteria ($\geq 10^5$ organisms per millilitre) either had low counts of conventional bacteria in bladder urine or chlamydial urethritis. Panja (1983) also found *C. trachomatis* in the urethra of 14 of 107 women investigated for frequency and dysuria. Whether these results can be transposed to other populations is doubtful, and chlamydial infection is likely to account for a smaller proportion of patients presenting to gynaecological or urological clinics.

Pelvic inflammatory disease

The association of *C. trachomatis* with PID is discussed below.

Pregnancy complications

The possible association of *C. trachomatis* with complications of pregnancy and the puerperium is discussed in Chapter 21.

Reiter syndrome

The combination of arthritis and/or conjunctivitis following a gastrointestinal or genital tract infection is much commoner in men than women. *Formes frustes* occur and sexually acquired reactive arthritis (SARA) is a term coined to denote a seronegative arthritis occurring following a sexually acquired genital tract infection. There is now convincing evidence that *C. trachomatis* is the aetiological agent in 50 per cent of cases and that the disease represents an abnormal response to the infection in genetically predisposed individuals. Controversy exists as to whether chlamydial antigen is detectable in joints (Keat *et al.* 1987). The sex difference is unexplained except that, at least in some cases, the genital tract infection may go undetected in some women who present with a seronegative arthritis.

Chlamydial eye disease

Chlamydial conjunctivitis occurs in adults by direct inoculation of the eye from a genital tract source. In a study from an ophthalmic casualty department, 9 per cent of 140 consecutive patients presenting with acute conjunctivitis had evidence of chlamydial infection (Wishart *et al.* 1984). Such patients and their partners need to be evaluated for chlamydial genital infection.

Cervical intraepithelial neoplasia

This possible association is discussed in Chapter 12.

Treatment

Numerous investigators have shown the efficacy of tetracyclines in eradicating *C. trachomatis* from the lower genital tract. One gram daily of oxytetracycline or equivalent in divided doses for seven days produces a cure rate approaching 100 per cent providing compliance has been acceptable and reinfection has not occurred. Regimens with less frequent administration, for example doxycycline 100 mg twice daily, may improve compliance. When tetracyclines cannot be used, for example in pregnancy, erythromycin 250 mg four times daily is an acceptable alternative, but cure rates are slightly lower, perhaps because side-effects may limit compliance (Sanders *et al.* 1986). Sulphonamides also have some activity against chlamydiae, but their use in genital tract infections is limited by poor activity against coexisting mycoplasma infections (Bowie *et al.* 1982, Johannisson *et al.* 1980).

Some of the new quinolones have reasonably good antichlamydial activity (Ahmed-Jushuf *et al.* 1988*a*), but it is difficult to justify the use of such expensive drugs when tetracyclines can produce acceptable results. Recently, a new macrolide antibiotic, azithromycin (Waugh 1991) showed good results in chlamydial infection when administered in a single dose of 1 g, it is also effective against *N. gonorrhoeae*. The possibility of treating gonorrhoea and chlamydial infection with a single dose regimen has its attractions and further studies are awaited with interest.

Tests of cure are not normally required for chlamydial infection since the organism does not acquire resistance to antibiotics. If, however, poor compliance or re-infection is suspected a test of cure is recommended. If an antigen detection test is to be used, a test of cure should be delayed several days after completion of treatment to avoid detecting non-viable particles.

Pelvic inflammatory disease (PID)

PID may be defined as inflammation of the upper genital tract.

Epidemiology

The increase in the numbers of cases of PID has mirrored the increased incidence of STDs in the last 30 years and supports the contention that PID is frequently a complication of an STD. The true incidence and prevalence are difficult to ascertain. Data which are available suggest an increase in cases over the last few years, although Westrom (1988) reported a decline in cases in Sweden in the 1980s. The incidence of PID in the UK, based on hospital in-patient statistics, doubled in the two decades up to 1980 and reached nearly 15 000 admissions in 1981, whilst in the USA, during the same period, it accounted for 212 000 admissions a year (Adler and Mindel 1988; Buchan and Vessey 1989). Data on the prevalence of asymptomatic and minimally symptomatic infection are not available, but serological studies of women presenting with tubal infertility suggest that asymptomatic chlamydial PID is commoner than frank clinical disease. PID is a disease of the young sexually active with a maximum incidence in the 20–24 age group. However, the highest age specific rates occur in sexually active girls under 20 (Buchan and Vessey 1989; Westrom 1980).

Pathogenesis

Although infectious microorganisms may reach the fallopian tubes by direct spread following appendicitis or another intraabdominal suppurative condition, or by haematogenous spread, for example in tuberculosis, the majority of cases follow ascending infection from a lower genital tract infection. Tuberculous PID was once a common cause of infertility but has been little discussed in the recent past as the incidence has declined. It will be interesting to see whether it reappears in the community as a result of HIV infection since infection with this and other mycobacteria is a common complication of HIV disease.

Ascending infection may arise *de novo* or following surgical or obstetric intervention and infection may spread canalicularly or via the lymphatics of the parametra as demonstrated by Moller *et al.* (1980) in animal models.

Microbiology

Assigning a microbiological cause to a particular case is difficult and hence rarely useful in management of that individual. Detailed studies of various sites and looking for a variety of microorganisms is required. Although taking swabs from the cervix is useful and may give the clinician some guidance it is not a substitute for obtaining swabs directly from the fallopian tubes by laparoscopy. Swab taking from tubes is technically difficult and produces a lower yield of potential pathogens than swabbing the cervix, yet it is from such detailed studies that our knowledge of the likely microbiological aetiology of PID comes. (Stacey *et al.* in press).

For many years it was believed that PID was invariably caused by *N. gonorrhoeae*, and, if the organism could not be detected, this was for technical reasons or because of the presence of superinfection. *C. trachomatis* was first isolated from a fallopian tube in 1976 (Hamark *et al.*), and since then evidence has accumulated to support the role of chlamydiae in PID. The majority of well-designed studies indicate that *C. trachomatis* is the most important cause of PID in the West and perhaps also in the developing world (Brihmer *et al.* 1987; Svensson *et al.* 1980). The proportion of cases due to *N. gonorrhoeae* depends on how well the infection is managed in the community. Thus if contact tracing is not performed and women cannot afford help for minor symptoms, hospital based studies are likely to include many cases of gonococcal PID (Cunningham *et al.* 1978). Conversely, when gonorrhoea becomes a rare disease because of efficient management, as in Scandinavia, the proportion of cases due

Table 6.3 Microorganisms detected in acute pelvic inflammatory disease

| | C. trachomatis % Isolation from: | | | N. gonorrhoeae % Isolation from: | |
	Cervix	Tubes	Serology	Cervix	Tubes
Europe	5–47	4–30	30–51	0–23	0–25
N. America	5–51	0–10	23–40	27–80	13–33

to *C. trachomatis* is greater. Most investigators believe that at least 60–70 per cent of cases are initiated by one or other of these two microorganisms, but in some cases secondary infection with other organisms, particularly anaerobes, may obscure the picture and give the impression of a polymicrobial infection (Cunningham *et al.* 1978). A summary of isolation and serology results from a number of European and North American studies is shown in Table 6.3.

Mycoplasma hominis was found in the tubes of some women with PID in the early 1970s (Mardh and Westrom 1970), but in these studies chlamydiae were not sought so the contribution of *M. hominis* to this condition is uncertain, although in at least some cases (Stacey *et al.* in press) the organism does appear to be a primary pathogen. *Mycoplasma genitalium* is a recently discovered mycoplasma which is difficult to culture. Some serological data suggest it may be an important cause in some cases (Moller *et al.* 1984). There is no evidence that *Ureaplasma urealyticum*, a mycoplasma found ubiquitously in the genital tract of sexually active women, plays any role in PID.

Anaerobes, in particular *Bacteroides* spp. and *Peptostreptococci*, are commonly found in the peritoneal fluid of severely ill patients (Monif *et al.* 1976). This often follows instrumentation of the uterus, (in the past to procure an illegal abortion) or may follow other infecting organisms.

Actinomyces israelii is often found in association with intrauterine contraceptive devices, particularly the old plastic ones, and may be associated with large inflammatory pelvic masses (Burkman *et al.* 1982).

Herpes simplex virus (Lehtinen *et al.* 1985) and a variety of respiratory bacteria, for example *Haemophilus influenzae* (Paavonen *et al.* 1985*a*) have occasionally been isolated from tubes, but their contribution to the syndrome is thought to be small.

PID and contraception

The associations between an increased incidence of PID and the use of an IUCD, and the decreased incidence of PID and the use of oral and barrier contraceptives are discussed in Chapter 5 (contraception).

Clinical features

The features of classical PID are well known, but it should be remembered that the disease may be mild with little or no abdominal or pelvic pain and no pelvic tenderness (Wolner-Hanssen *et al.* 1990). Research is needed to find a simple non-invasive test to identify such cases.

Diagnosis

Laparoscopy

Studies which are not based on a laparoscopic diagnosis of PID do not stand up to scientific scrutiny and this limits the reliance that may be placed on the results of many published studies. Jacobson and Westrom (1969) investigated 814 women with a clinical diagnosis of acute PID who underwent laparoscopy. The diagnosis was confirmed in 65 per cent, another significant condition was found in 12 per cent, and in 23 per cent no abnormality was detected. During the same period, 91 other patients had an unexpected diagnosis of PID. In a more recent study, laparoscopy confirmed the diagnosis of acute PID in 74 per cent of the patients in whom the condition was diagnosed clinically (Wolner-Hanssen *et al.* 1985). When women with less typical symptoms are considered, the likelihood of PID is even smaller, yet those who do have PID do not have pathognomonic clinical features (Jacobson and Westrom 1969). Laparoscopy is considered to be the 'gold standard' for making the diagnosis, but, except in Scandinavia where laparoscopy has been incorporated into protocols for the management of all women with abdominal pain, there is a reluctance to consider this investigation. Nevertheless it is cost-effective if a definite diagnosis can be achieved (Method *et al.* 1987), on the one hand sparing some patients courses of unnecessary and expensive antibiotics and on the other confirming, in some cases microbiologically, a diagnosis which if inappropriately treated would lead to expensive investigations and treatment for infertility (Westrom and Mardh 1990). If laparoscopy is not to be used to confirm all diagnoses of PID, it should certainly be used in cases of diagnostic doubt and also when conservative treatment has failed (Stacey *et al.* 1991). Laparoscopy is not without risk; in 1978, the results of a survey of over 50 000 laparoscopies notified to the Royal College of Obstetricians and Gynaecologists were published (Confidential Enquiry into Gynaecological Laparoscopy). Direct trauma to bowel occurred in 0.18 per cent, haemorrhage in 0.72 per cent, and death in four patients, a mortality rate of 8 per 100 000 laparoscopies. However, the laparoscopies described were performed at a time when many clinicians were learning the technique. Westrom and Mardh (1990), commenting on their personal series of over 3000 laparoscopies, recorded no deaths and only three serious perioperative complications requiring laparotomy. Clinicians will have to audit the place of laparoscopy for acute abdominal pain in their own practices.

Microbiology

Identification of *N. gonorrhoeae* or *C. trachomatis* in the cervix of a woman with abdominal pain supports the diagnosis of PID, but a considerable proportion of such women have no laparoscopic evidence of disease. Isolation of organisms from the tubes or Pouch of Douglas is a better indicator of the true cause but is more difficult. Culdocentesis has been popular in the past, but examination of fluid from the Pouch of Douglas is unlikely to identify *C. trachomatis* which is only found in specimens taken from epithelial surfaces.

Serological tests may be helpful in retrospect if appropriately timed, paired sera are obtained. Unfortunately, some have claimed that a diagnosis of PID can be made on the basis of finding a high titre of antichlamydial antibody in women with abdominal pain (see above), and there is no doubt that women who have had nothing more than a respiratory infection with *C. pneumoniae* in adolescence have been labelled as chronic PID sufferers on the basis of this test.

Other laboratory tests

The white cell count, erythrocyte sedimentation rate, and C-reactive protein are often elevated in women with PID. None of these markers is specific for PID and the sensitivity is low as many women with PID have normal results (Westrom and Mardh 1990).

Endometrial biopsy

Some have claimed a strong association between plasma cell endometritis and salpingitis (Paavonen *et al.* 1985*b*) and have used endometritis as a surrogate marker for tubal disease. Endometrial biopsy might also detect early cases before the development of salpingitis detectable at laparoscopy. This is an attractive outpatient technique which could replace laparoscopy but is not yet fully evaluated as far as sensitivity and specificity are concerned.

Pelvic ultrasound

Conventional ultrasound examination is only useful in confirming large inflammatory masses. Transvaginal ultrasound extends the sensitivity of the technique but cannot identify early or mild disease (Patten *et al.* 1990).

Complications and sequelae

(1) tubo-ovarian abscess;

(2) Fitz-Hugh–Curtis syndrome;

(3) tubal infertility;

(4) ectopic pregnancy;

(5) chronic pelvic pain.

Tubo-ovarian abscess

The frequency of this complication is very variable and may depend on the population studied. Landers and Sweet (1985) reviewed the literature and found this complication in up to one third of hospitalized patients with PID. In most cases the infection was polymicrobial with a predominance of anaerobes. Abscesses were bilateral in 54 per cent of cases. Sixty per cent responded to medical management but surgery was required to confirm the diagnosis, because of failure to respond to antibiotics or to treat a rupture in the remainder. In a series reported by Hager (1983), 35 per cent of 143 patients with PID had an abscess and 90 per cent required surgery. Brunham *et al.* (1988), however, found pelvic abscesses in 10 per cent of the women with PID whom they studied. The prognosis for fertility is poor, only 14 per cent of the patients reported by Landers and Sweet subsequently conceiving.

Fitz-Hugh–Curtis syndrome

Fitz-Hugh and Curtis independently described a condition of perihepatitis with 'violin string' adhesions between the liver surface and the anterior abdominal wall which they thought was caused by gonorrhoea. In 1978, Muller-Schoop and colleagues suggested that *C. trachomatis* might be an important cause, and it is now recognized that both *N. gonorrhoeae* and *C. trachomatis* may cause the syndrome (Wang *et al.* 1980). This is probably a very underdiagnosed condition, especially when it occurs in the absence of signs of pelvic infection. In one study, a number of admissions to a surgical ward of women with right upper quadrant pain, initially attributed to acute cholecystitis, were found to be due to chlamydial perihepatitis (Wood *et al.* 1982).

Tubal infertility

The likelihood of tubal infertility following treatment depends on the severity of the initial attack, the number of attacks of PID, and the nature of the aetiological agent. Thus Westrom (1975) found that 2 per cent of women were infertile after one episode of mild salpingitis compared to 29 per cent after one episode of severe disease. After one infection 12.8 per cent and after three or more 75 per cent of women were infertile. Furthermore, the outcome was worse after non-gonococcal than gonococcal PID. Many recent studies have shown that only a minority of women with tubal infertility have had a recognizable episode of PID in the past, and so many cases must be mild or asymptomatic (Cates and Wasserheit 1991; Sellors *et al.* 1988). Women who seek delay for their treatment of pelvic inflammatory disease may be three times more likely to experience tubal infertility or ectopic pregnancy than those promptly treated (Hillis *et al.* 1993).

Ectopic pregnancy

Westrom (1980) reported that a woman who has had PID has a 10-fold increased risk of a subsequent pregnancy being ectopic. Subsequent studies have shown a high prevalence of antichlamydial antibodies in women having ectopic pregnancies often in the absence of a history of PID or chlamydial infection (Brunham *et al.* 1986).

Chronic pelvic pain

Chronic pain and dyspareunia are well-recognized sequelae of PID. Westrom (1975) reported that 18 per cent of women with laparoscopically proven disease still complained of pain after a mean of 9.5 years of follow-up. Adler *et al.* (1982) followed 78 patients with presumed PID and 77 controls for 21 months. Chronic abdominal pain was reported by 74 per cent of patients and 23 per cent of controls, whilst dyspareunia was reported by 41 per cent of patients and 13 per cent of controls. Menstrual abnormalities were also common, being reported in 80 per cent of patients and 44 per cent of controls. The mechanism of pain production in chronic PID is poorly understood. In some cases division of adhesions may be helpful. In very extensive disease, pelvic clearance may be indicated, but it does not always guarantee a cure.

The assessment of pelvic pain after PID is extremely difficult particularly when the diagnosis of the initial infection is uncertain if laparoscopy has not been performed. Once a diagnosis of PID has been made it is customary to label every subsequent bout of pain in the same way so that such patients often have numerous courses of antibiotics without the diagnosis being confirmed. Yet endometriosis and pelvic congestion (Beard *et al.* 1988) are also common causes of chronic pelvic pain. Beard *et al.* pointed out that 46 per cent of women who were finally found to have pelvic congestion had previously had a presumably erroneous diagnosis of chronic or acute PID.

Treatment

Treatment should be aimed at eradicating the presumptive pathogens. In most cases, the specific cause of the infection is unknown and a regimen should be selected which has activity against *N. gonorrhoeae*, *C. trachomatis*, and anaerobic bacteria. General measures, such as bedrest and abstention from intercourse should not be forgotten (Westrom and Mardh 1990). Removal of an IUCD is indicated and appropriate contraceptive counselling should be given (Centers for Disease Control 1989).

Numerous antibiotic regimens have been studied with claims of excellent short-term cure rates. However few studies have been based on the outcome in terms of tubal patency and the achievement of an intrauterine pregnancy (Brunham 1984). Since the clinical diagnosis of PID is so inaccurate it is likely that the assessment of cure is equally inaccurate. For example, Sweet *et al.* (1983), found *C. trachomatis* in the tubes of patients who were apparently cured after treatment of their PID with a beta-lactam antibiotic.

The continued use of beta-lactam antibiotics, such as penicillin, can no longer be supported and regimens must include a tetracycline in appropriate dosage to eradicate chlamydiae and mycoplasmas and a drug active against anaerobes, such as metronidazole or cefoxitin. Many strains of *N. gonorrhoeae* are still sensitive to tetracycline but in areas where tetracycline resistance is common an appropriate drug active against such strains must be added. The Centers for Disease Control (1991*a*) recommendations are shown in Table 6.4.

The examination and treatment of sexual partners is controversial if no sexually transmitted pathogen has been identified. However, Gilstrap *et al.* (1977) found *N. gonorrhoeae* in the partners of 14 per cent of women with PID

Table 6.4 Pelvic inflammatory disease: CDC recommended regimens

---

In-patient treatment

    Cefoxitin 2 g i.v. 6 hourly or cefotetan 2 g i.v. 12 hourly

plus

    Doxycycline 100 mg orally or i.v. 12 hourly

or   Clindamycin 900 mg i.v. 8 hourly

plus

    Gentamicin 2 mg/kg i.v. loading dose followed by 1.5 mg/kg 8 hourly

Either regimen should be given for 48 hours or until clinical improvement and should then be replaced with:
Doxycycline 100 mg orally 12 hourly for 10–14 days

Out-patient treatment

    Cefoxitin 2 g i.m. or an equivalent cephalosporin plus probenecid 1 g orally

plus

    Doxycycline 100 mg orally 12 hourly or an equivalent tetracycline for 10–14 days

or

Erythromycin 500 mg orally 6 hourly for 10–14 days (if intolerant of tetracyclines)

---

thought to be non-gonococcal and Osser and Persson (1982) found *C. trachomatis* in the partners of 12 per cent of women thought to have non-chlamydial disease. These studies confirm that reliance cannot be placed on swabs taken from the patient to exclude absolutely a STD as the cause of her PID, and that screening of the partner provides additional diagnostic information as well as preventing re-infection if treatment is instituted. In fact the Centers for Disease Control (1991*a*) is more dogmatic stating:

The management of women with PID should be considered inadequate unless their sex partners have been appropriately evaluated and treated . . . After evaluation, sex partners should be empirically treated with regimens effective against *C. trachomatis* and *N. gonorrhoeae* infections.

Syphilis

Syphilis is a chronic sexually transmitted disease caused by a spirochaete, *Treponema pallidum*. In pre-antibiotic days, it was a much feared disease with significant morbidity resulting in serious cardiovascular and neurological disease. It is also a blood-borne disease and can be transmitted by blood transfusion and transplacentally.

Epidemiology

There has been a sharp decline in the number of cases of syphilis since the introduction of penicillin, although there is evidence that there was a decline in both incidence and morbidity over the previous century. Descriptions of syphilis in the fifteenth century when it first appeared in Europe were of a much more acute disease. By the 1960s and 70s syphilis was only rarely seen in heterosexuals and since the advent of AIDS there has been a precipitous decline in numbers. However, anecdotally, syphilis is now reappearing and a number of experts have expressed anxiety that concentration of efforts on HIV infection has distracted health care workers from traditional STDs like syphilis.

Natural history

The primary lesion (chancre) appears in the site exposed to the infection within 90 days. The usual incubation period is 2–6 weeks. In women, this site may be the vulva, but in some cases it is the cervix where it will probably remain undetected. Healing takes place even without treatment, but the organism spreads throughout the body and after an asymptomatic period of about three months the secondary stage appears. This is characterized by rashes, lymphadenopathy, mucous membrane lesions, and constitutional symptoms. Other organs such as the liver and kidneys are sometimes involved. These symptoms and signs again resolve without treatment and the patient enters a latent stage which may persist for many years. Approximately, one-third of infected patients eventually develop clinical manifestations of late syphilis, including parenchymatous disease (gummata), cardiovascular disease (aortitis and aneurysms of the ascending aorta), and neurological disease (meningovascular syphilis, tabes dorsalis, and general paralysis of the insane). Some patients present with late syphilis and have no history of any illness or lesion which could be compatible with the earlier stages. It must be assumed, therefore, that in some cases the disease is truly asymptomatic in the early stages.

Clinical features

The lesion of primary syphilis, the chancre, is a single painless ulcer with a well-defined margin and indurated base. It should be considered in the differential diagnosis of all genital ulcers, although other causes of ulceration such as genital herpes are much commoner today.

Secondary syphilis may mimic a wide range of conditions, but the constitutional symptoms frequently lead to a diagnosis of influenza, particularly if the patient is not examined. The symmetrical non-irritant rash may be macular, papular, pustular, or psoriaform and often involves the palms and soles. Other lesions include snail-track ulcers in the mouth and flat genital warts, condylomata lata, which may be mistaken for viral warts. Manifestations of late syphilis are outside the scope of this chapter.

Infectivity

Primary and secondary lesions are very infectious and the patient remains infectious for up to two years after the end of the secondary phase, during which time both sexual partners and fetuses may be infected.

Diagnosis

A high index of suspicion should be maintained to avoid the tragedy of fetal loss or late sequelae as a result of failure to consider this eminently treatable disease. The organism cannot be cultured but may be demonstrated by darkground microscopy of specimens obtained from primary or secondary lesions. This technique requires considerable experience.

Serological tests become positive during the primary stage, the first test to become positive being the fluorescent treponemal antibody test (FTA–ABS). A negative test does not, however, exclude primary syphilis in the presence of a suspicious lesion and should be repeated. The Venereal Disease Research Laboratory test (VDRL) and the *Treponema pallidum* haemagglutination assay (TPHA) are almost always positive in the secondary stage and negative tests exclude the diagnosis (Anderson *et al.* 1989). The VDRL is a quantitative but non-specific test which is useful for monitoring the progress of the disease. It usually becomes negative after successful treatment but may remain positive in low titre in some cases (Oates and FitzGerald 1988). The TPHA and FTA–ABS are specific treponemal tests and are only positive in treponemal diseases. They cannot, however, distinguish syphilis from other treponemal diseases such as Yaws and Pinta. Unless treatment is instituted very early in the course of the primary stage, the TPHA and FTA remain positive lifelong and make the diagnosis of re-infection difficult.

The interpretation of positive serological tests in asymptomatic patients found during routine screening (for example antenatally) is a complex task. Non-specific tests such as the VDRL may be positive in a wide range of conditions, including infectious mononucleosis and other acute febrile illnesses, rheumatoid arthritis and other autoimmune conditions, and occasionally simply as a result of pregnancy. These are known as biological false-positives (BFP). In 1972, Catterall noted that 98 per cent of positive serological tests for syphilis could be attributed to that disease, but because of the possibility of a BFP, the diagnosis should be confirmed using a specific treponemal antibody test. The persistence of positive test results means that it may be difficult to distinguish between old adequately treated infection and a new infection since re-infection is possible.

Treatment

Penicillin is the drug of choice and 40 years of experience in its use allows clinicians to be confident of longterm success (Anderson *et al.* 1989), although some have expressed anxiety when treponemes have been found in the CSF of patients who have been treated according to standard regimens (Tramont 1976). Because of the long division time of the organism, 30 hours in early lesions and longer in later disease (Rein 1983), it is important to maintain consistently treponemocidal levels of penicillin.

Idsoe *et al.* (1972) reported a 100 per cent seroconversion to negative (in a non-specific VDRL-like test) in 1381 patients with primary syphilis and a 98 per cent seroconversion in 783 patients with secondary syphilis, although some patients (3.2 per cent) were subsequently reinfected. Good results are obtained in late syphilis, but the antibiotic can only then halt the disease not reverse the effects of structural damage.

A number of regimens exist. The Centers for Disease Control (1989) recommend 2.4 million units benzathine penicillin intramuscularly for primary and secondary syphilis and latent syphilis of up to one year's duration. Kampmeier *et al.* (1981) showed that 0.6–1.2 megaunits of aqueous procaine penicillin given daily for 10 days was associated with an almost 100 per cent cure rate. Late latent syphilis and cardiovascular and neurosyphilis require prolonged treatment.

Patients who are allergic to penicillin may be treated with doxycycline (200 mg or 300 mg daily) or tetracycline (500 mg four times daily) for 14 days. Other alternatives include erythromycin (500 mg four times daily for 14 days) and ceftriaxone (250 mg intramuscularly daily for 10 days). Unfortunately, experience with these regimens is limited and compliance is more difficult to ensure with oral regimens.

Contact tracing is essential if this disease is to be controlled. All contacts of a case of primary syphilis in the previous three months should be tested. In the case of secondary syphilis, contacts for 12 months should be sought (Oates and Fitzgerald 1988).

Trichomoniasis

Trichomoniasis is caused by a motile flagellated protozoon, *Trichomonas vaginalis* (TV), approximately 10–20 μm in diameter, slightly larger than a pus cell.

Epidemiology

There are few studies of the prevalence of TV infection in defined populations, but the organism has been found in 7 per cent of women attending a gynaecological clinic, 5 per cent attending a family planning clinic, and 3 per cent in a General Practice setting (Adler *et al.* 1981). Trichomoniasis was formerly commonly seen in STD clinics (Fouts and Kraus 1980; McLellan *et al.* 1982) but appears to be declining in incidence according to Department of Health data for England where 19 511 cases were recorded in STD clinics in 1979 and 7753 in 1989. Since probably only a small proportion of cases are seen in this setting it is difficult to be sure whether this is a true decline.

Trichomoniasis is a sexually transmitted disease. Women with more than one sexual partner are more likely to have the condition than those with only one partner (McLellan *et al.* 1982), whilst the condition is also associated with non-use of barrier contraception and non-use of oral contraceptives (Wolner-Hanssen *et al.* 1989). There is no convincing evidence that transmission by fomites occurs.

Symptoms

Clinical suspicion is poor. A purulent frothy discharge is only present in up to 50 per cent of patients, pruritus in 17 per cent, and the classical 'strawberry' cervix is found in only 3 per cent of infected women (McLellan *et al.* 1982). Many women, however, have less dramatic symptoms and signs and may be asymptomatic. In these cases, differentiation from bacterial vaginosis may be difficult and studies which have not included assessment for this condition cannot be used to delineate the prevalence of particular clinical features in women with and without trichomoniasis (McLellan *et al.* 1982).

Diagnosis

Currently available methods of diagnosis include examination of a wet mount for motile trichomonads, culture in a variety of media, and staining of a fixed preparation with Papanicolaou or another stain. Wet films are of high specificity, the sensitivity being dependent on the expertise of the observer (Clay *et al.* 1988) identifying the organism in 23–80 per cent of cases diagnosed on culture (Fouts and Kraus 1980; Krieger *et al.* 1988). Use of a dark-ground or phase-contrast microscope improves the likelihood of diagnosis (Rein and Muller 1990).

All authors report a higher detection rate when a swab is cultured in a nutrient-rich medium and Feinberg–Whittington, Squires and McFadzean, and Diamond's media have all been promoted, but no one medium is unquestionably superior. Papanicalaou smears may also detect *T. vaginalis*. Thin *et al.* (1975) showed that this technique is as sensitive and specific as direct examination and culture, but others have disputed this (Krieger *et al.* 1988; Weinberger and Harger 1993).

Staining of fixed preparations by other methods has been evaluated but has no advantage in terms of sensitivity, specificity, and cost over wet preparations and culture. However (Krieger *et al.* 1988) investigated a monoclonal antibody stain and found it to be sensitive and specific. Other newer techniques include an ELISA (Yule *et al.* 1987) and a latex agglutination test (Carney *et al.* 1988).

The vaginal pH in trichomoniasis is almost invariably elevated at 5.5 or greater (Holmes 1990).

Treatment

Metronidazole is the treatment of choice and results in cure in up to 98 per cent of patients. (Centers for Disease Control 1989; Keighley 1971; Lumsden *et al.* 1988). A variety of multidose regimens exists, using 600–800 mg daily in divided doses for 5–7 days, although there is little to choose between these oral regimens (Evans and Catterall 1971; Hager *et al.* 1980; Keighley 1971; Thin *et al.* 1979). A 2 g single dose (Hager *et al.* 1980; Thin *et al.* 1979) is as effective as the multidose regimens and compliance is improved since ingestion of the tablets may be supervised. Austin *et al.* (1982) demonstrated that a 1 g single dose was insufficient. The use of rectal suppositories of metronidazole at a dose of 2 g is associated with a cure rate of 94 per cent (Panja 1982). However, metronidazole is difficult to tolerate and may lead to poor compliance especially with the single 2 g oral dose; its interaction with alcohol is an additional problem. Concern about carcinogenicity is probably unwarranted, at least in relation to short courses, but Rustia and Shubik (1972) did produce an excess of lung tumours in mice fed with metronidazole over long periods. No clinical case of malignancy has been reported in association with prolonged metronidazole therapy. Alternative imidazole drugs with trichomonicidal activity include nimorazole and tinidazole.

Treatment failure may be due to re-infection or poor compliance, but in some cases neither seems likely and management is difficult. *In vitro* resistance to metronidazole has been described (Lumsden *et al.* 1988) and may be useful in predicting those patients who may respond to increased doses of metronidazole (for example 800 mg three times daily for 10 days). Unfortunately, these tests are not widely available. Other possible mechanisms for treatment failure include poor absorption of the drug from the gastrointestinal tract which may be assessed by measuring serum metronidazole levels after an oral dose (Ahmed-Jushef *et al.* 1988*b*). This may be overcome by intravaginal or intravenous administration of metronidazole. Others have proposed competition for metronidazole in the vaginal ecosystem (Edwards *et al.* 1979) and the use of broad-spectrum antibiotics to eradicate other competing bacteria. Wilmott *et al.* (1983) proposed an association with low plasma levels of zinc.

Management of sexual partners

As the organism is difficult to detect in men, the need to treat asymptomatic and undetectable infection in male partners is controversial. Blind treatment with metronidazole should be deprecated and when possible such men should be examined to exclude other STDs and then treated epidemiologically if the organism cannot be identified. If assessment of the male is difficult it may be acceptable to treat the symptomatic patient, confirm cure, and wait to see if re-infection occurs following sexual intercourse.

Co-infection

Trichomoniasis often co-exists with other infections, including gonorrhoea (Wolner-Hanssen *et al.* 1989) and chlamydial infection but not candidiasis. Screening for other infections should be considered in any woman with trichomoniasis.

Candidosis/candidiasis

This common infection is generally caused by *Candida albicans*, but other yeasts, for example *C. glabrata* and *C. tropicalis*, may cause similar symptoms and signs (Oriel *et al.* 1972; Robertson 1988). *C. albicans* is a yeast which grows by producing budding yeast cells (spores) and hyphal filaments (mycelia).

Prevalence

Colonization with *C. albicans* is widespread and the results of various studies have suggested a prevalence of 5–55 per cent in asymptomatic healthy women of childbearing age, although most authorities suggest 15–20 per cent is more realistic (Sobel 1985). The fungus is rarely isolated from premenarchal and post-menopausal females indicating the importance of hormones in maintaining the infection. Colonization is often called candidosis to distinguish it from candidiasis or active infection when vaginitis is present.

Candidosis is not normally considered to be a sexually transmitted disease but the organism can be transmitted sexually (Davidson and Oates 1985). There is no relationship between the number of recent sexual partners and the occurrence of candidosis (Barbone *et al.* 1990).

Diagnosis

The organism may be detected by examining wet preparations (saline mounts) and Gram-stained fixed preparations, but both methods are relatively insensitive compared with culture (McLennan *et al.* 1972). Swabs should be taken from the mid or high vagina and inoculated directly on to Sabouraud's dextrose–peptone medium or similar, or sent to the laboratory in transport medium. The fungus can, however, survive for up to 24 hours on dry swabs (Odds 1982). Culture may identify as few as 1000 organisms per millilitre. Investigators have suggested that the number of organisms present may be related to the presence of symptomatic disease, and thus a very sensitive method of identification may pick up small numbers of organisms which are not clinically significant. However, in experimental models, vaginitis can be induced with as few as 100 organisms (Sobel 1985).

C. albicans has also been detected on Papanicalaou smears, but this method is not as sensitive as culture or examination of a Gram-stained smear and should be regarded as an opportunistic method of detecting the infection rather than a diagnostic technique of choice (Thin *et al.* 1975).

The vaginal pH in candidiasis is at the lower end of the normal range, around 3–4, and this may be a useful test when diagnostic facilities are limited or when the appearances are atypical (Holmes 1990).

Predisposing factors

(1) pregnancy;

(2) oral contraception;

(3) broad-spectrum antibiotics;

(4) clothing and other factors;

(5) diabetes mellitus and other medical conditions;

(6) immunosuppression.

Pregnancy

Vaginal colonization and symptomatic vaginitis are increased during pregnancy and maximal during the third trimester with 30–40 per cent of women carrying the organism asymptomatically (Milsom and Forssman 1985). It is likely that the increased proportion of glycogen-rich vaginal epithelial cells under the influence of increased oestrogen secretion in pregnancy is the predisposing factor, but other factors may be involved (Sobel 1985). Adding simple sugars to *C. albicans* in a culture medium increased its adhesion to monolayers of epithelial cells (Samaranayake and MacFarlane 1982).

Oral contraceptives

It was originally believed that oral contraceptives predisposed to vaginal candidiasis but later studies have not confirmed this view. Oriel *et al.* (1972) isolated vaginal yeasts from 32 per cent of 241 women attending an STD clinic and taking oral contraceptives and 18 per cent of 292 who were not using this method of contraception. The Royal College of General Practitioners (1974) found that candidiasis was twice as common in current oral contraceptive users as compared with non-users and ex-users.

However, Hilton and Warnock (1975) isolated yeasts from the vaginas of 28 per cent of 122 oral contraceptive users attending an STD clinic and 29 per cent of women not using an oral contraceptive. More recently, Davidson and Oates (1985) found genital candidosis in 28 per cent of women at three different STD clinics, regardless of the type of contraception used. Others have found candidosis as frequently in women using oral contraceptives as in sexually active women using other or no contraception (Barbone *et al.* 1990). These discrepancies may be due to the high oestrogen content of oral contraceptives used in the earlier studies. There is thus no reason to suggest that women suffering from repeated bouts of candidal infection should discontinue oral contraceptives.

Broad-spectrum antibiotics

In clinical practice, candidiasis is commonly observed after the administration of broad-spectrum antibiotics, and after such treatment both vaginal colonization and symptomatic vaginitis increases. Thus Leegaard (1984) found that 25 per cent of women who had taken antibiotics within the previous three months had vaginal candidosis compared with 12 per cent of those who had not, but a similar proportion of both groups was symptomatic. Oriel and Waterworth (1975) found increased colonization rates of 29 per cent as opposed to 13 per cent after administration of tetracyclines.

Antibiotics are thought to act by eliminating protective vaginal bacterial flora, in particular lactobacilli. Lactobacilli act by competing for nutrients, interference at receptor sites on vaginal epithelial cells, and perhaps by the elaboration of substances which directly inhibit yeast proliferation and germination (Sobel 1990).

Clothing and other local factors

Some evidence exists to implicate either tight clothing or the use of detergents as predisposing factors (Sobel 1985). Elegbe and Elegbe (1983) reported that *C. albicans* could be isolated more frequently and in larger numbers from Nigerian women who wore tight clothing compared with those who wore looser more traditional clothing. Rashid *et al.* (1984) showed that conventional laundering did not eradicate fungal elements from underwear.

Numerous other factors have been proposed as predisposing factors, such as bath additives, soaps, perfumed toilet paper, douches, intravaginal deodorants, and chlorinated swimming pools. There is no scientific evidence to support this, but some or all of these may alter the vaginal milieu or may cause local sensitivity reactions allowing asymptomatic colonization to develop into symptomatic vaginitis (Sobel 1990).

Diabetes mellitus and other medical conditions

Diabetic patients are generally considered to be at increased risk of candidiasis (Milsom and Forssman 1985). However, in a recent textbook Tattersall and Gale (1990) concluded that there was no evidence to support this. If there is an increased risk, it is probably only in uncontrolled diabetes (Sobel 1990).

Iron deficiency anaemia and thyroid dysfunction have been proposed as predisposing factors but there is no evidence to suggest that these conditions account for more than a small minority of cases. Indeed Davidson *et al.* (1977) found no association between acute or recurrent candidiasis and iron deficiency.

Immunosuppression

Women who are immunosuppressed for whatever reason are more likely to suffer persistent and recurrent vaginal candidiasis; oral and oesophageal candidiasis may occur and systemic infections are also found. These conditions occur in young women with HIV infection and this diagnosis should perhaps be considered in women with recurrent candidal infection in non-genital sites. Except in high-risk areas, recurrent vaginal candidiasis is most unlikely to be due to HIV infection in the absence of other clinical markers of the disease.

Treatment

Many authorities believe that treatment should not be instituted when the organism is identified in the absence of symptoms and signs (Mendling 1987). Treatment may be arbitrarily divided into treatment for single acute episodes and treatment for patients with persistent and recurrent disease.

Treatment of acute episodes

Local treatment with intravaginal tablets, pessaries, or cream has been in use for many years. These are either polyene antibiotics, of which nystatin and amphotericin B are examples, or imidazole derivatives, which include clotrimazole, econazole, miconazole, and isoconazole.

Odds (1977) reported a metaanalysis of 62 publications on the drug treatment of vaginal candidosis. The overall cure rates were 90 per cent for 4078 patients receiving an imidazole and 79 per cent of 2475 patients receiving a polyene antibiotic, suggesting that imidazoles should be the treatment of choice. Odds showed that the cure rates were not influenced by choice of imidazole drug nor by the vehicle, creams and ointments being similarly effective. Relapse rates were also similar, being 5 per cent with imidazoles and 4 per cent with polyenes.

Odds' data suggested that courses of treatment lasting less than six days were less successful than longer courses. However, over the last 15 years there has been a move towards shorter treatment courses with high doses to improve patient compliance. Masterton *et al.* (1976) noted that almost 50 per cent of patients did not complete a 14 day course of treatment, and that the results of a study in which a six day course of clotrimazole cured more patients than a 14 day course of nystatin could be explained by better patient compliance rather than a difference in efficacy between the two products. In another study, Masterton *et al.* (1977) found similar cure rates when a three day course of clotrimazole was compared with a six day course of the same drug. Bingham and Steele (1981) compared a three day course of econazole with a 14 day course of nystatin and found similar rates of cure in those who reattended. However, nearly twice as many patients prescribed nystatin failed to reattend for follow-up.

These multidose regimens have largely been superseded by the use of a single pessary. Milsom and Forssman (1982) compared the use of a single 500 mg pessary of clotrimazole with 200 mg inserted for three consecutive days and found similar cure and relapse rates in both groups. Many other studies have produced similar results with cure rates of 77–90 per cent after a single 500 mg clotrimazole pessary (Fleury *et al.* 1985; Lebherz *et al.* 1985). Interestingly, however, relapse rates in these studies of 18–24 per cent are considerably higher than those quoted by Odds (1977).

From these studies, it seems that a single treatment with a high-dose imidazole pessary is the optimal first-line treatment for vaginal candidosis.

Oral therapy may not be totally risk free. Lewis *et al.* (1984) reported that 33 patients treated with ketoconazole developed liver damage after a minimum of 11 days treatment and one died. This complication has not been reported in otherwise well patients treated with other orally active drugs such as fluconazole and itraconazole. Therapy with fluconazole or itraconazole has been promoted as an alternative to intravaginal therapy. An International Multicentre Trial (1989) compared a 150 mg single oral dose of fluconazole with 200 mg clotrimazole administered intravaginally for three days. Although both regimens had excellent short-term cure rates of 99 per cent and 97 per cent, respectively, recurrence rates were significantly higher after 27–62 days in those treated with clotrimazole compared with those treated with fluconazole.

Recurrent candidiasis

Relapse of infection is very common in a small group of women suffering very frequent episodes of symptomatic disease (Sobel 1990). A number of explanations have been proposed:

(1) failure to deal with predisposing factors (see above);

(2) re-infection from an intestinal reservoir;

(3) re-infection from an untreated sexual partner.

The intestinal reservoir theory (Milsom and Forssman 1985) was once popular, with many patients treated with a prolonged course of oral nystatin to eradicate *C. albicans* from this site. Hilton and Warnock (1975) reported that 71 per cent of 84 women who had yeasts in the vagina also had yeasts in the anorectal canal, and Miles *et al.* (1977) found *C. albicans* in the stools of all of the 51 women with recurrent candidiasis whom they studied. Finding the organism in the anorectum or stools does not, of course, necessarily indicate these as the source of re-infection and oral nystatin frequently neither eradicates the organism from the gastrointestinal tract nor results in relief of symptoms. Thus, a combination of oral nystatin with local treatment was studied by Milne and Warnock (1979) who concluded there was no advantage over single therapy.

Although studies have indicated that treatment of an asymptomatic male partner is unhelpful (Bisschop *et al.* 1986; Forssman and Milsom 1985), examination of men may be useful to exclude an alternative or associated diagnosis (such as non-gonococcal urethritis) and to treat men with obvious clinical disease.

In patients with frequent relapses, a variety of prophylactic regimens have been tried. Balsdon and Tobin (1988) studied 100 women who were treated with 100 mg miconazole pessary weekly after an initial treatment course. None of the 54 women who continued the treatment for six months had a relapse compared with 48 per cent of the 46 women who discontinued the treatment prematurely. Roth *et al.* (1990) reported that 30 per cent of 33 women who used a single clotrimazole vaginal tablet after each period had a recurrence compared with 79 per cent of 29 who had used a placebo.

Bacterial vaginosis

The term bacterial vaginosis (BV) was adopted at an international conference in Stockholm (Mardh and Taylor-Robinson 1984) for the common condition, first described by Gardner and Dukes in 1955 and then called non-specific vaginitis. Gardner and Dukes believed that the condition was caused by a microorganism, *Haemophilus vaginalis*, subsequently called *Corynebacterium vaginale* and now *Gardnerella vaginalis* (GV), but there is now good evidence that GV forms only part of the microbial flora of the vagina in this condition and is not the major aetiological agent. Indeed the predominance of anaerobic bacteria has led some to prefer the name 'anaerobic vaginosis' (Blackwell *et al.* 1983), a terminology which has not found widespread acceptance.

Epidemiology

The disease is common and in some surveys in the commonest cause of vaginal discharge. Gardner *et al.* (1957) found that amongst private patients, *H. vaginalis* infection was commoner (19 per cent) than trichomoniasis (8.1 per cent), or candidiasis (4.9 per cent), but amongst clinic patients, trichomoniasis was the commonest infection (40 per cent). Amsel *et al.* (1983), found non-specific vaginitis in 21 per cent, candidiasis in 16 per cent, and trichomoniasis in 2 per cent of 397 unselected college students whom they studied. BV is usually, but not exclusively, found in the sexually active (Bump and Bueschling 1988; Mead 1993).

Pathogenesis

The underlying pathological abnormality appears to be the replacement of the normal vaginal flora consisting predominantly of lactobacilli with a mixed flora containing GV, *Mycoplasma hominis*, and a variety of anaerobic organisms including *Bacteroides* spp. and the short curved rods of *Mobiluncus* spp. (Eschenbach 1993; Hill 1993; Taylor *et al.* 1982; Thomason *et al.* 1984). All these organisms may be found in asymptomatic women with no evidence of vaginal discharge, but usually in smaller numbers. BV is a vaginosis not a vaginitis and clinical and microbiological evidence of inflammation is absent. However, BV is often associated with other infections, especially gonorrhoea, trichomoniasis, and chlamydial infection (but not candidiasis) and the presence of inflammation should alert the observer to the possibility of other infections.

Clinical features

The pathognomonic feature is an offensive grey discharge, though many patients are reluctant to mention the smell unless questioned directly. This discharge was characterized as being malodorous in all the patients and grey in 85 per cent (Gardner and Dukes 1955). The malodour, sometimes described as 'fishy,' is due to the release of amines from the vaginal discharge (Chen *et al.* 1979). Symptoms are worse after intercourse and after menstruation. Pruritus has not been associated with BV (Eschenbach *et al.* 1988) but many patients complain of vulval soreness because of the presence of the discharge. The clinical features of BV are often found in asymptomatic women attending for examination for an unrelated reason. The need to treat in these circumstances is controversial for in most cases the abnormal physical signs disappear without therapy (Bump *et al.* 1984).

Diagnosis

The diagnosis is a clinical not a microbiological one (Eschenbach *et al.* 1988) and may be made if three of the following four features are present:

1. *Homogeneous grey offensive discharge* — this is often obvious when parting the labia to insert a speculum. Sometimes the discharge is frothy and may then be confused with trichomoniasis.

2. *Elevated vaginal pH* — this is usually ≥ 5.5 and may be detected using narrow-gauge pH paper, a simple bedside test used all too infrequently in gynaecological practice.

3. *Positive amine test* — the addition of potassium hydroxide to vaginal secretions produces a pungent fishy odour (Hillier *et al.* 1991).

4. *Clue cells* — examination of a 'wet prep' shows epithelial cells covered by adherent bacteria which obscure the cellular outline and nucleus. A Gram-stained smear shows numerous Gram-variable coccobacilli (Hillier *et al.* 1993).

Other diagnostic methods

1. *Culture for GV* — since the organism may be found, albeit in small numbers, in women with no clinical features of BV, culture should be abandoned except in research studies.

2. *Gas–liquid chromatography* — the ratio of succinate to lactate (S/L ratio) in vaginal fluid was ≥ 0.4 in women with BV in a study reported by Spiegel *et al.* (1980). These workers claimed the test correlated well with clinical features and response to therapy, but this method is not widely available.

3. *Papanicolaou staining* — Platz-Christensen *et al.* (1989) showed a good correlation between the presence of clue cells on Papanicolaou staining and evidence of BV using conventional criteria. However, clue cells are not

normally reported by cytologists and it is unlikely that this would be a useful routine method of diagnosis.

Complications

Several workers have associated bacterial vaginosis with preterm labour and this is considered in Chapter 22 (Preterm labour). There are some data to suggest that BV might predispose to PID (Eschenbach *et al.* 1988).

Treatment

Metronidazole, in a variety of regimens, is the mainstay of treatment with initial symptomatic cure rates of up to 99 per cent. (Centers for Disease Control 1989; Fischbach *et al.* 1993; Ledger 1993; Swedberg *et al.* 1985; Sweet 1993). Pheifer *et al.* (1978) found significantly better results with this drug when compared with sulfonamide creams, oral doxycycline, and oral ampicillin. Jones *et al.* (1985) found that a single oral dose of 2 g was as effective as a standard regimen of 500 mg twice daily for seven days. Swedberg *et al.* (1985), however, found a higher relapse rate after a 2 g dose. Unfortunately, at least 30 per cent of women successfully treated with metronidazole relapse within six weeks (Blackwell *et al.* 1983). Repeated courses of metronidazole are not recommended because of the theoretical risk of carcinogenicity, and management is difficult because the reason for the recurrence is unknown. Oral clindamycin may also cure up to 94 per cent of patients (Ledger 1993; Sweet 1993). Some have recommended routine simultaneous treatment of the sexual partner(s) (Brown 1984). However, Vejtorp *et al.* (1988) and Vutyavanich *et al.* (1993), in double-blind randomized trials, found that there was no benefit to the women from treatment of their partners. Swedberg *et al.* (1985) drew similar conclusions from their study. It is likely that topical treatments may be developed in the future, especially to treat the condition in pregnancy. Vaginal gels containing metronidazole or clindamycin seem to cure up to 87 per cent of patients and may be useful when oral therapy fails (Fischbach *et al.* 1993; Hillier *et al.* 1993; Livengood *et al.* 1990).

Non-specific vaginitis

Non-specific vaginitis is not uncommon in premenarchal children and postmenopausal women. In childhood, the vaginal pH is elevated, making children susceptible to infection with different microorganisms from those seen in adults. Coliforms, *Streptococcus pyogenes*, and *Shigella* species may cause vaginal discharge but will be detected if a swab is taken. Threadworms also occasionally cause discharge. Candidal infection is uncommon. The detection of a STD is prima facie evidence of sexual abuse, but further investigation will be required. Discharge in children is sometimes caused by poor hygiene and the association with a vaginal foreign body is well known.

In post-menopausal women, discharge is usually due to lack of oestrogens but STDs, though uncommon, do occur.

Since the delineation of the bacterial vaginosis syndrome, which in the past was a common cause of unexplained discharge, it is more unusual to see premenopausal women for whom a cause cannot be assigned to their discharge, particularly if they are examined on several occasions at different stages of the menstrual cycle. Nevertheless, this does occur and empirical therapy may be necessary. The following treatment modalities have been suggested:

(1) systemic antibiotics;

(2) local sulfonamides;

(3) antiseptics;

(4) acid preparations;

(5) oestrogens;

(6) removal of an IUCD;

(7) treatment of cervical ectopy.

Systemic antibiotics

Brunham *et al.* (1984) argued that mucopurulent cervicitis was the neglected equivalent of non-gonococcal urethritis (NGU). Since 50 per cent of cases of NGU are not caused by chlamydiae yet respond to tetracyclines and erythromycin, it was suggested that non-chlamydial cervicitis should be treated with these antibiotics. However, there are no data to support this.

Local sulphonamides

Local triple sulfonamide preparations are a well-established means of treating and preventing vaginal infections. Hodge and Murdoch (1963) reported relief of symptoms in 68 per cent of 50 patients treated for ten days with such pessaries compared with 38 per cent treated with placebo.

Antiseptics

Vaginal iodine preparations are commonly used for the treatment of non-specific vaginitis. Mayhew (1981) treated 80 patients, with a variety of conditions, with povidone iodine pessaries twice daily for 14 days, after which time 66 per cent were symptom-free but 6 per cent had ceased treatment because of vaginal 'burning'. This approach might be acceptable if facilities for making a microbiological diagnosis were not available, but is inappropriate under normal circumstances. For example, half the patients had candidiasis, the majority of whom would have been cured by a single antifungal pessary, yet 38 per cent carried the organism after the povidone iodine treatment.

Acid preparations

Re-establishing an acidic vagina in post-menopausal women may help to control vaginal discharge and is useful when oestrogens are contraindicated. Slater

(1950) suggested its use in post-menopausal women undergoing vaginal surgery to reduce the incidence of wound infections.

Oestrogens

Topical and systemic oestrogens are widely used in the management of atrophic vulvovaginitis. Speroff *et al.* (1989) reported that oestrogen replacement is 'invariably successful in reversing these atrophic problems', but there are no scientific studies to support the use of oestrogens in non-specific vaginitis in the older woman.

Removal of an IUCD

Vaginal discharge is a common complication of using an IUCD. Amsel *et al.* (1983) found a discharge with the characteristics of BV in 50 per cent of women with an IUCD as compared with 25 per cent of women without. Treatment with metronidazole is effective. However, recurrence is common and removal of the IUCD has to be weighed against other contraceptive needs. If pain accompanies the vaginal discharge, a possible diagnosis of PID should be considered.

Treatment of cervical ectopy

Endocervical cells secrete mucus and when a large area of cervical ectopy (erosion) is present, there may be a heavy mucoid discharge. Ectopy is common, and was found in 37 per cent of 1498 women attending a family planning clinic (Goldacre *et al.* 1978). In this study, there was no difference in the prevalence of a number of microorganisms between women with and without ectopy. However *C. trachomatis*, an important cause of ectopy, was not sought. Peck (1974) reported that 87 per cent of 15 patients with a cervical erosion became free of vaginal discharge after cryotherapy. Diathermy may also be used, but it is important to exclude important cervical and vaginal pathogens before treatment.

Genital herpes

This common infection is caused by herpes simplex virus (HSV) type 1 or type 2. HSV contains an inner core of double-stranded DNA surrounded by a glycoprotein envelope. The two types are distinguished by biochemical and immunological methods; at the molecular level there is 50 per cent homology between the two viruses. Although it was formerly thought that type 1 infection was restricted to the oral cavity and type 2 to the genitalia, it has become clear in recent years that either virus may be found in both sites. There is considerable geographical variation: in Seattle (Corey *et al.* 1983) 7 per cent of first attacks were due to type 1, whereas in N. Ireland (Lavery *et al.* 1986) and Sheffield (Kinghorn *et al.* 1986*a*) the proportions were 30 per cent and 49 per cent, respectively. As with all herpes viruses, infection is lifelong, and the virus is established in sensory ganglia within two to three days of acquisition. After the primary infection, recurrences may occur when the virus is reactivated from its latent state and travels along peripheral nerves to the skin surface where new lesions are produced.

Natural history

Primary infection occurs in patients with no pre-existing antibody to HSV 1 or 2 and usually produces severe symptoms lasting for up to three weeks if untreated. There may be marked constitutional symptoms. Initial genital herpes, which may be less severe, is a term used to describe a first attack of genital herpes in someone who has had orolabial herpes and thus has antibody to type 1 infection. Recurrences may occur frequently or infrequently, the mean number per year being three or four (Corey *et al.* 1983). HSV-2 is more likely to recur than HSV-1, 60-80 per cent of the former and 14-55 per cent of the latter recurring within a year of the initial attack (Corey *et al.* 1983; Reeves *et al.* 1981). The severity also varies, but recurrences are rarely as severe as the primary attack and neurological and systemic manifestations are unusual. Some patients, however, have very frequent attacks and significant psychological morbidity (Goldmeier *et al.* 1988).

Transmission of HSV requires close physical contact, which in practice implies sexual activity. Genital herpes acquired in stable relationships from symptomatic or asymptomatic oral lesions is increasingly common.

Epidemiology

The incidence of the condition is increasing; there was a 125 per cent increase in reported cases in England between 1978 and 1989. Some of this increase may, however, be due to an increase in attendances at STD clinics when acyclovir became available in the 1980s for treating this condition.

HSV has been isolated from 0.02-5 per cent of adult women (Ferrer *et al.* 1984). This is almost certainly an underestimate of the proportion of the population infected since not all infected patients would be shedding the virus at the time of any survey. Furthermore, recent serological surveys suggest that HSV antibody is very common. For example, Johnson *et al.* (1989) examined sera obtained from a nationwide survey of the US adult population and found type specific antibody in 16.4 per cent of those studied. This suggests that infection with HSV must be even commoner than previously thought and a large proportion of cases must be asymptomatic. Indeed, the phenomenon of acquisition of infection from an asymptomatic sexual partner has been well described (Barton *et al.* 1987; Rooney *et al.* 1986), and is undoubtedly very common in clinical practice. Furthermore, acquisition of infection which is asymptomatic, minimally symptomatic, or misinterpreted must account for the majority of infections.

Clinical features

Genital herpes is the commonest cause of genital ulceration in the West. Attacks begin with erythematous lesions which develop into blisters and then shallow ulcers. Eventually the ulcers crust over and scabs are shed leaving intact epithelia. In primary herpes there are numerous painful lesions of the labia, introitus, and perineum. The cervix is involved in 70 per cent of cases and when it is possible to pass a speculum, necrotic ulcers and a purulent discharge are observed. Bilateral tender inguinal lymphadenopathy is common. External dysuria is usual as a result of urine trickling over the ulcers and reflex retention of urine may occur. 'Flu-like symptoms often accompany the local disease and there may be neurological pain in the dermatomes involved. In men, lesions affect the glans and shaft of the penis. Severe attacks are more unusual in men than in women.

Recurrent herpes is much less severe with only a few lesions which may be very trivial, and constitutional and neurological symptoms are rare. The cervix is involved in 4 per cent of episodes. Recurrent herpes is often preceded by a prodrome lasting 24–48 hours which marks the onset of viral replication at the site of the recurrence. The frequency of recurrences varies between individuals and in any one individual over a period of time. Numerous factors have been proposed to account for the variation, but there is no doubt that stress is an important factor.

Asymptomatic viral shedding may occur from minor lesions not detected or misinterpreted by the patient, from internal sites (for example the cervix) and occasionally from intact epithelial surfaces (Barton *et al.* 1986*b*).

Complications

(1) aseptic meningitis;

(2) urinary retention;

(3) extragenital lesions;

(4) pelvic inflammatory disease;

(5) disseminated HSV infection;

(6) possible association with cervical neoplasia.

Aseptic meningitis

Symptoms suggestive of meningeal infection are not uncommon in primary disease but are rarely severe enough to require admission to hospital (Corey *et al.* 1983). HSV has been isolated from CSF in ≤ 3 per cent of cases of aseptic meningitis admitted to hospital (Skoldenberg *et al.* 1975).

Urinary retention

Urinary retention and constipation due to autonomic dysfunction occur in about 1 per cent of women, usually towards the end of the second week. Since the advent of acyclovir, admission to hospital for catheterization is rarely needed.

Extragenital lesions

These may occur in up to a quarter of primary attacks, presumably as a result of autoinoculation (Corey 1990).

Pelvic inflammatory disease

PID has been described in a few cases (Lehtinen *et al.* 1985) but is uncommon or unrecognized.

Disseminated HSV infection

This is extremely rare with a very high mortality, especially in the immunocompromised individual.

Cervical neoplasia

The possible association with cervical neoplasia is discussed in Chapter 12.

Diagnosis

Accurate diagnosis requires a swab taken from an active lesion to collect infected cells. The longer the duration of symptoms, the less likely is a swab to be positive, and, in recurrent episodes, a positive result can only be expected from a swab taken in the first 48 hours. However, positive results may sometimes be obtained from intact skin during the prodrome. It is important to remember that a negative result does not exclude a diagnosis of genital herpes in the presence of clinically suspicious lesions and the patient may need to return for further tests at the onset of the next attack. A number of techniques are available:

(1) tissue culture;

(2) ELISA and direct immunofluorescence;

(3) Papanicolaou staining;

(4) electron microscopy;

(5) DNA hybridization techniques and PCR;

(6) serology.

Tissue culture

HSV produces a specific cytopathic effect in many laboratory cell lines. This is a specific technique and produces results within 48–72 hours (Darougar *et al.* 1986); its sensitivity is dependent on the quality of the specimen obtained. Swabs must be taken into viral transport medium and held at +4 °C until inoculated into tissue culture.

ELISA and direct immunofluorescence

These antigen detection tests have shown good specificity (Alexander *et al.* 1985; Botcherby *et al.* 1987) with sensitivity compatible with culture if good specimens are obtained. No special precautions are required for the transportation of specimens.

Papanicolaou staining of cervical smears

Occasionally multinucleated giant cells typical of herpes infection are detected on a routine cervical smear. This technique should only be regarded as an opportunistic way of detecting cervical herpes virus infection since the diagnosis will only be suggested in 23 per cent of patients who undergo a smear but are culture positive (Vontver *et al.* 1979). Since a small proportion of women shed the virus only from the cervix and are usually unaware of the infection, the detection of change suggestive of HSV puts the clinician into a quandary. It would be unwise to make a diagnosis on this basis alone, but if swabs are taken from the patient, shedding may have ceased. However, if the possible diagnosis is not discussed with the patient, the clinician could be found liable if the woman unknowingly infects a subsequent sexual partner.

Electron microscopy

This is a useful technique if a rapid diagnosis is essential (for example in labour) but active lesions are necessary and the technique is of low sensitivity (Woodman *et al.* 1988).

DNA hybridization techniques and PCR

These new techniques are being developed and appear to have a sensitivity similar to antigen detection systems. PCR may be more sensitive than viral isolation (Rogers *et al.* 1992).

Serology

The development of serological tests has been bedevilled by the cross-reactivity between HSV 1 and 2, and many early studies purporting to distinguish between antibody to these two viruses can be criticized on technical grounds (Fife and Corey 1990). Since up to 80 per cent of the adult population have antibody to HSV 1 as a result of childhood orolabial infection, the specificity of the test is crucial. Furthermore, serology cannot distinguish between orolabial and genital infection caused by HSV 1. The test is, therefore, not useful for the individual patient in most cases, although the absence of antibody might be useful in excluding infection in the small proportion of the population not exposed to HSV 1. Newer tests which are type specific are not yet commercially available.

Table 6.5 Use of acyclovir in genital herpes simplex virus infection*

	Initial herpes		Recurrent herpes	
	Acyclovir	Placebo	Acyclovir	Placebo
No. of patients	17	14	41	42
Median duration (days)				
—symptoms	4	8	3	2.5
—time to healing	7	11.5	5	6
—viral shedding	1	13	1	2
% of patients with new vesicle formation	0	43	2	19

*From Nilsen *et al.* 1982

Treatment

First episode genital herpes

This is a severe systemic infection and should be treated with oral or, rarely, parenteral medication. Numerous studies have now shown that acyclovir in an oral dose of 200 mg five times daily for five days significantly reduces the duration of symptoms and viral shedding (Bryson *et al.* 1983; Centers for Disease Control 1989; Mertz *et al.* 1984; Mindel 1991; Nilsen *et al.* 1982). For example, Nilsen *et al.* (1982) reported a double-blind randomized trial of acyclovir (200 mg five times daily for five days) versus placebo in 31 patients with initial genital herpes. As can be seen from Table 6.5, acyclovir significantly reduced the duration of symptoms, the incidence of new vesicle formation, the duration of viral shedding, and the time to healing. Side-effects, including dizziness, nasal stuffiness, nausea, and diarrhoea, were no more common with acyclovir than with placebo. Acyclovir cream or ointment produced inferior results (Thin *et al.* 1983). The addition of co-trimoxazole (Kinghorn *et al.* 1986*a*) produced some benefit, a reduction in pain, and a shorter time to healing, presumably by controlling secondary infection, but concomitant oral and topical treatment did not (Kinghorn *et al.* 1986*b*).

Other drugs which have been investigated in first episode genital herpes include 3 per cent adenine arabinoside (Adams *et al.* 1976), topical surfactant (Vontver *et al.* 1979), topical idoxuridine in DMSO (Silvestri *et al.* 1982), and interferon alpha 2 (Mendelson *et al.* 1986). None has shown any significant benefit when compared with placebo. Treatment of a first episode does not prevent recurrences since the virus is already established in the ganglia at the onset of symptoms (Mindel *et al.* 1986).

In addition to drug therapy, patients with first episodes need rest and support; good counselling at this stage may prevent many of the more significant psychological sequelae.

Recurrent genital herpes

Since many recurrent attacks are associated with very minor symptoms, in assessing a patient requesting treatment it is important to discover the nature of the patient's concerns. In some patients lack of information or misinformation often generated by exaggerated media coverage underlies the consultation and good counselling can resolve many of the difficulties. Some patients are concerned about the risk of transmission to a partner or the risks in pregnancy and some have a fear of cervical cancer. A few patients have very frequent or prolonged attacks.

Treatment of short, single episodes with salt-water bathing is as effective as any other treatment. Acyclovir treatment may shorten a long attack and if used in the prodromal phase may abort some attacks, but for the majority of episodes it is little more than an expensive placebo (Nilsen *et al.* 1982). Other treatments which have been evaluated include topical adenine arabinoside (Adams *et al.* 1976), 'Intervir-A', a surfactant, (Goldberg 1986), phosphono-formate (Barton *et al.* 1986*a*), interferon alpha 2 (Mendelson *et al.* 1986), topical idoxuridine in DMSO (Silvestri *et al.* 1982), and a chlorous acid-releasing gel (Ruck *et al.* 1991). Goldberg claimed considerable benefits from 'Intervie-A' but there were methodological problems with this study rendering the conclusions questionable. All other studies failed to demonstrate any success.

Skinner *et al.* (1982) attracted considerable attention both from the scientific community and the media by producing a vaccine from HSV-1 which they claimed both prevented the acquisition of genital herpes and reduced the frequency of recurrences (Woodman *et al.* 1983). Unfortunately, later controlled studies in the United States failed to confirm these claims (Marsh 1990).

Oral acyclovir taken prophylactically in a daily divided dose of up to 800 mg has been shown to suppress herpes virus infection very effectively. Clinical episodes of disease and viral shedding are very rare (Mindel *et al.* 1989). In view of the expense of this treatment and the unknown longterm effects, treatment is reserved for those with very frequent recurrences and should be stopped periodically to see if the natural history of the disease has changed.

Resistance of HSV to acyclovir has been described (Burns *et al.* 1982). At least in the immunocompetent, resistant virus has not proved to be a clinical problem. HSV infection in the immunocompromised may be severe and persistent. Continuous prophylactic therapy is usually indicated.

Genital warts (Condylomata acuminata)

Genital warts are caused by the human papillomavirus (HPV), a DNA-containing papovavirus. There are at least 60 subtypes, classified by the degree of DNA hybridization. Since the virus cannot be cultured, there was little understanding of the biology and epidemiology of HPV infections until the genome was cloned in the late 1970s. Now a number of techniques have been developed to identify viral DNA in clinical material. Of the 60 or so types, types 6, 11, 16, and 18 are commonly found in anogenital lesions. The association of HPV infection with neoplasia is discussed in Chapter 12.

Epidemiology

There has been a dramatic rise in the number of cases of genital warts seen in departments of genitourinary medicine in the last decade, from 24 490 in 1979 to 78 146 in 1989 (Department of Health). Although this is almost certainly a true reflection of the increasing incidence of the condition, other factors, such as the association with premalignant disease of the cervix, may account for more patients seeking treatment for what was previously felt to be a trivial condition.

Genital warts are common in young sexually active adults, the peak age in females being 19 in the study reported by Oriel (1971) and 20–24 in that reported by Chuang *et al.* (1984). Warts are commonly found in association with other genital infections. Jenkins and Riley (1980) reported co-existing infections in 45 per cent of women with anogenital warts, the commonest being candidiasis, trichomoniasis, and gonorrhoea. However, had chlamydial infection been sought, the rate of associated infections would have been even higher. Griffiths (1989) screening women with warts attending an STD clinic found that 9 per cent had a chlamydial infection and commented that the prevalence of associated infections was no higher than in other young sexually active adults.

HPV is usually transmitted sexually through minute abrasions. Oriel (1971) found that 64 per cent of contacts of patients with genital warts developed warts themselves within nine months. However, HPV types characteristic of common skin warts have occasionally been found in genital lesions and in such cases autoinoculation is likely. Genital warts are not uncommon in children and have been the source of much controversy; in some cases, the virus has been transmitted from the mother's genital tract during pregnancy, but in other cases sexual abuse has occurred. Although, warts in childhood are not pathognomonic of abuse, such a possibility should always be considered (Oriel 1992; Sait and Garg 1985).

Natural history

All warts may resolve spontaneously, but this phenomenon is less common for genital warts than for skin warts (Oriel 1971). Spontaneous resolution is associated with a dense cellular inflammatory reaction suggestive of an immunological process (Tagami *et al.* 1985). Recurrence following both spontaneous resolution and treatment is common. Ferenczy *et al.* (1985) found virological evidence of HPV in the skin areas adjacent to excised genital warts more commonly in those patients who developed recurrences than in those who did not, and they hypothesized that recurrence was due to the presence of latent virus in untreated areas.

Clinical features

Warts may be flat and keratinized or florid and exophytic. In women, the commonest sites involved are the introitus (73 per cent), the labia minora and clitoris (32 per cent), the labia majora (31 per cent), and the perineum (23 per cent) (Oriel 1971). Perianal warts, either alone or in association with warts in other sites, are not uncommon in both men and women; they may be associated with anal intercourse but this is not invariable. Cervical lesions may be exophytic, but may also be non-condylomatous and then only detected by cytological examination and colposcopy (Meisels and Fortin 1976).

Diagnosis

The clinical appearance is usually characteristic but excision and histological examination may be necessary if the lesions are atypical, especially in the older patient when malignant change must be excluded.

The cytological changes associated with wart virus infection of the cervix were first described by Papanicolaou in 1960; typically there are large vacuolated cells called koilocytes, but other features including dyskeratosis and hyperchromasia are common. These changes are similar to those of minor degrees of cervical intraepithelial neoplasia and differentiation may be difficult (Meisels and Fortin 1976).

HPV DNA can now be detected and typed in exfoliated cells and in tissue biopsies using a number of molecular techniques including Southern blotting (generally regarded as the gold standard), Dot blot and *in situ* hybridization. The polymerase chain reaction can also be used to detect HPV DNA; it is extremely sensitive but laboratory contamination is a serious problem and spurious results may occur (Lorincz 1990).

Although identification and typing of HPV DNA is useful to study the epidemiology and natural history of wart virus infections (Wickenden *et al.* 1988), it is not clear whether such techniques currently have much value in the management of the individual patient. At one stage it was thought that the identification of certain types such as HPV 16 in particular lesions would help the clinician to evaluate the potential for progression and thus influence therapy; there are no data, as yet, to support this.

Treatment

The main aims of treatment are to remove visible warts and any associated symptoms, and also, as far as possible, to prevent transmission of the virus. Treatment may remove visible warts but cannot, at least using currently available techniques, eradicate latent virus. There is no evidence that treatment of a wart virus infection will prevent the subsequent development of cervical intraepithelial neoplasia. There are numerous treatment options but all may result in recurrence after apparent success.

(1) chemical applications;

(2) cryosurgery;

(3) electrocautery;

(4) surgical excision;

(5) laser treatment;

(6) interferon therapy;

(7) inosine pranobex;

(8) vaccination.

Chemical applications

Podophyllin is a cytotoxic agent which has been used as a first-line treatment for genital warts for many years. It is most successful in treating moist sessile warts of recent origin. Care must be taken to avoid painting adjacent skin when severe reactions may occur. The paint should be applied once or twice a week and this necessitates numerous visits to the physician which many patients find difficult. Although some men treat themselves successfully, women usually find difficulty in accurately applying the paint. Recently, preparations of podophyllotoxin have been licensed for self-application and are said to be less toxic to normal skin (Edwards *et al.* 1988). Stone *et al.* (1990) found a clearance rate of 41 per cent and a relapse rate of 17 per cent after six weekly treatments with podophyllin. Jenkins and Riley (1980) reported a cure rate of 45 per cent at one month and 75 per cent at three months.

Trichloracetic acid used alone or in combination with podophyllin (Gabriel and Thin 1983) is also relatively successful. It is more effective for keratinized warts than podophyllin. Other topical treatments include idoxuridine (Hasumi 1987).

Cryosurgery

Cryosurgery is an effective treatment method which does not require an anaesthetic. It is most successful with isolated warts and several treatments are usually necessary. Simmons *et al.* (1981) cured 63 per cent of male patients after a mean of 2.6 treatments. Stone *et al.* (1990) cured 79 per cent with a 21 per cent late recurrence rate. Cryotherapy is often used in association with other treatment modalities, such as the application of podophyllin or trichloracetic acid.

Electrocautery

Electrocautery requires a local anaesthetic and is suitable for a small number of larger warts. Simmons *et al.* (1981) cured 10 of 11 patients, evaluated after three months; Stone *et al.* (1990) cured 94 per cent with a 21 per cent late recurrence rate. In this randomized trial, electrocautery was more successful than either podophyllin or cryosurgery.

Surgical excision

This requires a local or general anaesthetic and may be appropriate if another procedure is to be undertaken simultaneously. Jensen (1985) cleared 93 per cent of his patients of perianal warts, but 29 per cent had recurred within 12 months. McMillan and Scott (1987), using a similar technique, had excellent early results (92 per cent cure rate) but two of 24 who returned for follow-up after three months had recurrences.

Laser treatment

A number of investigators have reported good results with laser vaporization. Bellina (1983) found that 14 per cent of patients had persistent lesions which he attributed to inadequate therapy and 3 per cent had a recurrence within a year of treatment. Ferenczy (1984) had an overall failure rate of only 5 per cent when treating pregnant patients. Billingham and Lewis (1982), however, had very high recurrence rates following laser treatment of extensive perianal warts. These rather atypical results may, in retrospect, have been due to undiagnosed HIV infection in these patients. These investigators also commented that laser treatment caused more post-operative discomfort that electrocautery.

Interferon therapy

Interferon has antiviral and antineoplastic activity and, therefore, is a logical treatment for HPV infections. It is, however, expensive and has unpleasant side-effects making it unsuitable for initial use. Intralesional, intramuscular, and local application of a gel formulation have all been tried with limited success. This topic has recently been reviewed by Main and Handley (1992).

Inosine pranobex

A preliminary study in 1986 (Mohanty and Scott) suggested that this immune modulator when used alone or in combination with conventional treatment resulted in improved results, especially when the warts had been present for a long time. Davidson-Parker *et al.* (1988) also found some benefit from the addition of this drug to conventional regimens for resistant warts.

Vaccination

Malison *et al.* (1982) studied an autogenous vaccine produced from the patients' own warts, but found no benefit when compared with a placebo vaccine.

Treatment of subclinical HPV infection

In the absence of CIN, the need to treat subclinical HPV infection is controversial. Some argue that such lesions are infectious but there is no convincing evidence that this is invariably so, nor is there evidence that any treatment modality is successful in eradicating subclinical infection. Thus, Boothby *et al.* (1990) failed to eradicate HPV infection with trichloracetic acid, and Riva *et al.* (1989) used extensive laser vaporization to treat multicentric disease with persistence of HPV infection in 88 per cent of cases.

HPV and HIV infection

In immunocompromised individuals, including those with HIV infection, both subclinical and clinical HPV infections may be extensive, multicentric, and resistant to treatment (Johnson *et al.* 1992). There is also some evidence that intraepithelial neoplasia involving cervix, vagina, vulva, and perianal areas progresses more rapidly that in immunocompetent women.

Human immunodeficiency virus (HIV) infection

The acquired immunodeficiency syndrome (AIDS) was first described in 1981 in previously healthy homosexual men who developed *Pneumocystis carinii* pneumonia and Kaposi's sarcoma, conditions only seen previously in severely immunosuppressed individuals (Gottleib *et al.* 1981). The condition was later described in intravenous drug abusers (Worsmer *et al.* 1983), transfusion recipients (Jett *et al.* 1983), haemophiliacs (Centers for Disease Control 1982), heterosexual contacts (Harris *et al.* 1983) and children of these people (Oleske *et al.* 1983), and residents of Central Africa (Plot *et al.* 1984).

These so-called 'risk groups' were the same as for hepatitis B infection, and this led to speculation that the disease was caused by an infectious agent, called LAV (lymphadenopathy associated virus) in Paris and HTLV-111 (human lymphotrophic virus type 111) in the USA. The term HIV was later introduced; two HIVs are now recognized, HIV-1 and HIV-2. HIV-2 originated in West Africa and is rare outside that region (*Lancet* 1988) and may be less infective (Kanki *et al.* 1994).

HIV is a RNA-containing retrovirus, characterized by an enzyme, reverse transcriptase, which converts RNA to DNA. It attacks T lymphocytes which are gradually depleted leaving the patient susceptible to conditions which are normally controlled by cell-mediated immunity. Antibody-mediated defence mechanisms are usually intact, although some antibody production may be abnormal. HIV probably also attacks other target cells including cells of the gastrointestinal tract and nervous system, accounting for diseases in these systems when no opportunistic pathogen can be found. There have also been recent reports of acquired immunodeficiency without evidence of HIV infection (McNulty *et al.* 1994).

Routes of transmission

There are three major routes of transmission, sexual, from infected blood or tissue, and *in utero* from mother to child (see Tables 6.6 and 6.7). In the West, homosexual transmission still accounts for the majority of cases of both HIV

Table 6.6 AIDS cases in UK to March 1992*

Diagnostic category	Male	Female
Homosexual/bisexual	4509	— men
Injecting drug use	187	76
Heterosexual contact		
—high-risk partner	17	38
—other partner abroad	249	133
—other partner UK	31	23
Haemophiliac	304	4
Other blood products		
—abroad	15	29
—UK	17	18
Mother to child	24	34
Other/undetermined	64	10
Total	5417	365

*From *Communicable Diseases Report*, 2, No. 17. 24th April 1992

infection (60 per cent) and clinical AIDS (78 per cent) whilst intravenous drug abuse provides a route of transmission into the heterosexual population. In Africa and other developing areas heterosexual transmission is the major mode of transmission. Even in the West, heterosexual transmission is now the fastest growing transmission category (Johnson 1992). Haemophiliacs were infected by batches of infected factor VIII and a number of people were infected by blood transfusion before a test was developed for HIV antibody which could be used to screen donated blood. Vertical transmission is discussed in Chapter 21.

Women still constitute a minority of cases (12 per cent of cases of HIV infection and 6 per cent of AIDS). Of those females with AIDS, 21 per cent were intravenous drug abusers and a further 47 per cent had either a 'high-risk' partner in the UK or were believed to have contracted the virus abroad. Only 6 per cent of women and 0.6 per cent of men developed AIDS after acquiring HIV during heterosexual activity with apparently 'low-risk' partners in the UK. AIDS statistics, however represent the end stage of an infection acquired perhaps more than a decade earlier and thus HIV statistics give a better estimate of more recent transmission. It can be seen in Table 6.7 that a larger proportion of HIV-infected individuals (compared to AIDS cases) are women and heterosexual transmission is more important. It is believed that the peak of the HIV infection epidemic has not yet been reached. Had transmission ceased in 1985, the peak of the AIDS epidemic would have been seen in the mid 1990s; it is now likely that secondary peaks will occur for the future (Biggar 1991; Brookmeyer 1991).

Sexual transmission is relatively inefficient and up to 50 per cent of the longterm partners of infected individuals remain uninfected even if condoms are not used (Al-Nozha *et al.* 1990). Although HIV infection has been reported

Table 6.7 HIV-1 infected persons in UK to March 1992*

Diagnostic category	Male	Female	NS[†]
Homosexual/bisexual men	10 570	—	—
Injecting drug use	1550	712	30
Heterosexual contact			
—high-risk partner	46	250	1
—other partner abroad	676	539	13
—other partner UK	60	83	2
—under investigation	147	168	
Haemophiliac	1258	9	—
Other blood products	78	81	1
Mother to child	55	60	1
Other/undetermined	844	177	83
Total	15 284	2079	131

[†] not specified
*From *Communicable Diseases Report*, 2, No. 17. 24th April 1992

after a single act of intercourse, for example as a result of rape, only 18–23 per cent of the regular female partners of HIV infected men become infected (Padian *et al.* 1987; Peterman *et al.* 1988). Factors which may predispose to transmission include genital ulceration, the presence of a non-ulcerative STD or the history of such a condition, coitus during menstruation, anal intercourse, and lack of circumcision (*Lancet* 1994; Mastro *et al.* 1994).

Prostitutes form a high-risk group for HIV infection in some areas. In Rwanda, 88 per cent of 33 female prostitutes were HIV positive (Van de Perre *et al.* 1985). In the West, HIV infection is commoner in prostitutes who are intravenous drug abusers than in others (Ward *et al.* 1993; Webster and Johnson, 1990). Recently, prostitution has been linked to the use of the drug 'crack' and the rapidly escalating HIV epidemic in many American urban areas has been attributed to the 'sex for drugs' subculture amongst the urban poor (Wolfe *et al.* 1992). Condom use has increased dramatically amongst prostitutes (Papaevangelou *et al.* 1988) yet many such women do not use them with regular or non-paying partners (Thomas *et al.* 1990).

The prevalence of HIV infection acquired by sharing needles varies dramatically in different cities. In Edinburgh, where infection was introduced into a relatively closed community in 1983/4 (Robertson *et al.* 1986), the prevalence was 51 per cent, whereas in London it was relatively rare (Webb *et al.* 1986). Attitudes to illegal drug use are very variable but there is a move now to damage-limitation policies, encouraging addicts to inject safely or to change to non-injectable drugs (Des Jarlais *et al.* 1985) and to use condoms (Ronald *et al.* 1993).

The risk of acquiring HIV infection as a result of blood transfusion is now very small in those countries where donated blood is tested for HIV antibody and where high-risk donors are asked not to donate blood. However, it is theoretically possible to be infected by blood from an individual who has been recently infected and is in the 'window period' before developing HIV antibody. Only one donation from a seronegative donor has transmitted HIV infection in the UK since screening started in 1985 (Barbara and Contreras 1990).

HIV has been transmitted by infected organ and semen donations (Stewart *et al.* 1985) and guidelines have been produced to prevent transmission by donated semen (Department of Health and Social Security 1986).

HIV has been found in blood, semen, saliva, tears, cervical secretions, breast milk, and urine. The titre of virus in some tissues and secretions is very low making them unlikely sources of infection. There is now very good evidence to confirm the fact that nosocomial spread does not occur. Mann *et al.* (1986) and Fischl *et al.* (1987*a*) could find no evidence for spread of the virus within households except by the established routes.

Epidemiology

Estimating the number of cases of HIV infection and AIDS and the future course of the epidemic is difficult. Reporting of AIDS is thought to be more complete than that of HIV infection, although the heavy work load and 'reporting fatigue' (B. G. Evans *et al.* 1991) in some large centres may result in an underestimate of current cases of AIDS by up to 20 per cent (Hickman *et al.* 1991).

Once a diagnosis of AIDS has been made, the patient had reached the attention of a physician and the case should be reported. HIV infection, however, is largely asymptomatic and detection is dependent on the infected individual being tested. Certainly in the early years of the epidemic, there was little incentive for a high-risk person to seek a test and the prejudice encountered by those who did, discouraged others. The advent of antiretroviral treatment has changed this somewhat, but widespread testing of low-risk individuals has not occurred. Estimates of numbers of cases of HIV infection are, therefore, widely variable.

In areas where HIV infection is common, such as New York, screening of high-risk groups failed to identify up to 86 per cent of HIV infected women (Krasinski *et al.* 1988). Furthermore, where voluntary screening was offered, the prevalence of infection amongst those who declined named testing was five times greater than amongst those who accepted testing (Hull *et al.* 1988.) Presumably in these areas, therefore, the epidemic is at a more advanced stage with spread beyond the risk groups into the general population.

Interestingly, at least until recently, testing of groups in the UK presumably at high risk of heterosexual transmission (such as STD clinic attenders) has revealed few cases of HIV infection outside the main risk groups (Evans *et al.* 1991; UK Collaborative Study 1989). This has led many to dismiss the risk of acquiring HIV infection heterosexually. A recent report (Evans *et al.* 1992), however, described transmission among young heterosexuals when no high-risk source could be identified. Heterosexual transmission is now the fastest growing transmission category.

Although in the West women and children still constitute a minority of cases of HIV infection and AIDS, in Africa, where heterosexual contact is the major mode of transmission, the sex ratio is 1:1 and the involvement of women has a major impact on the family. HIV infection and pregnancy is discussed in Chapter 21. The epidemic is developing along African lines in other parts of the world including South America and the Far East (Warden 1990).

The evidence suggests that most homosexually acquired HIV infection was acquired in the early 1980s and that, at least in the West, transmission of the virus by blood and blood products was virtually abolished with the introduction of the HIV test in 1985. The media campaigns of the mid and late 1980s ensured that there were few people who were unaware of AIDS. Many hoped that knowledge would be accompanied by a change in sexual behaviour, but it is clear that the message has had relatively little impact on young heterosexuals (see below). Furthermore, new cases of HIV infection are being seen in young homosexuals, suggesting that it is extremely difficult to modify behaviour on a longterm basis (Hunt *et al.* 1991).

Natural history

Within three months of acquisition, antibody develops and is detectable by the HIV antibody test. Seroconversion is sometimes accompanied by a 'flu-like illness with lymphadenopathy similar to infectious mononucleosis. Late seroconversion has been recorded but is exceedingly rare. The infection usually runs an asymptomatic course for many years. Sometimes persistent generalized lymphadenopathy (PGL) is present but this does not indicate a worse prognosis. Eventually, after a mean period of eight to ten years, depletion of T cells results in the development of symptoms and signs such as malaise, weight loss, persistent diarrhoea, and oral candidiasis, often known as the AIDS Related Complex (ARC). The diagnosis of AIDS is marked by the development of an 'indicator disease' such as *Pneumocystis carinii* pneumonia, Kaposi's sarcoma, atypical mycobacterial infections, central nervous system infections such as toxoplasmosis and cryptococcosis, disseminated cytomegalovirus infection, and others. Death is often preceded by severe wasting, incontinence, and dementia.

In women, an additional problem seems to be the high incidence of intraepithelial neoplasia which is multicentric involving the cervix, vagina, vulva, and perianal areas. Genital warts may also be particularly extensive and difficult to treat (Johnson *et al.* 1992).

It is now thought that between 75 per cent and 95 per cent of HIV infected individuals, without treatment, will develop AIDS which is almost invariably fatal (Lui *et al.* 1988; Moss *et al.* 1988). The mean survival time following a diagnosis of AIDS has increased from a few months in the early years to nearly two years now. During long periods of this time, the patient remains well and able to work. Approximately 55 per cent of all those diagnosed as having AIDS have died and this figure has been remarkably constant throughout the epidemic.

Diagnosis of HIV infection

The HIV antibody test becomes positive in almost all cases within three months of acquiring the infection and remains positive for the remainder of the individual's life. A few patients do lose antibody about the time that an AIDS indicator diagnosis is made. p24 antigen may be detected in the serum of some people before antibody appears and may occasionally be useful in early diagnosis. This antigen is also a marker of progression, although it is not invariably present as patients deteriorate. All the commercially available antibody tests are very well tested having high sensitivity and specificity. Before a positive result is given to a patient it is essential that the specimen has been tested using more than one method.

Since the diagnosis of HIV infection may have devastating effects on the individual, it is important that those who seek the test should have been appropriately counselled before undergoing the test (Barton and Roth 1992; Bor *et al.* 1991; *Lancet* 1991). A skilled counsellor should also be available when a positive result is given. Legal opinion obtained in the UK suggests that testing a patient without informed consent constitutes an assault. When the patient is unable or unwilling to give consent, but testing is thought appropriate, it is incumbent on the practitioner to justify his case which he may have to do in a court of law.

Prevention of HIV infection—safer sex?

It has long been accepted that barrier contraceptives provide some protection against STDs. Stone *et al.* (1986) reviewed a number of studies indicating that condoms reduce the likelihood of acquiring a wide range of STDs including gonorrhoea, NGU, and PID. It was postulated, therefore, that condoms might reduce HIV transmission. *In vitro* studies have demonstrated that HIV could not pass through five commercially available brands of condoms under experimental laboratory conditions (Conant *et al.* 1986). Krogsgaard *et al.* (1986) were unable to find evidence of HIV infection in 101 prostitutes whose clients always used condoms, and Mann *et al.* (1987) showed an inverse relationship between condom usage and the likelihood of prostitutes in Zaire being HIV positive (Table 6.8). In several studies of transmission rates when one partner in a stable relationship is infected and the other uninfected, condom use correlates with protection of the uninfected partner.

Safer sex practices also include reducing the numbers of sexual partners, ideally to one, and the avoidance of risky practices such as anal intercourse. Sexually active adolescents are a particularly vulnerable group as they appear to understand and be concerned about the risk but seem unable to modify their behaviour. Clarke *et al.* (1990) found that 63 per cent of sexually active

Table 6.8 Condom usage and HIV infection in prostitutes in Zaire*

Estimated partners using condoms %	No. of prostitutes	% HIV positive
0	288	26
0–25	55	35
26–49	22	32
50–4	2	0
75 +	6	0

*From Man et al. 1987

Table 6.9 Sexual behaviour of American college students*

| Behaviour | Proportion of students (%) in each year | | |
	1975	1986	1989
Sexually experienced	88	87	87
Using oral contraceptives	55	34	42
Using condoms for contraception	6	14	25
Using condoms plus other contraception	12	21	41

*From de Buono et al. 1990

adolescents had never used a condom. B. A. Evans *et al.* (1991) found that condom usage had increased in women attending a STD clinic between 1982 and 1989, but only from 3.6 to 16.2 per cent. The results of a study of college students' sexual behaviour (de Buono *et al.* 1990) are shown in Table 6.9.

Immunization might be one way of preventing HIV infection in the future. Despite a great deal of effort, the development of an effective vaccine is some way off (Schild and Stott 1993).

Treatment of HIV infection

Many of the indicator diseases of AIDS are treatable with very successful outcomes. The only drug currently licensed for the treatment of HIV infections *per se* is zidovudine (azidothymidine, AZT, Retrovir). Many of the early treatment trials have been widely criticized and in some cases were terminated prematurely, yet the results supporting the use of the drug in patients with AIDS and severe AIDS-related complex have been confirmed in clinical practice. Thus Fischl *et al.* (1987*b*) found that only one patient who received zidovudine died compared with 19 receiving placebo during a 24-week observation period. Others have produced similar results, although Dournon *et al.* (1988) found that the patients relapsed after six months of treatment and it is clear that eventually, zidovudine is unable to hold back the relentless progress of the disease.

The early studies used a large dose of zidovudine, 250 mg 4-hourly, which was associated with a high incidence of side-effects, in particular haematological toxicity. Lower-dose regimens are now in widespread use (Fischl *et al.* 1990*a*). Collier *et al.* (1990) reported that 300 mg daily was as effective as higher doses in improving clinical and laboratory parameters and was significantly less toxic.

Treating asymptomatic HIV infected individuals is much more controversial. In individuals with T-helper cell counts below 500/mm^3 Fischl *et al.* (1990*b*) found that progression to AIDS or ARC was significantly commoner in placebo-treated individuals as compared to zidovudine-treated individuals, and that haematological toxicity was much less common that in patients with more advanced disease. Graham *et al.* (1992) have shown that zidovudine reduces mortality significantly for all periods up to 24 months, but other studies have failed to demonstrate a benefit. The side-effects may, however, reduce the quality of life (Concord Co-ordinating Committee 1994; Oddone *et al.* 1993). In this study prophylaxis against PCP was also shown to reduce mortality rates. Unfortunately, some strains of HIV have developed resistance to zidovudine but the clinical significance of this finding is unknown as yet (Marx 1989).

Numerous other drugs have undergone or are undergoing evaluation and clinical trial. The most promising are perhaps DDI (dideoxyinosine) and DDC (dideoxycitidine), but their use is limited by peripheral neuropathy and, in some cases, acute pancreatitis (de Clercq 1991).

HIV and health-care workers

The only case so far of a health-care worker infecting a patient is of an American dentist, five of whose patients were found to be infected with an HIV strain matching that of the dentist (Centers for Disease Control 1991*b*). Several other cases of infected health care workers have been reported and when their patients have been tested, no unexpected case of HIV infection has been detected. The risk to the patient is, therefore, thought to be very low (Porter *et al.* 1990). In the US it is now an offence for a HIV infected health-care worker to fail to tell a patient of his infection before performing an invasive procedure (Morris 1991). In the UK, the General Medical Council has stated that 'it is unethical for doctors who know or believe themselves to be infected with HIV to put patients at risk by failing to seek appropriate counselling or to act upon it when given' (*British Medical Journal* 1987). It is likely that failure to observe these guidelines would result in disciplinary action for serious professional misconduct.

Conversely, the risk of a health-care worker becoming infected by a patient is small but real. Gazzard and Wastell (1990) estimate that the risk of infection is one case every 80 years in low-prevalence areas and one case every eight years in high-prevalence areas. Needlestick injuries constitute the greatest risk, although a few cases worldwide have been attributed to contamination of mucous membranes or broken skin. The risk of acquiring HIV infection after a significant needlestick injury with HIV positive blood is 0.36 per cent (Jeffries 1992).

Techniques to protect health-care workers include safer working practices and especially the safe handling of sharp instruments. Double gloving (Matta *et al.* 1988) reduces the number of exposures of surgeons' skin to patients' blood as a result of glove puncture by 72 per cent. Screening patients before surgery has been advocated by some, but this would not be possible before emergency surgery and would not identify patients who were infected but had not yet seroconverted. Furthermore, such testing would be likely to engender a false sense of security since many other infections can be transmitted in the same way and can only be prevented by attention to safe practices. Screening selected high-risk patients is also likely to be counterproductive. Those who support screening also claim that identification of infected patients would enable a surgeon to decline non-essential surgery thus reducing the risk to staff. The ethics of such an approach have not been fully debated and the legal situation has not been tested, but the General Medical Council has said that patients should not be denied treatment simply on account of being HIV positive.

Even were screening practically and ethically acceptable there is little evidence to support the claim that it would lead to less occupational accidents. In a study from San Francisco, knowledge of the patient's HIV status did not reduce the risk of surgical accidents (Gerberding *et al.* 1990).

It has been suggested that the use of zidovudine might prevent HIV infection if a percutaneous exposure to HIV positive blood has occurred. In primates, zidovudine failed to protect against exposure to simian immunodeficiency virus even when given prior to inoculation of the virus. If the drug were to be effective in humans it would need to be given very soon after the injury, before the first replicative cycle of the virus. There have been a few reported cases of failure of prophylaxis, in one case the drug being given less than an hour after the incident (Lange *et al.* 1990). Conversely, it would be very difficult to demonstrate that the drug had prevented infection, especially as the likelihood of infection after one exposure is so low. A planned double-blind placebo-controlled trial was abandoned because it was unlikely to reach a valid conclusion (Jeffries 1991). Since there are no data to support the use of zidovudine in occupational exposures, the decision to use the drug must be one for the individual concerned after full counselling has taken place. The possible advantages must be weighed against the short-term toxicity and the unknown longterm complications (Brown *et al.* 1991).

Those who are at risk would be wise to have thought about the issues concerned and attempted to make a decision before such an incident has occurred (Bird and Gore 1993; Joint Working Party 1992). Recent guidelines from the Department of Health have stated that zidovudine prophylaxis should not be considered a necessary part of the management of an individual exposed to HIV positive blood.

Conclusions

Sexually transmitted diseases and genital tract infections represent a not insignificant part of gynaecological practice. When complications such as tubal infertility, ectopic pregnancy, and cervical cancer are considered, it can be seen that improved management of early disease would be enormously beneficial. Thus close liason between gynaecologists, genitourinary physicians, and microbiologists will pay dividends in terms of the quality and outcome of patient care.

References

Adams, H. G., Benson, E. A., Alexander, E. R., Vontver, L. A., Remington, M. A., and Holmes, K. K. (1976). Genital herpetic infection in men and women: clinical course and effect of topical application of adenine arabinoside. *Journal of Infectious Diseases* **133S**, A151–9.

Adler, M. W. and Mindel, A. (1988). Epidemiological aspects of genital tract infection in the female. In *Genital tract infection in women* (ed. M. J. Hare), pp. 93–108. Churchill Livingstone, Edinburgh.

Adler, M. W., Belsey, E. M., and Rogers, J. S. (1981). Sexually transmitted diseases in defined population of women. *British Medical Journal* **283**, 29–32.

Adler, M. W., Belsey, E. H., and O'Connor, B. H. (1982). Morbidity associated with pelvic inflammatory disease. *British Journal of Venereal Diseases* **58**, 151–7.

Ahmed-Jushuf, I. H., Arya, O. P., Hobson, D., Pratt, B. C., Hart, C. A., How, S. J., *et al.* (1988*a*). Ciprofloxacin treatment of chlamydial infections of urogenital tracts of women. *Genitourinary Medicine* **64**, 14–17.

Ahmed-Jushuf, I. H., Murray, A. E., and McKeown, J. (1988*b*). Managing trichomonal vaginitis refractory to conventional treatment with metronidazole. *Genitourinary Medicine* **64**, 25–9.

Alexander, I., Ashley, C. R., Smith, K. J., Harbour, J., Roome, A. P. C. H., and Darville, J. M. (1985). Comparison of ELISA with virus isolation for the diagnosis of genital herpes. *Journal of Clinical Pathology* **38**, 554–7.

Al-Nozha, M., Ramia, S., Al-Frayh, A., and Arif, M. (1990). Female to male: an inefficient mode of transmission of HIV. *Journal of the Acquired Immune Deficiency Syndromes* **3**, 193–4.

Amsel, R., Totten, P. A., Spiegel, C. A., Chen, K. C. S., Eschenbach, D., and Holmes, K. K. (1983). Non-specific vaginitis. *American Journal of Medicine* **74**, 14–22.

Anderson, J., Mindel, A., Tovey, S. J., and Williams, P. (1989). Primary and secondary syphilis, 20 years' experience. *Genitourinary Medicine* **65**, 239–43.

Arya, O. P., Rees, E., Percival, A., Alergant, C. D., Annels, E. H., and Turner, G. C. (1978). Epidemiology and treatment of gonorrhoea caused by penicillinase-producing strains in Liverpool. *British Journal of Venereal Diseases* **54**, 28–35.

Arya, O. P., Rees, E., Turner, G. C., Percival, A., Bartzokas, C. A., Annels, E. H. *et al.* (1984). Epidemiology of penicillinase-producing *Neisseria gonorrhoeae* in Liverpool from 1977 to 1982. *Journal of Infection* **8**, 70–83.

Austin, T. W., Smith, E. A., Darwish, R., Ralph, E. D., and Pattison, F. L. M. (1982). Metronidazole in a single-dose for the treatment of trichomoniasis. *British Journal of Venereal Diseases* **58**, 121–3.

Balsdon, M. J. and Tobin, J. M. (1988). Recurrent vaginal candidosis. *Genitourinary Medicine* **64**, 124–7.

Barbara, J. A. J. and Contreras, M. (1990). Infectious complications of blood transfusions. *British Medical Journal* **300**, 450–2.

Barbone, F., Austin, H., Louv, W. C., and Alexander, W. J. (1990). A follow-up study of methods of contraception, sexual activity, and rates of trichomoniasis, candidiasis, and bacterial vaginosis. *American Journal of Obstetrics and Gynecology* **163**, 510–14.

Barlow, D. and Phillips, I. (1978). Gonorrhoea in women. *Lancet* **i**, 761–4.

Barlow, D. and Phillips, I. (1984). Cefotaxime in the treatment of gonorrhoea caused by beta-lactamase-producing *Neisseria gonorrhoeae*. *Journal of Antimicrobial Chemotherapy* **14**, supp. B, 291–3.

Barton, S. and Roth, P. (1992). Life insurance and HIV antibody testing. *British Medical Journal* **305**, 902–3.

Barton, S. E., Munday, P. E., Kinghorn, G. R., van der Meijden, W. I., Stolz, E., Notowicz, A., *et al.* (1986*a*). Topical treatment of recurrent genital herpes simplex virus infections with trisodium phosphonoformate (forscarnet): double-blind, placebo-controlled multicentre study. *Genitourinary Medicine* **62**, 247–50.

Barton, S. E., Wright, L. K., Link, C. M., and Munday, P. E. (1986*b*). Screening to detect asymptomatic shedding of herpes simplex virus (HSV) in women with recurrent genital HSV infection. *Genitourinary Medicine* **62**, 181–5.

Barton, S. E., Davies, J. M., Moss, V. W., Tyms, A. S., and Munday, P. E. (1987). Asymptomatic shedding and subsequent transmission of genital herpes simplex virus. *Genitourinary Medicine* **63**, 102–5.

Beard, R. W., Reginald, P. W., and Wadsworth, J. (1988). Clinical features of women with chronic lower abdominal pain and pelvic congestion. *British Journal of Obstetrics and Gynaecology* **95**, 153–61.

Bellina, J. H. (1983). The use of the carbon dioxide laser in the management of condylomata acuminatum with eight-year follow-up. *American Journal of Obstetrics and Gynecology* **147**, 375–8.

Bhattacharya, M. N., Jephcott, A. E., and Morton, R. S. (1973). Diagnosis of gonorrhoea in women: comparison of sampling sites. *British Medical Journal* **2**, 748–50.

Biggar, R. J. (1991). Preventing AIDS now. *British Medical Journal* **303**, 1150–1.

Billingham, R. P. and Lewis, F. G. (1982). Laser versus electrical cautery in the treatment of condylomata acuminata of the anus. *Surgery, Gynecology, and Obstetrics* **155**, 865–7.

Bingham, J. S. and Steele, C. E. (1981). Treatment of vaginal candidosis with econazole nitrate and nystatin: a comparative study. *British Journal of Venereal Diseases* **57**, 204–7.

Bird, A. G. and Gore, S. M. (1993). Revised guide-lines for HIV infected health care workers. *British Medical Journal* **306**, 1013–14.

Bisschop, M. P. J. M., Merkus, J. M. W. M., Scheygrond, H., and van Cutsem, J. (1986). Co-treatment of the male partner in vaginal candidosis: a double-blind randomized control study. *British Journal of Obstetrics and Gynaecology* **93**, 79–81.

Blackwell, A. L., Fox, A. R., Phillips, I., and Barlow, D. (1983). Anaerobic vaginosis (non-specific vaginitis): clinical, microbiological and therapeutic findings. *Lancet* **ii**, 1379–82.

Bleker, O. P., Smalbraak, D. J. C., and Schutte, M. F. (1990). Bartholin's abscess: the role of *Chlamydia trachomatis*. *Genitourinary Medicine* **66**, 24–5.

Boothby, R. A., Carlson, J. A., Rubin, M., Morgan, M., and Mikuta, J. J. (1990).

Single application treatment of human papillomavirus infection of the cervix and vagina with trichloracetic acid. *Obstetrics and Gynecology* **76**, 278–80.

Bor, R., Miller, R., and Johnson, M. (1991). A testing time for doctors: counselling patients before an HIV test. *British Medical Journal* **303**, 905–7.

Botcherby, M., Gilchrist, C., Bremner, J., Byrne, M. A., Harris, J. R. W., and Taylor-Robinson, D. (1987). Rapid diagnosis of genital herpes by detecting cells infected with virus in smears with fluorescent monoclonal antibodies. *Journal of Clinical Pathology* **40**, 687–9.

Bowie, W. R., Alexander, E. R., and Holmes, K. K. (1977). Chlamydial pharyngitis? *Sexually Transmitted Diseases* **4**, 13–14.

Bowie, W. R., Manzon, L. M., Borrie-Hume, C. J., Fawcett, A., and Jones, H. D. (1982). Efficacy of treatment regimes for lower vaginal *Chlamydia trachomatis* infection in women. *American Journal of Obstetrics and Gynecology* **142**, 125–9.

Brihmer, C., Kallings, I., Nord, C. E., and Brundin, J. (1987). Salpingitis: aspects of diagnosis and etiology: a 4-year study from a Swedish capital hospital. *European Journal of Obstetrics, Gynaecology and Reproductive Biology* **24**, 211–20.

British Medical Journal (1987). GMC warns doctors infected with HIV or suffering from AIDS. *British Medical Journal* **295**, 1500.

Brookmeyer, R. (1991). Reconstruction and future trends of the AIDS epidemic in the United States. *Science* **253**, 37–42.

Brown, E. M., Caul, E. O., Roome, A. P. C. G., Glover, S. C., Reeves, D. S., and Harling, C. C. (1991). Zidovudine after occupational exposure to HIV. *British Medical Journal* **303**, 990.

Brown, M. I. (1984). Anaerobic vaginosis. *Lancet* **i**, 337.

Brunham, R. C. (1984). Therapy for pelvic inflammatory disease: a critique of recent treatment trials. *American Journal of Obstetrics and Gynecology* **148**, 235–40.

Brunham, R. C., Paavonen, J., Stevens, C. E., Kiviat, N., Kuo, C. C., Critchlow, C. W., et al. (1984). Mucopurulent cervicitis. *New England Journal of Medicine* **311**, 106.

Brunham, R. C., Binns, B., McDowell, J., and Paraskevas, M. (1986). *Chlamydia trachomatis* infection in women with ectopic pregnancy. *Obstetrics and Gynecology* **67**, 722–6.

Brunham, R. C., Binns, B., Guijon, F., Damforth, D., Kosseim, M. L., Rand, F. et al. (1988). Etiology and outcome of acute pelvic inflammatory disease. *Journal of Infectious Diseases* **158**, 510–17.

Bryson, Y. J., Dillion, M., Lovett, M., Acuna, G., Taylor, S., Cherry, J. D., et al. (1983). Treatment of first episodes of genital herpes simplex virus infection with oral acyclovir. *New England Journal of Medicine* **308**, 916–21.

Buchan, H. and Vessey, M. (1989). Epidemiology and trends in hospital discharges for pelvic inflammatory disease in England 1975–85. *British Journal of Obstetrics and Gynaecology* **96**, 1219–23.

Bump, R. C. and Bueschling, W. J. (1988). Bacterial vaginosis in virginal and sexually active adolescent females: evidence against exclusive sexual transmission. *American Journal of Obstetrics and Gynecology* **158**, 935–9.

Bump, R. C. and Fass, R. J. (1985). Pelvic inflammatory disease. In *Sexually transmitted diseases* (ed. V. A. Spagna and R. B. Prior), pp. 187–220. Marcel Dekker, New York.

Bump, R. C., Zuspan, F. R., Bueschling, W. J., Ayers, L. W., and Stephens, T. J. (1984). The prevalence, six-month persistence, and predictive values of laboratory indicators of bacterial vaginosis (nonspecific vaginitis) in asymptomatic women. *American Journal of Obstetrics and Gynecology* **150**, 917–24.

Burkman, R., Schlesselman, S., McCaffrey, L., Gupta, P. K., and Spence, M. (1982). The relationship of genital tract actinomycetes and the development of pelvic inflammatory disease. *American Journal of Obstetrics and Gynecology* 143, 585-9.

Burns, W. H., Saral, R., Santos, G. W., Laskin, O. L., Lietman, P. S., McLaren, C., *et al.* (1982). Isolation and characterization of resistant herpes simplex virus after acyclovir therapy. *Lancet* i, 421-3.

Carney, J. A., Unadakat, P., Yule, A., Rajakumar, R., Lacey, C. N. J., and Ackers, J. P. (1988). New rapid latex test for diagnosis of *Trichomonas vaginalis* infection. *Journal of Clinical Pathology* 41, 806-8.

Chen, K. C. S., Forsyth, P. S., Buchanan, T. M., and Holmes, K. K. (1979). Amine content of vaginal fluid from untreated and treated patients with non-specific vaginitis. *Journal of Clinical Investigation* 63, 328-35.

Chuang, T. Y., Perry, H. U., Kurland, L. T., and Ilstrup, D. M. (1984). Condylomata acuminata in Rochester. *Archives of Dermatology* 120, 469-75.

Clarke, J., Abram, R., and Monteiro, E. F. (1990). The sexual behaviour and knowledge about AIDS in a group of young adolescent girls in Leeds. *Genitourinary Medicine* 66, 189-92.

Clay, J. C., Veeravanu, M., and Smyth, R. A. (1988). Practical problems of diagnosing trichomoniasis in women. *Genitourinary Medicine* 64, 115-17.

Collier, A. C., Judson, F. N., Murphy, V. L., Leach, L. A., Root, C. J., and Handsfield, H. H. (1984). Comparative study of ceftriaxone and spectinomycin in the treatment of uncomplicated gonorrhea in women. *American Journal of Medicine* 77(4C), 68-72.

Collier, A. C., Bozzette, E. S., Coombs, R. W., Causey, D. M., Schoenfeld, D. A., Spector, S. A., *et al.* (1990). A pilot study of low-dose zidovudine in human immunodeficiency virus infection. *New England Journal of Medicine* 323, 1015-21.

Cates, W. and Wasserheit, J. N. (1991). Genital chlamydial infections: epidemiology and reproductive sequelae. *American Journal of Obstetrics and Gynecology* 164, 1771-31.

Catterall, R. D. (1972). Systemic disease and the biological false-positive reaction. *British Journal of Venereal Diseases* 48, 1-12.

Centers for Disease Control (1982). *Pneumocystis carinii pneumonia among persons with hemophilia A. Morbidity and Mortality Weekly Report* 31, 365-7.

Centers for Disease Control (1989). Sexually transmitted diseases treatment guidelines. *Morbidity and Mortality Weekly Report* 38, supp 8, 4-43.

Centers for Disease Control (1991a). Pelvic inflammatory disease: guidelines for prevention and management. *Morbidity and Mortality Weekly Report* 40, supp RR5, 1-25.

Centers for Disease Control (1991b). Transmission of HIV infection during an invasive dental procedure. *Morbidity and Mortality Weekly Report* 40, 377-81.

Conant, M., Hardy, D., Sernatinger, J., Spicer, D., and Levy, J. A. (1986). Condoms prevent transmission of AIDS-associated retrovirus. *Journal of the American Medical Association* 255, 1706.

Concord Co-ordinating Committee (1994). MRC-ANRS randomized double blind control trial of immediate and deferred zidovudine in symptom-free HIV infection. *Lancet* 343, 871-81.

Confidential Enquiry into Gynaecological Laparoscopy (1978). In *The complications of laparoscopy* (ed. by G. Chamberlain and J. Carron-Brown), pp. 105-39. Royal College of Obstetricians and Gynaecologists, London.

Corey, L. (1990). Genital herpes. In *Sexually transmitted diseases* (2nd edn.), (ed. K. K. Holmes, P-A. Mardh, P. F. Sparling, P. P. Wiesner, W. Cates, S. M. Lemon, *et al.*), pp. 391-414. McGraw Hill, New York.

Corey, L., Adams, H. G., Brown, Z. A., and Holmes, K. K. (1983). Genital herpes simplex virus infections. clinical manifestations, course and complications. *Annals of Internal Medicine* **98**, 958–72.

Cunningham, F. G., Hauth, J. C., Gilstrap, L. C., Herbert, W. N. P., and Cappus, S. S. (1978). The bacterial pathogenesis of acute pelvic inflammatory disease. *Obstetrics and Gynecology* **52**, 161–4.

Darougar, S., Walpita, P., Thaker, U., Goh, B. T., and Dunlop, E. M. C. (1986). A rapid and sensitive culture test for the laboratory diagnosis of genital herpes in women. *Genitourinary Medicine* **62**, 93–6.

Davidson, F. and Oates, J. K. (1985). The pill does not cause 'thrush'. *British Journal of Obstetrics and Gynaecology* **92**, 1265–6.

Davidson, F., Hayes, J. P., and Hussein, S. (1977). Recurrent genital candidosis and iron metabolism. *British Journal of Venereal Diseases* **53**, 123–5.

Davidson-Parker, J., Dinsmore, W., Khan, M. H., Hicks, D. N., Morris, C. A., and Morris, D. F. (1988). Immunotherapy of genital warts with inosine pranobex and conventional treatment: double-blind placebo-controlled trial. *Genitourinary Medicine* **64**, 383–6.

De Buono, B. A., Zinner, S. H., Daamen, M., and McCormack, W. M. (1990). Sexual behaviour of college women in 1975, 1986, and 1989. *New England Journal of Medicine* **322**, 321–5.

De Clercq, E. (1991). Basic approaches to anti-retroviral treatnent. *Journal of the Acquired Immune Deficiency Syndromes* **4**, 207–18.

Department of Health (1989). New cases seen at NHS genitourinary medicine clinics in England and Wales. Circulated to genitourinary medicine departments.

Department of Health and Social Security (1986). Acquired immune deficiency syndrome (AIDS) and artificial insemination: Guidance for doctors and AI clinics. *DHSS Publications* **CMO (86)**, 12.

Des Jarlais, C. D., Friedman, S. R., and Hopkins, W. (1985). Risk reduction for the acquired immunodeficiency syndrome among intravenous drug users. *Annals of Internal Medicine* **103**, 755–9.

Dournon, E., Matheron, S., Rozenbaum, W., Gharakhanian, S., Mickon, C., Girard, P. M., *et al.* (1988). Effects of zidovudine in 365 consecutive patients with AIDS or AIDS-related complex. *Lancet* **ii**, 1297–1302.

Driscoll, A. M., McCoy, D. R., Nicol, C. S., and Barrow, J. (1970). Sexually transmitted disease in gynaecological out-patients with vaginal discharge. *British Journal of Venereal Diseases* **46**, 125.

Dunlop, E. M. C., Garner, A., Darougar, S., Treharne, J. D., and Woodland, R. M. (1989). Colposcopy, biopsy, and cytology results in women with chlamydial cervicitis. *Genitourinary Medicine* **65**, 22–31.

Edwards, A., Atma-Ram, A., and Thin, R. N. (1988). Podophyllotoxin 0.5 per cent versus podophyllin 20 per cent to treat penile warts. *Genitourinary Medicine* **64**, 263–5.

Edwards, D. I., Thompson, E. J., Tomusange, J., and Shanson, D. (1979). Inactivation of metronidazole by aerobic organisms. *Journal of Antimicrobial Chemotherapy* **5**, 315–16.

Elegbe, I. A. and Elegbe, I. (1983). Quantitative relationships of *Candida albicans* infections and dressing patterns in Nigerian women. *American Journal of Public Health* **73**, 450–2.

Eschenbach, D. A. (1993). History and review of bacterial vaginosis. *American Journal of Obstetrics and Gynecology* **169**, 441–5.

Eschenbach, D. A., Hillier, S., Critchlow, C., Stevens, C., DeRouen, T., and Holmes, K. K. (1988). Diagnosis and clinical manifestations of bacterial vaginosis. *American Journal of Obstetrics and Gynecology* **158**, 819–28.

Evans, B. A. and Catterall, R. D. (1971). Nitrimidazine compared with metronidazole in the treatment of vaginal trichomoniasis. *British Medical Journal* 4, 146-7.

Evans, B. A., McLean, K. A., Dawson, S. G., Teece, S. A., Bond, R. A., MacRae K. D., *et al.* (1989). Trends in sexual behaviour and risks factors for HIV infection among homosexual men, 1984-7. *British Medical Journal* 298, 215-18.

Evans, B. A., McCormack, S. M., Bond, R. A., and MacRae, K. D. (1991). Trends in sexual behaviour and HIV testing among women presenting at a genitourinary medicine clinic during the advent of AIDS. *Genitourinary Medicine* 67, 194-8.

Evans, B. C., Gill, O. N., and Emslie, J. A. N. (1991). Completeness of reporting of AIDS cases. *British Medical Journal* 302, 1351-2.

Evans, B. G., Noone, A., Mortimer, J. Y., Gilbart, V. L., Ig O.P., Picoll, A. *et al.* (1992). Peterosexually Gill, O. N., Nicoll, A., *et al.* (1992). Heterosexually .IG acquired HIV-1 infection: cases reported in England, Wales and Northern Ireland 1935-91. *Communicable Disease Report* 2, **Review 5**, 24th April 1992.

Faro, S. (1991). *Chlamydia trachomatis*: female pelvic infection. *American Journal of Obstetrics and Gynecology* 164, 1767-70.

Ferenczy, A. (1984). Treating genital condylomata during pregnancy with the carbon dioxide laser. *American Journal of Obstetrics and Gynecology* 148, 9-12.

Ferenczy, A., Mital, M., Nagai, N., Silverstein, S. J., and Crum, C. P. (1985). Latent papilloma virus and recurring genital warts. *New England Journal of Medicine* 313, 784-8.

Ferrer, R. M., Kraiselburd, E. N., and Kouri, Y. H. (1984). Inapparent genital herpes simplex infection in women attending a venereal disease clinic. *Sexually Transmitted Diseases* 11, 91-3.

Fife, K. H. and Corey, L. (1990). Herpes simplex virus. In *Sexually transmitted diseases* (2nd edn), (ed. K. K. Holmes, P. A. Mardh, P. F. Starling, P. P. Wiesner, W. Cates, S. M. Lemon, *et al.*), pp. 941-52. McGraw Hill, New York.

Fischbach, F., Petersen, E. E., Weissenbacher, E. R., Martius, J., Hosmann, J., and Mayer, H. (1993). Efficacy of clindamycin vaginal cream versus oral placebo in the treatment of bacterial vaginosis. *Obstetrics and Gynecology* 82, 405-10.

Fischl, M. A., Dickinson, G. M., Scott, G. B., Klimas, N., Fletcher, M. A., and Parks, W. (1987*a*). Evaluation of heterosexual partners, children, and household contacts of adults with AIDS. *Journal of the American Medical Association* 257, 640-4.

Fischl, M. A., Richman, D. D., Grieco, M. H., Gottlieb, M. S., Volberding, P. A., Laskin, L. L., *et al.* (1987*b*). The efficacy of (azidothymidine) AZT in the treatment of patients with AIDS and AIDS-related complex. *New England Journal of Medicine* 317, 185-91.

Fischl, M. A., Parker, C. B., Pettinelli, C., Wulfsohn, M., Hirsch, M. S., Collies, A. C., *et al.* (1990*a*). A randomized controlled trial of a reduced daily dose of zidovudine in patients with the acquired immunodeficiency syndrome. *New England Journal of Medicine* 323, 1009-14.

Fischl, M. A., Richman, D. D., Hassan, N., Collier, A. C., Corey, J. T., Param, F., *et al.* (1990*b*). Safety and efficacy of zidovudine in the treatment of subjects with midly symptomatic human immunodeficiency virus type I (HIV) infection. *Annals of Internal Medicine* 112, 727-37.

Fish, A. N. J., Robinson, G., Bounds, W., Fairweather, D. V. I., Guillebaund, J., Oriel, J. D., *et al.* (1987). *Chlamydia trachomatis* in various groups of contraceptors: preliminary observations. *British Journal of Family Planning* 13, 84-7.

Fleury, F., Hughes, D., and Floyd, R. (1985). Therapeutic results obtained in vaginal mycoses after single-dose treatment with 500 mg clotrimazole vaginal tablets. *American Journal of Obstetrics and Gynecology* 152, 968-70.

Forssman, L. and Milsom, I. (1985). Treatment of recurrent vaginal candidiasis. *American Journal of Obstetrics and Gynecology* **152**, 959-61.

Fouts, A. C. and Kraus, S. J. (1980). *Trichomonas vaginalis*: re-evaluation of its clinical presentation and laboratory diagnosis. *Journal of Infectious Diseases* **141**, 137-43.

Fox, H. (1983). Chlamydial cervicitis: a research study from general practice. *Journal of the Royal College of General Practitioners* **33**, 721-4.

Gabriel, and Thin, R. N. T. (1983). Treatment of anogenital warts. *British Journal of Venereal Diseases* **59**, 124-6.

Gardner, H. L. and Dukes, C. D. (1955). *Haemophilus vaginalis* vaginitis. *American Journal of Obstetrics and Gynecology* **69**, 62-76.

Gardner, H., Dampeer, T. K., and Dukes, C. D. (1957). The prevalence of vaginitis. *American Journal of Obstetrics and Gynecology* **73**, 1080-7.

Gazzard, B. G. and Wastell, C. (1990). HIV and surgeons. *British Medical Journal* **301**, 1003-4.

Gerberding, J. L., Littell, C., Tarkington, A., Brown, A., and Schecter, W. P. (1990). Risk of exposure of surgical personnel to patients' blood during surgery at San Francisco General Hospital. *New England Journal of Medicine* **322**, 1788-93.

Gilstrap, L. C., Herbert, W. N., Cunningham, F. G., Hauth, J. C., and Van Patten, H. G. (1977). Gonorrhea screening in male consorts of women with pelvic infection. *Journal of the American Medical Association* **238**, 965-6.

Goldacre, M. J., Loudon, N., Watt, B., Grant, G., Loudon, J. D. O., McPherson, K., *et al.* (1978). Epidemiology and clinical significance of cervical erosion in women attending a family planning clinic. *British Medical Journal* **1**, 748-50.

Goldberg, C. B. (1986). Controlled trial of 'Intervir-A' in herpes simplex virus infection. *Lancet* **i**, 703-6.

Goldmeier, D., Johnson, A., Byrne, M. A., and Barton, S. E. (1988). Psychosocial implications of recurrent genital herpes simplex virus infection. *Genitourinary Medicine* **64**, 327-30.

Gottleib, M. S., Schroff, R., Schanker, H. M., Weisman, J. D., Fan, P. T., Wolf, R. A., *et al.* (1981). *Pneumocystis carinii* pneumonia and mucosal candidiasis in previously healthy homosexual men. *New England Journal of Medicine* **305**, 1425-31.

Graham, N. M. H., Zeger, S. L., Park, L. P., Vermund, S. H., Detels, R., Rinaldo, C. R., *et al.* (1992). The effects on survival of early treatment of human immunodeficiency virus infection. *New England Journal of Medicine* **326**, 1037-42.

Griffiths, M. (1989). Genital warts and the need for screening. *Genitourinary Medicine* **65**, 339.

Hager, W. D. (1983). Follow-up of patients with tubo-varian abscess(es) in association with salpingitis. *Obstetrics and Gynecology* **61**, 680-4.

Hager, W. D., Brown, S. T., Kraus, S. J., Kleris, G. S., Perkins, G. J., and Henderson, M. (1980). Metronidazole for vaginal trichomoniasis. *Journal of the American Medical Association* **244**, 1219-20.

Hamark, B., Brorsson, J. E., Eilard, T., and Forssman, L. (1976). Salpingitis and chlamydiae subgroup A. *Acta Obstetrica et Gynaecologica Scandinavica* **S5**, 377-8.

Handsfield, H. H. (1983). Gonorrhea and uncomplicated gonococcal infection. In *Sexually transmitted diseases* (ed. K. K. Holmes, P-A. Mardh, P. F. Sparling, and P. P. Wiesner, W. Cates, S. M. Lemon, *et al.*), pp. 205-220. McGraw Hill, New York.

Harris, C., Small, C. B., Klein, R. S., Friedland, G. H., Moll, B., Emeson, E. E., *et al.* (1983). Immunodeficiency in female sexual partners of men with the acquired immunodeficiency syndrome. *New England Journal of Medicine* **308**, 1181-4.

Hasumi, K. (1987). A trial of topical idoxuridine for vulvar condyloma acuminatum. *British Journal of Obstetrics and Gynaecology* **94**, 366-8.

Hickman, M., Aldous, J., Porter, J., and Durman, L. (1991). HIV surveillance: the value of audit. *British Medical Journal* 302, 1376-7.

Hill, G. B. (1993). The microbiology of bacterial vaginosis. *American Journal of Obstetrics and Gynecology* 169, 450-4.

Hillier, S. L. (1993). Diagnostic microbiology of bacterial vaginosis. *American Journal of Obstetrics and Gynecology* 169, 455-9.

Hillier, S. L., Lipinski, C., Briselden, A. M., and Eschenbach, D. A. (1993). Efficacy of intravaginal metronidazole gel for the treatment of bacterial vaginosis. *Obstetrics and Gynecology* 81, 963-7.

Hillis, S. D., Joesoef, R., Marchbanks, P. A., Wassenheit, J. N., Cates, W., and Westrom, L. (1993). Delayed care of pelvic inflammatory disease as a risk factor for impaired fertility. *American Journal of Obstetrics and Gynecology* 168, 1503-9.

Hilton, A. L. and Warnock, D. W. (1975). Vaginal candidiasis and the role of the digestive tract as a source of infection. *British Journal of Obstetrics and Gynaecology* 82, 922-6.

Hilton, A. L., Richmond, S. J., Milne, J. D., Hindley, F., and Clarke, S. K. (1974). Chlamydia A in the female genital tract. *British Journal of Venereal Diseases* 50, 1-10.

Hodge, C. H. and Murdoch, R. (1963). Treatment of vaginal discharge by sulphonamide pessaries. *American Journal of Obstetrics and Gynecology* 36, 742-4.

Holmes, K. K. (1990). Lower genital tract infections in women: cystitis, urethritis, vulvovaginitis, and cervicitis. In *Sexually transmitted diseases* (2nd edn), (ed. K. K. Holmes, P-A. Mardh, P. F. Sparling, P. P. Wiesner, W. Cates, S. M. Lemon, *et al.*), pp. 527-45. McGraw Hill, New York.

Hull, H. F., Bettinger, C. J., Gallaher, M. M., Keller, N. M., Wilson, J., and Mertz, G. J. (1988). Comparison of HIV-antibody prevalence in patients consenting to and declining HIV antibody testing in an STD clinic. *Journal of the American Medical Association* 260, 935-8.

Hunt, A. J., Davies, P. M., Weatherburn, P., Coxon, A. P. M., and McManus, T. J. (1991). Changes in sexual behaviour in a large cohort of homosexual men in England and Wales, 1988-9. *British Medical Journal* 302, 505-6.

Idsoe, O., Guthe, T., and Wilcox, R. R. (1972). Penicillin in the treatment of syphilis. *Bulletin of the World Health Organization* 47, supp 5-68.

International Multicentre Trial (1989). A comparison of single-dose oral fluconazole with 3-day intravaginal clotrimazole in the treatment of vaginal candidiasis. *British Journal of Obstetrics and Gynaecology* 96, 226-32.

Ison, C. A. (1990). Laboratory methods in genitourinary medicine. Methods of diagnosing gonorrhoea. *Genitourinary Medicine* 66, 453-9.

Ison, C. A., Gedney, J., and Easmon, C. S. F. (1987). Chromosonal resistance of gonococci to antibiotics. *Genitourinary Medicine* 63, 239-43.

Ison, C. A., Bramley, N. S., Kirtland, K., and Easmon, C. S. F. (1991). Surveillance of antibody resistance in clinical isolates of *N. gonorrhoeae*. *British Medical Journal* 303, 1307.

Jacobson, L. and Westrom, L. (1969). Objectivized diagnosis of acute pelvic inflammatory disease. *American Journal of Obstetrics and Gynecology* 105, 1088-98.

Jeffries, D. J. (1991). Zidovudine after occupational exposure to HIV. *British Medical Journal* 302, 1349-51.

Jeffries, D. J. (1992). Doctors, patients, and HIV. *British Medical Journal* 304, 1258-9.

Jenkins, H. M. L. and Riley, V. C. (1980). A review of out-patient management of female genital warts. *British Journal of Clinical Practice* 34, 273-5.

Jensen, S. L. (1985). Comparison of podophyllin application with simple surgical excision in clearance and recurrence of perianal conlylomata acuminata. *Lancet* ii, 1146-8.

Jett, J. R., Kuritsky, J. N., Katzkmann, J. A., and Homburger, H. A. (1983). Acquired immunodeficiency syndrome associated with blood-product transfusions. *Annals of Internal Medicine* **99**, 621–4.

Johannisson, G., Lowhagen, G. B., and Lycke, E. (1980). Genital *Chlamydia trachomatis* infection in women. *Obstetrics and Gynecology* **56**, 671–5.

Johnson, A. M. (1992). Home grown heterosexually acquired HIV infection. *British Medical Journal* **304**, 1125–6.

Johnson, J. C., Burnett, A. F., Willet, G. D., Young, M. A., and Doniger, J. (1992). High frequency of latent and clinical papillomavirus cervical infections in immunocompromised human immunodeficiency virus-infected women. *Obstetrics and Gynecology* **79**, 321–7.

Johnson, R. E., Nahmias, A. J., Magder, L. S., Lee, F. K., Brooks, C. A., and Snowden, C. B. (1989). A seroepidemiologic survey of the prevalence of herpes simplex virus type 2 infection in the United States. *New England Journal of Medicine* **321**, 7–12.

Joint Working Party (1992). Risk to surgeons and patients from HIV and hepatitis. *British Medical Journal* **305**, 1337–43.

Jones, B. M., Geary, I., Alawattegama, A. B., Kinghorn, G. R., and Duerden, B. I. (1985). *In-vitro* and *in-vivo* activity of metronidazole against *Gardnerella vaginalis*, *Bacteroides* spp, and Mobiluncus spp in bacterial vaginasis. *Journal of Antimicrobial Chemotherapy* **16**, 189–97.

Kampmeier, R. H., Sweeney, E., Quinn, R. W., Lefkowitz, L. B., and Dupont, W. D. (1981). A survey of 251 patients with acute syphilis treated in the collaborative penicillin study of 1943–50. *Sexually Transmitted Diseases* **8**, 266–79.

Kanki, P. J., Travers, K. U., Boup, S. M., Hsieh, C. C., Marlink, R. G., Diaye, A. G. N., *et al.* (1994). Slower heterosexual spread of HIV-2 than HIV-1. *Lancet* **343**, 943–6.

Keat, A., Thomas, B., Dixey, J., Osborn, M., Sonnex, C., and Taylor-Robinson, D. (1987). *Chlamydia trachomatis* and reactive arthritis: the missing link. *Lancet* **i**, 72–4.

Keighley, E. E. (1971). Trichomoniasis in a closed community: efficacy of metronidazole. *British Medical Journal* **1**, 207–9.

Kinghorn, G. R., Abeywickreme, I., Jeavons, M., Rowland, M., Barton, I., Al-Hasani, G., *et al.* (1986*a*). Efficacy of oral treatment with acyclovir and co-trimoxazole in first episodo genital herpes. *Genitourinary Medicine* **62**, 33–7.

Kinghorn, G. R., Abeywickreme, I., Jeavons, M., Barton, I., Potter, C. W., Jones, D., *et al.* (1986*b*). Efficacy of combined treatment with oral and topical acyclovir in first episode genital herpes. *Genitourinary Medicine* **62**, 186–8.

Krasinski, K., Borkowsky, W., Bebenroth, D., and Moore, T. (1988). Failure of voluntary testing for human immunodeficiency virus to identify infected parturient women in a high-risk population. *New England Journal of Medicine* **318**, 185.

Krieger, J. N., Tam, M. R., Stevens, C. E., Nielsen, I. O., Hale, J., Kiviat, N. B., *et al.* (1988). Diagnosis of trichomoniasis. *Journal of the American Medical Association* **259**, 1223–7.

Krogsgaard, K., Gluud, C., Pedersen, C., Neilsen, J., Juhl, E., Gerstoft, J., *et al.* (1986). Widespread use of condoms and low prevalence of sexually transmitted diseases in Danish non-drug addict prostitutes. *British Medical Journal* **2**, 1473–4.

Lancet (1984). Disseminated gonococcal infection. *Lancet* **i**, 832–3.

Lancet (1988). HIV-2 in perspective. *Lancet* **i**, 1027–8.

Lancet (1991). HIV counselling in the 1990s. *Lancet* **337**, 950.

Lancet (1994). AIDS, the third wave. *Lancet* **343**, 186–8.

Landers, D. D. and Sweet, R. L. (1985). Current trends in the diagnosis and treatment of tubo-ovarian abscess. *American Journal of Obstetrics and Gynecology* **151**, 1098–110.

Lange, J. M. A., Boucher, C. A. B., Hollak, C. E. M., Wiltink, E. H. H., Reiss, P., van Royen, E. A., *et al.* (1990). Failure of zidovudine prophylaxis after accidental exposure to HIV-1. *New England Journal of Medicine* **322**, 1375–7.

Lavery, H. A., Connolly, J. H., and Russell, J. D. (1986). Incidence of herpes genitalis in Northern Ireland in 1973–83 and herpes simplex types 1 and 2 isolated in 1982–4. *Genitourinary Medicine* **62**, 24–7.

Lebherz, T., Guess, E., and Wolfson, N. (1985). Efficacy of single-versus multiple-dose clotrimazole therapy in the management of vulvovaginal candidiasis. *American Journal of Obstetrics and Gynecology* **152**, 965–8.

Ledger, W. J. (1993). Historical review of the treatment of bacterial vaginosis. *American Journal of Obstetrics and Gynecology* **169**, 474–8.

Leegaard, M. (1984). The incidence of *Candida albicans* in the vagina of healthy young women. *Acta Obstetrica et Gynaecological Scandinavica* **63**, 85–9.

Lehtinen, M., Rantala, I., Teisala, K., Heinonen, P. K., Lehtinen, T., Aine, R., *et al.* (1985). Detection of herpes simplex virus in women with acute pelvic inflammatory disease. *Journal of Infectious Diseases* **152**, 78–82.

Lewis, J. H., Zimmerman, H. J., Benson, G. D., and Iscak, K. G. (1984). Hepatic injury associated with ketoconazole treatment. *Gastroenterology* **86**, 503–13.

Livengood, C. H., Thomason, J. L., and Hill, G. B. (1990). Bacterial vaginosis: treatment with topical intravaginal clindamycin phosphate. *Obstetrics and Gynecology* **76**, 118–23.

Longhurst, H. J., Flower, N., Thomas, B. J., Munday, P. E., Elder, A., Constantinidou, M., *et al.* (1987). A simple method for the detection of *Chlamydia trachomatis* infections in general practice. *Journal of the Royal College of General Practitioners* **37**, 255–6.

Lorincz, A. T. (1990). Human papillomavirus detection tests. In *Sexually transmitted diseases* (2nd edn), (ed. K. K. Holmes, P-A. Mardh, P. F. Sparling, P. P. Wiesner, W. Cates, S.M. Holmes, *et al.*), pp. 953–60. McGraw Hill, New York.

Lui, K. J., Darrow, W. W., and Rutherford, G. W. (1988). A model-based estimate of the mean incubation period for AIDS in homosexual men. *Science* **240**, 1333–5.

Lumsden, W. H. R., Robertson, D. H. H., Heyworth, R., and Harrison, C. (1988). Treatment failure in *Trichomonas vaginalis* vaginitis. *Genitourinary Medicine* **64**, 217–18.

McLellan, R., Spence, M. R., Brockman, M., Raffel, L., and Smith, J. L. (1982). The clinical diagnosis of trichomoniasis. *Obstetrics and Gynecology* **60**, 30–4.

McLennan, M. T., Smith, J. M., and McLennan, C. E. (1972). Diagnosis of vaginal mycosis and trichomoniasis. *Obstetrics and Gynecology* **40**, 231–40.

McMillan, A. and Scott, G. R. (1987). Outpatient treatment of perianal warts by scissor excision. *Genitourinary Medicine* **63**, 114–15.

McNulty, A., Kaldor, J. M., McDonald, A. M., Baumgart, K., and Cooper, D. A. (1994). Acquired immunodeficiency without evidence of HIV infection. *British Medical Journal* **308**, 825–6.

Main, J. and Handley, J. (1992). Interferon: current and future clinical uses in infectious disease practice. *International Journal of STD and AIDS* **3**, 4–9.

Malison, M. D., Morris, R., and Jones, L. W. (1982). Autogenous vaccine therapy for condylomata acuminatum. *British Journal of Venereal Diseases* **58**, 62–5.

Mann, J. M., Quinn, T. C., Francis, H., Nzilambi, N., Bosange, N., Bila, K., *et al.* (1986). Prevalence of HTLV–III/LAV in household contacts of patients with confirmed AIDS and controls in Kinshasa, Zaire. *Journal of the American Medical Association* **256**, 721–4.

Mann, J. M., Quinn, T. C., Piot, P., Bosange, N., Izilambi, N., Kalala, M., et al. (1987). Condom use and HIV infection among prostitutes in Zaire. New England Journal of Medicine 316, 345.

Mardh, P-A. and Taylor-Robinson, D. (1984). Bacterial vaginosis. Introduction. Almqvist and Wiksell International, Stockholm.

Mardh, P-A. and Westrom, L. (1970). Tubal and cervical cultures in acute salpingitis with special reference to Mycoplasma hominis and T-strain mycoplasms. British Journal of Venereal Diseases 46, 179–86.

Marsh, P. (1990). Porton International, herpes vaccine, and the CA British Medical Journal 310, 1291.

Marx, J. (1989). Drug resistant strains of AIDS virus found. Science 243, 1551–2.

Maskell, R., Pead, L., and Allen, J. (1979). The puzzle of 'urethral syndrome': a possible answer? Lancet i, 1088–9.

Masterton, G., Henderson, J. N., Napier, I., and Moffett, M. (1976). Vaginal candidosis. British Medical Journal 1, 712–13.

Masterton, G., Napier, I. R., Henderson, J. N., and Roberts, J. E. (1977). Three-day clotrimazole treatment in candidal vulvovaginitis. British Journal of Venereal Diseases 53, 125–8.

Mastro, T. D., Satten, G. A., Nopkesorn, T., Sangkharomya, S., and Longini, I. M. (1994). Probability of female-to-male transmission of HIV-1 in Thailand. Lancet 343, 204–7.

Matta, M., Thompson, A. M., and Reiney, J. B. (1988). Does wearing two pairs of gloves protect operative staff from skin contamination? British Medical Journal, 297, 597–8.

Mayhew, S. R. (1981). Vaginitis: a study of the efficacy of povidone–iodine in unselected cases. Journal of International Medical Research 9, 157–9.

Mead, P. B. (1993). Epidemiology of bacterial vaginosis. American Journal of Obstetrics and Gynecology 169, 446–9.

Meisels, A. and Fortin, R. (1976). Condylomatous lesions of the cervix and vagina. Acta Cytologica 20, 505–9.

Mendelson, H., Clecner, B., and Eiley, S. (1986). Effect of recombinant interferon on clinical course of first episode genital herpes infection and subsequent recurrences. Genitourinary Medicine 62, 97–101.

Mendling, W. (1987). Vulvo-vaginal candidosis, p. 33. Springer–Verlag, Berlin.

Mertz, G. J., Critchlow, C. W., Benedetti, J., Reichman, R. C., Dolin, R., Connor, J., et al. (1984). Double-blind placebo controlled trial of oral acyclovir in first episode genital herpes simplex virus infection. Journal of the American Medical Association 252, 1147–51.

Method, M. W., Urnes, P., Casas, E. R., and Keith, L. (1987). Pelvic inflammatory disease, laparoscopy, and the expenditure of health care dollars. International Journal of Fertility 32, 17–37.

Miles, M. R., Olsen, L., and Rogers, A. (1977). Recurrent vaginal candidiasis. Journal of the American Medical Association 238, 1836–7.

Milne, J. D. and Warnock, D. W. (1979). The effect of simultaneous oral and vaginal treatment on the rate of cure and relapse in vaginal candidosis. British Journal of Venereal Diseases 55, 362–5.

Milsom, I. and Forssman, L. (1982). Treatment of vaginal candidosis with a single 500 mg clotrimazole pessary. British Journal of Venereal Diseases 59, 124–6.

Milsom, I. and Forssman, L. (1985). Repeated candidiasis: reinfection or recrudescene? American Journal of Obstetrics and Gynecology 152, 956–9.

Mindel, A. (1990). Reluctance to prescribe suppressive oral acyclovir for recurrent genital herpes. Lancet 335, 1107.

Mindel, A. (1991). Antiviral chemotherapy for genital herpes. *Reviews in Medical Virology* **1**, 111–18.

Mindel, A., Weller, I. V. D., Faherty, A., Sutherland, S., Fiddian, A. P., and Adler, M. W. (1986). Acyclovir in first attacks of genital herpes and prevention of recurrences. *Genitourinary Medicine* **62**, 28–32.

Mindel, A., Carney, O., Sonnex, C., Freris, M., Patou, G., and Williams, P. (1989). Suppression of frequently recurring genital herpes. *Genitourinary Medicine* **65**, 103–5.

Mohanty, K. C. and Scott, C. S. (1986). Immunotherapy of genital warts with inosine pranobex (Immunovir): preliminary study. *Genitourinary Medicine* **62**, 352–5.

Moller, B. R., Freundt, E. A., and Mardh, P-A. (1980). Experimental pelvic inflammatory disease provoked by *Chlamydia trachomatis* and *Mycoplasma hominis* in grivet monkeys. *American Journal of Obstetrics and Gynecology* **138**, 990–5.

Moller, B. R., Taylor-Robinson, D., and Furr, P. M. (1984). Serological evidence implicating *Mycoplasma genitalium* in pelvic inflammatory disease. *Lancet* **i**, 1102–3.

Moncada, J., Schachter, J., Bolan, C., Engelman, J., Howard, L., Musahwar, I., *et al.* (1990). Confirmatory assay increases specificity of the Chlamydiazyme test for *Chlamydia trachomatis* infection of the cervix. *Journal of Clinical Microbiology* **28**, 1770–3.

Monif, G. R. C., Welkos, S. R., Baer, H., and Thompson, R. J. (1976). Cul-de-sac isolates from patients with endometritis–salpingitis–peritonitis and gonococcal endocervicitis. *American Journal of Obstetrics and Gynecology* **126**, 158–61.

Morris, M. (1991). American legislation on AIDS. *British Medical Journal* **303**, 325–6.

Moss, A. R., Bacchetti, P., Osmond, D., Krampf, W., Chaisson, R. E., Stiten, D., *et al.* (1988). Seropositivity for HIV and the development of AIDS or AIDS-related condition. *British Medical Journal* **1**, 745–50.

Muller-Schoop, J. W., Wang, S. P., Munzinger, J., Schlapfer, H. U., Knoblauch, M., and Ammann, R. W. (1978). *Chlamydia trachomatis* as possible cause of peritonitis and perihepatitis in young women. *British Medical Journal* **1**, 1022–4.

Munday, P. E. (1983). Chlamydial infections in women. In *Progress in obstetrics and gynaecology*, vol. 3. (ed. J. Studd), pp. 231–45. Churchill Livingstone, Edinburgh.

Nilsen, A. E., Aasen, T., Halsos, A. M., Kinge, B. R., Tjotta, E. A. L., Wikstrom, K., *et al.* (1982). Efficacy of oral acyclovir in the treatment of initial and recurrent genital herpes. *Lancet* **ii**, 571–3.

Oates, J. K. and FitzGerald, M. R. (1988). Syphilis. In *Genital tract infections in women*. (ed. M. J. Hare), pp. 161–73. Churchill Livingstone, Edinburgh.

Oddone, E. Z., Cowper, P., Hamilton, J. D., Matchar, D. B., Hartigan, P., Samsa, G., *et al.* (1993). Cost effectiveness analysis of early zidovudine treatment of HIV infected patients. *British Medical Journal* **307**, 1322–5.

Odds, F. C. (1977). Cure and relapse with antifungal therapy. *Proceedings of the Royal Society of Medicine* **supp. 4**, 24–32.

Odds, F. C. (1982). Genital candidosis. *Clinical and Experimental Dermatology* **7**, 345–54.

Oleske, J. Minnefor, A., Cooper, R., Thomas, K., dela Cruz, A., Ahdieh, H., *et al.* (1983). Immune deficiency syndrome in children. *Journal of the American Medical Association* **249**, 2345–9.

Oriel, J. D. (1971). Natural history of genital warts. *British Journal of Venereal Diseases* **47**, 1–13.

Oriel, J. D. (1992). Sexually transmitted diseases in children: human papillomavirus infection. *Genitourinary Medicine* **68**, 80–3.

Oriel, J. D. and Waterworth, P. M. (1975). Effect of minocycline and tetracycline on the vaginal yeast flora. *Journal of Chemical Pathology* **28**, 403–6.

Oriel, J. D., Partridge, B. M., Denny, M. J., and Coleman, J. C. (1972). Genital yeast infections. *British Medical Journal* **4**, 761–4.

Oriel, J. D., Powis, P. A., Reeve, P., Miller, A., and Nicol, C. S. (1974). Chlamydial infections of the cervix. *British Journal of Venereal Diseases* **50**, 11–16.

Oriel, J. D., Johnson, A. L., Barlow, D., Thomas, B. J., Nayyar, K., and Reeve, P. (1978). Infection of the uterine cervix with *Chlamydia trachomatis*. *Journal of the Infectious Diseases* **137**, 443–51.

Osser, S. and Persson, K. (1982). Epidemiologic and serodiagnostic aspects of chlamydial salpingitis. *Obstetrics and Gynecology* **59**, 206–9.

Paavonen, J., Lehtinen, M., Teisala, K., Heinonen, P. K., Punnonen, R., Aine, R., et al. (1985a). *Haemophilus influenzae* causes purulent salpingitis. *American Journal of Obstetrics and Gynecology* **151**, 333–9.

Paavonen, J., Saikku, P., Vesterinen, E., Meyer, B., Vartiainen, E., and Saksela, E. (1978). Genital chlamydial infections in patients attending a gynaecological outpatient clinic. *British Journal of Venereal Diseases* **54**, 257–61.

Paavonen, J., Aine, R., Teisala, K., Heinonen, P. K., and Punnonen, R. (1985b). Comparison of endometrial biopsy and peritoneal fluid cytologic testing with laparoscopy in the diagnosis of acute pelvic inflammatory disease. *American Journal of Obstetrics and Gynecology* **151**, 645–50.

Pabst, K. M., Reichart, C. A., Knud-Hansen, C. R., Wasserheit, J. N., Quinn, T. C., Shah, K., et al. (1992). Disease prevalence among women attending a sexually transmitted disease clinic varies with reason for visit. *Sexually Transmitted Diseases* **19**, 88–91.

Padian, N., Marquis, L., Francis, D. P., Anderson, R. E., Rutherford, G. W., O'Malley. P. M., et al. (1987). Male-to-female transmission of HIV. *Journal of the American Medical Association* **258**, 788–90.

Palmer, H. M., Gilroy, C. B., Thomas, B. J., Hay, P. E., Gilchrist, C., and Taylor-Robinson, D. (1991). Detection of *Chlamydia trachomatis* by the polymerase chain reaction in swabs and urine from men with non-gonococcal urethritis. *Journal of Clinical Pathology* **44**, 321–5.

Panja, S. K. (1982). Treatment of trichomoniasis with metronidazole rectal suppositories. *British Journal of Venereal Diseases* **59**, 179–81.

Panja, S. K. (1983). Urethral syndrome in women attending clinic for sexually transmitted diseases. *British Journal of Venereal Diseases* **59**, 179–81.

Papaevangelou, G., Roumeliotou, A., Kallinikos, G., Papoutsakis, G., Trichopoulou, E., and Stefanou, Th. (1988). Education in preventing HIV infection in Greek registered prostitutes. *Journal of the Acquired Immune Deficiency Syndromes* **1**, 386–9.

Pariser, H. (1972). Asymptomatic gonorrhea. *Medical Clinics of North America* **56**, 1127–32.

Patten, R. M., Vincent, L. M., Wolner-Hanssen, P., and Thorpe, E. (1990). Pelvic inflammatory disease. *Journal of Ultrasound Medicine* **9**, 681–9.

Peck, J. E. (1974). Cryosurgery for benign cervical lesions. *British Medical Journal* **2**, 198–9.

Peterman, T. A., Stoneburner, R. L., Allen, J. R., Jaffe, H. W., and Curran, J. W. (1988). Risk of human immunodeficiency virus transmission from heterosexual adults with transfusion-associated infections. *Journal of the American Medical Association* **259**, 55–8.

Pheifer, T. A., Forsyth, P. S., Durfee, M. A., Pollock, H. M., and Holmes, K. K. (1978). Nonspecific vaginitis. Role of *Haemophilus vaginalis* and treatment with metronidazole. *New England Journal of Medicine* **298**, 1429–34.

Piot, P., Quinn, T. C., Taelman, H., Feinsod, F. M., Milangu, K. B., Wobin, O., et al. (1984). AIDS in a heterosexual population in Zaire. *Lancet* ii, 65–9.

Platz-Christensen, J. J., Larsson, P. G., Sundstrom, E., and Bondeson, L. (1989). Detection of bacterial vaginosis in Papanicolaou smears. *American Journal of Obstetrics and Gynecology* 160, 132–3.

Porter, J. D., Cruickshank, J. G., Gentle, P. H., Robinson, R. G., and Gill, O. N. (1990). Management of patients treated by a surgeon with HIV infection. *Lancet* 335, 113–14.

Rashid, S., Collins, M., Corner, J., and Morton, R. S. (1984). Survival of *Candida albicans* on fabric after laundering. *British Journal of Venereal Diseases* 60, 277.

Rees, E. and Annels, E. H. (1969). Gonococcal salpingitis. *British Journal of Venereal Diseases* 45, 205–15.

Reeves, W. C., Corey, L., Adams, H. G., Vontver, L. A., and Holmes, K. K. (1981). Risk of recurrence after first episode of genital herpes. *New England Journal of Medicine* 305, 315–19.

Rein, M. F. (1983). General principles of syphilotherapy. In *Sexually transmitted diseases* (1st edn), (ed. K. K. Holmes, P-A. Mardh, P. F. Sparling, and W. J. Wiesner), pp. 374–84, McGraw Hill, New York.

Rein, M. F. and Muller, M. (1990). *Trichomonas vaginalis* and trichomoniasis. In *Sexually transmitted diseases* (2nd edn), (ed. K. K. Holmes, P-A. Mardh, P. F. Sparling, W. J. Wiesner, W. Cates, and F. M. Lemon, *et al.*), pp. 481–92. McGraw Hill, New York.

Ripa, K. T. and Mardh, P-A. (1977). Cultivation of *Chlamydia trachomatis* in cyclohex-imide treated McCoy cells. *Journal of Clinical Microbiology* 6, 328–31.

Ripa, K. T., Svensson, L., Mardh, P-A., Westrom, L. (1978). *Chlamydia trachomatis* cervicitis in gynecologic outpatients Obstetrics and Gynecology 52, 698–702.

Riva, J. M., Sedlacek, T. V., Cunnane, M. F., and Mangan, C. (1989). Extended carbon dioxide laser vaporization in the treatment of subclinical papillomavirus infection of the lower genital tract. *Obstetrics and Gynecology* 73, 25–30.

Robertson, J. R., Bucknall, A. B. V., Welsby, P. D., Roberts, J. J. K., Inglis, J. M., Peutherer, J. F., *et al.* (1986). Epidemic of AIDS-related virus (HTLV-III/LAV) infection among intravenous drug abusers. *British Medical Journal* 292, 527–9.

Robertson, W. H. (1988). Mycology of vulvovaginitis. *American Journal of Obstetrics and Gynecology* 158, 989–91.

Rogers, B. B., Josephson, S. L., Mak, S. K., and Sweeney, P. J. (1992). Polymerase chain reaction amplification of herpes simplex virus DNA from clinical samples. *Obstetrics and Gynecology* 79, 464–9.

Ronald, P. J. M., Robertson, J. R., Wyld, R., and Weightman, R. (1993). Heterosexual transmission of HIV injecting drug users. *British Medical Journal* 307, 1184–5.

Rooney, J. F., Felser, J. M., Ostrove, J. M., and Straus, S. E. (1986). Acquisition of genital herpes from an asymptomatic sexual partner. *New England Journal of Medicine* 314, 1561–4.

Roth, A. C., Milsom, I., Forssman, L., and Wahlen, P. (1990). Intermittent prophylac-tic treatment of recurrent vaginal candidiasis by postmenstrual application of a 500 mg clotrimazole vaginal tablet. *Genitourinary Medicine* 66, 357–60.

Royal College of General Practitioners (1974). *Oral contraceptives and Health*, p. 62. Pittman Medical, New York.

Ruck, F. E., Banks, A., Munday, P. E., and Kross, R. D. (1991). Treatment of genital herpes with chlorous acid releasing gel. *Genitourinary Medicine* 67, 431.

Rustia, M. and Shubik, P. (1972). Induction of lung tumors and malignant lymphomas in mice by metronidazole. *Journal of the National Cancer Institute* 48, 721–9.

Sait, M. A. and Garg, B. R. (1985). Condylomata acuminata in children. *Genitourinary Medicine* **51**, 338–42.

Samaranayake, L. P. and MacFarlane, T. W. (1982). The effect of dietary carbohydrates on the *in vitro* adhesion of *Candida albicans* to epithelial cells. *Journal of Medical Microbiology* **15**, 511–17.

Sanders, L. L., Harrison, H. R., and Washington, A. E. (1986). Treatment of sexually transmitted chlamydial infections. *Journal of the American Medical Association* **255**, 1750–6.

Schachter, J., Cles, L., Ray, R., and Hines, P. A. (1979). Failure of serology in diagnosing chlamydial infections of the female genital tract. *Journal of Clinical Microbiology* **10**, 647–9.

Schild, G. S. and Stott, E. J. (1993). Where are we now with vaccines against AIDS? *British Medical Journal* **306**, 947–8.

Sellors, J. W., Mahony, J. B., Chernesky, M. A., and Rath, D. J. (1988). Tubal factor infertility: an association with prior chlamydial infection and asymptomatic salpingitis. *Fertility Sterility* **49**, 451–7.

Shanmugaratnam, K. and Pattman, R. S. (1989). Declining incidence of *Chlamydia trachomatis* in women attending a provincial genitourinary medicine clinic. *Genitourinary Medicine* **65**, 400.

Silyestri, D. L., Corey, L., and Holmes, K. K. (1982). Ineffectiveness of topical idoxyuridine in dimethyl sulfoxide for therapy for genital herpes. *Journal of the American Medical Association* **248**, 953–9.

Simmons, P. D., Langlet, F., and Thin, R. N. T. (1981). Cryotherapy versus electrocautery in the treatment of genital warts. *British Journal of Venereal Diseases* **57**, 273–4.

Sivakumar, K. and Basu-Roy, R. (1989). Falling prevalence of *Chlamydia trachomatis* infection among female patients attending the Department of Genito-Urinary Medicine, Bournemouth. *Genitourinary Medicine* **65**, 400.

Skinner, G. R. B., Woodman, C. B. J., Hartley, C. E., Buchan, A., Fuller, A., Durham, J., *et al.* (1982). Preparation and immunogenicity of vaccine AcNFU₁ (S−)MRC towards the prevention of herpes genitalis. *British Journal of Venereal Diseases* **58**, 381–6.

Skoldenberg, B., Jeansson, S., and Wolontis, S. (1975). Herpes simplex virus type 2 and acute aseptic meningitis. *Scandinavian Journal of Infectious Diseases* **7**, 227–32.

Slater, F. C. (1950). The effect of vaginal pH on wound healing. *American Journal of Obstetrics and Gynecology* **59**, 1089–94.

Sng, E. H., Lim, A. L., and Yeo, K. L. (1984). Susceptibility to antimicrobials of *Neisseria gonorrhoeae* isolated in Singapore. *British Journal of Venereal Diseases* **60**, 374–9.

Sobel, J. D. (1985). Epidemiology and pathogenesis of recurrent vulvovaginal candidiasis. *American Journal of Obstetrics and Gynecology* **152**, 924–35.

Sobel, J. D. (1990). Vulvovaginal candidosis. In *Sexually transmitted diseases* (2nd edn), (ed. K. K. Holmes, P-A. Mardh, P. F. Sparling, P. J. Wiesner, W. Cates, S. M. Lemon, *et al.*), pp. 515–526. McGraw Hill, New York.

Southgate, L. J., Treharne, J. D., and Forsey, T. (1983). *Chlamydia trachomatis* and *Neisseria gonorrhoeae* infections in women attending inner-city general practices. *British Medical Journal* **287**, 879–80.

Speroff, L., Glass, R. H., and Kase, N. G. (1989). *Clinical gynecologic endocrinology and infertility*, pp. 121–64, Williams and Wilkins, Baltimore.

Spiegel, C. A., Amsel, R., Eschenbach, D. A., Schoenknecht, F., and Holmes, K. K.

(1980). Anaerobic bacteria in non-specific vaginitis. *New England Journal of Medicine* **303**, 601–7.

Stacey, C. M., Barton, S. E., and Singer, A. (1991). Pelvic inflammatory disease. In *Progress in obstetrics and gynaecology*, vol. 9 (ed. J. Studd), pp. 259–71. Churchill Livingstone, Edinburgh.

Stacey, C. M., Munday, P. E., Taylor-Robinson, D., Thomas, B. J., Gilchrist, C., Ruck, F., *et al.* (1992). A longitudinal study of pelvic inflammatory disease. *American Journal of Obstetrics and Gynecology* **155**, 180–8.

Stamm, W. E., Whener, K. F., Amsel, R., Alexander, E. R., Turck, M., Counts, G. W., *et al.* (1980). Causes of the acute urethral syndrome in women. *New England Journal of Medicine* **303**, 409–15.

Stewart, G. J., Tyler, J. P. P., Cunningham, A. L., Barr, J. A., Driscoll, G. L., Gold, J., *et al.* (1985). Transmission of human T-cell lymphotrophic virus type III (HTLV-III) by artificial insemination by donor. *Lancet* **ii**, 581–4.

Stone, K. M., Grimes, D. A., and Magder, L. S. (1986). Personal protection against sexually transmitted diseases. *American Journal of Obstetrics and Gynecology*.

Stone, K. M., Becker, T. M., Hadgu, A., and Kraus, S. J. (1990). Treatment of external genital warts: a randomized clinical trial comparing podophyllin, cryotherapy, and electrodesiccation. *Genitourinary Medicine* **66**, 16–19.

Svensson, L., Westrom, L., Ripa, K. T., and Mardh, P-A. (1980). Differences in some clinical and laboratory parameters in acute salpingitis related to culture and serologic findings. *American Journal of Obstetrics and Gynecology* **133**, 1017–21.

Swedberg, J., Steiner, J. F., Deiss, F., Steiner, S., and Driggers, D. A. (1985). Comparison of single dose v one-week course of netranidazole for symptomatic bacterial vaginosis. *Journal of the American Medical Association* **254**, 1046–9.

Sweet, R. L. (1993). New approaches for the treatment of bacterial vaginosis. *American Journal of Obstetrics and Gynecology* **169**, 479–82.

Sweet, R. L. and Gibbs, R. S. (1990). *Infectious diseases of the female genital tract* (2nd ed), pp. 45–74. Williams and Wilkins, Baltimore.

Sweet, R. L., Schachter, J., and Robbie, M. O. (1983). Failure of beta-lactam antibiotics to eradicate *Chlamydia trachomatis* in the endometrium despite apparent clinical cure of acute salpingitis. *Journal of the American Medical Association* **250**, 2641–5.

Tagami, H., Oku, T., and Iwatsuki, K. (1985). Primary tissue culture of spontaneously regressing flat warts. *Cancer* **55**, 2437–41.

Talbot, M. D. and Kinghorn, G. R. (1985). Epidemiology and control of gonorrhoea in Sheffield. *Genitourinary Medicine* **61**, 230–5.

Tattersall, R. B. and Gale, E. A. M. (1990). *Diabetes: clinical management*, pp. 361–2. Churchill Livingstone, Edinburgh.

Taylor, E., Blackwell, A. L., Barlow, D., and Phillips, I. (1982). *Gardnerella vaginalis*, anaerobes, and vaginal discharge. *Lancet* **i**, 1376–9.

Taylor-Robinson, D. (1994). Chlamydia trachomatis and sexually transmitted disease. *British Medical Journal* **308**, 150–1.

Taylor-Robinson, D. and Thomas, B. J. (1991). Laboratory techniques for the diagnosis of chlamydial infections. *Genitourinary Medicine* **67**, 256–66.

Thin, R. N. T. (1988). Gonorrhoea. In *Genital tract infection in women* (ed. M. J. Hare), pp. 174–89. Churchill Livingstone, Edinburgh.

Thin, R. N. T., Atia, W., Parker, J. D. J., Nicol, C. S., and Canti, G. (1975). Value of Papanicolaou-stained smears in the diagnosis of trichomoniasis, candidiasis, and cervical herpes simplex virus infection in women. *British Journal of Venereal Diseases* **51**, 116–18.

Thin, R. N., Symonds, M. A. E., Booker, R., Cook, S., and Langlet, F. (1979). Double-blind comparison of a single-dose and a five-day course of metronidazole in the treatment of trichomoniasis. *British Journal of Venereal Diseases* **55**, 354–6.

Thin, R. N., Nabarro, J. M., Davidson-Parker, J., and Fiddian, A. P. (1983). Topical acyclovir in the treatment of initial herpes. *Genitourinary Medicine* **59**, 116–19.

Thomas, B. J., Evans, R. T., Hawkins, D. A., and Taylor-Robinson, D. (1984). Sensitivity of detecting *Chlamydia trachomatis* elementary bodies in smears by use of a fluorescein labelled monoclonal antibody: comparison with conventional chlamydial isolation. *Journal of Clinical Pathology* **37**, 812–16.

Thomas, R. M., Plant, M. A., Plant, M. L., and Sales, J. (1990). Risk of HIV infection among clients of the sex industry in Scotland. *British Medical Journal* **301**, 525.

Thomason, J. L., Schreckenberger, P. C., Spellacy, W. N., Riff, L. J., and LeBeau, L. J. (1984). Clinical and microbiological characterization of patients with nonspecific vaginosis associated with motile curved anaerobic rods. *Journal of Infectious Diseases* **149**, 801–9.

Tramont, E. C. (1976). Persistence of *Treponema pallidum* following penicillin G therapy. Report of two cases. *Journal of the American Medical Association* **236**, 2206–7.

Treharne, J. D., Darougar, S., and Jones, B. R. (1977). Modification of the microimmunofluorescence test to provide a routine serodiagnostic test for chlamydial infection. *Journal of Clinical Pathology* **30**, 515–17.

United Kingdon Collaborative Study (1989). HIV infection in patients attending clinics for sexually transmitted diseases in England and Wales. *British Medical Journal* **298**, 415–18.

Van de Perre, P., Clumeck, F., Carael, M., Nzabihimana, E., Guroff, M. R., De Mal, P., *et al.* (1985). Female prostitutes: a risk group for infection with human T-cell lymphotrophic virus type III. *Lancet* **ii**, 524–6.

Vejtorp, N., Bolerup, N. C., Vejtorp, L., Fanal, E., Nathan, N., Reiter, A., *et al.* (1988). Bacterial vaginosis: a double-bind randomized trial of the effect of treatment of the sexual partner. *British Journal of Obstetrics and Gynaecology* **95**, 920–6.

Vontver, L. A., Reeves, W. C., Rattray, M., Corey, L., Remmington, M. A., Tolentino, E., *et al.* (1979). Clinical course and diagnosis of genital herpes simplex virus infection and evaluation of topical surfactant therapy. *American Journal of Obstetrics and Gynecology* **133**, 548–54.

Vutyavanich, T., Pongsuthirak, P., Vannareumol, P., Ruangsri, R. A., and Luangsook, P. (1993). A randomized double blind trial of tridazole treatment for the sexual partners of women with bacterial vaginosis. *Obstetrics and Gynecology* **82**, 550–4.

Wang, S. P. and Grayston, J. T. (1970). Immunologic relationships between genital TRIC, lymphogranuloma venereum, and related organisms in a new microtiter indirect immunoflurescence test, *American Journal of Ophthalmology* **70**, 367–74.

Wang, S. P., Eschenbach, D. N., Holmes, K. K., Wager, G., and Grayston, J. F. (1980). *Chlamydia trachomatis* infection in Fitz-Hugh–Curtis syndrome. *American Journal of Obstetrics and Gynecology* **138**, 1034–8.

Ward, H., Day, S., Mezzone, J., Dunlop, L., Donegan, C., Farrar, S., *et al.* (1993). Prostitution and the risk of HIV. *British Medical Journal* **307**, 356–8.

Warden, J. (1990). AIDS in Thailand. *British Medical Journal* **300**, 415–16.

Waugh, M. A. (1991). Azithromycin in sexually transmitted diseases – an overview. *International Journal of STD and AIDS* **2**, 246–7.

Webb, G., Wells, B., Morgan, J. R., and McManus, T. J. (1986). Epidemic of AIDS-related virus infection among intravenous drug users. *British Medical Journal* **292**, 1202.

Webster, A. and Johnson, M. (1990). HIV infection. In *Progress in obstetrics and gynaecology* vol. 8, (ed. J. Studd), pp. 175–90. Churchill Livingstone, Edinburgh.

Weinberger, M. W. and Harger, J. H. (1993). Accuracy of the Pap smear in the diagnosis of asymptomatic infection with trichomonas vaginalis. *Obstetrics and Gynecology* **82**, 425-9.

Westrom, L. (1975). Effect of acute pelvic inflammatory disease on infertility. *American Journal of Obstetrics and Gynecology* **121**, 707-13.

Westrom, L. (1980). Incidence, prevalence, and trends of acute pelvic inflammatory disease and its consequences in industrialized countries. *American Journal of Obstetrics and Gynecology* **138**, 880-92.

Westrom, L. (1988). Decrease in incidence of women treated in hospital for acute salpingitis in Sweden. *Genitourinary Medicine* **64**, 59-63.

Westrom, L. and Mardh, P-A. (1990). Acute pelvic inflammatory disease (PID). In *Sexually transmitted diseases* (2nd edn.), (ed. K. K. Holmes, P-A. Mardh, P. F. Sparling, P. P. Wiesner, W. Cates, S.M. Lemon, *et al.*), pp. 593-614. McGraw Hill New York.

Wickenden, C., Hanna, N., Taylor-Robinson, D., Harris, J. R. W., Bellamy, C., Carroll, P., *et al.* (1988). Sexual transmission of human papillomaviruses in heterosexual and male homosexual couples, studied by DNA hybridization. *Genitourinary Medicine* **64**, 34-8.

Wilmott, F., Say, J., Downey, D., and Hookham, A. (1983). Zinc and recalcitrant trichomoniasis. *Lancet* **i**, 1053.

Wishart, P. K., James, C., Wishart, M. S., and Darougar, S. (1984). Prevalence of acute conjunctivitis caused by chlamydia, adenovirus, and herpes simplex virus in an ophthalmic casualty department. *British Journal of Ophthalmology* **68**, 653-5.

Witkin, S. S., Jeremias, J., Toth, M., and Ledger, W. J. (1993). Detection of Chlamydia trachomatis by the polymerase chain reaction in the cervices of women with acute salpingitis. *American Journal of Obstetrics and Gynecology* **168**, 1438-42.

Wolfe, H., Vranizan, K. M., Gorter, R. G., Keffelew, A. S., and Moss, A. R. (1992). Crack use and human immunodeficiency virus infection among San Francisco intravenous drug users. *Sexually Transmitted Diseases* **19**, 111-15.

Wolner-Hanssen, P., Svensson, L., Mardh, P. A., and Westrom, L. (1985). Laparoscopic findings and contraceptive use in women with signs and symptoms suggestive of acute salpingitis. *Obstetrics and Gynecology* **66**, 233-8.

Wolner-Hanssen, P., Krieger, J. N., Stevens, C. E., Kiviat, N. B., Koutsky, L., Critchlow, C., *et al.* (1989). Clinical manifestations of vaginal trichomoniasis. *Journal of the American Medical Association* **261**, 571-6.

Wolner-Hanssen, P., Kiviat, N. B., and Holmes, K. K. (1990). Atypical pelvic inflammatory disease: subacute, chronic or subclinical upper genital tract infection in women. In *Sexually transmitted diseases* (2nd edn), (ed. K. K. Holmes, P-A. Mardh, P. F. Sparling, P. J. Wiesner, W. Cates, S. M. Lemon, *et al.* pp. 615-20. McGraw Hill, New York.

Wood, J. J., Bolton, J. P., Cannon, S. R., Allan, A., O'Connor, B. H., and Darougar, S. (1982). Biliary-type pain as a manifestation of genital tract infection: the Curtis-Fitz-Hugh syndrome. *British Journal of Surgery* **69**, 251-3.

Woodman, C. B. J. (1998). Infection with herpes virus and cytomegalovirus. In *Genital tract infection in women* (ed. M. J. Hare), pp. 248-61. Churchill Livingstone, Edinburgh.

Woodman, C. D. J., Buchan, A., Fuller, A., Hartley, C., Skinner, G. R. P., Stocker, D., *et al.* (1983). Efficacy of vaccine $AcNFU_1(S-)MRC5$ given after an initial clinical epidose in the prevention of herpes genitalis. *British Journal of Venereal Diseases* **59**, 311-13.

Worm, A. M. and Petersen, C. S. (1987). Transmission of chlamydial infections to sexual partners. *Genitourinary Medicine* **63**, 19–21.

Wosmer, G. P., Krupp, L. B., Hanrahan, J. P., Gavis, G., Spira, T. J., and Cunningham-Rundles, S. (1983). Acquired immune deficiency syndrome in male prisoners. *Annals of Internal Medicine* **98**, 297–303.

Yule, A., Gellan, M. C. A., Oriel, J. D., and Ackers, J. P. (1987). Detection of *Trichomonas vaginalis* antigen in women by enzyme immunoassay. *Journal of Clinical Pathology* **40**, 566–8.

7 The management of menorrhagia

This chapter is concerned with menorrhagia, i.e. heavy or prolonged periods without any alteration in cycle length, occurring in the absence of overt pelvic pathology or exogenous hormonal therapy and endocrine disorders, namely dysfunctional uterine bleeding. This problem accounts for up to 40 per cent of all gynaecological out-patient consultations in the UK. It affects 40 women per 1000 in the UK annually, such that they seek the advice of their general practitioners, and results in 20 000 hysterectomies per year in England and Wales. In only 25 per cent of patients with menorrhagia can an underlying pathological diagnosis be found, the remaining 75 per cent being termed dysfunctional uterine bleeding.

What constitutes menorrhagia?

Menorrhagia due to dysfunctional uterine bleeding should probably be considered to be the right-hand end of the spectrum rather than an abnormality, for the difference in menstrual blood loss between 'normal' and 'menorrhagia' is based on a convention following cohort studies. Jacobs and Butler (1965) measured menstrual blood loss in 70 normal women and 15 women with iron deficiency anaemia. The normal women had a mean menstrual blood loss of 34.7 ml (range 3–87 ml), whilst the 15 anaemic women had a mean menstrual blood loss of 121.4 ml (range 21–624 ml). Hallberg *et al.* (1966) were responsible for the study upon which the conventional definition of menorrhagia (greater than 80 ml mean menstrual blood loss) was based. In a study of 474 women aged between 16 and 52 years, they reported that 75 per cent of women with a mean menstrual blood loss of less than 60 ml had a haemoglobin of 12 g per 100 ml or more. Of those women with a menstrual blood loss of between 60–80 ml, 61 per cent had a haemoglobin of 12 g per 100 ml or more, whilst only 33 per cent of women with a menstrual blood loss of greater than 80 ml had a haemoglobin of greater than 12 g per 100 ml. They concluded that the 11 per cent of women with a mean menstrual blood loss of greater than 80 ml per cycle should be considered to be the abnormal end of the menstrual spectrum.

Rybo (1966) reported that the average menstrual blood loss in nulliparous women was 38 ml and in multiparous women 45.5 ml. Some 79 per cent of this menstrual blood loss occurred within the first 48 hours and 92 per cent within the first three days. In women who had menorrhagia, 69 per cent of the blood loss occurred within the first 48 hours and 86 per cent within the first three days. There was, therefore, very little correlation between the duration of menstrual loss and the volume of menstrual loss. Similarly, Haynes *et al.* (1977) could find no correlation between the duration of menstruation and the menstrual blood loss in women with menorrhagia.

There would appear to be very little correlation between the amount of blood which is lost and the women's perception or description of that loss. Chimbira *et al.* (1980*a*) reported a series of 92 women in whom menstrual blood loss was measured. Sixty-eight of these women had menorrhagia, yet 23 of these (34 per cent) did not consider their periods to be heavy, whilst some 47 per cent of the 59 women in the series who did consider their periods to be heavy had a mean menstrual blood loss of less than 80 ml. There was also very little correlation between measured loss and the number of pads used. In general, more pads were used not in menorrhagia but in younger women of higher social class. Hysterectomy was performed in 40 of the women with menorrhagia. There was no correlation between uterine weight or endometrial surface area and menstrual blood loss.

The effect of previous sterilization

There is some evidence that sterilization procedures may result in heavier menses, although the evidence is not absolutely clearcut.

Williams *et al.* (1951) reported a series of 200 women who had undergone a previous sterilization procedure and whose subsequent medical records were analysed. Some 48 of these women (24 per cent) were diagnosed as having menorrhagia, and in 15 per cent it was considered to be dysfunctional, a diagnosis only made in 5 per cent of women attending their hospital and who had not had a previous sterilization. Although there was no attempt to make any allowance for the age of the patient, parity, or contraceptive use, the suggestion was made that sterilization may result in subsequent gynaecological problems. Similarly, Muldoon (1972) followed 374 patients for a mean of 10 years following tubal ligation. Menorrhagia occurred in 25 per cent of this population, 13 per cent undergoing hysterectomy, 6.4 per cent curettage alone, and 5.6 per cent hormonal therapy.

There are several possible explanations for this association, and it is likely that the aetiology is multifactorial. The patients may have developed dysfunctional uterine bleeding with time, an alteration in contraceptive practice will have occurred, and it is possible that sterilization does, in fact, result in menorrhagia in some women.

In a short-term prospective study, Kasonde and Bonnar (1976) measured menstrual blood loss in 25 women 3 months prior to sterilization and again some 6–12 months after sterilization. They found no significant difference in this blood loss. Neil *et al.* (1975) reported the results of a questionnaire on 257 women who had undergone a previous laparoscopic sterilization, 93 who had undergone a previous tubal ligation, and 143 whose husbands had had a vasectomy. The study suffers from the absence of a pre-operative questionnaire and takes no account of previous contraceptive use. There was an increased menstrual loss, on subjective assessment, in 39 per cent of women with a previous laparoscopic sterilization, 22 per cent with a previous tubal ligation, and in 13 per cent whose husbands had undergone a previous vasectomy.

Stock (1978) used pre-operative questionnaires in 233 women who were to undergo sterilization, and compared these to a post-operative questionnaire some 12.2 years following sterilization. On an initial audit, 68 per cent of women had heavier periods, but on attempting to exclude the effects of cessation of oral contraception, he estimated that the true incidence of menorrhagia following sterilization was only 6 per cent. Rulin *et al.* (1989) reported a prospective study based upon two interviews of 1107 women who intended to be sterilized and 498 controls. These groups were well matched for age, parity, race, religion, education, and social background. The second interview took place at a mean of 10 months after the first interview. Once the effects of either oral contraception or an IUCD were excluded, menstrual cycles, duration of menstrual flow, and the presence or absence of intermenstrual bleeding were unchanged in both groups.

The available evidence does not support a strong association between sterilization and menorrhagia. If sterilization is a true aetiological factor for menorrhagia, it is unlikely that any more than 6 per cent of women will develop menorrhagia because of this procedure.

The assessment before treatment

There is some debate as to whether dysfunctional uterine bleeding is more likely to be associated with ovulation or anovulation, although the bulk of current evidence suggests that ovulation is more usual. Taw (1975) reported 1520 women who underwent 1533 curettages. Only 382 specimens showed secretory endometrium (24.9 per cent), whereas Haynes *et al.* (1977) considered that the majority of people with dysfunctional menorrhagia were ovulating. Nedoss (1971) reported endometrial histopathology in 136 women with dysfunctional uterine bleeding, 16 per cent of whom were anovulatory. This discrepancy may, in part, be explained by the fact that accurate timing of curettage is not always possible. However, it would appear to be of little importance in that the purpose of the treatment for anovulatory menorrhagia is not, in general, ovulation-induction; progesterone or oral contraception may be used equally for anovulatory and ovulatory menorrhagia.

There is also growing evidence concerning a possible role for prostaglandins in endometrial pathology, with an increased concentration in prostaglandin E_2 in the endometrium of patients with menorrhagia, especially if complicated by dysmenorrhoea (Smith *et al.* 1981; Willman *et al.* 1976). It has been suggested that excessive bleeding may result from a shift in endometrial conversion from vasoconstrictory $PGF_2\alpha$ to vasodilatory PGE_2 with a subsequent effect upon the spiral arterioles (Cameron *et al.* 1987; Smith *et al.* 1981). There may also be an elevation in the ratio between vasodilatory prostacyclin and vasoconstrictory thromboxane, leading to, at least in theory, menorrhagia (Makarainen and Ylikorkala, 1986). However, the measured changes in prostaglandins and prostanoids in endometrial tissues do not give consistent results, perhaps because of variable laboratory techniques, hence further elucidation is required (Rees *et al.* 1984).

Having excluded non-gynaecological problems and overt pelvic pathology suggested by abnormal findings on pelvic examination, the major investigative procedure is dilatation and curettage. There are four reasons for this. First, endometrial carcinoma has to be excluded; secondly, other intrauterine pathology may be recognized, for example an endometrial polyp or submucous fibroid; thirdly, the absence of pathology may strongly reassure the patient; and finally, curettage may be therapeutic. The first two indications are discussed below, the third is almost impossible to assess scientifically, and the fourth will be discussed under 'Treatment'.

Endometrial carcinoma

Barter *et al.* (1968) reported all women with adenocarcinoma of the endometrium diagnosed, in Washington, over an 18-year period. There were 235 such women, whose ages ranged from 39 to 83 years, only two being below the age of 40 (0.85 per cent). Some 84.1 per cent of these women were post-menopausal and 15.9 per cent were still menstruating, suggesting the need for curettage in women with abnormal bleeding in the older (40 +) age group. MacKenzie and Bibby (1978) reported 1029 women who underwent a diagnostic curettage. Of 150 women with post-menopausal bleeding, 15 had an endometrial carcinoma (10 per cent) but, of 387 women with a menstrual disorder, and a further 193 women with either intermenstrual bleeding or postcoital bleeding, none had an endometrial carcinoma. They concluded that curettage was probably not indicated in women before the menopause, and certainly not before the age of 40 years. However, it may be that patients whose menorrhagia dates back from soon after the menarche should undergo curettage. Southam and Richart (1966) reported 291 'adolescent' women with menorrhagia, in half of whom the menstrual disorder returned to normal spontaneously. The other half continued with menstrual problems to varying degrees, and four of these women (1.37 per cent) developed carcinoma of the body of the uterus before the age of 33 years (age range 23–33 years).

Other intrauterine pathology

Benign endometrial pathology may be found on curettage in premenopausal women with a menstrual disorder. Thus, MacKenzie and Bibby (1978) reported endometrial polyps in 1.0 per cent of their patients with a menstrual disturbance, and in 3 per cent of the patients with intermenstrual bleeding.

It is possible that such pathological abnormalities may be discovered by, or reassurance given following, other techniques which do not require general anaesthesia. Thus, Varba aspiration of the uterine cavity provides an adequate histological specimen in between 85–99 per cent of samplings, as compared to curettage in 77–94 per cent (Grimes 1982). The Isaccs cell sampler was used in combination with curettage in 121 women by Hutton *et al.* (1978). They reported satisfactory tissue for histological examination following curettage in 79 per cent of patients, whereas they obtained satisfactory tissue for cytological examination in 91 per cent. Furthermore, cytology revealed seven patients with endometrial carcinoma, but only six of these would have been diagnosed on curettage alone.

There is very little indication to investigate premenopausal women with menorrhagia by means of hysterosalpingogram or laparoscopy unless other clinical indications exist, but the place of hysteroscopy may increase.

The treatment of menorrhagia

Although some women require only reassurance, explanation, and treatment of anaemia should it be present, the following drug or surgical treatment options are available.

Drug treatment

(1) progestogen therapy;

(2) oral contraceptive therapy;

(3) danazol;

(4) prostaglandin synthetase inhibitors;

(5) antifibrinolytic agents;

(6) ethamsylate;

(7) LHRH agonists.

Progestogen therapy

The place of progestogens in the treatment of dysfunctional uterine bleeding appears to have been established without the use of controlled drug trials, and before the days of objective measurement of menstrual blood loss was part of such a study. Thus, the evidence for the place of progestogen therapy is essentially anecdotal. Bishop and DeAlmeida (1966) reported that oral norethisterone arrested acute bleeding during metropathic episodes in five out of eight patients, and when given cyclically to 13 women with menorrhagia, 'normal cycles' then occurred in 34 out of 52 reported cycles (65 per cent). Conyngham (1965) reported that, when 121 patients with dysfunctional uterine bleeding were treated with norethisterone, the results were 'good' in 58 per cent, 'fair' in 25 per cent, and 'poor' in 16 per cent. Breakthrough bleeding occurred in 3.8 per cent of 571 treatment cycles.

Only recently has any objective study of progestogen therapy become available. Cameron *et al.* (1990) randomly allocated 32 women with objective evidence of menorrhagia to receive either norethisterone (5 mg twice daily on days 19–26 of the cycle, $n = 15$) or mefenamic acid (500 mg three times daily during menses, $n = 17$). The median blood loss was reduced by 16 per cent (from 109 ml to 92 ml) in the patients receiving norethisterone, which was not superior to mefenamic acid (see below). Some 73 per cent of patients treated with norethisterone complained of a side-effect (nausea, headache, abdominal pain) but only one (6.7 per cent) stopped taking the drug because of this. Cameron *et al.* (1987) had previously demonstrated a similar reduction in menstrual blood loss in a smaller series of patients allocated to receive danazol, mefenamic acid, a progesterone-impregnated coil, or norethisterone.

Progesterone and progestogen may also be administered via an IUCD for intrauterine release. Bergqvist and Rybo (1983) used a progesterone-releasing device in 12 women with menorrhagia, reducing the mean pretreatment menstrual blood loss by 64 per cent, from 138 ml to 49 ml, within 12 months. Other workers have demonstrated a reduction of menstrual blood loss in the region of 50 per cent using similar devices (Cameron *et al.* 1987). However, these devices are not recommended for clinical use because of the increased risk of ectopic pregnancy (please see Chapter 5 — Contraception).

Progesterone therapy acts, presumably, by inhibiting endometrial proliferation.

Oral contraceptive therapy

The mechanism of action of oral contraceptive therapy is presumed to be the induction of a relative endometrial atrophy. The value of oral contraceptive therapy depends upon a balance between the dosage of oestrogen and the side-effects; cycle control tending to be better in formulations containing 50 μg of oestrogen.

However, there is surprisingly little evidence to support the use of oral contraceptive therapy in menorrhagia. Nilsson and Rybo (1971) reported a series of 164 women whose mean pretreatment menstrual blood loss was 157.5 ml. Following oral contraceptive therapy, this was reduced by 52.6 per cent to a mean treatment blood loss of 74.7 ml, but, following cessation of the treatment, menstrual blood loss returned to its previous value. The Royal College of General Practitioners (1974) recorded that menorrhagia was reported at a rate of 12.5 per 1000 women-years by 23 611 oral contraceptive takers as opposed to a rate of 23.8 per 1000 women-years in 22 766 non-takers, suggesting a relative risk for menorrhagia of 0.52 for oral contraceptive takers. The only other series reported consisted of eight patients with menorrhagia whose mean menstrual blood loss was reduced by 72 per cent when treated with oral contraceptives (Dockeray 1988).

Danazol

Danazol is a derivative of 17-alpha ethyl testosterone, and probably acts in a multifactorial manner. There is evidence for a direct enzymatic inhibition of sex steroid synthesis coupled with a competitive inhibition of binding of sex hormones to cytoplasmic receptors, and a direct inhibitory effect upon endometrial proliferation (Jeppsson *et al.* 1984; Madanes and Farber 1982). Given a sufficient dosage, patients may be made amenorrhoeic, whereas a lower dosage will have a less dramatic effect on the periods but gives a lower incidence of side-effects, of which weight gain, skin rashes, and acne would appear to be the commonest ones.

Chimbira *et al.* (1979, 1980*b*) reported upon the efficacy of different dosages of danazol in a series of placebo-controlled trials and objective measurements of menstrual blood loss. The placebo did not alter menstrual blood loss. In a dosage of 100 mg of danazol per day, 16 women reduced their mean menstrual blood loss from 125 ml to 45 ml, but five of the 16 patients reported a significant shortening in the menstrual cycle which was unacceptable. At a dose of 200 mg per day, 16 women reported a reduction in their menstrual blood loss from a pretreatment mean of 182 ml to a mean blood loss on treatment of 26 ml. One woman became amenorrhoeic and there was no effect on the cycle length. At a dosage of 400 mg per day, 18 women reduced their mean menstrual blood loss from 231 ml before treatment to a loss of only 31 ml during the third month of treatment; however, two patients discontinued therapy, one because of a skin rash and the other because of weight gain. They conclude that danazol 200 mg per day was the 'best buy' for the menorrhagia of dysfunctional uterine bleeding.

Other workers have demonstrated a similar benefit in patients receiving 200 mg of danazol per day (Higham and Shaw 1993). Dockeray *et al.* (1989) demonstrated a 60 per cent reduction in mean measured blood loss in 20 women with menorrhagia taking 200 mg of danazol per day, but 75 per cent of the patients reported a side-effect of a 2 kg mean weight gain during treatment. When treatment was discontinued, weight returned to its pretreatment level.

Prostaglandin synthetase inhibitors

It has already been stated that prostaglandin metabolism may be disordered in primary dysfunctional uterine bleeding. It is, therefore, logical that prostaglandin synthetase inhibitors have been assessed as a treatment for menorrhagia.

The evidence suggests that these agents are effective methods of treatment. Anderson (1976) reported a fall from a mean pretreatment menstrual blood loss of 119 ml to a mean loss on treatment of 60 ml, in six women receiving mefenamic acid. Fraser *et al.* (1981), in a double-blind, randomized, placebo-controlled trial of mefenamic acid in 69 women with menorrhagia, demonstrated a mean reduction in menstrual blood loss of 28.1 per cent between placebo and active agent. Dockeray *et al.* (1989) reported an open randomized trial of mefenamic acid against danazol. The 19 women taking mefenamic acid (500 mg thrice daily for 3–5 days) showed a 20 per cent reduction in mean menstrual blood loss during treatment, whilst 20 women taking danazol (100 mg twice daily for 60 days) had a 60 per cent reduction in mean measured blood loss. Some 30 per cent of patients reported side-effects with mefenamic acid, especially nausea and diarrhoea. Cameron *et al.* (1990), in their randomized trial of norethisterone against mefenamic acid, demonstrated that both agents were equally effective in reducing menstrual blood loss. Mefenamic acid reduced the mean measured menstrual blood loss in 17 women by 24 per cent.

Antifibrinolytic agents

Substances such as epsilon aminocaproic acid (EACA) inhibit the activation of plasminogen to plasmin and may, therefore, reduce the enhanced fibrinolytic activity found within the endometrium of some women with menorrhagia.

Nilsson and Rybo (1971) demonstrated a mean reduction in blood loss of 47 per cent, from 164 ml to a mean of 87 ml in 172 women treated with EACA in a double-blind placebo-controlled trial of 37 patients. They reported that the only common side-effect was nausea. In a more recent study (Andersch *et al.* 1988), tranexamic acid, in a dose of between 2 and 4.5 g daily during the first five days of menstruation, reduced the total menstrual blood loss of 15 women by 47 per cent, from 295 to 155 ml. When this study was repeated (Milson *et al.* 1991) the total measured blood loss of 15 women with menorrhagia was reduced by 44 per cent using a similar drug regime.

However, serious side-effects have been reported, albeit rarely. These have included intracranial arterial thrombosis (Rydin and Lundberg 1976), and deaths from carotid artery thrombosis have also occurred (Davies and Howell 1977).

Ethamsylate

Ethamsylate is said to reduce capillary fragility, and, hence, may reduce menstrual blood loss by preventing the breakdown of the ground substance of the capillary wall by anti-hyaluronidase activity.

In a double-blind, cross-over trial comparing ethamsylate (Dicynene) with placebo in a series of nine women with dysfunctional uterine bleeding, there was a 50 per cent reduction in mean blood loss using the active agent compared with a placebo. The side-effects (see below) were slight, and were equally common between the active agent and placebo (Harrison and Campbell 1976). Chamberlain *et al.* (1991) demonstrated that 500 mg of ethamsylate four times daily during menstruation reduced the mean menstrual blood loss of 16 women with menorrhagia by 20 per cent, whilst the side-effects of nausea, a bloated abdomen, and headache were reported by five (31 per cent) patients.

LHRH agonists

The use of luteinizing hormone releasing hormone agonists was reported by Shaw and Fraser (1984) using buserelin, given by nasal spray, in four women. Pretreatment menstrual blood loss ranged from 95 to 198 ml per cycle compared with a range from 0 to 30 ml during treatment. Menstrual loss returned to the pretreatment values within two months. Longterm treatment is relatively contraindicated because of the risk of osteoporosis.

Table 7.1 Drug treatment for menorrhagia

Drug	Mean reduction in menstrual blood loss (%)
Danazol	60–86
OC*	52–72
Mefenamic acid	24–50
EACA[†]	47–52
Progestogens	20

*OC = oral contraception
[†]EACA = epsilon aminocaproic acid

Which drug?

Having excluded pathology, and having reassured the patient, drug treatment will generally be preferred to surgery in the first instance. Although Table 7.1. summarizes the results which can be anticipated using different drugs, the choice of agent will depend not only upon efficacy but also upon side-effects, the patients' wishes, and whether or not pain is also present. In general, the first line agents will be progestogens, danazol, or prostaglandin synthetase inhibitors. The latter are particularly useful when pain coexists, whilst danazol, although the most effective agent, is limited by side-effects and the need to take the tablets on a continuous rather than a cyclical basis. Progestogen therapy, whilst less effective than danazol, may be preferred by some patients because of the lower incidence of side-effects.

Surgical treatment

(1) curettage;

(2) hysterectomy;

(3) cryosurgery;

(4) laser endometrial ablation;

(5) endometrial resection;

(6) radiofrequency-induced thermal ablation.

Curettage

The therapeutic benefit from curettage would appear to be short-lived. Nilsson and Rybo (1971) demonstrated a mean reduction in menstrual blood loss of 48 per cent, from 144 to 44.6 ml, in 65 women in their first period following curettage. In the 30 women followed for three months, the mean reduction was only 8 per cent and in the 15 women followed for four periods, the mean reduction in menstrual blood loss was only 5 per cent. Haynes *et al.* (1977) reported that curettage only reduced the first period of 22 women with significant menorrhagia, with mean blood loss reverting to precurettage levels thereafter.

Table 7.2 The complications of hysterectomy

	Vaginal route	Abdominal route
No. of patients	586	1283
% With any complication	24.5	42.8
% With febrile morbidity	15.3	32.3
% Requiring transfusion	8.3	15.4
% With life-threatening complications	0	0.4
% With urinary retention	15	8
% With ileus	0.2	2.2
% With atelectasis	1.1	5.9
% With damage to other structures	1.8	0.6
Mean post-operative stay (days)	5	7

From Dicker *et al.* (1982)

Over and above the need for a general anaesthetic, curettage carries a risk of perforation in 0.7 per cent of patients, although virtually all such patients recover without incident (MacKenzie and Bibby 1978). The overall complication rate, including bleeding and infection, is 1.7 per cent.

Hysterectomy

Hysterectomy remains a common method of treatment for intractable menorrhagia. Some 20 per cent of women in the UK will have a hysterectomy during their lifetime, as will 40 per cent in Australia (Selwood and Wood 1978; Vessey *et al.* 1992). This means that in England and Wales each year, 2.4 per 10 000 women undergo hysterectomy, with a corresponding figure of 6.3 per 10 000 in the United States (Easterday 1983). Grant and Hussein (1984), in a retrospective survey of 205 women undergoing abdominal hysterectomy, reported that no macroscopic pathology was apparent in 60 per cent of these patients.

The mortality associated with hysterectomy has been reported by Wingo *et al.* (1985). They reported 46 deaths in 119 972 vaginal hysterectomies, giving an incidence of 3.8 per 10 000 procedures. They reported 477 deaths in 317 389 abdominal hysterectomies, giving a mortality of 15 per 10 000 procedures. However, the mortality following abdominal hysterectomy is complicated by the fact that some of these procedures were associated with pregnancy or malignant disease, both known to impose additional mortality upon the procedure. If pregnancy and malignant disease are excluded, the mortality rate for abdominal hysterectomy becomes 4.6 per 10 000 procedures as compared with a mortality of 53.4 per 10 000 procedures when the operation is associated with pregnancy and 102.6 per 10 000 procedures when it is associated with malignant disease.

The morbidity following hysterectomy was reported in a prospective multicentre study of 1851 women (Dicker *et al.* 1982). The results are detailed in Table 7.2. It should be noted that 42.8 per cent of patients undergoing abdominal hysterectomy had a complication, however slight, as compared with 24.5 per cent of patients undergoing vaginal hysterectomy. Life-threatening complications occurred in 0.4 per cent of patients undergoing abdominal hysterectomy and none undergoing vaginal hysterectomy. No patient in this series died. Only 1.1 per cent of patients in whom a vaginal hysterectomy was planned required an abdominal approach to complete the procedure.

When hysterectomy for dysfunctional uterine bleeding in the presence of a normal sized uterus is to take place, it may be possible that the morbidity can be reduced by the performance of the increasingly popular laparoscopically-assisted vaginal hysterectomy (LAVH) (Fernandez *et al.* 1992; Magos *et al.* 1991*b*; Nezhat *et al.* 1990; Reich *et al.* 1989; Scrimgeour *et al.* 1991). These authors have reported small series of patients who would have ordinarily undergone an abdominal hysterectomy but in whom the round ligaments and infundibulopelvic ligaments were divided by a laparoscopic technique. Some authors advocate that the laparoscopic technique should also be used to divide the round ligament, separate the bladder from the uterus, and ligate the uterine vessels (Nezhat *et al.* 1990; Reich *et al.* 1989; Scrimgeour *et al.* 1991). It is too early to say whether or not this potentially attractive technique will stand the test of time with regard to the potential reduction in morbidity but ureteric injury is described and the incidence of incisional hernia is 3.1 per cent following the use of a 12 ml trocar compared with 0.23 per cent with the 10 ml trocar (Hunter and McCartney 1993; Kadar *et al.* 1993).

Hysterectomy and depression

A major controversy related to the prevalence of depression following hysterectomy, although it is now accepted that post-hysterectomy depression is not a specific complication.

The evidence which claimed to link hysterectomy with depression was retrospective and based upon poorly-matched case-control studies. Barker (1968) compared the notes of 729 women undergoing hysterectomy with 280 women undergoing cholecystectomy over a 4.5-year period in Dundee, where the expected referral rate for women with depressive incidence over a 2-year period would have been 1.2 per cent. Of those patients undergoing cholecystectomy, 3 per cent required psychiatric referral at some stage post-operatively, with a referral rate of 1.1 per cent within the first two years. Following hysterectomy, 7 per cent required psychiatric referral over the period of study, with a referral rate of 3.2 per cent within two years of the operation. There was no difference in the need for psychiatric referral in those patients who had undergone bilateral oophorectomy when compared to those who had not. Richards (1973) compared 200 women who had undergone hysterectomy with 200 women who had undergone another operation at a similar time, these women were matched for age, marital status, and parity, but not for the presence or absence of malignant disease, nor for the incidence of pre-operative depression. Of those patients who had undergone hysterectomy, 33 per cent had consulted their general practitioners with depression within the first three years following the operation compared to 7 per cent of the controls. Psychiatric admission was required for 6 per cent of the hysterectomy patients as compared to 0.5 per cent of the controls. In a further study, Richards (1974) compared the three years following hysterectomy in 56 women with the three years following comparable major surgery at a similar time in a further 56 matched controls. Some 21 per cent of the controls had consulted their general practitioner with a depressive illness at some stage before the operation, and this rose to 30 per cent in the first three years after surgery. Of the patients undergoing hysterectomy 36 per cent had consulted their general practitioner at some stage pre-operatively with a depressive illness, as compared to 70 per cent of the hysterectomy group within the first three years following their operation.

When prospective studies were performed, the association between hysterectomy and depression no longer becomes apparent. Gath *et al.* (1982) reported a prospective study of 156 women with menorrhagia due to benign disease who were interviewed prior to hysterectomy. At six months following hysterectomy, 147 were reinterviewed and at 18 months following hysterectomy, 148 were reinterviewed. There was evidence of psychiatric morbidity in 58 per cent of these patients pre-operatively, but in only 26 per cent at six months, and 29 per cent at 18 months. There appeared to be no association between the mental state at 18 months following operation and either the pre-operative mental state, the previous psychiatric history, or the presence or absence of functioning ovarian tissue. There was, however, a less good psychiatric outcome in patients with dysfunctional uterine bleeding when compared with fibroids or endometriosis, and this may have represented either a reduced tolerance of the menstrual disorder by these patients or some degree of regret for their surgery. It is unlikely, therefore, that there is any association between hysterectomy and depression.

Hysterectomy and ovarian conservation

In patients undergoing hysterectomy for benign disease there is debate as to whether the ovaries should be removed as a method of preventing carcinoma of the ovary. The arguments for and against prophylactic oophorectomy in the prevention of ovarian cancer are debated in Chapter 13 (on ovarian cancer), but a further debate remains as to the length of time to ovarian failure in ovaries preserved at the time of hysterectomy.

There is also evidence that when ovaries are conserved at the time of hysterectomy, they continue to function for a shorter period of time than if hysterectomy had not taken place. Beavis *et al.* (1969) measured the urinary oestrogen excretion in 69 women undergoing abdominal hysterectomy with ovarian conservation for dysfunctional uterine bleeding. The patients were aged 25–48 years at the time of surgery, and urinary oestrogens were measured on a regular basis for 2.5 years after the surgery. The authors concluded that the ovaries continued to function normally after hysterectomy in 75 per cent of 48 patients with total conservation of the ovaries, whilst 10 per cent were anovulatory and 15 per cent inactive. However, Siddle *et al.* (1987) determined, retrospectively and by symptoms, the age of ovarian failure in 90 women who had undergone abdominal hysterectomy with bilateral ovarian conservation and in 226 women who had undergone a spontaneous menopause. The mean age at ovarian failure in the hysterectomized group was 45.4 years, statistically significantly lower than that in the spontaneous group of 49.5 years. There was also a significant correlation between the age at hysterectomy and the age at ovarian failure, 34 per cent of patients undergoing ovarian failure within two years of hysterectomy, suggesting the possibility of a causal relationship.

The likeliest explanation, should this causal relationship exist, is of a mechanical effect on the ovaries rather than a stress effect. Stone *et al.* (1975) reported a significant, but transient, fall in the mean plasma levels of oestrogen during the first five days in all eight patients undergoing abdominal hysterectomy, in five patients undergoing vaginal hysterectomy, but in none of six patients undergoing laparoscopy. Plasma oestrogen levels, however, recovered within four weeks of surgery. Janson and Jansson (1977) measured ovarian stromal blood flow by xenon clearance in five women immediately before and after abdominal hysterectomy, in which the adnexae were preserved. The mean rate of xenon clearance was reduced by between 52 and 89 per cent in four women who were premenopausal, and by 29 per cent in the one woman who was post-menopausal, suggesting an acute decrease in ovarian blood flow following hysterectomy.

Cryosurgery

Cryosurgery of the uterine cavity was reported as curing five out of six patients with intolerable menorrhagia without any particular morbidity (Cahan and Brockunier 1967), but there have been few further reports of this treatment.

Laser endometrial ablation

Goldrath *et al.* (1981) reported the use of photo-evaporation of the endometrium using neodymium–yttrium aluminium garnet (Nd–YAG) laser ablation. The thickened myometrium provides a protective coat, and 22 women with dysfunctional bleeding were all discharged within 48 hours following laser ablation under hysteroscopic vision. The uterus was perforated by the hysteroscope in one patient and all patients had a serosanguinous vaginal discharge for up to three weeks. Some 21 of the 22 women (95 per cent) became amenorrhoeic or hypomenorrhoeic. Lomano (1988) reported a 50 per cent incidence of amenorrhoea in 62 women undergoing endometrial ablation with the Nd–YAG laser using a blanching technique, but a much lower success rate using a draging technique. Davis (1989) reported 25 patients who underwent laser ablation of the endometrium for menorrhagia. The overall success rate was only 52 per cent, but the rate was increased to 83 per cent of 12 patients by increasing the power levels. Goldfarb (1990) reported that after laser endometrial ablation, 60 per cent of 35 patients became amenorrhoeic, 31 per cent resumed menstruation but at acceptable levels, and 9 per cent had an unsatisfactory result.

In the largest trial so far, Garry *et al.* (1991) treated 859 women using the Nd–YAG laser. The technique appeared to be safe, without any major complications. Perforation of the uterus occurred in 0.3 per cent of patients, but no patient required either a laparotomy or a blood transfusion. The mean stay in hospital was less than 24 hours and the mean duration of laser ablation was

24 minutes. Of 479 women followed for six months, 60 per cent had complete amenorrhoea, 32 per cent had reduced menstruation, and 8 per cent failed to improve of whom 3 per cent underwent hysterectomy. It would seem that in selected patients this may be an acceptable alternative to hysterectomy although longterm follow-up is required.

Absorption of irrigating fluid occurs during laser surgery. In a study of 12 women undergoing laser ablation, the mean duration of surgery was 92 minutes and the mean deficit of irrigation fluid was 2.5 litres (Morrison *et al.* 1989). This is discussed in greater detail below under 'Endometrial resection'.

Endometrial resection

There is currently great interest in this technique with increasing numbers of surgeons performing the resection. De Cherney *et al.* (1987) reported the use of a modified urological resectoscope which has the advantages of being faster than laser ablation, cheaper, and may require only a minor alteration in equipment which is already available. The initial series of patients involved a high incidence of women with blood dyscrasias, three of the 21 patients dying from their blood disease. However, 17 of the 18 survivors (94 per cent) became amenorrhoeic. Danazol is generally prescribed (200 mg thrice daily) for some 4–8 weeks pre-operatively to inhibit endometrial proliferation (Magos *et al.* 1989*b*).

The results of this method of treatment have recently been reported (Dwyer *et al.* 1993; Magos *et al.* 1989*a*, 1989*b*, 1991*a*). Magos *et al.* (1991*a*) reported a series in which 234 women underwent 250 endometrial resections for menorrhagia. General anaesthesia was used in 63 per cent of the procedures and sedation with local anaesthetic was used in the rest. The main complications included uterine perforation (1.6 per cent) and absorption of greater than 2 litres of irrigation fluid (2.8 per cent). Some 93 per cent of patients left hospital within 24 hours of the procedure. Of 113 women followed for one year, 27 per cent reported amenorrhoea and a further 27 per cent reported that their periods were 'much decreased'. In addition, 25 per cent reported that their periods were 'decreased', suggesting that some 79 per cent of patients had some benefit from this procedure. Hysterectomy was performed for menorrhagia in 4 per cent of the patients.

However, colleagues working in the unit from which the above series originated reported a further eight patients who had undergone hysterectomy following persistent symptoms after endometrial resection, yet had not been included in the above series. This would mean that the minimal incidence of hysterectomy for continuing unacceptable menorrhagia was 7.2 per cent (Slade *et al.* 1991). Slade *et al.* (1991) also reported that only 19.5 per cent of their 220 patients became amenorrhoeic, suggesting that the enthusiasm of initial results should be tempered, whilst 94 per cent of patients undergoing hysterectomy were very satisfied compared with 89 per cent after resection (Dwyer *et al.* 1993).

The major problems would appear to be the risk of fluid overload and haemolysis from the distension medium. Baumann *et al.* (1990) reported the effects of the 1.5 per cent glycine solution used to distend and irrigate the uterus in 10 women undergoing endometrial resection (mean operating time of 39 minutes). There was a linear negative correlation between the volume of irrigant absorbed and the change in plasma sodium concentration, such that significant hyponatraemia (plasma sodium less than 130 mmol/l) occurred in 20 per cent of patients, associated with an excess of fluid absorption (greater than one litre of glycine). The mean deficit in irrigating fluid at the end of the procedure was 630 ml (range 100–2030 ml). Such changes responded to the use of a diuretic. In a larger series from the same unit, Magos *et al.* (1990) reported that the range of fluid deficit was 0–4350 ml in 56 women, and that there was no statistically significant difference between the fluid deficit in women who had undergone a previous sterilization ($n = 22$), compared with women who had not been previously sterilized ($n = 34$), suggesting that the fluid absorption takes place through the venous network of the uterus and not via the peritoneum. West and Robinson (1989) reported that the mean glycine deficit was 298 ml (range 0–1500 ml) in 16 patients undergoing endometrial resection.

Not all menorrhagic patients are suitable for endometrial resection. Rutherford *et al.* (1991) estimated that 29 per cent of 375 hysterectomies performed over a period of time in their unit would have been suitable for endometrial resection, in that the indication was menorrhagia in the absence of a concomitant secondary indication for hysterectomy or any significant uterine pathology. It may be that endometrial resection is specifically indicated in patients in whom hysterectomy is considered to be undesirable, dangerous, or impossible (Lockwood *et al.* 1990).

On the results available so far, it would seem that endometrial resection is not as successful a procedure as is laser ablation, which in turn is not so successful a procedure as hysterectomy in the management of menorrhagia. However, longterm follow-up is mandatory if the place of these procedures is to become established within clinical practice. The need for prospective comparative studies has been stressed by several authors (Magos *et al.* 1991*a*; Stirrat *et al.* 1990). The need for caution has been demonstrated by the longterm study of transurethral resection of the prostate. (Roos *et al.* 1989). Transurethral resection of the prostate is the current 'operation of choice' for benign prostatic hypertrophy yet, after 20 years of wide-use, the above series reported a retrospective study of over 54 000 men who had undergone prostatectomy, approximately 39 000 by TURP and 15 000 by an open operation. In all three centres of study (Oxford, Manitoba, and Denmark) there was an unexpected excess mortality in the TURP group, corrected for age, with a relative risk of death of 1.45 compared with open operations.

There are now two randomized trials comparing endometrial resection with abdominal hysterectomy for the treatment of menorrhagia reported in the literature (Dwyer *et al.* 1993; Gannon *et al.* 1991).

As can be seen from Table 7.3, the mean stay in hospital and return to work was significantly lower after endometrial resection than after abdominal

Table 7.3 Endometrial resection versus abdominal hysterectomy

	Endometrial resection		Abdominal hysterectomy	
	a	b	a	b
Mean operating time (minutes)	31	35	51	45
Mean stay in hospital (days)	1.4	2	7.1	6
Mean time to return to work (days)	14.9	—	67.6	—

From: (a) Gannon *et al.* (1991) and (b) Dwyer *et al.* (1993)

hysterectomy and there is a greatly reduced need for post-operative analgesia. To assess the benefits and deficits of endometrial resection, larger trials and longer term follow-up are required.

There is a variant on transurethral resection which utilizes electrodiathermy using a roller ball. The combined results from the two series reported so far suggest that, some 6–12 months after treatment, 50 per cent of 40 patients became amenorrhoeic, 45 per cent became hypomenorrhoeic, and 5 per cent of patients required hysterectomy (Townsend *et al.* 1990; Vancaille 1989).

Radiofrequency-induced thermal ablation

RITA has recently been described as a treatment for menorrhagia. Theoretically, this technique should have an advantage over other minimally invasive methods of surgery in that a medium to distend the uterine cavity is not required.

Phipps *et al.* (1990*a*) reported the treatment of 42 patients with menorrhagia and described the 'optimal dose'. When 33 patients were treated with this 'optimal dose', 33 per cent became amenorrhoeic and a further 55 per cent had a reduced menstrual blood flow at short-term follow-up. Some 94 per cent of patients were discharged on the same day of treatment. All patients experienced some degree of lower abdominal pain within the first 48 hours of treatment and all patients experienced a bloodstained vaginal discharge for up to four weeks after treatment. Some 6 per cent of patients required hysterectomy (Phipps *et al.* 1990*b*). However, two patients who received greater than the 'optimal dose' developed a vesicovaginal fistula (Phipps *et al.* 1990*b*). It is, therefore, not possible to assess the place of this technique without further studies.

Conclusions

There are numerous methods of treatment for the patient with dysfunctional uterine bleeding. The place of management and drug therapy has already been discussed. The major advance would appear to be in the field of minimally invasive surgery. Should these techniques find a place in the clinical practice of the future, they offer a significant potential saving both in terms of finance to the health services (Boike *et al.* 1993; Macdonald 1990; Rutherford and Glass 1990) together with the benefits to the patient of a reduced hospital stay and a shorter time to reach full recovery. However, it would seem that new surgical techniques can be introduced into practice with significantly less assessment and far fewer comparative studies than would be allowed for a new drug. In order that the place of these minimally invasive techniques as an alternative to hysterectomy may be established, the importance of randomized prospective comparative studies cannot be overstressed.

References

Andersch, B., Milson, I., and Rybo, G. (1988). An objective evaluation of flurbiprofen and tranexamic acid in the treatment of idiopathic menorrhagia. *Acta Obstetrica et Gynaecologica Scandinavica* **67**, 645–8.

Anderson, A. B. M. (1976). Reduction in menstrual blood flow by prostaglandin synthetase inhibitors. *Lancet* **i**, 744–6.

Barker, M. G. (1968). Psychological illness after hysterectomy. *British Medical Journal* **2**, 91–5.

Barter, R. H., Brennon, G., Newman, W., and Merrill, K. W. (1968). The place of curettage in the diagnosis of cancer of the endometrium. *American Journal of Obstetrics and Gynecology* **100**, 696–702.

Baumann, R., Magos, A. L., Kay, J. D. S., and Turnbull, A. C. (1990). Absorption of glycine irrigating solution during transcervical resection of endometrium. *British Medical Journal* **300**, 304–5.

Beavis, E. L. G., Brown, J. B., and Smith, M. A. (1969). Ovarian function after hysterectomy with conservation of the ovaries in pre-menopausal women. *Journal of Obstetrics and Gynaecology of the British Commonwealth* **76**, 969–78.

Bergqvist, A. and Rybo, G. (1983). Treatment of menorrhagia with intrauterine release of progesterone. *British Journal of Obstetrics and Gynaecology* **90**, 255–8.

Bishop, P. M. F. and De Almeida, J. C. C. (1960). Treatment of functional menstrual disorders with norethisterone. *British Medical Journal* **1**, 1103–5.

Boike, G. M., Elfstrand, E. P., Delpriore, G., Schumock, D., Holley, H. S., and Lurain, J. R. (1993). Laparoscopically assisted vaginal hysterectomy in a university hospital. *American Journal of Obstetrics and Gynecology* **168**, 1690–701.

Cahan, W. G. and Brockunier, A. (1967). Cryosurgery of the uterine cavity. *American Journal of Obstetrics and Gynecology* **99**, 138–53.

Cameron, I. T., Leask, R., Kelly, R. W., and Baird, D. T. (1987). The effects of danazol, mefenamic acid, norethisterone, and a progesterone-impregnated coil on endometrial prostaglandin concentrations in women with menorrhagia. *Prostaglandins* **34**, 99–110.

Cameron, I. T., Haining, R., Lumsden, M. A., Thomas, V. R., and Smith, S. K. (1990). The effects of mefenamic acid and norethisterone on measured menstrual blood loss. *Obstetrics and Gynecology* **76**, 85–8.

Chamberlain, G., Freeman, R., Price, F., Kennedy, A., Green, D., and Eve, L. (1991). A comparative study of ethamsylate and mefenamic acid in dysfunctional uterine bleeding. *British Journal of Obstetrics and Gynaecology* **98**, 707–11.

Chimbira, T. H., Cope, E., Anderson, A. B. M., and Bolton, F. G. (1979). The efficacy of danazol on menorrhagia. *British Journal of Obstetrics and Gynaecology* **86**, 46–50.

Chimbira, T. H., Anderson, A. B. M., and Turnbull, A. C. (1980a). Relationship between measured menstrual blood loss and patients' objective assessment of loss. *British Journal of Obstetrics and Gynaecology* **87**, 603–9.

Chimbira, T. H., Cope, E., and Turnbull, A. C. (1980b). Reduction of menstrual blood loss by danazol in unexplained menorrhagia. *British Journal of Obsetrics and Gynaecology* **87**, 115–28.

Conyngham, R. B. (1965). Norethisterone in menorrhagia. *New Zealand Medical Journal* **64**, 697–701.

Davies, D. and Howell, D. A. (1977). Tranexamic acid and arterial thrombosis. *Lancet* **i**, 49.

Davis, J. A. (1989). Hysteroscopic endometrial ablation with the neodynium–YAG laser. *British Journal of Obstetrics and Gynaecology* **96**, 928–32.

De Cherney, A. H., Diamond, M. P., Lavy, G., and Polan, M. L. (1987). Endometrial ablation for intractable uterine bleeding. *Obstetrics and Gynecology* **70**, 668–70.

Dicker, R. C., Greenspan, J. R., Strauss, L. T., Cowart, M. R., Scally, M. J., Peterson, H. B., *et al.* (1982). Complications of abdominal and vaginal hysterectomy. *American Journal of Obstetrics and Gynecology* **144**, 841–8.

Dockeray, C. J. (1988). The medical treatment of menorrhagia. In *Contemporary obstetrics and gynaecology* (ed. G. Chamberlain), pp. 299–314. Butterworths, London.

Dockeray, C. J., Sheppherd, B. L., and Bonnar, J. (1989). Comparison between mefenamic acid and danazol in the treatment of established menorrhagia. *British Journal of Obstetrics and Gynaecology* **96**, 840–8.

Dwyer, N., Hutton, J., and Stirrat, G. M. (1993). Randomized controlled trial comparing endometrial resection with abdominal hysterectomy for the surgical treatment of menorrhagia. *British Journal of Obstetrics and Gynaecology* **100**, 237–43.

Easterday, C. L. (1983). Hysterectomy in the United States. *Obstetrics and Gynecology* **62**, 203–12.

Fernandez, H., Lelaidier, C., and Frydman, R. (1992). Laparoscopically-assisted vaginal hysterectomy. *Lancet* **339**, 123.

Fraser, I. S., Pearse, C., Shearman, R. P., Elliott, P. M., McIlveen, J., and Markham, R. (1981). Efficacy of mefenamic acid in patients with menorrhagia. *Obstetrics and Gynecology* **58**, 543–51.

Gannon, M. J., Holt, E. M., Fairbank, J., Fitzgerald, M., Milne, M .A., Crystal, A. M., *et al.* (1991). A randomized trial comparing endometrial resection and abdominal hysterectomy for the treatment of menorrhagia. *British Medical Journal* **303**, 1362–4.

Garry, R., Erian, J., and Grochmal, S. A. (1991). A multicentre collaborative study in the treatment of menorrhagia by Nd–YAG laser ablation of the endometrium. *British Journal of Obstetrics and Gynaecology* **98**, 357–62.

Gath, D., Cooper, P., and Day, A. (1982). Hysterectomy and psychiatric disorders. *British Journal of Psychiatry* **140**, 335–50.

Goldfarb, H. A. (1990). A review of 35 endometrial ablations using the Nd–YAG laser for recurrent menometrorrhagia. *Obstetrics and Gynecology* **76**, 833–5.

Goldrath, M. H., Fuller, T. A., and Segal, S. (1981). Laser photo-evaporation of endometrium for treatment of menorrhagia. *American Journal of Obstetrics and Gynecology* **140**, 14–29.

Grant, J. M. and Hussein, I. Y. (1984). An audit of abdominal hysterectomy over a decade in a district hospital. *British Journal of Obstetrics and Gynaecology* **91**, 73–7.

Grimes, D. A. (1982). Diagnostic D and C: a reappraisal. *American Journal of Obstetrics and Gynecology* **142**, 1–6.

Hallberg, L., Hogdhal, A. M., Nilsson, L., and Rybo, G. (1966). Menstrual blood loss—a population study. *Acta Obstetrica et Gynaecologica Scandinavica* **45**, 320–51.

Harrison, R. F. and Campbell, S. (1976). A double-blind trial of ethamsylate. *Lancet* **ii**, 283–5.

Haynes, P. J., Hodgson, H. M., Anderson, A. M. B., and Turnbull, A. C. (1977). Measurement of menstrual blood loss in patients complaining of menorrhagia. *British Journal of Obstetrics and Gynaecology* **84**, 763–8.

Higham, J. M. and Shaw, R. W. (1993). A comparative study of danazol and norethindrone in the treatment of objectively proven unexplained menorrhagia. *American Journal of Obstetrics and Gynecology* **169**, 1143–9.

Hunter, R. W. and McCartney, A. J. (1993). Can laparoscopic assisted hysterectomy safely replace abdominal hysterectomy? *British Journal of Obstetrics and Gynaecology* **100**, 932–4.

Hutton, J. D., Morse, A. R., Anderson, M. C., and Beard, R. W. (1978). Endometrial assessment with Isaacs cell sample. *British Medical Journal* **1**, 947–9.

Jacobs, A. and Butler, E. B. (1965). Menstrual blood loss in iron-deficiency anaemia. *Lancet* **ii**, 407–9.

Janson, P. O. and Jansson, I. (1977). The acute effect of hysterectomy on ovarian blood flow. *American Journal of Obstetrics and Gynecology* **127**, 349–52.

Jeppson, S., Mellquist, P., and Rannevik, G. (1984). Short-term effects of danazol on endometrial histology. *Acta Obstetrica et Gynaecologica Scandinavica* Supp. **123**, 41–4.

Kadar, N., Reich, H., Liu, C. Y., Manko, G. F., and Gimpelson, R. (1993). Incisional hernia after major laparoscopic gynecological procedures. *American Journal of Obstetrics and Gynecology* **168**, 1493–5.

Kasonde, J. M. and Bonnar, J. (1976). Effects of sterilization on menstrual blood loss. *British Journal of Obstetrics and Gynaecology* **83**, 572–5.

Lockwood, M., Magos, A. L., Baumann, R., and Turnbull, A. C. (1990). Endometrial resection when hysterectomy is undesirable, dangerous, or impossible. *British Journal of Obstetrics and Gynaecology* **97**, 656–8.

Lomano, J. M. (1988). Dragging technique versus blanching technique for endometrial ablation with the Nd–YAG laser. *American Journal of Obstetrics and Gynecology* **159**, 152–5.

Macdonald, R. (1990). Modern management of menorrhagia. *British Journal of Obstetrics and Gynaecology* **97**, 3–7.

MacKenzie, I. Z. and Bibby, J. G. (1978). Critical assessment of dilatation and curettage of 1029 women. *Lancet* **ii**, 566–8.

Madanes, A. E. and Farber, M. (1982). Danazol. *Annals of Internal Medicine* **96**, 625–30.

Magos, A. L., Baumann, R., and Turnbull, A. C. (1989a). Transcervical resection of endometrium in women with menorrhagia. *British Medical Journal* **298**, 1209–12.

Magos, A. L., Baumann, R., Cheung, K., and Turnbull, A. C. (1989b). Intra-uterine surgery under intravenous sedation as an alternative to hysterectomy. *Lancet* **ii**, 925–6.

Magos, A. L., Baumann, R., and Turnbull, A. C. (1990). Safety of transcervical endometrial resection. *Lancet* **i**, 44.

Magos, A. L., Baumann, R., Lockwood, G. M., and Turnbull, A. C. (1991a). Experience with the first 250 endometrial resections for menorrhagia. *Lancet* **337**, 1074–8.

Magos, A. L., Broadbent, J. A. M., and Amso, N. N. (1991b). Laparoscopically-assisted vaginal hysterectomy. *Lancet* **338**, 1091–2.

Makarainen, L. and Ulikorkala, O. (1986). Primary and myoma-associated menor-rhagia: a possible role for prostaglandins. *British Journal of Obstetrics and Gynecology* **93**, 934–8.

Milson, I., Anderson, K., Andersch, B., and Rybo, G. (1991). A comparison of flur-biprofen, tranexamic acid, and a levonorgestrel-releasing intrauterine contraceptive device in the treatment of idiopathic menorrhagia. *American Journal of Obstetrics and Gynecology* **164**, 879–83.

Morrison, L. M. M., Davis, J., and Sumner, D. (1989). Absorption of irrigating fluid during laser photocoagulation of the endometrium in the treatment of menorrhagia. *British Journal of Obstetrics and Gynaecology* **96**, 346–52.

Muldoon, M. J. (1972). Gynaecological illness after sterilization. *British Medical Journal* **1**, 84–5.

Nedoss, B. R. (1971). Dysfunctional uterine bleeding: relation of endometrial histology to outcome. *American Journal of Obstetrics and Gynecology* **109**, 103–7.

Neil, J. R., Hammond, G. T., Noble, A. D., Rushton, L., and Letchworth, A. T. (1975). Late complications of sterilization by laparoscopy or tubal ligation. *Lancet* **ii**, 699–700.

Nezhat, C., Nezhat, F., and Silfen, S. L. (1990). Laparoscopic hysterectomy and bilateral salpingo-oophorectomy using multifire GIA surgical stapler. *Journal of Gynecologic Surgery* **6**, 287–8.

Nilsson, L. and Rybo, G. (1971). The treatment of menorrhagia. *American Journal of Obstetrics and Gynecology* **110**, 713–20.

Phipps, J. H., Lewis, B. V., Roberts, T., Prior, M. V., Hand, J. W., Elber, M., *et al.* (1990*a*). Treatment of functional menorrhagia by radiofrequency-induced thermal endometrial ablation. *Lancet* **335**, 374–6.

Phipps, J. H., Lewis, B. V., Prior, M. V., and Roberts, T., (1990*b*). Experimental and clinical studies with radiofrequency-induced thermal endometrial ablation for func-tional menorrhagia. *Obstetrics and Gynecology* **76**, 876–81.

Rees, M. C. P., Anderson, A. B. M., Deners, L. M., and Turnbull, A. C. (1984). Endometrial and myometrial prostaglandin release during the menstrual cycle in rela-tion to menstrual blood loss. *Journal of Clinical Endocrinology and Metabolism* **58**, 813–18.

Reich, H., De Caprio, J., and McGlynn, F. (1989). Laparoscopic hysterectomy. *Journal of Gynecologic Surgery* **5**, 213–16.

Richards, D. H. (1973). Depression after hysterectomy. *Lancet* **ii**, 430–2.

Richards, D. H. (1974). A post-hysterectomy syndrome. *Lancet* **ii**, 983–5.

Roos, N. P., Wennberg, J. E., Malenka, D. J., Fisher, E. S., McPherson, K., Anderson, T. F., *et al.* (1989). Mortality and re-operation after open and transurethral resection of the prostate for benign hypertrophy. *New England Journal of Medicine* **320**, 1120–4.

Royal College of General Practitioners (1974). *Oral contraceptives and health*, pp. 61–4. Pittman Medical, London.

Rulin, M. C., Davidson, A. R., Philliber, S. G., Graves, W. L., and Cushman, L. F. (1989). Changes in menstrual symptoms amongst sterilized and comparison women. *Obstetrics and Gynecology* **74**, 149–54.

Rutherford, A. J. and Glass, M. R. (1990). Management of menorrhagia. *British Medical Journal* **301**, 290–1.

Rutherford, A. J., Glass, M. R., and Wells, M. (1991). Patient selection for hysteroscopic endometrial resection. *British Journal of Obstetrics and Gynaecology* **98**, 228–30.

Rybo, G. (1966). Clinical and experimental studies upon menstrual blood loss. *Acta Obstetrica et Gynaecologica Scandinavica* **Supp. 7**, 1–45.

Rydin, E. and Lundberg, P. O. (1976). Tranexamic acid and intracranial thrombosis. *Lancet* **ii**, 49.

Scrimgeour, J. B., Ng, K. B., and Gaudoin, M. R. (1991). Laparoscopically-assisted vaginal hysterectomy. *Lancet* **338**, 1465–6.

Selwood, T. and Wood, C. (1978). Incidence of hysterectomy in Australia. *Medical Journal of Australia* **2**, 201–4.

Shaw, R. W. and Fraser, H. M. (1984). Use of a superactive luteinizing hormone releasing hormone (LHRH) agonist in the treatment of menorrhagia. *British Journal of Obstetrics and Gynaecology* **91**, 913–16.

Siddle, N., Sarrel, L., and Whitehead, M. (1987). The effect of hysterectomy on the age at ovarian failure. *Fertility Sterility* **47**, 94–100.

Slade, R. J., Ahmed, A. I. H., and Gillmar, M. D. G. (1991). Problems with endometrial resection. *Lancet* **337**, 1473.

Smith, S. K., Abel, M. H., Kelly, R. W., and Baird, D. T. (1981). Prostaglandin synthesis in the endometrium of women with ovular dysfunctional uterine bleeding. *British Journal of Obstetrics and Gynaecology* **88**, 432–42.

Southam, A. L. and Richart, R. M. (1966). The prognosis for adolescents with menstrual abnormality. *American Journal of Obstetrics and Gynecology* **94**, 637–45.

Stirrat, G., Dwyer, N., and Browning, J. (1990). Planned trial of transcervical resection of the endometrium versus hysterectomy. *British Journal of Obstetrics and Gynaecology* **97**, 459.

Stock, R. J. (1978). Evaluation of sequelae of tubal ligation. *Fertility Sterility* **29**, 169–74.

Stone, S. C., Dickey, R. P., and Mickal, A. (1975). The acute effect of hysterectomy on ovarian function. *American Journal of Obstetrics and Gynecology* **121**, 193–7.

Taw, R. L. (1975). Review of menstrual disorders in which secretory endometrium was found. *American Journal of Obstetrics and Gynecology* **122**, 490–7.

Townsend, D. E., Richart, R. M., Paskowitz, R. A., and Woolfork, R. E. (1990). Roller ball coagulation of the endometrium. *Obstetrics and Gynecoloay* **76**, 310–13.

Vancaille, T. G. (1989). Electrocoagulation of the endometrium with the ball-end resectoscope. *Obstetrics and Gynecology* **74**, 425–7.

Vessey, M. P., Villard-Mackintosh, L., McPherson, K., Coulter, A., and Yeates, D. (1992). The epidemiology of hysterectomy. *British Journal of Obstetrics and Gynaecology* **99**, 402–7.

Villard-Mackintosh, L., McPherson, K., Coulter, A., and Yeates, D. (1992). The epidemiology of hysterectomy: findings in a large cohort study. *British Journal of Obstetrics and Gynaecology* **99**, 402–7.

West, J. H. and Robinson, D. A. (1989). Endometrial resection and fluid absorption. *Lancet* **ii**, 1387–8.

Williams, E. L., Jones, H. E., and Merrill, R. E. (1951). The subsequent course of patients sterilized by tubal ligation. *American Journal of Obstetrics and Gynecology* **61**, 423–6.

Willman, E. A., Collins, W. P., and Clayton, S. G. (1976). Studies in the involvement of prostaglandins and uterine symptomatology. *British Journal of Obstetrics and Gynaecology* **83**, 337–41.

Wingo, P. A., Huezo, C. M., Rubin, G. L., Ory, H. W., and Peterson, H. B. (1985). The mortality risk associated with hysterectomy. *American Journal of Obstetrics and Gynecology* **152**, 883–8.

8 The premenstrual syndrome

Premenstrual syndrome (PMS) is defined as the cyclical recurrence of psychological behavioural or somatic symptoms in the luteal phase of the menstrual cycle (O'Brien 1987). The symptoms must be relieved by the end of menstruation when there should be a symptom-free interval. To distinguish between the normal physiological changes associated with the menstrual cycle and the syndrome itself, the symptoms must be of sufficient severity to disrupt the woman's normal functioning. Such debilitating severity occurs in some 5 per cent of women (O'Brien 1987).

When making a diagnosis of premenstrual syndrome, the point which must be stressed is that it is the timing of the symptoms and not the symptoms themselves which is important. Patients should be asked to document their symptoms precisely and prospectively in some form which would demonstrate that they do fulfil the above conditions for the diagnosis of premenstrual syndrome. This assessment of the accurate timing of symptoms may be made using a menstrual distress questionnaire (Moos 1968), by the use of a self-assessment chart or disc (Magos and Studd 1988), or by the completion of a calendar (Mortola *et al*. 1990, Smith and Schiff 1989). Whichever technique is used, it should be stressed that the documentation of symptoms should be prospective and taken over at least two cycles (Watson and Studd 1990).

There are some relationships between premenstrual syndrome and psychological disorders. A significant percentage of patients presenting to a gynaecologist with premenstrual syndrome have a past history of psychiatric illness. In one series, some 39 per cent of patients gave such a past history (West 1989); in another, 38 per cent (Plouffe *et al*. 1993). Patients currently complaining of premenstrual syndrome may in fact have a major psychiatric disorder and this has been reported in up to 45 per cent of such patients (De Jong *et al*. 1985). The clinician may, therefore, have to distinguish between these conditions. This may be made more complicated by the observation that some patients with an affective mood disorder may have an increase in the severity of that disorder premenstrually (Pariser *et al*. 1985). When PMS exists without any underlying condition this is termed primary PMS; when an underlying condition is exacerbated premenstrually this is secondary PMS.

The prevalence of PMS in the female population, as reported in the scientific literature, would seem to vary widely, being 25 per cent of 500 women (Kessel and Coppen 1963), 50 per cent of women (K. Dalton 1984), or 73 per cent (Hallman 1986). Whilst minor changes preceding menstruation may, therefore, be so common as to be considered normal physiological premenstrual changes, severe and even disabling changes occur in 3.5 per cent of women (Reid 1991). The prevalence of PMS would also appear to be age-related, in that 20 per cent of patients with PMS develop their symptoms before the age of 20 years, whereas 64 per cent have symptoms by 30 years; the symptoms also seem to increase in severity with time (Sampson 1989). Not all women with PMS seek medical help; only 7.5 per cent of 1124 women with PMS felt the need for a physician's assistance (Hallman 1986).

The ramifications of premenstrual syndrome may be wide ranging, affecting the quality of academic work, the performance of industry, and even criminal activity. Thus, 45 per cent of 269 regularly menstruating female employees who used the sick-bay at work did so during their paramenstruum (K. Dalton 1964); the examination results for 34 girls sitting 68 examinations showed a pass rate of 74 per cent if the papers were written premenstrually, 84 per cent during menstruation, and 87 per cent intermenstruum (K. Dalton, 1968); 49 per cent of crimes committed by 156 regularly menstruating women prisoners occurred during the 30 per cent of the cycle which included the premenstruum and the early days of menstruation (K. Dalton, 1961). Although such statements may have some truth in them, the scientific approach of these studies is not suficiently rigorous for them to be accepted without question.

Following hysterectomy, the diagnosis of premenstrual syndrome may be more difficult, and can only be made after reliable charting of symptoms. There is some evidence that the syndrome persists but with a 'small but significant improvement' (Backstrom *et al.* 1981). It may be that this is a transient placebo effect.

Symptoms

Well over 150 symptoms have been associated with premenstrual syndrome (O'Brien 1987).

The percentages of patients with PMS complaining of the commonest symptoms are shown in Table 8.1. In general, the symptoms of premenstrual syndrome may be classified into three groups: psychological (tension, irritability, depression, restlessness, anxiety, tiredness, mood swings, decreased libido, lack of concentration, and decreased appetite); somatic (mastalgia, hot flushes, dizziness, nausea palpitations, bloating, sensation of weight gain, and visual disturbances); behavioural (agoraphobia, decreased work performance, accidents, suicide, and criminal behaviour); (Watson and Studd, 1990).

Aetiological factors

The aetiology of premenstrual syndrome is not known. Much has been written by way of explanation of the cause, but much of the evidence has either not been reproduced or has been contradicted, especially when open trials have been followed by controlled studies (Rubinow and Roy-Byrne, 1984). The following aetiological factors should be considered:

Table 8.1 Symptoms in premenstrual syndrome

Symptoms	% Of patients
Depression	71
Irritability	56
Tiredness	35
Headache	33
Bloatedness	31
Breast tenderness	21
Tension	19
Violence	13
Suicidal	6
Anxiety	5
Food cravings	5

(1) oestrogen and progesterone;

(2) sex-hormone binding globulin;

(3) prolactin;

(4) fluid retention;

(5) vitamin deficiency;

(6) hypoglycaemia;

(7) psychological factors;

(8) genetic factors;

(9) endorphin theory.

Oestrogen and progesterone

Since the basic characteristic of premenstrual syndrome is the cyclical variance in symptoms, it is reasonable that the ovarian cycle should have been considered to be the key to aetiology. However, no convincing explanation has been forthcoming (O'Brien 1993).

That progesterone deficiency during the luteal phase of the cycle was important was advoctated by Morton (1950). Morton reported that, as a group, women with premenstrual syndrome had either no rise or a poorly sustained rise on basal body temperature charting, no evidence of luteal activity on endometrial biopsy, evidence of unopposed oestrogen secretion on a vaginal smear, and subnormal or absent pregnanediol excretion in urine. However, none of these features was present in all 29 of the patients on whom these observations were based, the incidence for each of these findings being applicable to the group varying from 71 to 96 per cent. The same author was then able to reproduce PMS-like symptoms in three women following injection of 'a large dose' of oestrogen.

Other workers have produced either conflicting results or, at least, less clear-cut ones. Munday *et al.* (1981) reported that whilst 20 patients studied with PMS 'apparantly ovulated', in that progesterone appeared during the luteal phase, the mean luteal plasma levels of progesterone were lower than in 10 controls. Taylor (1979) could find no such correlation between progesterone levels and PMS, whilst O'Brien *et al.* (1980) found higher levels of plasma progesterone in the luteal phase of 18 women with PMS compared with 10 asymptomatic controls. Watts *et al.* (1985) found that whilst the maximum concentrations of progesterone and oestradiol were similar in 35 patients with PMS and 11 controls, the former ovulated prematurely, on average some 17 days prior to menstruation rather than 14.

If some form of progesterone deficiency was an aetiological factor, then it might be expected that the use of an antiprogesterone would reproduce the symptoms of PMS. Schmidt *et al.* (1991) administered the antiprogesterone mifepristone to 14 women with PMS without any alteration in the timing or severity of the syndrome. It would, therefore, seem unlikely that the aetiology will relate to some defect simply in progesterone levels.

The occurrence of a high premenstrual oestrogen–progesterone ratio has been implicated (Backstrom and Carnstein, 1974). Such a theory is supported by the association between oestrogen-dominated oral contraceptives and some adverse reactions, including anxiety, tension, and depression (Cullberg, 1972). Munday *et al.* (1981) reported higher mean luteal phase plasma oestradiol levels in 20 patients with PMS compared with 10 controls, but Taylor (1979) was unable to find any correlation between luteal phase levels of plasma oestradiol and the occurrence or severity of PMS.

It would, therefore, also seem unlikely that any alteration in the premenstrual oestrogen–progesterone ratio is an aetiological factor for PMS. If progesterone therapy does have a place in the treatment of premenstrual syndrome, it is unlikely that it is a progesterone deficiency which is being treated.

Sex-hormone binding globulin (SHBG)

It has been suggested that a deficiency in SHBG may be an aetiological factor in PMS. M. E. Dalton (1981) found that day 21 serum levels of SHBG in 50 women with severe PMS were significantly lower than in 50 age-matched controls, and proposed that this reduction might be the aetiological factor in causing an increase in free oestradiol at tissue level and, hence, an oestrogen–progesterone imbalance. Furthermore, when 31 such women were given progesterone suppositories, the SHBG binding capacities rose. Conversely, Backstrom and Aakvaag (1981) found a significantly higher mean binding capacity of SHBG in luteal phase blood taken from 15 women with PMS when compared with 17 controls.

Prolactin

It seems unlikely that variations in prolactin levels are the aetiological factor. Halbreich *et al.* (1976) found that the prolactin level of 28 women with PMS were significantly higher throughout the menstrual cycle compared with 21 controls, but the levels generally remained within the normal range and may have represented stress rather than pathology. Backstrom and Aakvaag (1981) were unable to find any significant difference in prolactin levels between 15 women with PMS and 17 controls, conversely O'Brien and Symonds (1982) were unable to find any differences between the prolactin levels in 18 subjects with PMS compared with 10 without, as were Watts *et al.* (1985).

Fluid retention

Although fluid retention occurs in some women with PMS, there is no good evidence to suggest that this is either a consistent or an aetiological factor (O'Brien 1993). Moreover, symptoms such as bloating, mastalgia, headache, and weight gain are not necessarily associated with fluid retention or relieved by diuretics (Reid and Yen 1981). Hahn *et al.* (1978) calculated total body water using an isotope dilution technique in 20 women with severe PMS and in 20 controls, during both follicular and luteal phases of their cycles. No significant difference could be found in the total body water of patients with PMS or controls for either phase of the cycle, or even between their follicular and luteal phases. More recent work has demonstrated no luteal phase changes in plasma volume, total body water, or total exchangable sodium in either symptomatic or asymptomatic women (Hussain and O'Brien, unpublished data).

Vitamin deficiency

There is a dearth of evidence to link vitamin B_6 (pyridoxine) deficiency with PMS. Biskind and Biskind (1943) demonstrated that a deficiency of vitamin B complex in female rats impaired their ability to inactivate oestrogen, but not testosterone, with a resultant increase in the absolute levels of body oestrogen. This has been extrapolated, together with the known associations between pyridoxine, tryptophan metabolism, and depression in oral contraceptive use (Adams *et al.* 1973), to presume a similar mechanism as an aetiological factor in PMS. There is no satisfactory evidence for this.

Hypoglycaemia

Altered glucose tolerance and reactive hypoglycaemia, resulting in hunger, fatigue, anxiety, and irritability, were proposed by Morton (1950) as a possible aetiological factor, but there is no evidence that women with PMS actually reduce their blood glucose levels into the hypoglycaemic range, nor is there evidence that the clinical changes in glucose tolerance in women with PMS differ from those cyclical changes in women without PMS. It now seems most unlikely that hypoglycaemia is an aetiological factor in premenstrual syndrome. Reid *et al.* (1986) examined the glucose, insulin, and glucagon responses to an oral glucose challenge at different stages in the menstrual cycle in normal women and in women with alleged hypoglycaemic attacks. The responses did not differ, either between normal women and women with PMS, or between the luteal and proliferative phases of the cycle.

Psychological factors

Whilst PMS is clearly associated with psychological symptoms, and normal women may also show a cyclical variation in mood throughout the menstrual cycle (Sampson, 1989), it is not clear whether there is any psychological element to the aetiology of PMS. Such women are more likely to have higher anxiety trait scores (Watts *et al.* 1980) and higher levels of neuroticism on testing (Slade and Jenner, 1980) than do normal women, but the criticism has been levelled that such studies only test those who complain of their premenstrual syndrome as opposed to those who suffer it without complaint. The features may, therefore, be features of women who complain of premenstrual syndrome to a physician rather than those of women who suffer from premenstrual syndrome (Sampson, 1989).

There is evidence that women with affective disorders have a higher incidence of PMS than does the normal female population. De Jong *et al.* (1985) reported that 45 per cent of 33 women with PMS had a past history of a psychiatric disorder of which a major depressive illness was the commonest (30 per cent).

Genetic factors

There is a familial tendency towards premenstrual syndrome, in that 70 per cent of the adolescent daughters of women who complain of PMS had similar symptoms compared with 37 per cent if their mothers were asymptomatic (Magos and Studd, 1984). K. Dalton *et al.* (1987) suggested that this relationship is genetic rather than evironmental. They reported 15 pairs of monozygous twins and 16 pairs of dizygous twins, no sibling having been brought up separated. They reported that both siblings had PMS in 93 per cent of the monozygous twins and 44 per cent of the dizygous twins. They also reported that 31 per cent of the non-twin sisters of women with PMS also experienced PMS.

Endorphin theory

There is current interest in the theory, or perhaps it should still be termed a hypothesis, that alterations in the central effects of endorphins may be an aetiological factor in premenstrual syndrome.

Endorphins are endogenous opioid peptides which are known to have some function as both neurotransmitters and neuromodulators. It has been proposed that luteal phase sensitivity to, and withdrawal from, the central effects of beta-endorphins may result in a cascade of central nervous system changes which result in premenstrual syndrome (Reid and Yen 1981). Several studies have demonstrated that plasma beta-endorphin levels are lower during the luteal phase in patients with premenstrual syndrome than in controls (Chuong *et al.* 1985; Tulenheimo *et al.* 1987). However, this does not necessarily mean that this is an aetiological factor, nor does it necessarily reflect what is happening inside the central nervous system. However, this hypothesis has allowed for the trial of a new range of therapeutic agents (please see 'Methods of treatment' section). The evidence in support of this hypothesis has been summarized by Lurie and Borenstein (1990).

Methods of treatment

Numerous forms of treatment for patients with premenstrual syndrome have been advocated, assuming that the patient wishes treatment. From the wealth of scientific literature available, two major observations are clear. Firstly, there are large numbers of different drugs that have been advocated in the treatment of premenstrual syndrome, and none would appear to be outstandingly superior to any other. Secondly, the placebo effect is very significant. The following treatment suggestions have been made:

(1) general measures;

(2) placebo;

(3) progestogens and progesterones;

(4) pyridoxine;

(5) diuretics:

(6) bromocriptine;

(7) danazol;

(8) oral contraception;

(9) oestradiol implants and patches;

(10) prostaglandin inhibitors;

(11) GnRH analogues;

(12) opiate antagonists;

(13) serotonin reuptake inhibitors;

(14) oophorectomy.

General measures

Some patients may only require an explanation of their symptoms and a reassurance about the absence of pathology, whilst others respond to general measures designed to be 'self-help', such as weight control, exercise, dietary manipulation, stress counselling, and information (Sampson, 1989).

There have been numerous suggestions of advice to patients concerning their diets. For instance, Wurtman *et al.* (1989) reported a group of women with PMS who reduced their premenstrual symptoms by an increased consumption of carbohydrate-rich, protein-poor food during the late luteal phase of the menstrual cycle. Reid *et al.* (1986) suggested that there was no real benefit from an increased carbohydrate intake in the treatment of PMS, but rather there might be an increased satisfaction of satisfying hunger in a patient already anxious because of PMS. There is no benefit from the increased intake of essential fatty acids compared with placebo (Collins *et al.* 1993).

The use of tranquillizers have been advocated. Carstairs and Talbot (1981) reported a cross-over study of 62 patients with PMS treated with either placebo or bendrofluazide, 2.5 mg daily, or meprobamate, 200 mg daily, or a combination of bendrofluazide and meprobamate, all taken three times a day for the seven days prior to menstruation. Relief of symptoms occurred in 48 per cent of patients taking placebo, 36 per cent taking bendrofluazide, 42 per cent taking meprobamate, and 63 per cent taking the drug combination.

Antidepressants have also been advocated, of which lithium seems to have been the most popular for premenstrual syndrome. It is suggested that the capacity of lithium to affect water and electrolytes makes it useful in cyclical disorders. Singer *et al.* (1974) compared lithium (750–1000 mg per day) to placebo in a double-blind, cross-over study of 19 patients with premenstrual syndrome. Lithium was not superior to placebo.

Some benefit is claimed from reflexology (Oleson and Flocco 1993).

Placebo

There is no doubt that a placebo is effective in treating premenstrual syndrome; the only debate relates to the size of the placebo response. Mattsson and Schoultz (1974) have reported a placebo success rate of 89 per cent in 18 women with premenstrual syndrome in the placebo arm of a double-blind study, 10 women being 'much better' and a further six 'somewhat better'. Sampson *et al.* (1988) reported a placebo response of 50 per cent of 64 patients, whilst Magos *et al.* (1986) reported an initial response of 94 per cent for 35 women with premenstrual syndrome treated with a placebo implant. The importance of this placebo response is that it becomes almost impossible to interpret the value of non-placebo controlled studies in assessing modes of treatment in this condition. It is not unusual to find that the apparently significant effect of a therapeutic agent in a non-controlled study is almost totally explicable by its placebo effect.

Progestogens and progesterone

There is now general agreement that progestogens are of very limited value, if any, in the treatment of premenstrual syndrome. Originally Greene and Dalton (1953), in a totally open study, found that oral norethisterone completely

Table 8.2 Progesterone treatment

	Progesterone 200 mg twice daily	Progesterone 400 mg twice daily
No. of patients	35	26
Progesterone better than place than placebo (%)	31	27
Placebo better than progesterone (%)	43	35
Both equally helpful (%)	6	15
Neither helpful (%)	20	23

From Sampson (1979)

relieved symptoms of 48 per cent of 46 women with premenstrual syndrome. However, Jordheim (1972) treated 21 patients with premenstrual syndrome in a double-blind cross-over study comparing progesterones with placebo. He found there was a 'good effect' in 21 per cent of progesterone-treated cycles and 19 per cent of placebo-treated cycles. Similarly, Sampson *et al.* (1988) found no difference in the efficacy of treatment of premenstrual syndrome in a double-blind cross-over study involving 65 patients receiving either placebo or dihydrogesterone, 10 mg twice daily for the 14 days premenstrually.

Progesterone, which is inactive orally (unless micronized) and is, therefore, given by injection, nasal administration, or vaginal or rectal pessaries, is in common use. Greene and Dalton (1953) found that an intramuscular injection of progesterone completely relieved the premenstrual syndrome of 84 per cent of 61 women, whilst K. Dalton (1984) recommended progesterone pessaries in dosages of between 400 and 3200 mg daily without adverse effect, but the results were largely anecdotal. She further claimed that the lack of success claimed by other authors related to their use of insufficient progesterone pessaries.

Sampson (1979) reported two controlled studies of progesterone against placebo, both by pessary or suppository. The results for both 200 mg and 400 mg, twice daily, of progesterone are shown in Table 8.2, suggesting that progesterone and placebo were equally effective in the treatment of premenstrual syndrome. Dennerstein *et al.* (1985) reported a double-blind randomized cross-over trial of oral micronized progesterone, 300 mg per day, and placebo for 23 women with premenstrual syndrome, each agent being taken for two cycles. Using self-assessment records, they showed that symptoms were less on active treatment than placebo, although both were effective. Furthermore, side-effects were commonly reported by both groups, 22 side-effect symptoms being reported in the progesterone group and 19 in the placebo. Maddocks *et al.* (1986) compared progesterone, 200 mg vaginally twice daily for 12 days premenstrually for three cycles, with a placebo in a cross-over trial involving a further three cycles in 20 women with premenstrual syndrome. Detailed self-reporting questionnaires were completed by the patients who found that vaginal progesterone was no more effective than vaginal placebo.

It is, therefore, an interesting observation that the only studies which have suggested any value for these agents have been uncontrolled trials. Whenever a controlled trial is reported, progesterone treatment, even in dosages of 800 mg per day, fails to be superior to placebo (Freeman *et al.* 1990). Despite this, the advocates of progesterone therapy still advocate its use without any statistical support for their claims (Mackenzie and Holten 1991). O'Brien (1993) states 'the widespread use of progesterone probably results from the enthusiasm of its advocacy rather than its pharmacotherapeutic efficacy'.

Pyridoxine

Pyridoxine is a popular treatment for premenstrual syndrome, partly because it is easily available without the need for a prescription. The evidence for its value is, however, inconclusive, yet the side-effects at very high doses may be significant.

Stokes and Mendels (1972) reported a double-blind comparison of pyridoxine, 50 mg per day, and placebo in 13 women with PMS, alternating cycles between the two agents for up to one year. The results showed that five patients preferred placebo, four pyridoxine, three found no improvement, and one became worse. Barr (1984) reported a double-blind trial of 48 women with PMS given a two-month supply of pyridoxine, 100 mg per day, or placebo and then crossed over for a further two months. There was a statistically significant advantage for pyridoxine over placebo. Williams *et al.* (1985) assessed 434 patients treated with pyridoxine or placebo in a double-blind randomized trial. Some 82 per cent of 204 women taking pyridoxine improved compared with 70 per cent of 230 taking placebo, this result being statistically significant. However, Kjeijnen *et al.* (1990) reviewed 12 controlled trials of vitamin B_6 therapy in the treatment of premenstrual syndrome, and concluded that the evidence for a positive effect over placebo was weak. Some three trials gave a positive result, five were ambiguous, and four gave a negative result. It is even possible that these trials represent an artificially beneficial view of pyridoxine in that neutral or negative trials could have been subject to a negative publication bias.

Pyridoxine not free of side-effects. Schaumburg *et al.* (1983) reported seven patients (six women) with severe sensory neuropathy (four severely disabled) related to pyridoxine therapy. All patients improved on cessation of the treatment. The maximum daily dose used by the patients was up to 6 g for between 4 and 40 months. Two patients received a prescription from a gynaecologist and five initiated the treatment themselves, either to improve premenstrual syndrome, or general health, or both.

Diuretics

Diuretics have been used in view of the mistaken association between bloatedness, weight gain, and the premenstrual syndrome. There is only limited evidence for their value.

O'Brien *et al.* (1979) gave spironolactone to 18 women with premenstrual syndrome in a double-blind cross-over trial of either spironolactone, 25 mg four times a day, or placebo, four times a day, during the luteal phase of four cycles. Some 80 per cent of patients felt that the treatment cycles were less symptomatic than the placebo ones. Similarly Vellacott *et al.* (1987) reported a double-blind placebo-controlled trial of 100 mg daily of spironolactone from day 12 of the cycle until menstruation compared with placebo. Of the 27 patients who received spironolactone, 56 per cent considered the treatment to have been a 'global success' as compared with 30 per cent of the 27 patients who received the placebo. There were no differences in weight or blood pressure between the active and placebo treatment groups.

Mattsson and Schoultz (1974) reported a double-blind cross-over study of 18 women given either a diuretic (chlorthalidone 25–50 mg daily), or lithium carbonate, or placebo. The results demonstrated that the placebo was the most effective form of treatment. Hahn *et al.* (1978) could find no significant benefit for the use of the diuretic bumetanide compared with placebo.

Bromocriptine

Ghose and Coppen (1977) reported a double-blind cross-over study of 13 women with premenstrual syndrome randomized to receive either bromocriptine, 2.5 mg daily, or placebo. There was no significant difference in improvement between the bromocriptine-and placebo-treated cycles. Andersen *et al.* (1977) treated 21 patients with premenstrual syndrome with placebo or bromocriptine, 2.5 mg twice daily, in a double-blind cross-over study. Medication, either active or placebo, improved the premenstrual symptoms of all women. The only subgroup in which bromocriptine was statistically significant to placebo related to breast tenderness, and there was a relationship between the severity of breast tenderness and the prolactin level even though the prolactin level was never high enough to be abnormal, although Benedek-Jaszmann and Hearn-Sturtevant (1976) reported 34 women with premenstrual syndrome who were given complete relief of their symptoms, based on self-assessment, when given bromocriptine 2.5 mg twice daily.

Andersch (1983) surveyed 14 double-blind placebo-controlled trials of bromocriptine in premenstrual syndrome, and concluded that the only benefit over placebo occurred in women with premenstrual breast pain, providing a dose of at least 5 mg daily was used.

Danazol

Since danazol may render a patient amenorrhoeic by depressing the ovarian cycle, it is logical that this drug has been tried in premenstrual syndrome. There is some evidence that it is superior to placebo in dosages which are not high enough to cause amenorrhoea.

Gilmore *et al.* (1989) reported a double-blind cross-over study of 36 patients

Table 8.3 The influence of age

	% Prevalence of premenstrual syndrome by age (years)				
Age	18	25	32	39	46
Users	70.0	62.9	60.0	75.0	76.5
Non-users (n = 595)	67.8	80.6	76.9	79.3	78.1

From Andersch and Hahn (1981)

with premenstrual syndrome, allocated to danazol, 400 mg daily, or placebo. This study demonstrated a statistically significant improvement with danazol compared with either placebo or the pretreatment state for the symptoms of breast tenderness, tension, and irritability. Some three of the 25 patients receiving danazol reported side-effects (12 per cent). Similarly, Sarno *et al.* (1987), in a double-blind cross-over study of 40 women with premenstrual syndrome receiving either placebo or danazol, 200 mg daily, found that 11 of the 14 patients improved significantly with danazol (79 per cent), without side-effects, whilst the other 21 per cent felt better on the placebo. The authors concluded that danazol was statistically significantly superior to placebo.

Providing that the patients do not stop taking danazol because of its side-effects (weight gain, hot flushes, and increased hair growth being the major ones), it would appear to be an effective treatment for premenstrual syndrome. The dose may have to be titrated against effect and some patients will need to be rendered amenorrhoeic.

Oral contraception

Whereas K. Dalton (1984) advocated that oral contraception should be stopped in patients with premenstrual syndrome, the Royal College of General Practitioners' (1974) study on 23 611 oral contraceptive takers and 22 766 controls (1974) found that takers reported premenstrual syndrome 29 per cent less often than did controls. Similarly, Kutner and Brown (1972) also found premenstrual syndrome to be less common in oral contraceptive users than non-users in a survey of 5151 women, but with a subgroup of previous oral contraceptive users in whom there was an excess of premenstrual syndrome, this being a factor for their cessation of oral contraception. Andersch and Hahn (1981) compared the premenstrual syndromes of 217 women taking oral contraception with 595 age-matched women who were not. As can be seen in Table 8.3, the prevalence of premenstrual syndrome was lower in oral contraceptive users when compared with non-users throughout most of the ages reported, but not at the younger end of the age scale. If this result is valid, then cohort studies will have to be corrected for age.

Placebo-controlled studies involving oral contraception are not common, largely because of the potential side-effect of pregnancy in the control group. However, Morris and Udry (1972) reported a double-blind randomized trial

Table 8.4 Oral contraceptive treatment

| | % Patients with symptoms of | | |
	Nervousness	Depression	Weight gain
Placebo	8	9	30
OC 1	4	1	19
OC 2	16	8	20
OC 3	10	5	28
OC 4	11	7	31

From Goldzeiher *et al.* (1971)

or oral contraception or placebo in 51 women, and found that premenstrual syndrome was equally likely to occur in both group. Goldzeiher *et al.* (1971) reported a placebo-controlled trial of four oral contraceptive agents in 398 women over 1523 cycles. Although this study looked at 'nervousness and depression' at any time of the cycle and not just premenstrually, the results, shown in Table 8.4, lend some support to the view that oral contraception is just as likely to be associated with nervousness, depression, or even weight gain as is a placebo.

Although one might have expected some benefit from oral contraceptive use, all the evidence is that all oral contraceptive preparations (monophasic, biphasic, or triphasic) do not play an effective role in the treatment of premenstrual syndrome (Watson and Studd, 1990). However, there is no data relating to studies of the newer oral contraceptives.

Oestradiol implants and patches

There is evidence that the use of oestradiol implants and patches are superior to placebo.

Magos *et al.* (1986) treated 61 women with premenstrual syndrome, randomly allocated to receive either a 100 mg implant of oestradiol and 5 mg oral norethisterone for seven days per cycle ($n = 33$), or a placebo implant and 5 mg of oral placebo ($n = 35$). The same implant was repeated five months later. Assessment was by questionnaire and daily symptom ratings. Although the authors reported an initial response to placebo pellets in 94 per cent of 35 women, the response was weaker and of shorter duration than the active agent. The authors attributed the effect to a relative suppression of cyclical ovarian function by oestradiol. Similarly, Watson *et al.* (1990) reported a continued improvement in PMS patients receiving longterm oestradiol implants. This response occurred in between 74 and 96 per cent of patients, although only 42 per cent of patients became fully symptom-free. In a randomized, cross-over study of oestradiol vs. placebo transdermal patches, both active and placebo groups improved, but the improvement deteriorated in those patients who changed from the active to the placebo group (Watson *et al.* 1989). Those symptoms which improved on the cross-over from placebo to oestradiol patches

Table 8.5 Symptoms improving with oestradiol patches

Bloating
Difficulty concentrating
Depression
Loss of efficiency
Irritability
Mood swings
Tension
Tiredness
Weight gain

From Watson *et al.* (1989)

Table 8.6 Treatment with the prostaglandin inhibitors metenamic acid

Symptom	No. with symptom	% Relieved
Depression	60	88
Irritability	54	87
Tension	18	94
Headache	39	92
Nausea	21	95
Loss of concentration	18	94
Mastalgia	21	71

From Jakubowicz *et al.* (1984)

are shown in Table 8.5. Since oestradiol patches are contraceptive, they may be particularly suited to the women with PMS who need birth control (Watson *et al.* 1989).

There would appear to be a benefit from oestradiol therapy, but it is difficult to assess the size of this benefit over a placebo effect.

Prostaglandin inhibitors

Prostaglandin synthetase inhibitors are of limited value in the treatment of premenstrual syndrome, although they are superior to placebo.

Jakubowicz *et al.* (1984) reported a trial of 80 patients treated with mefenamic acid, 1500–2000 mg per day during the luteal phase. The effects, shown in Table 8.6, were as good as any other treatment, with up to 95 per cent of some symptoms relieved, although 26 per cent of patients complained of side-effects (dyspepsia, nausea, diarrhoea, and skin rashes). Wood and Jakubowicz (1980) treated 37 women with premenstrual syndrome using mefenamic acid, 1500 mg per day, or a placebo in a randomly allocated double-blind cross-over trial. Of the 37 women, 62 per cent preferred mefenamic acid, 16 per cent placebo, and 22 per cent were not helped by either drug. Mira *et al.* (1986) reported a randomly allocated double-blind cross-over study of 15 women with PMS, using mefenamic acid or placebo. The authors analysed 39 mefenamic acid cycles and 35 placebo cycles. They found that mefenamic acid was superior to placebo in alleviating mood symptoms, but no better than placebo in alleviating breast or abdominal symptoms, or food cravings.

Most patients seem to know of Oil of Evening Primrose. This is a nutritional supplement containing two polyunsaturated fatty acids which are early metabolites in prostaglandin synthesis. Evening Primrose Oil has, therefore, been used on the assumption that it may correct a defect in prostaglandin metabolism which may itself have caused the PMS.

There have been few controlled clinical trials of Evening Primrose Oil (O'Brien and Massil, 1990; Puoloakka *et al.* 1985). In both studies, the PMS scores were reduced to a significantly greater degree by Evening Primrose Oil than by placebo, suggesting that there is good evidence for the use of this agent in premenstrual syndrome. However, the volume of scientific information is limited.

GnRH analogues

GnRH, given intranasally or subcutaneously, has been used in the treatment of endometriosis, menorrhagia, and subfertility. Muse *et al.* (1984) in a cross-over study, conducted over six months, relieved symptoms in all eight women using GnRH, but to a lesser extent following placebo, as judged by a patient questionnaire. However, the inconvenience of subcutaneous or intranasal administration, the potential longterm risk of osteopenia, and the reappearance of symptoms immediately that treatment is discontinued make this an unlikely choice for longterm treatment (Hussain *et al.* 1992).

Opiate antagonists

Since a withdrawal of endorphins has been implicated in the aetiology of PMS, opiate antagonists have been used on the assumption that the withdrawal would be inhibited (Chuong *et al.* 1988).

In a double-blind placebo-controlled cross-over study, the above authors assessed the effect of either placebo or the potent oral opiate antagonist naltrexone, 25 mg twice daily from the 9th to the 18th day of the cycle. Some 87 per cent of 16 patients had a lower PMS score during the cycles in which naltrexone was used compared with the cycles in which placebo was used, suggesting a possible clinical benefit. Side-effects were few, and included nausea, decreased appetite, and dizziness, but no patient withdrew because of side-effects. The need for larger studies is clear.

Serotonin reuptake inhibitors

It has been recently suggested that a reduction in brain serotonin (5-hydroxytryptamine) could lead to symptoms very reminiscent of PMS, and that clomipramine, a tricyclic inhibitor of serotonin reuptake inactivation, is superior to placebo in the reduction of both premenstrual irritability and carbohydrate craving (Eriksson *et al*. 1990; Sundblad *et al*. 1992).

Oophorectomy

Since PMS may be alleviated by danazol, GnRH analogues, pregnancy, and the menopause, it seems logical that bilateral oophorectomy, with or without hysterectomy, should have been tried in some women with intractable, severe PMS. Hysterectomy without oophorectomy is not associated with a significantly high improvement (Backstrom *et al*. 1981). Casper and Hearn (1990) and Casson *et al*. (1990) both reported a series of 14 women with severe PMS treated by abdominal hysterectomy, bilateral salpingo-oophorectomy, and continuous oestrogen hormone replacement therapy. All patients in both series became free of symptoms following this treatment, although longterm results need to be collected in order that a realistic place for this therapy may be assessed.

In patients who are being counselled for hysterectomy for other benign indications, it is important to consider (amongst other considerations) the occurrence and severity of premenstrual syndrome before deciding whether to remove or conserve the ovaries.

Conclusions

There can be no doubt that premenstrual syndrome is a common problem, and it is likely that the cause is neither exclusively hormonal nor psychogenic but is multifactorial. It may even be that PMS is not a homogenous condition (Gath and Iles, 1988). Similarly, whilst many treatments are offered, only a few have been shown to be convincingly superior to placebo in appropriate trials, and all drugs used to treat this condition should be subject to such studies. Although side-effects need to be taken into account, it would seem that danazol is the most active single medical agent in this condition, and that bilateral oophorectomy should be considered in patients whose symptoms are severe enough to warrant further intervention should drug treatment fail.

The future of PMS research rests on accepting that differences in ovarian hormones will probably never be found and that the normal ovarian cycle is no more than the 'triggering event' for abnormal neurotransmission within the brain; perhaps involving endorphins or serotonin. Until the central abnormality is found, the gynaecologist can only hope to modulate or eliminate the ovarian cycle. Identification of such a substance that will be free from side-effects and avoid surgery will be the key to future success in treatment.

References

Adams, P. W., Rose, D. P., Folkard, J., Wynn, V., Seed, M., and Strong, R. (1973). The effect of pyridoxine hydrochloride upon depression associated with oral contraceptives. *Lancet* **i**, 897-904.

Andersch, B. (1983). Bromocriptine and premenstrual symptoms: a survey of double-blind trials. *Obstetric and Gynecological Survey* **38**, 643-6.

Andersch, B. and Hahn, L. (1981). Premenstrual complaints. *Acta Obstetrica et Gynaecologica Scandinavica* **60**, 579-83.

Andersen, A. N., Larsen, J. F., Steenstrup, O. R., Svendstrup, B., and Neilsen, J. (1977). The effect of bromocriptine upon the premenstrual syndrome. *British Journal of Obstetrics and Gynaecology* **84**, 370-4.

Backstrom, T. and Aakvaag, A. (1981). Plasma prolactin and testosterone during the luteal phase in women with premenstrual tension syndrome. *Psychoneuroendocrinology* **6**, 245-51.

Backstrom, T. and Carnstein, H. (1974). Oestrogen and progesterone in plasma in relation to premenstrual syndrome. *Journal of Steroid Biochemistry* **5**, 257-60.

Backstrom, C. T., Boyle, H., and Baird, D. T. (1981). Persistence of symptoms of premenstrual tension in hysterectomised women. *British Journal of Obstetrics and Gynaecology* **88**, 530-6.

Barr, W. (1984). Pyridoxine supplements in the premenstrual syndrome. *Practitioner* **228**, 425-7.

Benedek-Jaszmann, L. J. and Hearn-Sturtevant, M. D. (1976). Premenstrual tension and functional infertility. *Lancet* **i**, 1095-8.

Biskind, M. S. and Biskind, G. R. (1943). Inactivation of testosterone propionate in the liver during vitamin B complex deficiency. *Endocrinology* **32**, 97-102.

Carstairs, M. W. and Talbot, D. J. (1981). A placebo-controlled trial of Tenavoid in the management of premenstrual syndrome. *British Journal of Clinical Practice* **35**, 403-9.

Casper, R. F. and Hearn, M. T. (1990). The effect of hysterectomy and bilateral oophorectomy in women with severe premenstrual syndrome. *American Journal of Obstetrics and Gynecology* **162**, 105-9.

Casson, P., Hahn, P. M., Vugh, D. A. V., and Reid, R. L. (1990). Lasting response to ovariectomy in severe intractable premenstrual syndrome. *American Journal of Obstetrics and Gynecology* **162**, 99-105.

Chuong, C. J., Coulam, C. B., Kao, P. C., Bergstralh, E. J., and Go, V. L. W. (1985). Neuropeptide levels in premenstrual syndrome. *Fertility Sterility* **44**, 760-5.

Chuong, C. J., Coulam, C. B., Bergstralh, E. J., O'Fallon, W. M., and Steinmerz, G. I. (1988). Clinical trial of naltrexone in premenstrual syndrome. *Obstetrics and Gynecology* **72**, 332-6.

Collins, A., Cerin, A., Coleman, G., and Landgren, D. M. (1993). Essential fatty acids in the treatment of PMS. *Obstetrics and Gynecology* **81**, 93-8.

Cullberg, J. (1972). Mood changes and menstrual symptoms with different gestogen-oestrogen combinations. *Acta Psychiatrica Scandinavica* **Supp. 236**, 1-86.

Dalton, K. (1961). Menstruation and crime. *British Medical Journal* **2**, 1752-3.

Dalton, K. (1964). The influence of menstruation on health and disease. *Proceedings of the Royal Society of Medicine* **57**, 262-4.

Dalton, K. (1968). Menstruation and examinations. *Lancet* **ii**, 1386-8.

Dalton, K. (1984). *The premenstrual syndrome and progesterone therapy* (2nd edn), pp. 3-9; 45-59. 127-140; 228-39. Heinemann Medical, London.

Dalton, K., Dalton, M. E., and Guthrie, K. E. (1987). Incidence of the premenstrual syndrome in twins. *British Medical Journal* 295, 1027-8.

Dalton, M. E. (1981). Sex hormone binding globulin concentrations in women with severe premenstrual syndrome. *Postgraduate Medical Journal* 57, 560-1.

De Jong, R., Rubinow, D. R., Roy-Byrne, P., Hoban, M. C., Grover, G. N., and Post, R. M. (1985). Premenstrual disorder and psychiatric illness. *American Journal of Psychiatry* 142, 1359-61.

Dennerstein, L., Spencer-Gardner, T., Gotts, G., Brown, J. B., Smith, M. A., and Burrows, G. D. (1985). Progesterone and the premenstrual syndrome, a double-blind cross-over trial. *British Medical Journal* 290, 1617-21.

Eriksson, E., Lisjo, P., Sundblad, C., Andersson, K., Andersch, B., and Modigh, K. (1990). Clomipramine in the premenstrual syndrome. *Acta Psychiatrica Scandinavica* 82, 87-8.

Freeman, E., Rickels, K., Sondheimer, S. J., and Polansky, M. (1990). Ineffectiveness of progesterone suppository treatment for premenstrual syndrome. *Journal of the American Medical Association* 264, 349-53.

Gath, D. and Iles, S. (1988). Treating the premenstrual syndrome. *British Medical Journal* 297, 237-8.

Ghose, K. and Coppen, A. (1977). Bromocriptine and premenstrual syndrome: a controlled study. *British Medical Journal* 1, 147-8.

Gilmore, D. H., Hawthorn, R. J. S., and Hart, D. M. (1989). Treatment of premenstrual syndrome. *Journal of Obstetrics and Gynaecology* 9, 318-22.

Goldzeiher, J. W., Moses, L. E., Averkin, E., Scheel, C. and Taber, B. A. (1971). Nervousness and depression attributed to oral contraception. *American Journal of Obstetrics and Gynecology* 111, 1013-20.

Greene, R. and Dalton, K. (1953). The premenstrual syndrome. *British Medical Journal* 1, 1007-14.

Hahn, L., Andersson, N., and Isaksson, B. (1978). Body water and weight in patients with premenstrual tension. *British Journal of Obstetrics and Gynaecology* 85, 546-50.

Halbreich, U., Assael, M., Ben-David, M., and Bornstein, R. (1976). Serum prolactin in women with premenstrual syndrome. *Lancet* ii, 564-6.

Hallman, J. (1986). The premenstrual syndrome—an equivalent of depression? *Acta Psychiatrica Scandinavica* 73, 403-11.

Hussain, S., Massil, H., Matta, W. H., Shaw, R. W., and O'Brien, P. M. S. (1992). Buserelin in premenstrual syndrome. *Gynecologic Endocrinology* 6, 1-8.

Jarubowicz, O. L., Godurd, E., and Dewhurst, J. (1984). The treatment of premenstrual tension with mefenamic acid. *British Journal of Obstetrics and Gynaecology* 91, 78-84.

Jordheim, O. (1972). The premenstrual syndrome. *Acta Obstetrica et Gynaecologica Scandinavica* 51, 77-80.

Kessel, N. and Coppen, A. (1963). The problem of common menstrual symptoms. *Lancet* ii, 61-6.

Kjeijnen, J., Riet, G. T., and Knipschild, P. (1990). Vitamin B_6 in the treatment of the premenstrual syndrome—a review. *British Journal of Obstetrics and Gynaecology* 97, 847-52.

Kutner, S. J. and Brown, W. L. (1972). Types of oral contraception, depression, and premenstrual syndrome. *Journal of Nervous and Mental Health* 155, 153-62.

Lurie, S. and Borenstein, R. (1990). The premenstrual syndrome. *Obstetric and Gynecologic Survey* 45, 220-8.

Mackenzie, N. and Holten, W. (1991). Premenstrual syndrome and progesterone suppositories. *Journal of the American Medical Association* **265**, 26.

Maddocks, S., Hahn, P., Moller, F., and Reid, R. L. (1986). A double-blind placebo controlled study of progesterone vaginal suppositories in the treatment of premenstrual syndrome. *American Journal of Obstetrics and Gynecology* **154**, 573–81.

Magos, A. and Studd, J. (1984). The premenstrual syndrome. In *Progress in obstetrics and gynaecology*, Vol. 4, (ed. J. Studd), pp. 334–50. Churchill Livingstone, Edinburgh.

Magos, A. L. and Studd, J. W. W. (1988). A simple method for the diagnosis of premenstrual syndrome by use of a self-assessment disc. *American Journal of Obstetrics and Gynecology* **158**, 1024–8.

Magos, A. L., Brincat, M., and Studd, J. W. W. (1986). Treatment of the premenstrual syndrome by subcutaneous oestradiol implants and cyclical oral norethisterone: placebo controlled study. *British Medical Journal* **292**, 1629–33.

Mattsson, B. and Schoultz, B. (1974). A comparison between lithium, placebo, and a diuretic in premenstrual tension. *Acta Psychiatrica Scandinavica* **Supp. 255**, 75–84.

Mira, M., McNeil, D., Fraser, I. S., Vizzard, J., and Abraham, S. (1986). Mefenamic acid in the treatment of premenstrual syndrome. *Obstetrics and Gynecology* **68**, 395–8.

Moos, R. H. (1968). The development of a menstrual distress questionnaire. *Psychosomatic Medicine* **30**, 853–67.

Morris, N. M. and Udry, J. R. (1972). Contraceptive pills and day-by-day feelings of well-being. *American Journal of Obstetrics and Gynecology* **113**, 763–5.

Mortola, J. F., Girton, L., Beck, L., and Yen, S. S. (1990). Diagnosis of premenstrual syndrome by a simple improved prospective and reliable instrument. *Obstetrics and Gynecology* **76**, 302–7.

Morton, J. H. (1950). Premenstrual tension. *American Journal of Obstetrics and Gynecology* **60**, 343–52.

Munday, M. R., Brush, M. G., and Taylor, R. W. (1981). Correlations between progesterone, oestradiol, and aldosterone levels in the premenstrual syndrome. *Clinical Endocrinology* **14**, 1–9.

Muse, K. N., Cetal, N. S., Futterman, L. A., and Ien, S. S. C. (1984). The premenstrual syndrome. *New England Journal of Medicine* **311**, 1345–9.

O'Brien, P. M. S. (1987). *The premenstrual syndrome*, pp. 5–37. Blackwell Scientific Publications, Oxford.

O'Brien, P. M. S. (1993). Helping women with premenstrual syndrome. *British Medical Journal* **307**, 1471–5.

O'Brien, P. M. S. and Massil, H. Y. (1990). Premenstrual syndrome – clinical studies on essential fatty acids. In *Essential fatty acids – pathophysiology and roles in clinical medicine* (ed D. F. Horrobin), pp. 523–45. Wiley-Liss, New York.

O'Brien, P. M. S. and Symonds, E. M. (1982). Prolactin levels in the premenstrual syndrome. *British Journal of Obstetrics and Gynaecology* **89**, 306–8.

O'Brien, P. M. S., Craven, D., Selby, C., and Symonds, E. M. (1979). Treatment of premenstrual syndrome by spironolactone. *British Journal of Obstetrics and Gynaecology* **86**, 142–7.

O'Brien, P. M. S., Selby, C., and Symonds, E. M. (1980). Progesterone, fluid, and electrolytes in premenstrual syndrome. *British Medical Journal* **2**, 1161–3.

Oleson, T. and Flocco, W. (1993). Randomized control study of premenstrual symptoms treated with ear, hand, and foot reflexology. *Obstetrics and Gynecology* **82**, 906–11.

Pariser, S. F., Stern, S. L., Shank, M. L., Falko, J. O., O'Shaughnessy, R. W., and Friedman C. I. (1985). Premenstrual syndrome: concerns, controversies, and treatment. *American Journal of Obstetrics and Gynecology* **153**, 599–604.

Plouffe, L., Stewart, K., Craft, K. S., Maddox, M. S., and Rausch, J. L. (1993). Diagnostic and treatment results from a southeastern academic centre based premenstrual syndrome clinic. *American Journal of Obstetrics and Gynecology* **169**, 295–307.

Puoloakka, J., Makarainen, L., Viinikka, L., and Ylikorkala, O. (1985). Biochemical and clinical effects of treating the premenstrual syndrome with prostaglandin synthesis precursors. *Journal of Reproductive Medicine* **30**, 149–53.

Reid, R. L. (1991). Premenstrual syndrome. *New England Journal of Medicine* **324**, 1208–10.

Reid, R. L. and Yen, S. S. C. (1981). Premenstrual syndrome. *American Journal of Obstetrics and Gynecology* **139**, 85–104.

Reid, R. L., Greenaway-Coates, A., and Hahn, P. M. (1986). Oral glucose tolerance during the menstrual cycle in normal women and women with alleged premenstrual 'hypoglycaemic' attacks: effects of naloxone. *Journal of Clinical Endocrinology and Metabolism* **62**, 1167–72.

Royal College of General Practioners (1974). *Oral contraceptions and health*. Pittmun Medical, London.

Rubinow, D. R. and Roy-Byrne, P. (1984). Premenstrual syndrome: an over view. *American Journal of Psychiatry* **141**, 163–72.

Sampson, G. A. (1979). Premenstrual syndrome: a double-blind controlled trial of progesterone and placebo. *British Journal of Psychiatry* **135**, 209–15.

Sampson, G. A. (1989). Premenstrual syndrome. *Clinical Obstetrics and Gynaecology* **3**, 687–704.

Sampson, G. A., Heathcote, P. R. M., Wordsworth, J., Prescott, P., and Hodgson, A. (1988). A double-blind cross-over study of treatment with dihydrogesterone and placebo. *British Journal of Psychiatry* **153**, 232–5.

Sarno, A. P., Miller, M. J., and Lundblad, E. G. (1987). Premenstrual syndrome: beneficial effects of periodic low-dose danazol. *Obstetrics and Gynecology* **70**, 33–6.

Schaumburg, H., Kaplan, J., Windebank, A., Vick, N., Rasmus, S., Pleasure, D., *et al.* (1983). Sensory neuropathy from pyridoxine abuse. *New England Journal of Medicine* **309**, 445–8.

Schmidt, P. J., Nieman, L. K., Grover, G. N., Muller, K. L., Merriam, G. R., and Rubinow, D. R. (1991). Lack of effect of induced menses on symptoms in women with premenstrual syndrome. *New England Journal of Medicine* **324**, 1474–9.

Singer, K., Cheng, R., and Schoo, M. (1974). A controlled evaluation of lithium in the premenstrual syndrome. *British Journal of Psychiatry* **124**, 50–1.

Slade, P. and Jenner, F. A. (1980). Attitudes to female roles, aspects of menstruation and complaining of menstrual symptoms. *British Journal of Social and Clinical Psychology* **19**, 109–13.

Smith, S. and Schiff, I. (1989). The premenstrual syndrome. *Fertility Sterility* **52**, 527–43.

Stokes, J. and Mendels, J. (1972). Pyridoxine and premenstrual tension. *Lancet* **i**, 117–18.

Sundblad, C., Modigh, K., Andersch, B., and Eriksson, E. (1992). Clomipramine effectively reduces premenstrual irritability and dysphoria: a placebo controlled trial. *Acta Psychiatrica Scandinavica* **85**, 39–47.

Taylor, J. W. (1979). Plasma progesterone, oestradiol-17β and premenstrual symptoms. *Acta Psychiatrica Scandinavica* **60**, 76–86.

Tulenheimo, A., Laatikainen, T., and Salminen, K. (1987). Plasma beta-endorphin immunoreactivity in premenstrual tension. *British Journal of Obstetrics and Gynaecology* **94**, 26–9.

Vellacott, I. D., Shroff, N. E., Pearce, M. Y., Stratford, M. E., and Akbar, F. A.

(1987). A double-blind placebo controlled evaluation of spironolactone in the premenstrual syndrome. *Current Medical Research and Opinion* **10**, 450–6.

Watson, N. R. and Studd, J. W. W. (1990). Premenstrual syndrome. *British Journal of Hospital Medicine* **44**, 286–92.

Watson, N. R., Studd, J. W. W., Savvas, M., Garnett, T., and Baber, J. R. (1989). Treatment of severe premenstrual syndrome with oestradiol patches and cyclical norethisterone. *Lancet* **ii**, 730–4.

Watson, N. R., Studd, J. W .W., Savvas, M., and Baber, J. R. (1990). The long-term effects of oestradiol implant therapy for the treatment of premenstrual syndrome. *Gynecological Endocrinology* **4**, 99–107.

Watts, S., Dennerstein, L., and Horne, D. J. (1980). The premenstrual syndrome: a psychological evaluation. *Journal of Affective Disorders* **2**, 257–66.

Watts, J. F., Butt, W. R., Logan-Edwards, R., and Holder, G. (1985). Hormonal studies in women with premenstrual tension. *British Journal of Obstetrics and Gynaecology* **92**, 247–55.

West, C. P. (1989). The characteristics of 100 women presenting to a gynaecological clinic with premenstrual complaints. *Acta Obstetrica et Gynaecologica Scandinavica* **68**, 743–7.

Williams, M. J., Harris, R. I., and Dean, B. C. (1985). Controlled trial of pyridoxine in the premenstrual syndrome. *Journal of International Medical Research* **13**, 174–9.

Wood, C. and Jakubowicz, D. (1980). The treatment of premenstrual syndrome with mefenamic acid. *British Journal of Obstetrics and Gynaecology* **87**, 627–30.

Wurtman, J. J., Brzezinski, A., Wurtman, R. J., and Laferrere, B. (1989). Effect of nutrient intake on premenstrual depression. *American Journal of Obstetrics and Gynecology* **161**, 1228–34.

9 The management of the menopause

The menopause is a loose term which really means the last period of a woman's menstrual career, but has become synonymous with the climacteric. The average age at which Caucasian women reach the menopause is 50.5 years and has probably been constant throughout this century (Brambilla and McKinlay 1989; McKinlay et al. 1985). Some 6 per cent of women undergo a surgical menopause. The age at menopause appears to be unrelated to the age at menarche or the number of pregnancies. In Britain, some 95 per cent of women survive to beyond the menopause and 50 per cent survive to reach 75 years. The management of the menopause, especially in terms of the potential benefits and risks of longterm hormonal therapy, is perhaps the single most important public health issue in the western world today. Quality of life studies suggest significant improvement in post-menopausal women on hormone replacement therapy (Daly et al. 1993).

The basic endocrine feature of the menopause is that the ovaries are no longer able to respond to endogenous or exogenous gonadotrophins. The ovarian theca cells are still able to produce low levels of dehydroepiandrosterone, testosterone, and progesterone. Levels of FSH and, to a lesser extent, LH tend to rise approximately one year before the menopause, presumably reflecting deteriorating ovarian function, whilst maximum levels of gonadotrophins are reached some three to five years beyond the menopause, and then fall progressively thereafter (Chakravarti et al. 1976).

The assessment of menopausal symptoms is sometimes difficult in that 20 per cent of women attending a menopause clinic are still menstruating (Studd et al. 1977). The only satisfactory confirmatory test is the measurement of FSH. The assessment of serum oestrogen is poorly correlated with symptoms, and vaginal cytological examination is unsatisfactory, in that correlation between circulating levels of oestrogen and the vaginal cytology is poor. Although a poorly proliferative vaginal smear is generally associated with low circulating levels of oestrogen, the converse cannot be assumed. James et al. (1984) were unable to demonstrate any convincing association between vaginal cytology, plasma hormonal estimations, and the severity of menopausal symptoms in 96 women.

Genitourinary symptoms and sexual symptoms

The pathological changes that occur in the pelvic organs after the menopause are well recognized. Vulval and vaginal skin atrophy may result in loss of both distensibility and lubrication within the vagina. Vaginal dryness, a common finding in post-menopausal women, may lead to dyspareunia. In one series, 14 per cent of women reported dyspareunia (Studd *et al.* 1977). Local and systemic oestrogen therapy has a place in the treatment of dyspareunia.

Masters and Johnson (1966) noted that post-menopausal women had diminished clitoral response, decreased Bartholin's gland secretion, decreased vaginal secretions, and weaker muscle contractions during orgasm compared with regularly menstruating women. Sexual interest would seem to decrease beyond the menopause, the effect being more closely related to menopausal status than age (Montgomery and Studd 1991). This loss of libido may occur even in the presence of a well-oestrogenized vagina and tends to be multi-factorial in origin (Hallstrom 1977; Studd *et al.* 1977). These authors quote an incidence of reduced libido in 50 per cent of post-menopausal women.

There is interest in the effect of decreased local blood flow to the vagina resulting in sexual dysfunction. Morrell *et al.* (1984) measured sexual arousal as judged by the amplitude of vaginal pulse whilst subjects were watching erotic films (alternating with Sesame Street) and found it to be lower in post-menopausal than in premenopausal women. Exogenous oestrogen increases uterine blood flow and vulval blood flow in post-menopausal women (Bourne *et al.* 1990; Sarrel 1990).

Oestrogen alone may have a small therapeutic effect on diminished libido. There is debate about the effect of testosterone implants combined with oestrogen in the treatment of decreased libido. One retrospective cross-sectional study showed an improvement in 80 per cent of patients treated (Studd *et al.* 1977), whilst a prospective study showed no difference between oestrogen implants and combined oestrogen and testosterone implants (Dow *et al.* 1983).

Since the trigone and urethra are derived from the urogenital sinus, oestrogen dependence of these tissues might be assumed. However, although lower urinary tract symptoms are more common in women beyond the menopause, these symptoms, which include frequency, nocturia, urgency, and dysuria, tend not to be associated with a specific pathological condition or with a degree of atrophic changes (Brocklehurst *et al.* 1972; Smith 1972). There is a proven increased incidence in urinary tract infection beyond the menopause. Microbiologically confirmed urinary tract infection occurred in 5 per cent of women before the menopause, in 7 per cent of women between the ages of 55 and 65 years, and in 20 per cent of women above the age of 65 years (Brocklehurst *et al.* 1972).

Oestrogen therapy is superior to placebo in relieving lower urinary tract symptoms when an exact diagnosis is difficult (Brown 1977), but it is of limited value in the management of patients with urinary incontinence (see Chapter 10 – 'Management of urinary incontinence').

Vasomotor symptoms

Vasomotor symptoms were reported by 75 per cent of post-menopausal women, of whom 50 per cent had the symptoms for between 2 and 5 years after the menopause (McKinlay and Jeffreys 1974). The cause of vasomotor instability is not well understood, and does not seem to be due to low or falling oestrogen levels since vasomotor symptoms are not associated with prepuberty, hypophysectomized women, or those with primary ovarian failure, although some anti-oestrogenic drugs are associated with flushing (for example clomiphene). The role of raised gonadotrophins is also uncertain for there is little correlation between the gonadotrophin levels and flushes. Moreover, women given gonadotrophins in order to induce ovulation do not usually complain of vasomotor symptoms (Ravnikar 1990). Some authors believe that the hot flushes are triggered from within the hypothalamus (Freedman *et al*. 1990).

There is good evidence that oestrogen replacement therapy relieves vasomotor symptoms. Coope *et al*. (1975) reported a randomized, double-blind, cross-over study, in which 30 post-menopausal women receiving either equine oestrogen or a placebo for a three-month period and who were then crossed over to receive the other agent. During the first three months, 50 per cent of those women receiving oestrogen reported that their flushes were abolished, whilst 20 per cent of those receiving placebo also reported an absence of flushes. Following cross-over, all flushes were abolished in the oestrogen-treated group, whereas the patients in the placebo-treated group reverted to their pretreatment level of flushing. It would seem that the placebo effect was only of benefit to those women who had not previously experienced oestrogen replacement. An oestrogen transdermal patch has also been proven to be superior to placebo for flushes, as are progestogens (such as medroxyprogesterone acetate), alpha-adrenergic agonists (such as clonidine), and the synthetic steroid tibolone (Albrecht *et al*. 1981; *Drug and Therapeutics Bulletin* 1991; Haas *et al*. 1988; Ravnikar 1990).

Psychological problems

There is no specific psychological syndrome associated with the menopause and, in addition to the change in endogenous hormones, numerous exogenous factors may exert their effect on the psychological well-being of post-menopausal women. Although the incidence of depression is approximately 50 per cent higher in post-menopausal women than in premenopausal women, there is no evidence that the menopause *per se* can precipitate a depressive illness severe enough to warrant psychiatric therapy. Life stress is a more significant aetiological factor in depression in women of this age group than is the menopause (Gath *et al*. 1987; Greene and Cooke 1980; McKinlay *et al*. 1987).

There are some biochemical changes which could predispose to depression.

There is an association between depression and a deficit in brain 5-hydroxytryptamine (5-HT) (Shaw 1973). The synthesis of 5-HT is dependent upon the availability of free, non-protein bound, plasma L-tryptophan, and lower levels of free L-tryptophan have been found in some depressed patients. There is controversy regarding the relationship between serum tryptophan and depression with one study showing decreased L-tryptophan levels in depressed patients (Coppen and Wood 1978), while other studies produce contradictory results (Niskanen *et al.* 1976; Peet *et al.* 1976). Oestrogen is able to displace L-tryptophan from its plasma protein binding site, thus increasing the levels of free tryptophan in the circulation (Aylward and Maddock 1973). Although there is a marked placebo response, several placebo-controlled trials of oestrogen in post-menopausal depression have demonstrated a beneficial effect upon the depression, but the effect may be short-lived. The response is equally good with or without added testosterone (Montgomery *et al.* 1987).

Osteoporosis

Albright *et al.* (1941) reported an association between the menopause and osteoporosis in a series of crush fractures of the vertebrae in 42 post-menopausal patients. The importance of osteoporotic bone disease is the increased incidence of fractures in post-menopausal women. There are three classical sites of fracture in osteoporotic bone. Colles' fracture and vertebral fractures occur in bones of high trabecular content. The incidence of Colles' fracture increases beyond the menopause until the age of 65 years when it reaches a plateau, whereas the incidence of vertebral fractures continues to rise (Riggs and Melton 1986). The proximal femur, the third classical site, contains substantial amounts of both cortical and trabecular bone, which might explain the delayed incidence of fractures in the intertrochanteric area. Fractures of the proximal femur begin to rise significantly in incidence beyond the age of 60 years, then rise almost exponentially thereafter (Riggs and Melton 1986), often occurring after only minimal trauma (Aitken 1984). Such a fracture is associated with an excess mortality of up to 20 per cent and a loss of independence in up to 50 per cent of patients (Lindsay and Cosman 1990).

Bone density studies have shown that the loss of bone begins approximately 10 years before the menopause and continues gradually until the menopause. There is then a rapid loss of bone during the first 5–10 years after the menopause, following which bone loss slows again. The mean decrease in bone density has been estimated as 2.7 per cent per year for the first three years, then decreasing to a steady mean loss of 0.7 per cent per year (Lindsay *et al.* 1976). By this process, some women have lost between 30 and 40 per cent of bone mass before the age of 65 years, although some women lose bone at faster rates than others (Hansen *et al.* 1991). This loss appears to affect trabecular bone in greater quantities than cortical bone, perhaps because of the greater metabolic activity of trabecular bone. This leaves the less dense honeycomb structure at risk of fracture (Riggs and Melton 1986). Women who have undergone an oophorectomy prior to the menopause lose bone at a rate approaching that of the post-menopausal population (Richelson *et al.* 1984).

Oestrogen appears to antagonize the effect of parathyroid hormone on bone, resulting in a hypophosphataemia, hyperphosphaturia, and hypocalcuria (Lindsay *et al.* 1976). In view of the fact that it is the loss of bone in general, as opposed to specific bone constituents, some authors prefer to use the term osteopenia rather than osteoporosis (Riggs and Melton 1986; Watts *et al.* 1990).

Risk factors

Although the menopause is the major risk factor for the development of osteoporosis in women, not all women are at equal risk for the development of this complication (Hansen *et al.* 1991). Stevenson and Whitehead (1982) have estimated that up to 40 per cent of women aged 65 or more will have an osteoporotic fracture in one of the three classical sites. Those factors which are thought to influence the development of osteoporosis in post-menopausal women are discussed below:

(1) initial bone mass;

(2) race;

(3) heredity;

(4) cigarette smoking;

(5) alcohol consumption;

(6) body build;

(7) exercise;

(8) amenorrhoea.

Initial bone mass   Bone mass reaches a peak at between 30 and 35 years of age. Thereafter, women will ultimately lose up to 35 per cent of their cortical bone and 50 per cent of their trabecular bone (Riggs and Melton 1986). As a basic premise, those women with a greater initial bone mass may be the ones who are less likely to develop osteoporosis and its complications in later life, or, at least, have that development delayed. Mazess (1982) reviewed ten published series involving 11 365 women, in which age changes in bone had been studied. He reported that bone mass reached its peak during the mid-thirties followed by a slow decline of 0.3 per cent per year until the menopause, at which stage there was an accelerated decline of 0.9 per cent per year for the first 'few years'.

Race   Racial studies in the United States have demonstrated that Caucasian and Asian women are at a greater risk of developing osteoporosis and osteoporotic fractures than are Negro women (Goldsmith *et al.* 1973). Cohn *et al.* (1977) reported that 26 black women had a greater mean bone mineral content and skeletal mass than did 79 age-matched and height-matched white women. They proposed that this was a major factor in the apparent resistance

Table 9.1 The risk of fracture

	Relative risk
Obese, non-smoker	1.0
Obese, smoker	0.5
Average, non-smoker	1.6
Average, smoker	3.4
Thin, non-smoker	2.3
Thin, smoker	7.1

From Williams *et al.* (1982)

to osteoporosis and fracture of their skeletons. Negroes are prone to keloid formation, a reflection of increased skin collagen, and there is evidence that skin collagen content reflects bone mass since collagen is an important constituent of bone. This may well explain their increased bone mass. It has been shown that oestrogen withdrawal following the menopause will result in a decrease of both skin collagen and bone mass (Brincat *et al.* 1987).

Heredity   The premenopausal daughters of post-menopausal women with osteoporosis have reduced bone mass in both lumbar spine and femoral neck as compared with other age-matched premenopausal women, suggesting that a reduction in peak bone mass may put some women at greater risk of developing osteoporosis (Seeman *et al.* 1989). There is also a greater concordance in bone density studies between monozygotic twins than between dizygotic twins (Pocock *et al.* 1987, Smith *et al.* 1973).

Cigarette smoking   Smokers have a lower bone density and a higher risk of osteoporosis and osteoporotic fractures than do non-smokers (Daniell 1976). This change is especially noticeable in vertebrae (Stevenson *et al.* 1989). Williams *et al.* (1982) studied the risk factors in 426 post-menopausal women with osteoporotic fractures in a comparison with 626 control women without fractures. This study demonstrated (Table 9.1) that smoking was a specific risk factor for the development of an osteoporotic fracture. Although the average weight of smokers was less, in this study, than the average weight of non-smokers, smoking was a significant risk factor even when allowances were made for body build.

There is also evidence that smokers reach the menopause at approximately 22 months earlier than do non-smokers (Brambilla and McKinlay 1989; McKinlay *et al.* 1985) possibly because of toxic effects of tobacco products upon ovarian function (Mattison and Thorgeirsson 1978). Metabolites from tobacco may also interfere with the bioconversion of androgens to oestrogens in subcutaneous adipose tissue. Everson *et al.* (1986), in a small study, reported that passive smokers reached the menopause earlier than non-smokers.

Alcohol consumption   There is an increased incidence of osteoporosis in chronic alcoholics. Saville (1975) reported a small group of chronic alcoholics who showed a loss of vertebral bone mass in the region of 42 per cent after ten years of alcohol abuse. This would appear to be a direct effect of alcohol upon bone rather than an effect mediated by either nutrition or parathyroid hormone (Baran *et al.* 1980; Bikle *et al.* 1985).

There is conflicting evidence concerning the risk of osteoporosis in moderate drinkers. Paganini-Hill *et al.* (1981) were unable to find any statistically significant risk of osteoporosis related to alcohol intake in a study of 83 post-menopausal women with a past history of fracture of the hip and 166 age-matched controls. However, Stevenson *et al.* (1989) reported reduced bone density in 19 women who had two or more units of alcohol per day compared with 25 who had one or two units; the bone density of these latter subjects was, in turn, lower than that in 64 women who had less than one unit of alcohol daily. Others have suggested an increase in bone mineral density in women classed as 'social drinkers' (Holbrook and Barrett-Connor 1993).

Body build   Thin women are at a greater risk of osteoporosis than are fat women (Williams *et al.* 1982). The relative risks of developing osteoporotic hip fracture are shown in Table 9.1. It would seem that smoking is a greater risk factor than is thinness, but the thin smoker has a risk of an osteoporotic fracture seven times higher than that found in the obese non-smoker. Kiel *et al.* (1987) reported that 6.2 per cent of a cohort of 2873 post-menopausal women suffered a fracture of the proximal femur at some stage. The relative risk of this fracture in overweight women was 0.54 that of women of an ideal weight for height.

In addition to adipose tissue acting as a cushion in order to protect bones against trauma, obesity increases the amount of biologically available oestrogen by the conversion of androstenedione to oestrone in adipose tissue. MacDonald *et al.* (1978) reported a statistically significant correlation between mean urinary oestrone levels following an intravenous infusion of androstenedione in 50 post-menopausal women and their excess body weight. Additionally, the concentration of sex hormone binding globulin is lower in obese women, and this will tend to increase the amount of available oestrogen (Davidson *et al.* 1982).

Exercise   Exercise is able to reduce (and may even reverse) bone loss in post-menopausal women. Lane *et al.* (1986) demonstrated that the lumbar vertebrae of post-menopausal long-distance runners had a 40 per cent greater bone mineral content than did the vertebrae of age-matched controls. This is said to relate to the effect of muscular pull upon bony insertions. However, exercise-induced amenorrhoea, as found in high-level female athletes, may be associated with stress fractures; ballet dancers have also been demonstrated to be prone to stress fractures and scoliosis (Jonnavithula *et al.* 1993; Lindberg *et al.* 1984; Warren *et al.* 1986).

Prolonged bedrest may have a negative effect upon bone mass. Donaldson *et al.* (1970) reported that urinary calcium, phosphate, and hydroxyproline excretions were elevated during prolonged bedrest and bone calcium demineralization was observed.

Amenorrhoea   Amenorrhoea, from any cause, may result in premature bone loss. The effect of exercise-induced amenorrhoea has already been discussed. Aitken *et al.* (1973*a*) reported that 25 per cent of 66 women, who had undergone bilateral oophorectomy at the time of hysterectomy for benign disease before the age of 45 years, had radiological evidence of osteoporosis within six years of surgery. Anorexia nervosa is associated with a significant decrease in bone mass and an incidence of vertebral crush fractures (Savvas *et al.* 1988*a*; Szmukler *et al.* (1985). Kliplanski *et al.* (1980) described decreased bone density in 14 women with hyperprolactinaemia. The degree of osteoporosis correlated more closely with the reduced level of oestrogen than with the raised level of prolactin. Davies *et al.* (1990) reported a mean reduction in bone mineral density in 15 per cent of 200 women, aged 16–40 years, with amenorrhoea of any cause when compared with 57 age-matched menstruating controls. Greenblatt *et al.* (1967) reported an association between primary gonadal dysgenesis and osteoporosis, whilst Cann *et al.* (1984) reported a decrease of 20.9 per cent in bone density in 16 women with premature ovarian failure compared with age-matched menstruating controls.

Pregnancy, lactation, and the taking of oral contraceptives do not have any significant effect upon bone density (Christiansen *et al.* 1976; Goldsmith and Johnston 1975; Stevenson *et al.* 1989). However, should the patient be osteoporotic before pregnancy, pregnancy and lactation may increase the risk of fractures (Dent and Friedman 1965).

From the above, it is clear that not all women are at equal risk of osteoporosis. Ideally, it would be more appropriate to assess individual risk rather than treat all women in order to prevent osteoporosis. Specifically, thin smokers with either a family history of osteoporosis or with an earlier than average menopause are at particular risk.

The assessment of bone density

Many techniques have been used in order to measure bone mass. These include:

(1) radiographs;

(2) single photon absorptiometry;

(3) dual photon absorptiometry;

(4) computerized tomography;

(5) neutron activation analysis;

(6) bone biopsy.

Radiographs

Radiographs have the advantage of being relatively inexpensive and may allow some measurement to be made on the dimensions of cortical bone, but the assessment of trabecular bone tends to be subjective. They will obviously detect fractures and deformities.

Single photon absorptiometry

Single photon absorption, especially of the forearm, is also relatively inexpensive, but may provide a more precise measurement of changes in bone mass than will radiography (Cummings *et al.* 1985).

Dual photon absorptiometry

This has been used to measure the mineral content of bone surrounded by soft tissue where single photon studies would be inaccurate. It is, therefore, especially useful for vertebral and proximal femoral assessment. The technique is more expensive and more time consuming than the above techniques, however, it does provide a relatively accurate measurement of both cortical and trabecular mineral content (American College of Physicians 1984). Newer generation dual photon absorption machines, using an X-ray source rather than a nucleotide (dual energy X-ray absorptiometry or DEXA) may allow a less expensive and more rapid screen than did the early technology, and it may be that this will become the technique used for population screening should such be indicated (Office of Health Economics 1990). A lower than average bone density may then become an indication for offering specific advice upon the prevention of further osteoporosis. The investigation may then be repeated some three to five years later (Fogelman 1988), although the benefit from such population screening is not yet proven (Cummings and Black 1986). Such techniques have also been used to monitor the efficacy of therapy (Mazess *et al.* 1989).

Computerized tomography

Computerized tomography may also be used to measure bone mineral density, but this involves a greater dose of radiation than does dual photon absorptiometry.

Neutron activation analysis

Neutron activation analysis can measure bone calcium levels, but it is rarely used in clinical practice for the radiation involved is even higher than in computerized tomography (American College of Physicians 1984).

Bone biopsy

Biopsy of the iliac crest will provide an accurate histological assessment of bone mineral content but, being invasive, is rarely used. It has yet to be shown whether the assessment of bone mass will be of clinical value in selecting patients in whom primary prevention of osteoporosis is indicated (Ott 1994).

The non-hormonal prevention of osteoporosis

In clinical practice, the prevention of osteoporosis should not be synonymous, necessarily, with the prescribing of oestrogen. Several non-hormonal techniques have been advocated and will be discussed below. The use of the hormone calcitonin, which is able to prevent bone resorption by the inhibition of osteoclast activity has rarely been used in clinical practice since the route of administration is intramuscular, although calcitonin is as effective as oestradiol in the prevention of post-menopausal bone loss (MacIntyre *et al.* 1988). However, the introduction of an intranasal calcitonin preparation may offer greater potential for use (Overgaard *et al.* 1989).

Those non-hormonal techniques which will be discussed include:

(1) exercise;

(2) calcium supplementation;

(3) fluoride supplementation;

(4) vitamin D supplementation;

(5) etidronate;

(6) tibolone.

Exercise

Whilst it has already been discussed that exercise may be beneficial in increasing bone mass Chow *et al.* 1987; Dalsky *et al.* 1988), it is unlikely that exercise alone will prevent osteoporosis. In a recent study, exercise, with or without calcium supplementation, reduced, but did not prevent, post-menopausal bone loss (Prince *et al.* 1991). There is no evidence that an exercise programme alone will prevent osteoporotic fractures (Block *et al.* 1987) but weight-bearing exercise is thought to be the most important type (Lindsay 1993).

Calcium supplementation

The evidence from the literature concerning calcium supplementation is probably best summarized by stating that high doses of calcium have some benefit in the deceleration of post-menopausal bone loss, but are not as efficient as oestrogen (Nordin and Heaney 1990; Reid *et al.* 1993).

There is good evidence that a supplemented daily calcium intake of up to a level of 2 g per day will reduce post-menopausal bone loss in some patients (Recker *et al.* 1977; Riis *et al.* 1987) but not in all patients (Nilas *et al.* 1984). Whereas calcium supplementation may reduce the rate of bone loss, a combination of calcium and oestrogen (1500 mg calcium and 0.625 mg conjugated oestrogen daily) has been shown to increase bone mass by 2.3 per cent (Ettinger *et al.* 1987). Milk consumption is able to influence bone mineral density (Murphy *et al.* 1994).

It would be expected from the above that calcium supplementation would not be as efficient as oestrogen in the prevention of fractures. Nordin *et al.*

Table 9.2 The treatment of osteoporosis

	No. of patients	Person-years of observation	Fracture rate per 1000 person-years
No treatment	45	91	834
Calcium (± vitamin D)	27	74	419
Fluoride and calcium	33	138	304
Oestrogen and calcium	32	144	181
Fluoride, calcium, and oestrogen	28	113	53

From Riggs *et al.* (1982)

(1980) reported a series of post-menopausal women with radiological evidence of compressed or wedged vertebrae managed by any one of seven different regimes. Those 41 patients who were untreated continued to lose bone, with further episodes of wedging and compression. The administration of calcium, with or without vitamin D, was of some benefit in 43 patients in *reducing* the risk of subsequent crush fractures, whereas oestrogen *arrested* the risk of subsequent crush fractures in 35 patients (Chapuy *et al.* 1992).

Fluoride supplementation

Some authors claim that fluoride supplementation is capable of depressing the incidence of vertebral osteoporotic fractures by up to 25 per cent (Kanis 1990). Mamelle *et al.* (1988) reported a prospective study in which 257 patients with at least one osteoporotic vertebral fracture were randomized to receive sodium fluoride 25 mg twice daily, elemental calcium 1 g daily, and vitamin D_2 800 IU per day, whilst 207 similar patients were randomized to receive the calcium and vitamin D but not the fluoride. During a mean follow-up period of 24 months, one or more new fractures occurred in 39.2 per cent of the fluoride group, and 50.8 per cent of the non-fluoride group, this difference being statistically significant. The side-effects of fluoride included pain in the lower limbs due to fluoridation of tendons, anaemia due to gastrointestinal tract bleeding, and new bone formation which causes back pain (Thorneycroft 1989).

In a non-randomized trial of patients with post-menopausal osteoporosis treated by different regimes, as can be seen in Table 9.2, a combination of fluoride and calcium was less likely to be associated with fractures than calcium alone or no treatment. However, the best regimes contained oestrogen (Riggs *et al.* 1982). In a randomized placebo-controlled trial of sodium fluoride, 75 mg per day, in post-menopausal women, bone density was greater in the fluoride group than the placebo group, but the overall rate of vertebral fractures did not decrease, suggesting that the new bone was structurally unsound (Riggs *et al.* 1990).

Fluoride is, therefore, only of limited value, has side-effects, and is not as effective as oestrogen (Lindsay 1990).

Table 9.3 The treatment of osteoporosis

	No. of patients	Mean % change in bone density	Rate of new fractures per 1000 patient-years
Placebo	104	no change	68.0
Phosphate	107	no change	57.7
Etidronate	105	+ 4.2	44.2
Etidronate and phosphate	147	+ 5.2	14.8

From Watts et al. (1990)

Vitamin D supplementation

Vitamin D therapy alone is generally considered not to be helpful in the prevention of osteoporosis, although vitamin D combined with oral calcium may increase calcium absorption from the gastrointestinal tract (Nordin et al. 1980). However, a recent study involving vitamin D_3 (calcitriol) administration resulted in a significantly lower incidence of subsequent fractures when given to women with a previous osteoporotic vertebral fracture when compared with calcium supplementation (Tilyard et al. 1992).

Etidronate

Etidronate is an organic diphosphonate able to inhibit osteoclast-mediated bone resorption. Heaney and Saville (1976) reported that administration of this drug resulted in a positive calcium balance, with reduced bone resorption, in ten osteoporotic patients. Watts et al. (1990) reported a prospective double-blind placebo-controlled study of 423 women with one or more vertebral compression fractures and osteoporosis. The patients were randomly assigned to treatment with placebo, phosphate, etidronate, or phosphate and etidronate. Bone density measurements of the spine were made by dual photon absorptiometry over a two-year period. As can be seen from Table 9.3, etidronate 400 mg daily, with or without added phosphate, resulted in a net increase in spinal bone density but, more significantly, reduced the rate of new spinal compression fractures by over 50 per cent. Other authors found similar results (Storm et al. 1990). Adverse drug reactions were mild, generally infrequent, and included nausea and diarrhoea. Etidronate tends to be given as an intermittent cyclical therapy (for instance, two weeks in six) in order to prevent the risk of hyperphosphataemia (Heaney and Saville 1976).

Tibolone

The synthetic steroid, tibolone, was more effective than placebo in preventing post-menopausal osteoporosis (Lindsay et al. 1980b). These results have been confirmed in other studies, but the drug is not licensed for the prevention of menopausal osteoporosis and hence its use will remain limited until additional information is available (Drug and Therapeutics Bulletin 1991).

The prevention of osteoporosis by oestrogen

The evidence that oestrogen is able to prevent post-menopausal osteoporosis is overwhelming. Aitken *et al.* (1973*b*) randomized 114 women who had undergone previous hysterectomy and bilateral salpingo-oophorectomy for benign disease to a controlled double-blind trial of oestrogen and placebo. Initial and annual radiological metacarpal mineral studies were performed; the placebo group experienced a 4 per cent annual decrease in bone density, whilst the bone density in the oestrogen treated group fell by only 0.1 per cent per annum. In a subgroup of 17 women who commenced hormone replacement therapy within six years of their surgical menopause, there was an increase in bone density of 2.4 per cent per annum. No patient in the oestrogen group suffered a fracture, but two fractures were reported by patients in the placebo group. Quigley *et al.* (1987) studied 397 post-menopausal women, divided into age decades of 50–60 years and 71–80 years. They found that in oestrogen non-users the bone density continued to fall up to age 70, but not beyond. The bone loss in non-users declined at three times the rate of that in oestrogen users. When oestrogen users ceased oestrogen treatment, even at age 65 or older, their bone densities decreased at 2.5 per cent per annum compared with the 0.5 per cent per annum whilst they were taking oestrogen. These results suggest that the rate of bone loss can be reduced in all women given oestrogen provided that they are less than 70-years-old, and that the degree of bone preservation will be greater the nearer to the menopause that oestrogen is commenced.

Numerous other trials now support this concept. Nachtigall *et al.* (1978) reported 168 post-menopausal women randomly allocated to oestrogen or placebo. After ten years of treatment, the oestrogen group showed no significant decrease in bone mass, and those patients who received oestrogen within three years of the menopause actually increased their bone mass. The placebo-treated group showed a decrease in mean bone mass of between 9 and 12 per cent at the end of ten years. Lindsay *et al.* (1980*a*) reported 100 oophorectomized women who entered a prospective trial of oestrogen or placebo for nine years in order to assess the effect of oestrogen replacement on vertebral osteoporosis. Some 32 per cent of 50 patients in the placebo group lost a mean height of 0.9 cm, and 28 per cent had radiological evidence of vertebral crush or collapse. Only 4 per cent of 50 patients in the oestrogen group had any evidence of spinal osteoporosis, and none had evidence of vertebral crush or collapse.

Several studies have specifically addressed the incidence of fractures in women receiving homone replacement therapy. Hutchinson *et al.* (1979) reported a case-controlled study in order to assess the potential benefits of hormone replacement therapy upon the prevention of fracture of the proximal femur. Some 4.2 per cent of patients with this fracture had taken oestrogen, whereas 16.9 per cent of 71 matched controls had not. Using a similar case-controlled study, Paganini-Hill *et al.* (1981) demonstrated that the risk of fracture of the proximal femur in post-menopausal non-oestrogen takers was

Table 9.4 The prevention of osteoporosis

	Annual rate of fractures per 1000 women		
	Age group 50–59	60–69	70–74
Lower arm			
Oestrogen	1.2	2.0	2.0
No oestrogen	3.0	5.0	5.0
Proximal femur			
Oestrogen	0.2	0.6	2.0
No oestrogen	0.5	1.5	5.0

From Weiss *et al.* (1980)

2.4 times that for oestrogen takers. A recent large study from Sweden (133 022 women-years of observation) demonstrated that the relative risk for a fracture of the hip in women on hormone replacement therapy was 0.8 that for age-matched women not on hormone replacement therapy (Naessen *et al.* 1990). For Colles' fracture, the same authors reported a trend towards a decreased incidence of fractures in oestrogen takers compared with non-takers, but the results did not reach statistical significance, possibly because there were only nine patients with a Colles' fracture.

Weiss *et al.* (1980) calculated the differences in the annual incidence of fracture of the lower forearm and proximal femur between oestrogen takers and non-takers over different age groups, based on 327 women with fractures and 567 controls. It can be seen from Table 9.4 that the oestrogen takers had less than half the incidence of fractures of the non-takers. Ettinger *et al.* (1985) reported that the total incidence of osteoporotic fractures of all types in 245 oestrogen takers over a 17-year period was 10 per cent compared with 34 per cent in 245 case-matched non-oestrogen taking controls.

Moreover, oestrogen will protect against post-menopausal osteoporosis when administered either subcutaneously or percutaneously, as well as orally (Holland *et al.* 1994). In a non-randomized trial, Savvas *et al.* (1988*b*) compared bone density, by dual photon absorptiometry, in 37 women at a median time of 8.75 years from the last menstrual period who were receiving oral oestrogen, with 41 women at a median time of 9.5 years from the last menstrual period and who were given oestrogen implants. Mean bone density was greater in the women receiving implants, suggesting that this method is at least as effecive as oral therapy in the protection against osteoporosis. Stevenson *et al.* (1990) randomly allocated 66 early post-menopausal women to receive oral oestrogen, percutaneous oestrogen, or no treatment, and measured urinary bone meta-bolites and bone density in the vertebrae and proximal femora over an 18-month period. Both oral oestrogen and oestrogen patches were equally effective in preserving bone density compared with the control group, and equally effective in reducing bone turnover based on urinary calcium excretion.

In the primary prevention of osteoporosis, it would seem that oestrogen is able to reduce post-menopausal bone loss to such small levels that there is a significant decrease in the incidence of osteoporotic fractures. It is clear that not all women will become severely osteoporotic and it may be that high-risk patients could be selected by means of premenopausal peak bone density studies. Those patients who have a reduced peak bone density could then be offered oestrogen therapy, assuming there were no contraindications, together with calcium supplementation and advice concerning exercise and smoking. It is unlikely that oestrogen will reverse bone loss unless it is given within the first three years of the menopause, but it may arrest osteoporotic changes and, hence, be of value in secondary prevention. No other treatment 'stops the disease in its tracks' (Smith 1987).

Arterial disease

Arteriosclerotic vascular disease affecting the coronary, cerebral, and, to a lesser extent the peripheral circulations, is a major cause of death in western society. There is marked difference in the onset of arteriosclerotic disease between men and women with a lag of about 10–15 years in women. Thus premenopausal women are less likely to suffer from arteriosclerotic disease than either men of the same age or post-menopausal women. The protective factor was felt to be oestrogen and in view of this, in the late 1960s, a trial of exogenous oestrogen given to men who had a myocardial infarct was undertaken. Unfortunately, the trial had to be abandoned due to increased reinfarction, pulmonary emboli, and thrombophlebitis in a group of men prescribed conjugated oestrogens (Coronary Drug Project Research Group 1970).

There is good evidence for the protective nature of oestrogen replacement therapy against cardiovascular disease in post-menopausal women. Nearly all the studies performed have used premarin and were conducted in the USA. When allowance has been made for other known risk factors (especially smoking) there has been a reduction of cardiovascular disease in approximately 50 per cent of the treated women. For instance, in the Boston Nurses Health Study which involved 48 000 nurses being followed for up to ten years of observation, the overall relative risk of major coronary heart disease in women currently taking oestrogen was 0.6 compared with non-takers, and the mortality was 0.7, a reduction in mortality of 30 per cent (Stampfer *et al.* 1991). Only one study (Wilson *et al.* 1985) has shown a negative effect of oestrogen replacement therapy on cardiovascular disease. In a recent review of 11 studies published since 1980, the relative risk of coronary heart disease, stroke, or death from cardiovascular disease in women taking hormone replacement therapy was 0.3–0.5 that observed in non-users (Gorsky *et al.* 1994; Hunt and Vessey 1991).

It is important to emphasize that these studies have looked at unopposed oestrogen therapy only and that studies of combined oestrogen and progestogen

Table 9.5 Hormone replacement therapy and coronary artery disease

	Relative risk	
	Never users	Ever users
Death from any cause	1.0	0.8
Death from myocardial infarction	1.0	0.59
Death from myocardial infarction (current users)	1.0	0.47
Death from myocardial infarction (past users)	1.0	0.62
Hospital admission for coronary heart disease	1.0	0.72

From Stampfer *et al.* 1991

treatment have yet to be reported in sufficient detail for conclusions to be drawn.

One of the possible mechanisms for the apparent protection of oestrogen on cardiovascular disease is the effect of endogenous and exogenous oestrogen on lipoprotein metabolism. Prior to the menopause, women have relatively higher levels of HDL (high-density lipoprotein) and lower levels of LDL (low-density lipoprotein) than men and post-menopausal women. HDL levels are inversely proportional to cardiovascular risk, whilst LDL levels are directly related to risk (Egeland *et al.* 1990). After the menopause, LDL levels tend to rise to similar levels as those seen in men, although there is little change in HDL levels. It is difficult to show a direct effect of the menopause on lipoprotein levels totally separate from the effect of age.

Oestrogen given to post-menopausal women will produce a beneficial lipo-protein profile by lowering LDL levels and increasing HDL levels (Walsh *et al.* 1991). Even percutaneous oestrogen will lower LDL levels and either leave HDL levels unchanged or increase them (Crook *et al.* 1992; Jensen *et al.* 1987). The important issue here is the effect of progestogens on lipoprotein metabolism. In general, most progestogens will negate the beneficial effect of oestrogen on lipids. However, this effect will depend upon the type of progestogen used, the route of administration, and the dose. One should aim to use the lowest dose needed to protect the endometrium yet not influence the apparently beneficial lipoprotein changes induced by oestrogen (Christiansen and Reis 1990; Miller *et al.* 1991; Montgomery and Crook 1990; Siddle *et al.* 1990).

The effect of oestrogen on lipoproteins is only one of the possible mechanisms by which oestrogen appears to protect against cardiovascular disease. Recently, there has been interest in the proposed direct protective effect of oestrogen upon coronary arterial vessels (Gangar *et al.* 1991). Other theories include the alteration of glucose and insulin handling by oestrogen as well as a direct effect on some haemostatic factors, all of which may contribute to the cardioprotection afforded by oestrogen (Collins *et al.* 1993).

Most of the research relating to arterial disease and hormone replacement therapy has concentrated upon coronary artery disease. There is, however, good evidence that oestrogen replacement therapy may half the incidence of cerebrovascular accidents (Hunt *et al.* 1990; Paganini-Hill *et al.* 1988).

Hormone replacement therapy has either no effect on blood pressure or produces a slight lowering of both the systolic and diastolic pressures (Barrett-Connor *et al.* 1979 and 1989; Lind *et al.* 1979).

With the current state of knowledge, women should be advised that unopposed hormone replacement therapy is associated with a reduction in mortality from arterial disease of up to 50 per cent. Further information is required before it can be stated that the progestogen in combined therapies does not negate the cardiovascular benefits of unopposed oestrogen.

The benefits of hormone replacement therapy in practice

There is no doubt that morbidity and mortality due to osteoporosis is reduced by hormone replacement therapy. Similarly, there is a reduction of between 30 and 50 per cent in cardiovascular disease and a reduction in strokes by 50 per cent with oestrogen replacement therapy.

However, it is just possible that women who receive a prescription for hormone replacement therapy may be 'subtly healthier' and the need for randomized trials rather than case-controlled studies is clear (Vandenbroocke 1991). In the meantime, two cohort studies have demonstrated a reduced mortality from all causes for women taking oestrogen replacement therapy. In California, the mortality from all causes in post-menopausal women receiving hormone replacement therapy was 0.8 that expected from an age-adjusted population of non-users (Henderson *et al.* 1991), whilst the UK study demonstrated that death from all causes was 0.6 that expected from the national statistics (Hunt *et al.* 1990).

Proven oestrogen dangers

When considering the evidence for potentially serious side-effects associated with longterm oestrogen therapy, it is important that the evidence is based on oestrogen use for longterm hormone replacement therapy, and is not extrapolated from the evidence relating to oestrogen use in oral contraception. Over and above the non-scientific nature of such an extrapolation, the following points should be observed:

1. The oestrogen used in oral contraceptives is synthetic, whilst virtually all oestrogen hormone replacement therapy now given uses a natural oestrogen, such as piperazine oestrone sulfate, oestradiol valerate, or conjugated equine oestrogen.
2. The metabolic effects of natural oestrogens are not necessarily those of synthetic oestrogens.

3. Metabolic effects may be dose-related, and significantly lower doses of oestrogen are used for hormone replacement therapy than for oral contraception.

4. Percutaneous or subcutaneous oestrogen may have advantages over oral oestrogen. Oral oestrogen is metabolized in the gut and, to a lesser extent, in the liver where oestradiol is partially converted into oestrone with a resulting high bolus on 'first pass' through the liver. Since this 'first pass' cannot occur with percutaneous or subcutaneous administration, those potentially important oestrogenic side-effects which depend upon the induction of liver enzymes (for example an increase in prothrombin production or an increase in renin substrate production) should be reduced (Belchetz 1989; Chetkowski *et al.* 1986; Holst *et al.* 1983).

The three major risks from oestrogen replacement therapy which require discussion are thromboembolism, endometrial adenocarcinoma, and carcinoma of the breast.

Hormone replacement therapy and thromboembolism

There is good evidence that synthetic oestrogen, when used for hormone replacement therapy, increases the risk of thromboembolic disease. Gow and MacGillivary (1971) reported a prospective study using a synthetic oestrogen (mestranol) as post-menopausal hormone replacement therapy. Some 16 per cent of 25 patients developed thromboembolic complications (12 per cent having a deep venous thrombosis and 4 per cent a superficial thrombophlebitis). The authors concluded that the 'gravity of the adverse effects far outweighs any beneficial ones'. Beller *et al.* (1972) also demonstrated that a statistically significant alteration in the clotting mechanisms towards thrombogenesis occurred when synthetic oestrogen was used for hormone replacement therapy. There were increased levels of plasminogen and antithrombin III. Synthetic oestrogen is, therefore, not acceptable for hormone replacement therapy.

Natural oestrogens have a significantly smaller effect on the clotting mechanisms (Studd *et al.* 1978) and it is likely that this is not clinically significant. Menopausal women have elevated levels of antithrombin III compared with men of a similar age or premenopausal women, suggesting some protection against thrombosis, especially venous, beyond the menopause (Meade *et al.* 1990). This may offer some degree of protection against venous thromboembolism to women receiving hormone replacement therapy. There is no good evidence of increased thromboembolic phenomenon in post-menopausal women receiving natural oestrogen in the absence of a past history of thromboembolic disease (Saleh *et al.* 1993).

Table 9.6 Hormone replacement therapy and endometrial stimulation

Duration of progestogen (days)	Total (n)	Cystic hyperplasia (n)	Adenomatous hyperplasia (n)	Atypical hyperplasia (n)	Total abnormal (%)
0	67	23	1	0	56
5	156	7	4	1	8
7	45	5	0	0	13
10	34	1	0	0	3
>10	23	0	0	0	0

From Paterson *et al.* (1980)

Hormone replacement therapy and endometrial carcinoma

There have been over 20 case-controlled studies published since 1975 which suggest that the use of exogenous oestrogen without a progestogen in post-menopausal women who have a uterus is associated with an increased risk of endometrial cancer. Although some of these studies have been criticized (Cooke 1976) in that there might have been a higher social class bias (they consisted largely of middle class American ladies in private medical insurance schemes), and because they did not examine any other known risk factors for endometrial carcinoma (such as parity, obesity, age at menopause, diabetes, hypertension, or previous anovulation) the evidence was nevertheless strong enough to alter clinical practice. The four classical studies of 1975 and 1976 may be consulted (Mack *et al.* 1976; Quint 1975; Smith *et al.* 1975; Ziel and Finkle 1975), but a recent study has shown a relative risk of 5.7 for endometrial carcinoma in women using unopposed oestrogen compared with no hormones (Voigt *et al.* 1991).

That progestogen therapy may help to avoid the risk endometrial carcinoma was a logical step. Hustin (1970) had already shown that progestogens had an adverse effect on endometrial carcinoma, with histological evidence of necrosis, squamous metaplasia, and a general reduction in adverse histological features in women who received progestogens for one week prior to hysterectomy. The protective benefit of sequential oestrogen and progestogen compared with cyclical oestrogen alone in women with an intact uterus is well documented (Paterson *et al.* 1980; Whitehead *et al.* 1989). Paterson *et al.* (1980) performed endometrial biopsies on 745 post-menopausal women receiving various forms of hormone replacement therapy. There was a 7 per cent incidence of cystic hyperplasia in women receiving low-dose unopposed cyclical oestrogen, a 15 per cent incidence in women taking high-dose unopposed cyclical oestrogen, while women receiving combined oestrogen and progestogen therapy had a 1.2 per cent incidence of hyperplasia. The duration of the progestogen course also affected the incidence of hyperplasia, in that a course lasting more than ten days was associated with no cases of hyperplasia. These results are shown in Table 9.6. Moreover, the endometrium of women with hyperplasia following cyclical oestrogen alone who were then given sequential therapy reverted to normal, suggesting that progestogen therapy will reverse, as well as prevent, oestrogen-induced endometrial atypia (Whitehead *et al.* 1979). Similarly, G. Lane *et al.* (1986) demonstrated that the protective effect of a progestogen is dependent upon both the dosage of progestogen given and the number of days in each cycle for which it is taken. They were able to demonstrate secretory changes on endometrial biopsy in 100 per cent of patients who received dydrogesterone, 20 mg per day for 12 days each month, in addition to natural oestrogen replacement therapy.

Recently, oestrogen and progestogen have become available for routine clinical practice in a transdermal therapeutic system. Preliminary results in a small number of patients have suggested that this transdermal combination will prevent endometrial stimulation (Whitehead *et al.* 1990), but greater clinical experience is required before the benefits of this regimen are proved.

Thus, so long as progestogens are combined with oestrogen for hormone replacement therapy for at least ten days in women with an intact uterus, the relative risk for endometrial carcinoma becomes 0.9 that expected from women who do not receive hormone replacement therapy (Hunt *et al.* 1990; Persson *et al.* 1989; Voigt *et al.* 1991).

Hormone therapy and breast cancer

Carcinoma of the breast will affect one woman in twelve. If any scientific report is going to show an effect upon this statistic, then either the causative agent must be very powerful or else the series very large. It would not be unexpected for cancer of the breast to be associated with hormone replacement therapy, since the disease is already known to be associated with an early menarche, a late menopause, and nulliparity.

There are numerous studies which have examined the relationship between hormone replacement therapy and carcinoma of the breast. These studies vary greatly in size, in the methodology by which relative risk is assessed, in the length of oestrogen usage, in the dosage of oestrogen, and in the inclusion or exclusion of women who have received progestogen therapy. G. J. J. has been able to identify 35 studies which, generally on a case-controlled basis, have examined the relative risk of carcinoma of the breast in women receiving hormone replacement therapy. These studies have been summarized in Table 9.7. There have also been five recent meta-analyses but the studies used in these meta-analyses have, for various reasons, not included all 35 studies (Armstrong 1988; Colditz *et al.* 1993; Dupont and Page 1991; Sillero-Arenas *et al.* 1992; Steinberg *et al.* 1991). In summary, 11 of these studies demonstrate a neutral risk, 13 a decreased risk, and 11 an increased risk for carcinoma of the breast in women receiving hormone replacement therapy. From the meta-analyses, the following conclusions may be drawn:

1. *Overall*, these studies have demonstrated a neutral risk for carcinoma of the breast in women receiving hormone replacement therapy, or at most a small relative risk of 1.06.

Table 9.7 Hormone replacement therapy and breast cancer

Primary author and year of publication	Journal, Vol., page	Relative risk
Boston Collab. (1974)	*NEJM*, **290** 15	1.0
Henderson (1974)	*JNCI*, **53**, 609	0.8
Mack (1975)	*NEJM*, **292**, 1366	1.6
Hoover (1976)	*NEJM*, **295**, 401	1.3
Casagrande (1976)	*JNCI*, **56**, 839	3.1
Byrd (1977)	*Ann. Surg.*, **189**, 574	1.4
Sartwell (1977)	*JNCI*, **58**, 1589	0.8
Wynder (1978)	*Cancer*, **41**, 2341	1.1
Hammond (1979)	*Am. JOG*, **133**, 537	1.1
Ravnikar (1979)	*Eur. J. Clin. Onc.*, **15**, 395	0.6
Jick (1980)	*Am. J. Epi.*, **112**, 586	3.4
Ross (1980)	*JAMA*, **243**, 1635	1.1
Hoover (1981)	*JNCI*, **67**, 815	1.4
Kelsey (1981)	*JNCI*, **67**, 327	0.9
Thomas (1982)	*JNCI*, **69**, 1017	1.8
Hulka (1982)	*Am. JOG*, **143**, 638	1.3
Vakil (1983)	*Can. Det. Prev.*, **6**, 415	0.7
Gambrell (1983)	*O. & G.*, **62**, 435	0.7
Sherman (1983)	*Cancer*, **51**, 1527	0.7
Kaufman (1984)	*JAMA*, **252**, 63	0.9
Hurwitz (1984)	*Am. J. Med.*, **76**, 192	0.5
Hiatt (1984)	*Cancer*, **54**, 139	0.7
Nomura (1986)	*Int. J. Can.*, **37**, 49	1.0
Brinton (1986)	*Br. J. Can.*, **54**, 825	1.0
La Vecchia (1986)	*Int. J. Can.*, **38**, 853	1.9
McDonald (1986)	*Breast Can. Res. Tr.*, **7**, 193	0.7
Buring (1987)	*Am. J. Epi.*, **125**, 939	1.1
Hunt (1987)	*BJOG*, **94**, 620	0.6
Wingo (1987)	*JAMA*, **257**, 209	0.8
Ewertz (1988)	*Int. J. Can.*, **42**, 832	1.4
Rohan (1988)	*Med. J. Austr.*, **148**, 217	1.0
Bergkvist (1989)	*NEJM*, **321**, 293	1.1
Dupont (1989)	*Cancer*, **63**, 948	0.5
Mills (1989)	*Cancer*, **64**, 591	1.7
Hunt (1990)	*BJOG*, **97**, 1080	0.8

2. There is no increased risk for carcinoma of the breast in women receiving hormone replacement therapy and who have a past history of benign breast disease.

3. There is a statistically insignificant increased relative risk of carcinoma of the breast in women receiving hormone replacement therapy and who have a family history of carcinoma of the breast (range 0.83–2.3).

4. Although there was a trend towards an increased relative risk with an increased oestrogen dosage, the range of relative risks was so wide that no firm conclusion could be drawn.

5. There was no convincing evidence for a relationship between the duration of treatment and carcinoma of the breast. Although Hunt and Vessey (1991)

have estimated that the risk of carcinoma of the breast *may* be doubled by taking hormone replacement therapy for 15 years, Buring *et al.* (1987) were unable to find an increased risk following low-dose hormone replacement therapy taken for 20 years. The consensus opinion is that there is not a dose-duration response.

At the current state of knowledge, patients should be reassured that there is no convincing evidence for an increased risk of carcinoma of the breast in women receiving long-term hormone replacement therapy, but they should be counselled that this conclusion may need to be altered with the accumulation of further information, and perhaps all women receiving hormone replacement therapy should be offered regular (? every three years) mammography.

Hormone replacement therapy and other tumours

There is no evidence for an increased risk of carcinoma of the cervix in hormone replacement therapy users. Indeed, those few studies which have addressed this relationship demonstrated a reduced risk (Adami *et al.* 1989; Hunt *et al.* 1987), but this may represent an increased incidence of cervical cytology screening and a higher socio-economic class in oestrogen users compared with non-users.

The available evidence would suggest that there is no increased risk of carcinoma of the ovary in women receiving hormone replacement therapy (Adami *et al.* 1989; Hammond *et al.* 1979; Hunt *et al.* 1987; Kaufman *et al.* 1989). However, there may be an increased risk of *endometroid* tumours of the ovary in women receiving hormone replacement therapy (La Vecchia *et al.* 1982; Weiss *et al.* 1982). The incidence of endometroid ovarian cancer would appear to be some three times that noted in women who do not use hormone replacement therapy and this may therefore, also, be an area for increased vigilance. There is no increased risk of benign breast tumours in women who receive hormone replacement therapy when compared with women who do not (Boston Collaborative Drug Surveillance Program 1974).

The clinical situation arises in which a woman with a past history of ovarian cancer which was not endometroid is considered for hormone replacement therapy. There is no evidence that such women are at an increased risk of recurrence (Eeles *et al.* 1991).

Conclusions

Potentially, the prevention of mortality and serious morbidity in post-menopausal women is an issue of huge importance. The current advice strongly favours a benefit from the prevention of osteoporotic fractures and a probable benefit from the prevention of coronary arterial disease. The major potential risk, that of breast cancer, must await more well-controlled data. Yet, only 10 per cent of post-menopausal women in the UK have ever taken hormone replacement therapy, and then not longterm. Moreover, even women at particular risk from the complications of the menopause because of oophorectomy before the age of 40 years are commonly not offered hormone replacement therapy (Barlow *et al.* 1989).

It is not just the doctors who are reluctant to offer and prescribe hormone replacement therapy. A significant percentage of patients are relatively reluctant to take this treatment. Draper and Roland (1990) surveyed 84 women, aged 50–52 years, of whom 77 per cent would consider taking hormone replacement therapy if they knew more, 61 per cent were worried about side-effects, and 18 per cent considered that continued 'menstruation' was unacceptable. Patient compliance may, therefore, be improved by reducing the number of withdrawal bleeds by giving oestrogen continuously for six months followed by a single 10-day course of progestogen resulting in only one withdrawal bleed every six months. However, some 2 per cent of patients so treated developed endometrial hyperplasia, albeit mild, and this would seem to be an inappropriate regime (Kemp *et al.* 1989). This incidence of endometrial hyperplasia may be reduced by a longer progestogen course (Casper and Chapdelaine 1993; Rees 1994). The need for withdrawal bleeding should not occur in post-menopausal women with the synthetic steroid tibolone, but it is not yet clear whether this drug is as effective as oestrogen in the prevention of osteoporosis and coronary heart disease (*Lancet* 1991).

It is essential that patients and doctors understand the benefits, risks, and alternative treatments available for women both with menopausal symptoms and those in need of primary prevention in high-risk groups. There is considerable uncertainty amongst doctors in general, and general practitioners in particular, as to the balance of beneficial and harmful effects from longterm hormone replacement therapy (Wilkes and Meade 1991).

References

Adami, H. O., Persson, I., Hoover, R., Schairer, C., and Bergkvist, L. (1989). Risk of cancer in women receiving hormone replacement therapy. *International Journal of Cancer* **44**, 833–9.

Aitken, J. M. (1984). Relevance of osteoporosis in women with fracture of the femoral neck. *British Medical Journal* **288**, 596–601.

Aitken, J. M., Hart, D. M., Anderson, J. B., Lindsay, R., Smith, D. A., and Speirs, C. F. (1973*a*). Osteoporosis after oophorectomy for non-malignant disease in premenopausal women. *British Medical Journal* **2**, 325–8.

Aitken, J. M., Hart, D. M., and Lindsay, R. (1973*b*). Oestrogen replacement therapy for prevention of osteoporosis after oophorectomy. *British Medical Journal* **3**, 515–18.

Albrecht, B. H., Schiff, I., Tulchinsky, D., and Ryan, K. J. (1981). Objective evidence that placebo and oral medroxyprogesterone acetate therapy diminish menopausal vasomotor flushes. *American Journal of Obstetrics and Gynecology* **139**, 631–5.

Albright, F., Smith, P. H., and Richardson, A. M. (1941). Postmenopausal osteoporosis — its clinical features. *Journal of the American Medical Association* **116**, 2465–74.

American College of Physicians (1984). Radiologic methods to evaluate bone mineral content. *Annals of Internal Medicine* **100**, 908–11.

Armstrong, B. K. (1988). Oestrogen therapy after the menopause—boon or bane? *Medical Journal of Australia* **148**, 213–14.

Aylward, M. and Maddock, J. (1973). Total and free plasma tryptophan concentrations in rheumatoid disease. *Journal of Pharmacy and Pharmacology* **25**, 570–2.

Baran, D. T., Teitebaum, S. L., Berfield, M. A., Parker, G., Curvant, E. M., and Avioli, L. V. (1980). Effect of alcohol ingestion on bone and mineral metabolism in rats. *American Journal of Physicians* **238**, E507–10.

Barlow, D. H., Grosset, K. A., Hart, H., and Hart, D. M. (1989). A study of the experience of Glasgow women in the climacteric years. *British Journal of Obstetrics and Gynaecology* **96**, 1192–7.

Barrett-Connor, E., Brown, V., Turner, J., Austin, M., and Criqui, M. H. (1979). Heart disease risk factors and hormone use in postmenopausal women. *Journal of the American Medical Association* **241**, 2167–9.

Barrett-Connor, E., Wingard, D. L., and Criqui, M. H. (1989). Postmenopausal oestrogen use and heart disease risk factors in the 1980s. *Journal of the American Medical Association* **261**, 2095–100.

Belchetz, P. (1989). Hormone replacement therapy. *British Medical Journal* **298**, 1467–8.

Beller, F. K., Nachtigall, L., and Rosenberg, M. (1972). Coagulation studies of menopausal women taking oestrogen replacement. *Obstetrics and Gynecology* **39**, 775–8.

Bikle, D. D., Genant, H. K., Cann, C., Recker, R. R., Halloran, B. P., and Strewler, G. J. (1985). Bone disease in alcohol abuse. *Archives of Internal Medicine* **103**, 42–8.

Block, J. E., Smith, R., Black, D., and Genant, H. K. (1987). Does exercise prevent osteoporosis? *Journal of the American Medical Association* **257**, 3115–16.

Boston Collaborative Drug Surveillance Program (1974). Surgically confirmed gall bladder disease, venous thromboembolism, and breast tumors in relation to postmenopausal oestrogen therapy. *New England Journal of Medicine* **290**, 15–19.

Bourne, T., Hillard, T. C., Whitehead, M. I., Crook, D., and Campbell, S. (1990). Oestrogens, arterial status, and postmenopausal women. *Lancet* **335**, 1470–1.

Brambilla, D. J. and McKinlay, S. M. (1989). A prospective study of factors affecting age at menopause. *Journal of Clinical Epidemiology* **42**, 1031–9.

Brincat, M., Kabalan, S., Studd, J. W. W., Moniz, C. F., Trafford, J., and Montgomery, J. C. (1987). A study of the decrease of skin collagen content, skin thickness, and bone mass in the postmenopausal woman. *Obstetrics and Gynecology* **70**, 840–5.

Brinton, L. A. (1986). Menopausal oestrogen and breast cancer risk—an expanded case control study. *British Journal of Cancer* **54**, 825–32.

Brocklehurst, J. C., Fry, J., Griffiths, L. L., and Kalton, G. (1972). Urinary infection and symptoms of dysuria in women aged 45–64 years. *Age and Aging* **1**, 41–7.

Brown, A. D. G. (1977). Postmenopausal urinary problems. *Clinics in Obstetrics and Gynaecology* **4**, 181–206.

Buring, J. E., Hennekens, C. H., Lipnick, R. J., Willett, W., Stampfer, M. J., Rosner, B., *et al.* (1987). A prospective cohort study of postmenopausal hormone use and risk of breast cancer in US women. *American Journal of Epidemiology* **125**, 939–47.

Cann, C. E., Martin, M. C., Genant, H. K., and Jaffe, R. B. (1984). Decreased spinal mineral content in amenorrhoeic women. *Journal of the American Medical Association* **251**, 626–9.

Casper, R. F. and Chapdelaine, A. (1993). Oestrogen and interrupted progestogen. *American Journal of Obstetrics and Gynecology* **168**, 1189–96.

Chakravarti, S., Collins, W. P., Forecast, J. D., Newton, J. R., Oram, D. H., and

Studd, J. W. W. (1976). Hormonal profiles after the menopause. *British Medical Journal* **2**, 784-7.

Chapuy, M. C., Arlot, M. E., Duboeuf, F., Brun, J., Crouzet, B., Arnaud, S., *et al.* (1992). Vitamin D and calcium to prevent hip fractures in elderly women. *New England Journal of Medicine* **327**, 1637-42.

Chetkowski, R. J., Meldrum, D. R., Steingold, K. A., Randle, D., Lu, J. K., Eggena, P., *et al.* (1986). Biologic effects of transdermal estradiol. *New England Journal of Medicine* **314**, 1615-20.

Chow, R., Harrison, J. E., and Notarious, C. (1987). Effect of two randomized exercise programmes on bone mass of healthy postmenopausal women. *British Medical Journal* **295**, 1441-4.

Christiansen, C. and Riis, B. J. (1990). Five years with continuous combined oestrogen-progestogen therapy. *British Journal of Obstetrics and Gynaecology* **97**, 1087-92.

Christiansen, C., Rodbro, P., and Heinilid, B. (1976). Unchanged body calcium in normal human pregnancy. *Acta Obstetrica et Gynaecologica Scandinavica* **55**, 141-3.

Cohn, S. H., Abesamis, C., Yasumura, S., Aloia, J. F., Zanzi, I., and Ellis, K. J. (1977). Comparative skeleton mass and radiological bone mineral content in black and white women. *Metabolism* **26**, 171-8.

Colditz, G. A., Egan, K. M., and Stampfer, M. J. (1993). Hormone replacement therapy and risk of breast cancer. *American Journal of Obstetrics and Gynecology* **168**, 1473-80.

Collins, P., Rosano, G. M. C., Jiang, C., Lindsay, D., Sarrel, P. M., and Poole-Wilson, P. A. (1993). Cardiovascular protection by oestrogen — a calcium antagonist effect? *Lancet* **341**, 1264-5.

Cooke, I. D. (1976). Oestrogens as a cause of endometrial carcinoma. *British Medical Journal* **1**, 1209-10.

Coope, J., Thomson, J. M., and Poller, L. (1975). The effects of natural oestrogen replacement therapy on menopausal symptoms and blood clotting. *British Medical Journal* **4**, 139-43.

Coppen, A. and Wood, K. (1978). Trytophan and depressive illness. *Psychological Medicine* **8**, 49-57.

Coronary Drug Project Research Group (1970). The coronary drug project. *Journal of the American Medical Association* **214**, 1303-13.

Crook, D., Cust, M. P., Ganger, K. F., Worthington, M., Hillard, T. C., Stevenson, J. C., *et al.* (1992). Comparison of transdermal and oral estrogen-progestin replacement therapy: effects on serum lipids and lipoproteins. *American Journal of Obstetrics and Gynecology* **166**, 950-5.

Cummings, S. R. and Black, D. (1986). Should perimenopausal women be screened for oesteoporosis? *Annals of Internal Medicine* **104**, 817-23.

Cummings, S. R., Kelsey, J. L., Nevitt, M. C., and O'Dowd, K. J. (1985). Epidemiology of osteoporosis and osteoporosis fractures. *Epidemiologic Review* **7**, 178-208.

Dalsky, G. P., Stocke, K. S., Ehsani, A. A., Slatopolsky, E., Lee, W. C., and Birge, S. J. (1988). Weight-bearing exercise training and lumbar bone mineral content in postmenopausal women. *Annals of Internal Medicine* **108**, 824-8.

Daly, E., Gray, A., Barlow, D., McPherson, K., Roche, M., and Vessey, M. (1993). Measuring the impact of menopausal symptoms on quality of life. *British Medical Journal* **307**, 836-40.

Daniell, H. W. (1976). Osteoporosis of the slender smoker. *Archives of Internal Medicine* **136**, 298-304.

Davidson, B. J., Ross, R. K., Paganini-Hill, A., Hammond, G. D., Siteri, P. K., and Judd, H. L. (1982). Total and free oestrogens and androgens in post-menopausal women with hip fractures. *Journal of Clinical Endocrinology and Metabolism* **54**, 115-20.

Davies, M. D., Hall, M. L., and Jacobs, H. S. (1990). Bone mineral loss in young women with amenorrhoea. *British Medical Journal* **301**, 790-3.

Dent, C. E. and Friedman, M. (1965). Pregnancy and idiopathic osteoporosis. *Quarterly Journal of Medicine* **34**, 341-57.

Donaldson, C. L., Hulley, S. B., Vogel, J. M., Hartner, R. S., Bayers, J. H., and McMillan, D. E. (1970). Effect of prolonged bedrest on bone mineral. *Metabolism* **19**, 1071-84.

Dow, M., Hart, E. M., and Forrest, C. A. (1983). Hormonal treatments of sexual unresponsiveness in postmenopausal women. *British Journal of Obstetrics and Gynaecology* **90**, 361-6.

Draper, J. and Roland, M. (1990). Perimenopausal women's views on taking hormone replacement therapy to prevent osteoporosis. *British Medical Journal* **300**, 786-8.

Drug and Therapeutics Bulletin (1991). Tibolone, **29**, 77-8.

Dupont, W. D. and Page, D. L. (1991). Menopausal estrogen replacement therapy and breast cancer. *Archives of Internal Medicine* **151**, 67-72.

Eeles, R. A., Tan, S., Wiltshaw, E., Fryatt, I., A'Hern, R. P., Shepherd, J. H., *et al.* (1991). Hormone replacement therapy and survival after surgery for ovarian cancer. *British Medical Journal* **302**, 259-62.

Egeland, G. M., Kuller, L. H., Mathews, K. A., Kelsey, S. F., Cauley, J., and Guzick, D. (1990). Hormone replacement therapy and lipoprotein changes during early menopause. *Obstetrics and Gynecology* **76**, 776-82.

Ettinger, B., Genant, H. K., and Cann, C. C. (1985). Long-term estrogen replacement therapy prevents bone loss and fractures. *Annals of Internal Medicine* **102**, 319-24.

Ettinger, B., Genant, H. K., and Cann, C. C. (1987). Post-menopausal bone loss is prevented by treatment with low-dose estrogen and calcium. *Annals of Internal Medicine* **106**, 40-5.

Everson, R. B., Sandler, D. P., Wilcox, A. J., Schreinenachers, D., Shore, D. L., and Weinberg, C. (1986). Effect of passive exposure to smoking on age at natural menopause. *British Medical Journal* **293**, 792.

Fogelman, I. (1988). The case for routine bone mass measurements. *Nuclear Medicine Communications* **9**, 541-3.

Freedman, R. R., Woodward, S., and Sabharwal, S. C. (1990). Alpha-adrenergic mechanism in menopausal hot flushes. *Obstetrics and Gynecology* **76**, 573-8.

Gangar, K. F., Vyas, S., Crook, D., Meire, H., and Whitehead, M. I. (1991). Pulsatility index in internal carotid artery in relation to transdermal oestradiol and time since menopause. *Lancet* **338**, 839-42.

Gath, D., Osborne, M., Bungay, G., Iles, S., Day, A., Bond, A., *et al.* (1987). Psychiatric disorder and gynaecological symptoms in middle-aged women. *British Medical Journal* **294**, 213-18.

Goldsmith, N. F. and Johnston, J. O. (1975). Bone mineral effects of oral contraceptives, pregnancy, and lactation. *Journal of Bone and Joint Surgery* **57A**, 657-81.

Goldsmith, N. F., Johnston, J. O., Picetti, G., and Garcia, C. (1973). Bone mineral in the radius and vertebral osteoporosis in an insured population. *Journal of Bone and Joint Surgery* **55A**, 1276-93.

Gorsky, R. D., Koplan, J. P., Peterson, H. B., and Thacker, S. B. (1994). Relative risks and benefits of long term oestrogen hormone replacement. *Obstetrics and Gynecology* **63**, 161-6.

Gow, S. and MacGillivary, I. (1971). Metabolic, hormonal, and vascular changes after synthetic oestrogen therapy. *British Medical Journal* **2**, 73-7.

Greenblatt, R. B., Byrd, J. R., and McDonough, P. G. (1967). The spectrum of gonadal dysgenesis. *American Journal of Obstetrics and Gynecology* **98**, 151-72.

Greene, J. G. and Cooke, D. J. (1980). Life stress and symptoms at the climacteric. *British Journal of Psychiatry* **136**, 849-91.

Haas, S., Walsh, B., Evans, S., Crache, K., Ravnikar, V., and Schiff, I. (1988). The effect of transdermal estradiol on hormone and metabolic dynamics. *Obstetrics and Gynecology* **71**, 671-6.

Hallstrom, T. (1977). Sexuality in the climacteric. *Clinics in Obstetrics and Gynaecology* **4**, 227-39.

Hammond, C. B., Jelovsek, F. R., Lee, K. L., Creasman, W. T., and Parker, R. T. (1979). Effect of long-term estrogen replacement. *American Journal of Obstetrics and Gynecology* **133**, 537-47.

Hansen, M. A., Overgaard, K., Riis, B. J., Christiansen, C. (1991). Role of peak bone mass and bone loss in postmenopausal osteoporosis. *British Medical Journal* **303**, 961-4.

Heaney, R. P. and Saville, P. D. (1976). Etidronate disodium in postmenopausal osteoporosis. *Clinical Pharmacology and Therapeutics* **20**, 597-604.

Henderson, B. E., Paganini-Hill, A., and Ross, R. K. (1991). Decreased mortality in users of estrogen replacement therapy. *Archives of Internal Medicine* **151**, 75-8.

Holbrook, T. L. and Barrett-Connor, E. (1993). A prospective study of alcohol consumption and bone mineral density. *British Medical Journal* **306**, 1506-9.

Holland, E. F. N., Leather, A. T., and Studd, J. W. W. (1994). The effects of 25 mg percutaneous oestrogen implants on bone mass of post-menopausal women. *Obstetrics and Gynecology* **83**, 43-6.

Holst, J., Cajander, S., Carlstrom, K., Damber, M. G., and Schoultz, B. (1983). A comparison of liver protein induction in postmenopausal women during oral and percutaneous oestrogen replacement therapy. *British Journal of Obstetrics and Gynaecology* **90**, 355-60.

Hunt, K. and Vessey, M. (1991). The risks and benefits of hormone replacement therapy. *Current Obstetrics and Gynaecology* **1**, 21-7.

Hunt, K., Vessey, M., McPherson, K., and Coleman, M. (1987). Long-term surveillance of mortality and cancer incidence in women receiving hormone replacement therapy. *British Journal of Obstetrics and Gynaecology* **94**, 620-35.

Hunt K., Vessey, M. and McPherson, K. (1990). Mortality in a cohort of long-term users of hormone replacement therapy. *British Journal of Obstetrics and Gynaecology* **97**, 1080-6.

Hustin, J. (1970). Endometrial carcinoma and synthetic progestogens. *Journal of Obstetrics and Gynaecology of the British Commonwealth* **77**, 915-22.

Hutchinson, T. A., Polansky, S. M., and Feinstein, A. R. (1979). Postmenopausal oestrogens protect against fractures of hip and distal radius. *Lancet* ii, 705-9.

James, C. E., Breeson, A. J., Kovacs, G., Hill, J. G., Grant, C., Allen, K. M., *et al.* (1984). The symptomatology of the climacteric in relation to hormonal and cytological factors. *British Journal of Obstetrics and Gynaecology* **91**, 56-62.

Jensen, J., Riis, B. J., Strom, V., Nilas, L., and Christiansen, C. (1987). Long-term effects of percutaneous estrogen and oral progestogen on serum lipoproteins in postmenopausal women. *American Journal of Obstetrics and Gynecology* **156**, 66-71.

Jonnavithula, S., Warren, M. P., Fox, R. P., and Lazaro, M. I. (1993). Bone density is compromised in amenorrheic women. *Obstetrics and Gynecology* **81**, 669-74.

Kanis, J. A. (1990). Effect of fluoride on postmenopausal osteoporosis. *New England Journal of Medicine* **323**, 416.

Kaufman, D. W., Kelly, J. P., Welch, W. R., Rosenberg, L., Stolley, P., Warshauer,

M. E., *et al.* (1989). Non-contraceptive estrogen use and epithelial ovarian cancer. *American Journal of Epidemiology* **130**, 1142-51.

Kemp, J. F., Fryer, J. A., and Baber, R. J. (1989). An alternative regimen of hormone replacement therapy to improve patient. compliance. *Australian and New Zealand Journal of Obstetrics and Gynaecology* **29**, 66-9.

Kiel, D. P., Felson, D. T., Anderson, J. J., Wilson, P. W. F., and Moskowitz, M. A. (1987). Hip fracture and the use of estrogen in postmenopausal women. *New England Journal of Medicine* **317**, 1169-74.

Klaiber, E. L., Broverman, D. M., Vogel, W., and Kobayashi, Y. (1979). Oestrogen therapy for severe persistent depression in women. *Archives of General Psychiatry* **36**, 550-4.

Klipanski, A., Neer, R. M., Bietens, I. Z., Ridgway, E. C., Zervas, N. T., and McArthur, J. W. (1980). Decreased bone density in hyperprolactinaemic women. *New England Journal of Medicine* **303**, 1511-14.

La Vecchia, C., Liberati, A., and Franceschi, S. (1982). Non-contraceptive oestrogen use and the occurrence of ovarian cancer. *Journal of the National Cancer Institute* **69**, 1207.

Lancet (1991). More than hot flushes. *Lancet* **338**, 917-18.

Lane, G., Siddle, N. C., Ryder, T. A., Pryse-Davies, J., King, R. J. B., and Whitehead, M. I. (1986). Effects of dydrogesterone on the oestrogenized postmenopausal endometrium. *British Journal of Obstetrics and Gynaecology* **93**, 55-62.

Lane, N. E., Block, D. A., Jones, H. H., Marshall, W. H., Wood, P. D., and Fries, J. F. (1986). Long distance running, bone density, and osteoporosis. *Journal of the American Medical Association* **255**, 1147-51.

Lind, T., Cameron, E. C., Hunter, W. M., Leon, C., Moran, P. F., Oxley, A., *et al.* (1979). A prospective, controlled trial of six forms of hormone replacement therapy given to postmenopausal women. *British Journal of Obstetrics and Gynaecology* **86**, Supp. 3, 1-29.

Lindberg, J. S., Fears, W. B., Hunt, M. M., Powell, M. B., Ball, D., and Wade, C. E. (1984). Exercise induced amenorrhoea and bone density. *Annals of Internal Medicine* **101**, 647-8.

Lindsay, R. (1990). Fluoride and bone—quantity versus quality. *New England Journal of Medicine* **322**, 845-6.

Lindsay, R. (1993). Prevention and treatment of osteoporosis. *Lancet* **341**, 801-6.

Lindsay, R. and Cosman, F. (1990). Epidemiology of osteoporosis. In *Hormone replacement therapy and osteoporosis* (ed. J. O. Drife and J. W. W. Studd), pp. 75-86. Springer-Verlag, London.

Lindsay, R., Hart, D. M., Aitken, J. M., MacDonald, E. B., Anderson, J. B., and Clark, A. C. (1976). Long-term prevention of postmenopausal osteoporosis by oestrogen. *Lancet* **i**, 1038-40.

Lindsay, R., Hart, D. M., Forrest, C., and Baird, C. (1980*a*). Prevention of spinal osteoporosis in oophorectomized women. *Lancet* **ii**, 1151-3.

Lindsay, R., Hart, D. M., and Kraszewski, A. (1980*b*). Prospective double-blind trial of synthetic steroid for preventing postmenopausal osteoporosis. *British Medical Journal* **280**, 1207-9.

MacDonald, P. C., Edman, E. D., Hamsell, D. L., Porter, J. C., and Siteri, P. K. (1978). Effect of obesity on conversion of plasma androstenedione to estrone in postmenopausal women with and without endometrial cancer. *American Journal of Obstetrics and Gynecology* **130**, 448-55.

MacIntyre, I., Stevenson, J. C., Whitehead, M. I., Wimalawansa, S. J., Banks, L. M., and Healy, M. J. R. (1988). Calcitonin for prevention of postmenopausal bone loss. *Lancet* **i**, 900-2.

Mack, T. M., Pike, M. C., Henderson, B. E., Pfeffer, R. I., Gerkins, V. R., and

Arthur, M. (1976). Estrogens and endometrial cancer in a retirement community. *New England Journal of Medicine* **294**, 1262–7.

McKinlay, J. B., McKinlay, S. M., and Brambilla, D. J. (1987). Health status and utilization behavior associated with the menopause. *American Journal of Epidemiology* **125**, 110–21.

McKinlay, S. M. and Jeffreys, M. (1974). The menopause syndrome. *British Journal of Preventative and Social Medicine* **28**, 108–15.

McKinlay, S. M., Bifano, N. L., and McKinlay, J. B. (1985). Smoking and age at menopause. *Annals of Internal Medicine* **105**, 350–6.

Mamelle, N., Meunier, P. J., Dusan, R., Guillaume, M., Martin, J. L., Gaucher, A., *et al.* (1988). Risk benefit ratio of sodium fluoride treatment in primary vertebral osteoporosis. *Lancet* **ii**, 361–5.

Masters, W. H. and Johnson, V. E. (1966). *Human sexual response*, pp. 223–47. Boston, Little, Brown, and Company, Chicago.

Mattison, D. R. and Thorgeirsson, S. S. (1978). Smoking and industrial pollution, and their effects on menopause and ovarian cancer. *Lancet* **i**, 187–8.

Mazess, R. B. (1982). On aging bone loss. *Clinical Orthopedics* **165**, 239–52.

Mazess, R. B., Gallagher, J. C., Notelovitz, N., Schiff, I., and Utian, W. (1989). Monitoring skeletal response to estrogen. *American Journal of Obstetrics and Gynecology* **161**, 843–8.

Meade, T. W., Dyer, S., Howarth, D. J., Imeson, J. D., and Sterling, J. Y. (1990). Antithrombin III and procoagulant activity: sex differences and effects of the menopause. *British Journal of Haematology* **74**, 77–81.

Miller, V. T., Muesing, R. A., La Rosa, J., Stoy, D. B., Phillips, E. A., and Stillman, R. J. (1991). Effects of conjugated equine oestrogen with and without different progestogens on lipoproteins, high density lipoprotein subfractions, and apolipo-protein. *Obstetrics and Gynecology* **77**, 235–40.

Montgomery, J. C. and Crook, D. (1990). Progestagens: symptomatic and metabolic side-effects. In *Hormone replacement therapy and osteoporosis* (ed. J. O. Drife and J. W. W. Studd), pp. 197–208. Springer–Verlag, London.

Montgomery, J. C. and Studd, J. W. W. (1991). Psychological and sexual aspects of the menopause. *British Journal of Hospital Medicine* **45**, 300–2.

Montgomery, J. C., Appleby, L., Brincat, M., Versi, E., Tapp, A., Fenwick, P. B. C., *et al.* (1987). Effect of oestrogen and testosterone implants on psychological disorders in the climacteric. *Lancet* **i**, 297–9.

Morrell, M. J., Dixen, J. M., Carter, S., and Davidson, J. M. (1984). The influence of age and cycling status on sexual arousability in women. *American Journal of Obstetrics and Gynecology* **148**, 66–71.

Murply, S., Khaw, K. T., May, H., and Compston, J. E. (1994). Milk consumption and bone mineral density in middle aged and elderly women. *British Medical Journal* **308**, 939–41.

Nachtigall, L. E., Nachtigall, R. H., Nachtigall, R. D., and Beckman, E. M. (1978). Estrogen replacement therapy: a 10 year prospective study in the relationship to osteoporosis. *Obstetrics and Gynecology* **53**, 277–81.

Naessen, T., Persson, I., Adami, H. O., Bergstrom, H., and Bergkvist, L. (1990). Hormone replacement therapy and the risk for first hip fracture. *Annals of Internal Medicine* **113**, 95–103.

Nilas, L., Christiansen, C., and Rodbro, P. (1984). Calcium supplementation and postmenopausal bone loss. *British Medical Journal* **284**, 1103–6.

Niskanen, P., Huttunen, M., Tamminen, T., and Jaaskelainen, J. (1976). The daily rhythm of plasma tryptophan and tyrosine in depression. *British Journal of Psychiatry* **128**, 255–8.

Nordin, B. E. C. and Heaney, R. P. (1990). Calcium supplementation of the diet: justified by present evidence. *British Medical Journal* **300**, 1056-60.

Nordin, B. E. C., Horsman, A., Crilly, R. G., Marshall, B. H., and Simpson, M. (1980). Treatment of spinal osteoporosis in postmenopausal women. *British Medical Journal* **280**, 451-4.

Office of Health Economics (1990). Osteoporosis and the risk of fracture. *Office of Health Economics* **no. 94**, pp. 40-1, London.

Ott, S. M. (1994). Bone mass measurements—reasons to be cautious. *British Medical Journal* **308**, 931-2.

Overgaard, K., Riis, B. J., Christiansen, C., Podenphant, J., and Johansen, J. S. (1989). Nasal calcitonin for treatment of established osteoporosis. *Clinical Endocrinology* **30**, 435-42.

Paganini-Hill, A., Ross, R. K., Gerkins, V. R., Henderson, B. E., Arthur, M., and Mack, T. M. (1981). Menopausal estrogen treatment and hip fractures. *Annals of Internal Medicine* **95**, 28-31.

Paganini-Hill, A., Ross, R. K., and Henderson, B. E. (1988). Postmenopausal oestrogen treatment and stroke: a prospective study. *British Medical Journal* **297**, 519-22.

Paterson, M. E. L., Wade-Evans, T., Sturdee, D. W., Thom, M., and Studd, J. W. W. (1980). Endometrial disease after treatment with oestrogens and progestogens in the climacteric. *British Medical Journal* **i**, 822-4.

Peet, M., Moody, J. P., Worrall, E. P., Walker, P., and Naylor, G. J. (1976). Plasma tryptophan concentration in depressive illness and mania. *British Journal of Psychiatry* **128**, 255-8.

Persson, I., Adami, H. O., Bergkvist, L., Lindgren, A., Petterson, B., Hoover, R., et al. (1989). Risk of endometrial carcinoma after treatment with oestrogen alone or in conjugation with progestogens. *British Medical Journal* **298**, 147-51.

Pocock, N. A., Eisman, J., Hopper, J. L., Yeates, M. G., Sambrooke, P. N., et al. (1987). Genetic determinance of bone mass in adults. *Journal of Clinical Investigation* **80**, 706-10.

Poller, L., Thomson, J. M., and Coope, J. (1977). Conjugated equine oestrogens and blood clotting. *British Medical Journal* **1**, 935-6.

Prince, R. L., Smith, M., Dick, I. M., Price, R. T., Webb, P. J., Henderson, N. K., et al. (1991). Prevention of postmenopausal osteoporosis. *New England Journal of Medicine* **325**, 1189-95.

Quigley, M. E. T., Martin, P. L., Burnier, A. P., and Brooks, P. (1987). Estrogen therapy arrests bone loss in elderly women. *American Journal of Obstetrics and Gynecology* **156**, 1516-23.

Quint, B. C. (1975). Changing patterns in endometrial adenocarcinoma. *American Journal of Obstetrics and Gynecology* **122**, 498-501.

Ravnikar, V. (1990). Physiology and treatment of hot flushes. *Obstetrics and Gynecology* **75**, Supp. 3S-8S.

Recker, R. P., Saville, P. D., and Heaney, R. P. (1977). Effect of oestrogen and calcium carbonate on bone loss in postmenopausal women. *Annals of Internal Medicine* **87**, 649-55.

Rees, M. (1994). On menstrual bleeding with hormone replacement therapy. *Lancet* **343**, 250.

Reid, I. R., Ames, R. W., Evans, M. C., Gamble, G. D., and Sharpe, S. J. (1993). Effect of calcium supplementation on bone loss in postmenopausal women. *New England Journal of Medicine* **328**, 460-4.

Richelson, L. S., Wahner, H. W., Melton, L. J., and Riggs, B. L. (1984). Relative contribution of aging and oestrogen deficiency to postmenopausal bone loss. *New England Journal of Medicine* **311**, 1273–5.

Riggs, B. L. and Melton, L. J. (1986). Involutional osteoporosis. *New England Journal of Medicine* **314**, 1676–86.

Riggs, B. L., Seeman, E., Hodgson, S. F., Taues, D. R., and O'Fallon, W. M. (1982). Effect of the fluoride-calcium regimen on vertebral fracture occurrences in post-menopausal osteoporosis. *New England Journal of Medicine* **306**, 446–50.

Riggs, B. L., Hodgson, S. F., O'Fallon, W. M., Chao, E. Y. S., Wahner, H. Z., Muhs, J. M., *et al.* (1990). Effect of fluoride treatment on the fracture rate in post-menopausal women with osteoporosis. *New England Journal of Medicine* **322**, 802–9.

Riis, B., Thomsen, K., and Christiansen, C. (1987). Does calcium supplementation prevent postmenopausal bone loss? A double-blind controlled study. *New England Journal of Medicine* **316**, 173–7.

Saleh, A. A., Dorey, L. G., Dombrowski, M. P., Ginsberg, K. A., Hirokawa, S., *et al.* (1993). Thrombosis and hormone replacement therapy in postmenopausal women. *British Journal of Obstetrics and Gynaecology* **169**, 1554–7.

Sarrel, P. M. (1990). Ovarian hormones and the circulation. *Maturitas* **12**, 287–98.

Saville, P. D. (1975). Alcohol-related skeletal disorders. *Annals of the New York Academy of Science* **252**, 287–91.

Savvas, M., Treasure, J., Studd, J., Fogelman, I., Moniz, C., Brincat, M., *et al.* (1988*a*). The effect of anorexia nervosa on skin thickness, skin collagen, and bone density. In *Recent research on gynaecological endocrinology* (ed. A. R. Genazzani, F. Petraglia, A. Volpe, and F. Facchinetti), pp. 178–82, Parthenon Publishing Group, Lancaster.

Savvas, M., Studd, J. W. W., Fogelman, I., Dooley, M., Montgomery, J., and Murby, B. (1988*b*). Skeletal effects of oral oestrogen compared with subcutaneous oestrogen and testosterone in postmenopausal women. *British Medical Journal* **297**, 331–3.

Seeman, E., Hooper, J. L., Back, L. A., Cooper, M. E., Parkinson, E., McKay, J., *et al.* (1989). Reduced bone mass in daughters of women with osteoporosis. *New England Journal of Medicine* **320**, 554–8.

Shaw, D. M. (1973). Biochemical basis of affective disorders. *British Journal of Hospital Medicine* **10**, 609–10.

Siddle, N. C., Jesinger, D. K., Whitehead, M. I., Turner, P., Lewis, B., and Prescott, P. (1990). Effect on plasma lipids and lipoprotein of postmenopausal oestrogen therapy with added dydrogesterone. *British Journal of Obstetrics and Gynaecology* **97**, 1093–100.

Sillero-Arenas, M., Delgardo-Rodriguez, M., Rodriguez-Canteras, R., Bueno-Cavanillas, A., and Galvez-Vargas, R. (1992). Menopausal hormone replacement therapy and breast cancer. *Obstetrics and Gynecology* **79**, 286–92.

Smith, D. C., Prentice, R., Thompson, D. J., and Herrman, W. L. (1975). Association of exogenous oestrogen and endometrial carcinoma. *New England Journal of Medicine* **293**, 1164–7.

Smith, D. M., Nance, W. E., Kary, K. W., Christian J. C., and Johnston, C. C. (1973). Genetic factors in determining bone mass. *Journal of Clinical Investigation* **52**, 8200–8.

Smith, P. (1972). Age changes in the female urethra. *British Journal of Urology* **44**, 667–76.

Smith, T. (1987). Consensus on preventing osteoporosis. *British Medical Journal* **295**, 872.

Stampfer, M. J., Colditz, G. A., Willett, W. C., Manson, J. E., Rosner, B., Speizer, F. E., *et al.* (1991). Postmenopausal estrogen therapy and cardiovascular disease. *New England Journal of Medicine* **325**, 756–62.

Steinberg, K. K., Thacker, S. B., Smith, S. J., Stroup, D. F., Zack, M. N., Flanders, D., *et al.* (1991). A meta-analysis of the effect of estrogen replacement therapy on the risk of breast cancer. *Journal of the American Medical Association* **265**, 1985–90.

Stevenson, J. C. and Whitehead, M. I. (1982). Post-menopausal osteoporosis. *British Medical Journal* **285**, 585–8.

Stevenson, J. C., Lees, B., Davenport, M., Cust, M. P., and Ganger, K. F. (1989). Determinance of bone density in normal women: risk factors for future osteoporosis. *British Medical Journal* **298**, 924–8.

Stevenson, J. C., Cust, M. P., Ganger, K. F., Hillard, T. C., Lees, B., and Whitehead, M. I. (1990). Effect of transdermal versus oral hormone replacement therapy on bone density in spine and proximal femur in post-menopausal women. *Lancet* **ii**, 265–9.

Storm, T., Thamsborg, G., Steinisch, E. T., Genant, H. K., and Sorensen, O. H. (1990). Effect of intermittent cyclical etidronate therapy on bone mass and fracture rate in women with postmenopausal osteoporosis. *New England Journal of Medicine* **322**, 1265–71.

Studd, J., Collins, W. P., Chakravarti, S., Newton, J. R., Oram, D., and Parsons, J. (1977). Oestradiol and testosterone implants in the treatment of psychiatric problems in the postmenopausal woman. *British Journal of Obstetrics and Gynaecology* **84**, 314–15.

Studd, J., Dubiel, M., Kakkar, V. V., Thom, M., and White, P. J. (1978). The effect of hormone replacement therapy on glucose tolerance, clotting factors, fibrinolysis, and platelet function in postmenopausal women. In *The role of oestrogen-progestogen in the management of the menopause* (ed. I. D. Cooke), pp. 41–59, MTP, Lancaster.

Szmukler, G. I., Brown, S. W., Parsons, V., and Darby, A. (1985). Premature bone loss in chronic anorexia nervosa. *British Medical Journal* **290**, 26–7.

Thorneycroft, I. H. (1989). The role of estrogen replacement therapy in the prevention of osteoporosis. *American Journal of Obstetrics and Gynecology* **60,** 1306–10.

Tilyard, M. W., Spears, G. F. S., Thompson, J., and Dovey, S. (1992). Treatment of postmenopausal osteoporosis with calcitrol or calcium. *New England Journal of Medicine* **326**, 357–62.

Vandenbroocke, J. P. (1991). Postmenopausal oestrogen and cardioprotection. *Lancet* **337**, 833–4.

Voigt, L. F., Weis, N. S., Chu, J., Daling, J. R., McKnight, B., and von Belle, G. (1991). Progestogen supplementation of exogneous oestrogens and the risk of endometrial cancer. *Lancet* **338**, 274–7.

Walsh, B. W., Schiff, I., Rosner, B., Greenberg, L., Ravnikar, V., and Sacks, F. M. (1991). Effect of post-menopausal estrogen replacement therapy on the concentrations and metabolism of plasma lipoproteins. *New England Journal of Medicine* **325**, 1196–204.

Warren, M. P., Brooks'Gunn, J., Hamilton, L. H., Warren, L. F., and Hamilton, W. G. (1986). Scoliosis and fracture in young ballet dancers. *New England Journal of Medicine* **314**, 1348–53.

Watts, N. B., Harris, S. T., Genant, H. K., Wasnich, R. D., Miller, P. D., Jackson, R. D., *et al.* (1990). Intermittent cyclical etidronate treatment of postmenopausal osteoporosis. *New England Journal of Medicine* **323**, 73–9.

Weiss, N. S., Ure, C. L., Ballard, J. H., Williams, A. R., and Daling, J. R. (1980). Decreased risk of fracture of the hip and lower forearm with postmenopausal use of estrogen. *New England Journal of Medicine* **303**, 1195–8.

Weiss, N. S., Lyon, J. L., Krishnamurthy, S., Dietert, S. E., Liff, J. M., and Daling,

J. R. (1982). Non-contraceptive oestrogen use and the occurrence of ovarian cancer. *Journal of the National Cancer Institute* **68**, 95-8.

Whitehead, M. I., King, R. J. B., McQueen, J., and Campbell, S. (1979). Endometrial histology and biochemistry in climacteric women during oestrogen and oestrogen–progestogen therapy. *Journal of the Royal Society of Medicine* **72**, 322-7.

Whitehead, M. I., Fraser, D., Schenkel, L., Crook, D., and Stevenson, J. C. (1990). Transdermal administration of oestrogen–progestogen hormone replacement therapy. *Lancet* **335**, 310-12.

Wilkes, H. C. and Meade, J. W. (1991). Hormone replacement therapy in general practice. *British Medical Journal* **302**, 1317-20.

Williams, A. R., Weiss, N. S., Ure, C. L., Ballard, J. H., and Daling, J. R. (1982). Effect of weight, smoking, and estrogen use on the risk of hip and forearm fractures in postmenopausal women. *Obstetrics and Gynecology* **60**, 695-9.

Wilson, P. W. F., Garrison, W. J., and Castelli, W. P. (1985). Postmenopausal estrogen use, cigarette smoking, and cardiovascular morbidity in women over 50. *New England Journal of Medicine* **313**, 1038-43.

Ziel, H. K. and Finkle, W. D. (1975). Increased risk of endometrial carcinoma among users of conjugated estrogens. *New England Journal of Medicine* **293**, 1167-70.

10 The management of urinary incontinence

Urinary incontinence is defined as the condition in which involuntary loss of urine is a social or hygienic problem which and is objectively demonstrable. This definition, recommended by the International Continence Society (1990), makes no mention of either volume or frequency of loss. An insignificant volume to one woman may be devastating to another. The degree of interference with her comfort, hygiene, self-image, work, or social activity may be judged clinically or quantified by pad testing (see below).

Basic statistics

The prevalence of incontinence in the female population is surprisingly high. Various estimates are available and suggest that between 8 and 25 per cent of all women between the ages of 15 and 65 years may leak urine involuntarily, this figure being surprisingly consistent for all age groups up to the age of 85 years, the incidence increasing thereafter (Brocklehurst 1993; Jarvis 1993; Thomas *et al*. 1980). In a recent study, 16 per cent of all women aged 35–64 years had some degree of urinary incontinence (O'Brien *et al*. 1991). Clearly, therefore, only a minority of women seek medical advice about their incontinence, perhaps because many accept this as 'normal'. All women should be asked about their urinary symptoms as part of a standard gynaecological history taking, for some will wish to accept further advice.

Women with urinary incontinence generally delay seeking medical advice either because they hope that the symptoms will go away, or because of embarrassment, or because they believe their symptoms to be normal. Thus Norton *et al*. (1988) found that only 40 per cent of 201 women attending their incontinence clinic saw their general practitioners within the first year of symptoms, 25 per cent delaying in excess of five years.

The anatomy of urinary incontinence

Sphincter mechanisms

Continence is maintained by the pressure in the urethra exceeding the pressure in the bladder at all times, except during voluntary micturition. No single anatomical structure may be identified to correspond to this sphincter mechanism, and, indeed, the sphincter mechanism itself is really a group of interrelated but separate mechanisms which act in unison. Only when all mechanisms 'fail' will incontinence result.

If radio-opaque medium is placed in the bladder and a woman asked to stand and strain whilst being screened radiologically, the medium remains in the bladder; thus the proximal sphincter is in the region of the bladder neck and proximal urethra. The difference between the intravesical pressure and the pressure in the proximal urethra is in the region of 40 cm of water. There is considerable biological variation, but this pressure tends to reduce with age and is lower in patients with genuine stress incontinence than in the normal population (Edwards and Malvern 1974). This is termed the proximal spincter mechanism. The anatomical basis for this spincter has been hotly debated. It does *not* appear to be the orientation of smooth muscle in the urethra, for this is mainly in a longitudinal or oblique direction and contraction of this would shorten the urethra and open the bladder neck. There is, however, a rich mucosal and subepithelial vascular bed in the urethra (including arteriovenous anastamoses), far more than would seem necessary for the usual vascular functions. The effect of the turgor pressure exerted by this vasculature upon the soft, compressable, hollow urethra throughout its circumference would be urethral closure, thus forming a hermetic seal. This is the likely mechanism of the proximal sphincter, and may also be the mechanism by which age and oestrogen status exert their effects (Hilton 1990).

The proximal sphincter mechanism is augmented by the distal sphincter mechanism. The existence of a distal sphincter mechanism may be demonstrated by measuring the pressure differences between the bladder and the urethra along its length (urethral pressure profile). The maximum difference, called the maximal urethral closure pressure, is found in the mid-urethra and is in the region of 110 cm of water, and is reduced with increasing age. The importance of the sphincter mechanism may be demonstrated by the observation that 50 per cent of continent, perimenopausal women and 21 per cent of nulliparous women have an incompetent proximal sphincter but maintain continence by use of the distal sphincter mechanism (Chapple *et al.* 1989; Versi *et al.* 1986).

The distal sphincter mechanism, sometimes known as the rhabdosphincter, is a sleeve of striated, slow-twitch muscle fibres found within the wall of the urethra, being of maximal thickness in the mid-urethra, especially anteriorly. Although it is situated in the region of levator ani, it is anatomically distinct from it and has the characteristic of being able to maintain tone over a relatively long period of time without fatigue. It is innervated by the pudendal nerve.

The medial parts of levator ani are related to the urethral wall, but anatomically distinct from it. They consist of both slow-twitch and fast-twitch striated muscle fibres and may provide an additional occlusive force to the urethra, especially as a reflex component during episodes of raised intra-abdominal pressure, as well as providing support for the pelvic viscera.

In its normal anatomical position, the proximal urethra is an intraabdominal structure. It is maintained in this position by the combination of the muscles of the pelvic floor and the endopelvic fascia (De Lancey 1986). So long as the

Table 10.1 The causes of urinary incontinence

Diagnosis	Percentage
Genuine stress incontinence (g.s.i)	47.5
Detrusor instability (d.i)	37.7
Mixed g.s.i. and d.i.	5.2
Primary vesical sensory urgency	3.7
No satisfactory diagnosis	4.4
Chronic retention	1.2
Fistula	0.3

proximal urethra remains above the pelvic floor, any rise in intraabdominal pressure, caused by activity, will be transmitted to both the bladder and the proximal urethra, hence the pressure difference between the two remains unchanged, and the woman remains continent. In women with genuine stress incontinence, the pressure transmission is significantly reduced and may collapse totally following a series of coughs (Hilton and Stanton 1983*a*).

Neurological components

The bladder has a dual function, storage and micturition. In order to store, the bladder must be able to increase in volume by stretch of the detrusor without significant elevation of intravesical pressure, that is, it is compliant. If functional bladder capacity is reduced, for example following radiation, tuberculosis, or interstitial cystitis, then frequency and incontinence may ensue. Similarly, a bladder already near its maximum capacity due to a large residual urine volume will overflow.

The motor component of the detrusor reflex, in response to the afferent proprioceptor stimulus, is mediated by the parasympathetic nerve fibres. The preganglionic fibres originate in the grey columns of the sacral spinal cord (S3, S4), and run in the pelvic splanchnic nerves through the pelvic plexus into ganglia throughout the bladder wall; post-ganglionic cholinergic fibres then supply the detrusor cells. Central inhibition of the detrusor reflex originates within the cerebral cortex, and, hence, the detrusor should only contract during voluntary micturition, that is the bladder muscle is stable. Involuntary detrusor contractions will occur secondary to neurological disease or injury, or as a phenomenon to produce an unstable bladder.

Clinical features of incontinence

The major causes of urinary incontinence and their relative incidences in women are shown in Table 10.1. The diagnoses were made following a clinical and urodynamic assessment of 1000 consecutive incontinent patients. It should be

Table 10.2 Symptoms and diagnosis

Symptom	Genuine stress incontinence (n = 100)	Detrusor instability (n = 100)
Frequency	57	86
Nocturia	29	80
Urgency	46	92
Urge incontinence	37	88
Stress incontinence	99	26

Data from Leeds Urodynamic Clinic

noticed that there is a small, but significant, percentage of women (4.4 per cent) who claim to have urinary incontinence but in whom no abnormality or leakage may be demonstrated.

Genuine stress incontinence is the accepted diagnostic term for the condition in which involuntary loss of urine occurs when the intravesical pressure exceeds the maximal urethral pressure in the absence of a detrusor contraction. The term stress incontinence should be used only for the symptom or physical sign and not as a diagnosis (International Continence Society Committee on Standardization of Terminology 1990).

An unstable bladder is one that is shown to contract, spontaneously or on provocation, during the filling phase while the patient is attempting to inhibit micturition. Urgency, the strong desire to void, may be sensory, that is unassociated with a detrusor contraction, or motor, that is an unstable bladder. Urge incontinence is thus a symptom and not a diagnosis, being the involuntary loss of urine associated with the strong desire to void.

The presence or absence of prolapse may be important in planning treatment but is not of diagnostic relevance in incontinence. Jeffcoate (1961) reported that the incidence of incontinence amongst women with prolapse was 33 per cent, the same as that amongst women of similar age and parity without prolapse but attending a gynaecological clinic.

Since stress incontinence is not pathognomonic of genuine stress incontinence and urge incontinence is not pathognomonic of detrusor instability, there is an imperfect association between symptoms and diagnosis in urinary incontinence. Table 10.2 compares the symptoms between 100 women with genuine stress incontinence and 100 with detrusor instability (Jarvis 1990). Similarly, symptom complexes are poorly discriminatory. The patient who complains of stress incontinence without any other urinary symptom has between a 63 per cent and 90 per cent chance of having genuine stress incontinence, but, therefore, a 10–27% chance of having either detrusor instability alone or both detrusor instability and genuine stress incontinence (Jarvis 1990; Sand *et al.* 1988). Similarly, if a patient complains of both stress incontinence and urge incontinence, she has a 67 per cent chance of having genuine stress incontinence

Table 10.3 Urodynamic investigations

Pad weighing

Cystometry

(Video) cystourethrography

Vaginal ultrasound

Urethral pressure profilometry
   resting
   stress

Fluid bridge test

Urethral electrical conductance

Pressure flow studies

Residual urine assessment

Electromyography

Sacral nerve studies

alone, a 10 per cent chance of detrusor instability alone, and a 23 per cent chance of both diagnoses (Jarvis 1990; Sand *et al.* 1988). Only the patient who complains of urgency and urge incontinence without stress incontinence allows for an accurate diagnosis to be made.

These statistics demonstrate that an inaccurate diagnosis will be made should clinical features alone be used. Several authors have demonstrated that, using symptoms and signs, between 19 and 26 per cent of patients will be incorrectly diagnosed unless a urodynamic investigation is performed (Jarvis *et al.* 1980; Lagro-Janssen *et al.* 1991; Sand *et al.* 1988; Versi *et al.* 1991).

It would seem that symptoms give a better guide to severity than to diagnosis. Only the patient who complains of urgency and urge incontinence without stress incontinence should be treated clinically. No patient should undergo surgery for genuine stress incontinence based upon a history in the absence of a urodynamic investigation (Byrne *et al.* 1987; Haylen *et al.* 1989).

Urodynamic studies

Urodynamic studies involve the assessment of the function and dysfunction of the urinary tract by any appropriate method. They are dynamic investigations since continence and incontinence are dynamic processes. Static investigations such as intravenous urography and cystoscopy are not indicated, unless there is either another appropriate clinical indication or perhaps in the difficult refractory patients. Every patient does not require every test; a critical review of the indications for, and the limitation of, each test should be used in order to allow the most appropriate selection to be made for each patient. The list of available tests is shown in Table 10.3.

Pad weighing

This test is designed to quantify urine loss under standard and reproducable conditions. Having emptied her bladder, the patient wears a preweighed absorbent pad or nappy, drinks 500 ml of liquid over a 15-minute period, and then performs a series of tasks, including walking, climbing stairs, coughing, and hand-washing, over a 60-minute period. The pad is then reweighed and the urine loss recorded in grams. Sometimes the diuresis is delayed and the test results are expressed at both 60 and 120 minutes. Any voluntary voiding should be avoided, but measured and recorded separately should it occur. This test allows an accurate quantification of incontinence (Haylen *et al.* 1988; Sutherst *et al.* 1981).

Cystometry

Cystometry is the method by which the pressure/volume relationship of the bladder is measured, assessing detrusor activity, sensation, capacity, and compliance. In general, the bladder is filled with sterile saline or radio-opaque medium via a urethral catheter at approximately 100 ml per minute. Both bladder pressure and rectal pressure are measured throughout using either a fluid-filled line or microtransducer. As the total bladder pressure equals the rectal (abdominal) pressure together with the detrusor pressure, dual channel electronic subtraction will result in a continuous read-out of detrusor pressure. The patient should assume a standing position at some stage during the test and provocations to elicit positive changes, for example coughing, should occur (Bates *et al.* 1970).

Cystometry is especially useful in distinguishing between the different causes of incontinence, or identifying whether more than one cause exists, as it does in over 5 per cent of patients. It is the single most useful urodynamic investigation (Jarvis *et al.* 1980; Sand *et al.* 1988). The use of ambulatory urodynamics may increase the incidence of diagnosis of detrusor instability and reduce the percentage of patients in whom no diagnosis is made (Davila 1994).

(Video) cystourethrography

In this test, a cystometrogram is performed coincidentally with radiological screening of the bladder and urethra using an image intensifier (Bates *et al.* 1970). Although the combined test is not better than a cystometrogram alone in distinguishing between genuine stress incontinence and detrusor instability (based on a study of 150 incontinent women), it has the advantages of easier visualization of leakage, the assessment of the position and mobility of the bladder neck (especially after previous surgery), the estimation of residual 'urine', and an opportunity to diagnose morphological abnormalities, such as bladder or urethral diverticulae, urethral stenosis, or vesicoureteric reflux which may be present in up to 7 per cent of incontinent patients (Benness *et. al.* 1989). In current practice, therefore, VCUs could be safely reserved for more complicated cases, such as failed previous surgery and urological abnormalities.

Vaginal ultrasound

Transvaginal ultrasonography allows the bladder neck opening during a cough to be clearly demonstrated. It is simpler and quicker than VCU and is better accepted by the patients (Quinn *et al.* 1988). However, since detrusor instability may only be implied by this study, its use will be limited unless a cystometrogram is performed as an additional procedure.

Urethral pressure profilometry

The urethral pressure measures intraluminal pressure along the length of the urethra. The test is usually performed using dual catheter-tipped micro-transducers, one inside the bladder to act as a 'zero' and the second micro-transducer at a known position in the urethral lumen. The pressure exerted by the proximal sphincter mechanism and by the rhabdosphincter (maximum urethral closure pressure) may be noted, together with that length of urethra with a pressure in excess of intravesical pressure, that is the functional urethral length.

Although both the functional urethral length and the maximum urethral closure pressure are generally lower in patients with genuine stress incontinence than in detrusor instability, the degree of overlap both with continent patients and between these two conditions is too great for the technique to be diagnostic (Edwards and Malvern 1974; Versi 1990).

Urethral pressure profilometry has been used in the assessment of successful and unsuccessful surgery for genuine stress incontinence. Weil *et al.* (1984) reported 86 such patients, of whom 59 became continent and 27 remained incontinent. The mean increases in maximum urethral closure pressure and functional length, as shown in the urethral pressure profile of the continent patients, was greater than the increase in these parameters in the incontinence patients when a post-operative urethral pressure profile was compared with a pre-operative one. However, it has not proved of help in the choice of operative procedure, nor as a guide to intraoperative technique.

Fluid bridge test

This test is designed to identify the presence of urine in the proximal urethra in the presence of a cough and an incompetent proximal sphincter mechanism. When this occurs, fluid forms a bridge between the bladder and the proximal urethra, hence if pressures are measured at both these positions, they will be identical at that moment. This test was designed to diagnose genuine stress incontinence, but is of limited value since it has already been stated that continence may be maintained using the distal sphincter mechanism and that bladder neck incontinence is not necessarily synonymous with genuine stress incontinence. Moreover, Sutherst and Brown (1980), who designed the test, found a 28 per cent false-positive diagnostic rate.

Urethral electrical conductance

This test uses a probe with two gold-plated brass electrodes, each 1 mm wide and 1 mm apart. In the presence of a conducting fluid (saline) there will be an increased conductance, but in the absence of a conducting fluid there is a fall. If saline is placed in the bladder and the probe is placed in the urethra, then the leakage of saline from bladder to urethra will be detected. This test is able to detect small volumes of fluid in any part of the urethra which the operator chooses, and may distinguish between the short spurts of urine which tend to be found with genuine stress incontinence and the longer periods of leakage which tend to be associated with detrusor instability. This investigation is more useful when combined with a cystometrogram since it only correlates with the cystometric diagnosis in up to 55 per cent of patients (Creighton *et al.*; Peattie *et al.* 1988*a*).

Pressure-flow studies

These studies assess the dynamics of urine flow, measuring detrusor pressure during voiding, the maximal urine flow rate in millilitres per second, and time during which flow occurred, the latter two using a collecting vessel with a metal strip capacitor. The volume voided should also be measured, as voiding parameters are inconsistent if the volume is below 200 ml.

The vast majority of women will have a maximum flow rate of 20–30 ml/second; a rate of less than 15 ml would indicate voiding dysfunction, due to either increased outflow resistance or a hypotonic detrusor. A hypotonic detrusor, perhaps related to neurological problems or longterm outflow obstruction, will be characterized by a detrusor contraction inadequate to affect bladder emptying. Furthermore, as there is a short delay between voluntary interruption of the urine stream and even a poor detrusor contraction relaxing, asking the patient with a poor stream to attempt to inhibit micturition produces only a small additional increase in intravesical pressure if the cause is a hypotonic detrusor but produces a large rise if the cause is outflow obstruction. Detrusor instability is often associated with a high flow rate and rapid flow-time.

The importance of a voiding study lies in the observation that up to 16 per cent of 600 women attending with incontinence have coexisting voiding dysfunction, 14 per cent having some of the classical symptoms of hesitancy, poor stream, difficulty in voiding or incomplete emptying, whilst 2 per cent are asymptomatic. Such patients are particularly likely to develop overt voiding problems following surgery for genuine stress incontinence and, in addition to the forewarning, the choice of operation may be modified (Bergman and Bhatia 1985; Stanton *et al.* 1983).

Residual urine assessment

Residual urine is defined as the volume of fluid remaining in the bladder immediately following micturition. Its recognition is of importance either as evidence of a voiding dysfunction, a predisposing factor to infection or as evidence of a bladder diverticulum or vesicoureteric reflux. It may be estimated by catheter, radiography, ultrasound, or bimanual examination. Ravichandran (1983) reported that ultrasound tended to underestimate residual urine when compared to a catheter, whilst Norton *et al.* (1989) reported that bimanual palpation correctly estimated residual urine in excess of 50 ml in 84 per cent of patients, suggesting that this is a comfortable alternative to catheterization in the estimation of post-operative, post-voiding residual volumes.

Electromyography

Electromyography is the study of electric potentials generated by the depolarization of muscles. It may be measured either by placing needle electrodes directly into the muscle mass or by placing the electrode on to an epithelial surface as close as possible to the muscle under study, in this situation being pelvic sphincteric striated muscle. The techniques have no place in routine practice, but are of value either as research tools or in the assessment of myological disease or damage (Craggs and Stephenson 1976; Eardley and Fowler 1993).

Sacral nerve studies

These studies assess the integrity of the sacral reflex arc by measuring the speed of response, that is the latency following the stimulation of a peripheral nerve and the time taken for a given muscle to respond. Reflex latencies can also be measured, as can evoked responses from central nervous system stimulation. Such highly specialized studies help to distinguish between neuropathic and myopathic disorders (Massey and Abrams 1985).

Urodynamic studies in clinical practice

The urodynamic tests used in clinical practice should be those most likely to answer the question being asked. It has already been argued that no patient should undergo surgery for genuine stress incontinence without a preliminary cystometrogram. This will distinguish between genuine stress incontinence and detrusor instability. If further information about the bladder neck is required, a VCU or an ultrasound study should be performed. When the choice of operative procedures is debated later in this chapter, it will be shown that operations are associated with varying degrees of outlet obstruction and hence if a potentially obstructive procedure is to be performed, it would seem desirable to know whether or not some degree of undiagnosed obstruction is already present since the combination may cause longterm voiding problems. A pressure-flow study would, therefore, seem to be desirable. If neurological disease or damage is present, an electromyograph or sacral nerve study will be appropriate.

A cystometrogram is an invasive procedure and between 2–7 per cent of all patients undergoing this will develop a urinary tract infection (Carter *et al.* 1991; Coptcoat *et al.* 1988). It has been debated whether prophylactic antibiotics should be given to cover this procedure. Several randomized trials have failed to show any significant reduction in the incidence of urinary tract infection following the use of prophylactic antibiotics, but this observation almost certainly relates to the small number of patients in each of these trials (Carter *et al.* 1991; Coptcoat *et al.* 1988). The need for a larger trial (200–300) is clear. At the current time, patients should either be given prophylactic antibiotics or advised to report symptoms suggestive of a post-investigation urinary tract infection.

Genuine stress incontinence

Genuine stress incontinence is the condition in which urinary incontinence occurs when the intravesical pressure exceeds the maximum urethral closure pressure in the absence of detrusor activity. It requires some degree of weakness of both the proximal and distal sphincter mechanisms, and is the commonest form of urinary incontinence in women, accounting for at least 47.5 per cent of patients.

Aetiology

No one cause may be identified, but numerous factors exist and may coexist:

(1) age;
(2) pregnancy;
(3) prolapse;
(4) menopause;
(5) support;
(6) denervation;
(7) obesity.

Age

Age appears to be important only in that older women are more likely either to be parous or to be post-menopausal as compared to younger women. There is also a reduction in maximum urethral closure pressure with age.

Pregnancy

Genuine stress incontinence is more common in multiparous women, over and above the increased prevalence of multiparity in the general population. Debate exists as to whether it is the pregnancy or the delivery which is the major factor.

The early evidence suggested that both pregnancy and delivery were separate aetiological factors in the onset of genuine stress incontinence (Beck and Hsu 1965; Francis 1960).

More recent evidence has suggested that it is vaginal delivery rather than pregnancy which is the main aetiological factor. Several studies have now demonstrated that after vaginal delivery, there is a reduction in either the size of a maximum pelvic floor contraction as measured with a perineometer or a reduction in the maximal urethral closure pressure as measured by urethral pressure profilometry (Allen *et al.* 1990; Tapp *et al.* 1988; van Geelen *et al.* 1982). Such studies have demonstrated, prospectively, a reduction in pelvic floor function following vaginal delivery compared with the antenatal period but no reduction following Caesarean section. It is hypothesized that denervation is the major mechanism for this observation (please see below).

Prolapse

It has already been stated that the proximal urethra should remain as an intra-abdominal structure in order that continence may be maintained during those times when the intraabdominal pressure is raised. However, this subtle positioning of the proximal urethra should not necessarily be equated with the more gross appearances of a prolapse, this condition being no more common in patients with genuine stress incontinence than in the total parous population (Jeffcoate 1961). Some degree of anterior vaginal wall prolapse may be observed in 63 per cent of women with detrusor instability and 86 per cent of women with genuine stress incontinence (Walter and Oleson 1982).

The presence or absence of anterior vaginal wall prolapse may influence the treatment options for an incontinent patient but does not aid the diagnosis.

Menopause

Some patients date the onset of their symptoms of genuine stress incontinence from the menopause (Beck and Hsu 1965; Onuora *et al.* 1991). There is also a decrease in maximal urethral closure pressure with age (Edwards and Malvern 1974). It seems likely that this reduction in maximal urethral closure pressure after the menopause allows incontinence to occur in a woman in whom the proximal and distal sphincter mechanisms have already been compromised. The role of oestrogen in therapy will be discussed later.

Support

It has already been observed that the position of the bladder neck and proximal urethra as intraabdominal structures, supported by the posterior pubourethral ligaments and the pubocervical fascia, enables rises in intraabdominal pressure to be transmitted to the proximal urethral lumen. If this transmission is reduced, for example by trauma, prolapse, or surgical fibrosis, then genuine stress incontinence may result (Hilton and Stanton 1983*a*). Successful surgery is generally associated with a repositioning of the bladder neck anteriorly and upwards towards the symphysis pubis, and is associated with an enhancement of pressure transmission (Quinn *et al.* 1989).

The urethra and the pelvic floor are rich in collagen and there is thought to be an association between urethral collagen content and the urethral pressure profile (Versi *et al.* 1988). There is also histological evidence that the collagen from the pelvis in women with genuine stress incontinence and prolapse is different, and perhaps weaker, than in asymptomatic women (Warrell 1989).

Denervation

Denervation of pelvic floor musculature is an aetiological factor in faecal incontinence (Parks *et al.* 1977). The pudendal nerve not only innervates the distal sphincter mechanism and the pubococcygeus muscle but, via the inferior rectal nerve, innervates the external sphincter suggesting, at least in some patients, a common aetiology for genuine stress incontinence and faecal incontinence.

Neurophysiological studies have demonstrated a reduced rate of conduction of nerve impulses in the pudendal nerve in women with genuine stress incontinence compared with women without pelvic pathology (Smith *et al.* 1989*a*; Snooks *et al.* 1985; Varma *et al.* 1988). Single fibre EMG studies of the pubococcygeus muscle have suggested changes compatible with both denervation and reinnervation of this muscle, whilst histological and histochemical studies of biopsy samples have shown evidence compatible with a denervation injury (Gilpin *et al.* 1989; Smith *et al.* 1989*b*).

Obesity

There is no good evidence to suggest that obesity is either an aetiological factor in genuine stress incontinence, a predictor of poor surgical outcome, or an influence on urodynamic variables (Dwyer *et al.* 1988).

Warrell (1989) has hypothesized that genuine stress incontinence without prolapse may be a denervation problem whilst genuine stress incontinence with prolapse is likely to be a mixture of denervation and a collagen abnormality. The cause of a denervation injury is thought to be childbirth (Sultan *et al.* 1994). In a study of women with genuine stress incontinence or prolapse or both, and who had evidence of a denervation injury, the major factors appear to be the duration of pushing in the second stage of labour and the size of the baby. The length of the first stage of labour and the type of vaginal delivery were unimportant. It is, therefore, possible, at least theoretically, that these conditions may be avoided by Caesarean section (Smith 1991; Sultan *et al.* 1994). Faecal incontinence may coexist in approximately 17 per cent of women with genuine stress incontinence (Spence-Jones *et al*. 1994).

The treatment of genuine stress incontinence

Treatment may be conservative, using some form of pelvic floor exercises or oestrogen, or surgical. The choice of treatment may depend upon the patient's wishes, her wishes for further children, the social effect of the symptom, and the presence or absence of other pathology.

Pelvic floor physiotherapy

The rationale behind pelvic floor physiotherapy relates to the improved efficacy in the ability of the slow-twitch striated muscle within the urethra and the adjacent, but separate, striated muscle of the pelvic floor to occlude the urethra during episodes of raised intraabdominal pressure.

There is no doubt that pelvic floor physiotherapy will improve some women with genuine stress incontinence in the short-term (Elia and Bergman 1993; Mouritsen 1994; Wall and Davidson 1992). Thus, Henalla *et al*. (1988) reported that 67 per cent of patients treated in this way were cured or improved. Similarly, Wilson *et al*. (1987*a*) reported that 27 per cent of such patients were 'dry' or 'almost dry'. Neither of these series distinguished between continence and significant improvement. There was no benefit from adding interferential therapy or faradic stimulation to the regime of pelvic floor exercises (Wilson *et al*. 1987*a*).

Peattie *et al*. (1988*b*) advocated the use of vaginal weighted cones as a technique to ensure that the patient contracted pelvic floor muscles rather than performed a Valsalva manoeuvre. Such a regime resulted in a subjective cure or improvement rate of 70 per cent, although the objective cure or improvement rate was only 23 per cent. Some 37 per cent of the patients in this group subsequently opted for surgery. In a randomized study which compared weighted vaginal cones with interferential therapy, there were no differences between the cure rates or the cure with improvement rate between the two groups. Some 40 per cent of the patients were cured whilst using cones, whereas 40 per cent were cured whilst receiving interferential therapy (Olah *et al*. 1990). This series did distinguish between 'cure' and 'improvement', and would suggest that earlier series which did not distinguish between these terms probably overestimated the benefit of pelvic floor physiotherapy by 50 per cent.

It is also probably inappropriate to use the term 'cure' when debating physiotherapy since the treatment requires a longterm commitment by the patient. When physiotherapy ceases, the incontinence is likely to return. Ferguson *et al*. (1990) reported that only 35 per cent of patients still exercise one year after ceasing a course of pelvic floor physiotherapy despite the fact that they had improved during treatment and relapsed off the treatment. Moreover, in a randomized study comparing pelvic floor physiotherapy with colposuspension, the objective cure rate relating to pelvic floor physiotherapy

Table 10.4 The choice of operation

First or repeat surgery

Presence of other pathology
    cystocoele
    uterine prolapse
    menstrual disorder
    fibroid uterus

Fitness or age of patient

Mobility of bladder neck

Maximum urethral closure pressure

Objective success rate of the operation

Surgeon's own expertise

Incidence of post-operative instability

Incidence of post-operative voiding problems

Incidence of other complications

---

was 19 per cent compared with an objective cure rate of 75 per cent following colposuspension, demonstrating that the technique was not as efficacious as surgery (Tapp *et al.* 1989).

It is likely that pelvic floor physiotherapy should be offered to women whilst on a waiting-list for surgery for genuine stress incontinence or to women who prefer this treatment modality to surgery, but it is unlikely to replace surgery as the primary treatment for the majority of patients.

Oestrogen

There is evidence that the use of oestrogen, either vaginally or orally, in post-menopausal women with genuine stress incontinence will result in the restoration of continence to some patients (Fantl *et al.* 1994). Such a regime, in various series taken from the literature, rendered continent 21, 22, 55, and 70 per cent of patients, respectively (Rub 1980; Hilton and Stanton 1983*b*; Bhatia *et al.* 1989; Onuora *et al.* 1991). However, even intermediate term results from this method of treatment are not available and the total number of patients included in all of these series was small. In a randomized, double-blind, placebo-controlled trial of oestrogen in post-menopausal women with genuine stress incontinence, Wilson *et al.* (1987*b*) were unable to find any difference between oestrogen and placebo, although a weak oestrogen was used.

It would seem that the benefit of oestrogen is mediated via the urethra, several authors demonstrating a mean increase in the maximum urethral closure pressure of between 4 and 7 per cent (Hilton and Stanton 1983*b*; Karram *et al.* 1989; Rud 1980). This relatively poor increase in maximum urethral closure pressure together with the modest results from treatment, which presumably must have to be continued longterm, suggests that the place of oestrogen in the treatment of genuine stress incontinence is very limited.

Surgery

There are numerous operations advocated for genuine stress incontinence, demonstrating that no operation is universally successful. The choice of operation may depend upon the factors shown in Table 10.4. The five most popular procedures in current practice are the bladder buttress, the colposuspension, the Marshall–Marchetti–Krantz, the endoscopic bladder neck suspension procedure (Stamey), and the bladder sling. Comparisons between the various procedures are sometimes difficult as patient selection is variable, the length of follow-up is inconsistent, statistics for subjective and objective reporting of cure rates must be distinguished, and there is a paucity of randomized trials.

These procedures will now be discussed. Only objective results will be given. The relative incidence of complications will be compared and the relative place of each procedure in clinical practice suggested.

Bladder buttress   The anterior repair with bladder buttress is the classical procedure for genuine stress incontinence. It has the advantage of simplicity and a low complication rate, but the disadvantage of lower continence rates than some of the other procedures discussed. The objective cure rates reported in the literature vary between 31–96 per cent (Bergman *et al.* 1989; Green 1975; Obrink *et al.* 1978; Stanton *et al.* 1982; Thunedburg *et al.* 1990). This writer has assessed the overall results from the literature which demonstrate an objective cure rate of 72 per cent for this procedure. Following repeat surgery, the cure rate falls to 65 per cent suggesting that this procedure should only be used when no previous surgery for genuine stress incontinence has been performed (Lockhart *et al.* 1990).

The complications of this procedure are minimal. The largest study of complications reported a 1 per cent 'serious complication rate' (Beck *et al.* 1991). The incidence of detrusor instability arising as a consequence of the bladder buttress procedure is rare, as are voiding difficulties (Jarvis 1981*a*; Stanton *et al.* 1983).

Colposuspension   The colposuspension operation involves the approximation, with sutures, of the paravaginal tissue of the lateral vaginal fornices to the ipsilateral ileopectineal ligaments on the pelvic side wall. The procedure is performed suprapubically, it will elevate a cystocoele, and may be combined with other procedures such as abdominal hysterectomy. The continence rates quoted in the literature vary between 59 and 100 per cent (Caspi and Langer 1991; Eriksen *et al.* 1990; Galloway *et al.* 1987; Sand *et al.* 1987; van Geelen 1988). From a study of the published literature, the author is able to report an overall continence rate of 84 per cent following this procedure. However, the cure rate is again significantly higher if the operation is performed in the absence of previous surgery (87 per cent) compared with the cure rate following previously failed surgery (69 per cent) (Korda *et al.* 1989*a*).

Although colposuspension is a particularly successful operation for the cure of genuine stress incontinence, it is associated with a considerable incidence of complications. These complications include wound pain (12 per cent, Galloway *et al.* 1987), ureteric injury (Applegate *et al.* 1987), and dyspareunia (4 per cent, Galloway *et al.* 1987). Specific attention should be drawn to the high incidence of post-operative prolapse, which may be a cystocoele, rectocoele, or enterocoele, following colposuspension in between 7 and 20 per cent of patients (Eriksen *et al.* 1990; Shull and Baden 1989). The incidence of longterm voiding disorders following colposuspension has been variously reported as between 3 and 23 per cent with most studies quoting a figure of between 12 and 16 per cent (Eriksen *et al.* 1990; Galloway *et al.* 1987; Lose *et al.* 1987). These results suggest that the colposuspension operation is a relatively obstructive procedure. The incidence of detrusor instability arising following this surgical procedure is variously reported as being between 3 and 18 per cent of patients (Lose *et al.* 1987; Stanton and Cardozo 1979; Steel *et al.* 1985).

Marshall–Marchetti–Krantz procedure This is a suprapubic operation in which the bladder neck and proximal urethra are sutured in close proximity to the posterior surface of the pubic bone. The range of cure rates quoted in the literature vary between 71 and 100 per cent (Henriksson and Ulmsten 1978; Milani *et al.* 1985). A recent meta-analysis has shown an overall cure rate of 86 per cent, rising to 92 per cent when the procedure is performed in the absence of previous surgery, but falling to 84 per cent when previous operations have failed (Mainprize and Drutz 1988). Longterm voiding disorders occur in 3.6 per cent of patients and detrusor instability in 1 per cent (Mainprize and Drutz 1988).

The complication of osteitis pubis occurs in 2.5 per cent of patients who undergo this procedure (Mainprize and Drutz 1988) and is one of the major reasons why the procedure is not performed as commonly in the UK as it is in the USA. This complication generally becomes apparent within eight weeks of surgery and presents as an acute onset of pain in the pubic region. There is tenderness over the pubic bone and a hazy appearance to the borders of the pubic symphysis as seen radiologically. This is due to lytic changes in the bone. Treatment is generally by antibiotics, sometimes with drainage if an abscess has formed, and occasionally curettage of bone is needed.

Bladder neck suspension Stamey (1980) described the modification of the bladder neck suspension procedure in which the position of sutures, inserted on a long needle carrier, was as close as possible to the bladder neck as judged via a cystoscope. The overall cure rate quoted in the literature varies between 39 and 93 per cent (Ashken 1990; Peattie and Stanton 1989; Stamey *et al.* 1975). The overall objective cure rate from the literature is 70 per cent with a cure rate reaching 67 per cent following previous surgery but 100 per cent in the absence of previous surgery (Jones *et al.* 1989). The incidence of longterm outlet obstruction following this procedure is generally reported at between 0 and 5 per cent (Ashken 1990; Hilton and Mayne 1991; Vordermark *et al.* 1979). The incidence of detrusor instability following a bladder neck suspension procedure is generally quoted at between 2 and 7 per cent of patients (English and Fowler 1988; Hilton and Mayne 1991). The commonest reported complication following bladder neck suspension procedures is suture removal, either because of pain or infection, occurring in up to 9 per cent of patients (Kirby and Whiteway 1989).

Bladder sling　Suburethral sling procedures were one of the earliest and most effective methods of surgical treatment described for genuine stress incontinence and, surgically, is the largest of the operations described here. For this reason, the sling is used essentially as a treatment after previous failed surgery. However, there is good evidence that it is one of the most effective procedures for the cure of genuine stress incontinence in patients who have not undergone previous surgery, in these women a cure rate of 100 per cent has been reported (Morgan *et al.* 1985). Following previous surgery, cure rates in the region of 78–91 per cent have been reported (Hodgkinson 1978; Jarvis and Fowlie 1985). Most series report a 2–4 per cent incidence of obstruction following the bladder sling procedure, (Jarvis and Fowlie 1985; Raz *et al.* 1989), although one series has reported an incidence of voiding disorders approaching 37 per cent of patients (Korda *et al.* 1989*b*). The incidence of detrusor instability following bladder sling surgery ranges between 7 and 27 per cent, whilst the incidence of sling erosion into the bladder is generally less than 3 per cent (Kersey 1983).

From these statistics, it becomes clear that those procedures which carry the highest continence rates also seem to carry the highest incidence of complications, hence the treatment offered will need to be structured to the individual patient referring to the list of factors shown in Table 10.4. It should be stated specifically that poor mobility of the bladder neck or a low maximum urethral closure pressure are indications for a bladder sling procedure (Kohorn 1989; Penttinen *et al.* 1989). In other situations, the surgeon will make a decision as indicated above, but has very few randomized trials in which the various operative procedures have been compared for aiding this decision. The largest and best of these trials reported an objective cure rate after 12 months of 69 per cent for the bladder buttress, 70 per cent for the bladder neck suspension procedure, and 87 per cent for the colposuspension (Bergman *et al.* 1989). A recent review of the world literature has suggested that colposuspension, endoscopic bladder neck suspension, and bladder sling procedures are superior to other procedures in terms of objective cure rates for either primary or recurrent genuine stress incontinence (Jarvis 1994).

The mechanism by which surgical procedures restore continence is not clear, but they do not necessarily mimic normal continence mechanisms. The anatomical feature associated with successful surgery would appear to be the elevation of the bladder neck into a position closer to the posterior surface of the symphysis pubis whilst, physiologically, this new anatomical position facilitates the transmission of raised intraabdominal pressure to the proximal urethra, presumably causing momentary compression of this structure against the symphysis pubis (Penttinen *et al.* 1989; Quinn *et al.* 1989).

Post-operatively, bladder drainage will almost always be required after surgery for genuine stress incontinence. Some 50 per cent of patients will be voiding satisfactorily within 10 days, but up to 15 per cent will still require catheter drainage at 14 days. The suprapubic route is to be preferred to the urethral route because of comfort, the ease of checking residual urine, the ease of releasing acute urinary retention, the lower incidence of infection, and the reduced psychological effects of voiding difficulties with repeated catheterization (Bergman *et al.* 1987).

The unstable bladder

The unstable bladder is essentially a urodynamic diagnosis; its presence can only be inferred clinically, but requires a cystometrogram for its confirmation. The symptoms may include frequency, nocturia, urgency, urge incontinence, stress incontinence, nocturnal enuresis, incontinence at orgasm, and even voiding problems (Wiskind *et al.* 1994). There may be a history of childhood nocturnal enuresis in up to 7 per cent of patients. Detrusor instability accounts for incontinence in 38 per cent of incontinent women, but may occur in up to 10 per cent of asymptomatic women. It is not known whether this is a variant of normal or whether these women will ultimately become symptomatic. However, once detrusor instability is demonstrable cystometrically, the finding is consistent (Jarvis *et al.* 1980; Turner-Warwick 1979).

Aetiology

The proposed aetiological factors include:

(1) idiopathic;

(2) psychosomatic;

(3) neuropathic;

(4) outlet obstruction;

(5) incontinence surgery.

These aetiological factors have been the subject of a recent detailed review (Brading and Turner 1994).

Idiopathic

This accounts for over 90 per cent of patients with detrusor instability, but other factors should first be excluded. It may relate to spontaneous detrusor muscle activity (Kinder and Mundy 1987).

Psychosomatic

There is accumulating evidence that dysfunction instability may have psychogenic features, at least in some women.

1. Mosso and Pellacani demonstrated the relationship between emotion, or the sound of running water, and bladder contraction (Macauley 1988).
2. Frewen (1978 and 1984) suggested that a strong emotive event in the patient's life was the initial trigger.
3. Patients with detrusor instability have a higher neuroticism score on formal testing than do patients with genuine stress incontinence (Hafner *et al.* 1977).
4. There is a relationship between detrusor instability and hysterical personality traits (Stone and Judd 1978).
5. Patients with detrusor instability are more likely to have psychosexual problems than patients with genuine stress incontinence (Sutherst 1979).
6. Behavioural forms of therapy, for example bladder drill, hypnosis, are very effective methods of treatment (see below).
7. Treatment is associated with a strong placebo effect, in the region of 25 per cent (see below).

Neuropathic

Overt or covert neurological disorders or spinal cord trauma may result in detrusor instability.

Outlet obstruction

Although up to 50 per cent of men with prostatic enlargement have detrusor instability, there is no good evidence to suggest that detrusor instability is any more common in women with bladder obstruction than in those who are unobstructed (Farrar *et al.* 1976).

Incontinence surgery

The association between surgery for genuine stress incontinence and the post-operative onset of detrusor instability is well recognized (Jarvis 1981*a*), and is associated with different incidences in different procedures, as discussed above. The mechanism by which surgery may be followed by detrusor instability is unclear and may be due either to the presence of an outlet obstruction in a minority of patients, the coexistence of unrecognized detrusor instability pre-operatively (unlikely), or to a mechanism not yet explained.

Treatment of detrusor instability

(1) exclude other pathology;
(2) drug treatment;

(3) bladder drill;

(4) biofeedback;

(5) hypnosis;

(6) acupuncture;

(7) surgery.

Exclude other pathology

Other causes for the patient's symptoms should be excluded, but cystoscopy need only be performed if there is a formal indication. However, 23 per cent of patients with detrusor instability will be rendered symptom-free and their bladders will revert to stability following cystoscopy and urethral dilation (Jarvis and Millar 1980).

Drug treatment

Anticholinergic drugs   The most successful drug treatment involves the use of either anticholinergic drugs, or drugs which are partly anticholinergic but have additional pharmacological activity. Drugs are unlikely to be 100 per cent successful, in that not all detrusor motor activity depends upon the release of acetylcholine, and there is evidence for the existence of other neurotransmitters, for example purinergic nerves with adenosine triphosphate and peptidergic nerves with vasoactive intestinal polypeptides (Cardozo *et al.* 1978). Placebo success rates of up to 47 per cent are reported (Meyhoff *et al.* 1983).

Probanthine is an anticholinergic agent, a synthetic analogue of atropine. It would seem to improve (but not necessarily cure) between 31 and 48 per cent of patients in dosages which range between 45–145 mg per day, often a larger dose being required for a response (Blaivas *et al.* 1980; Holmes *et al.* 1989*a*; Thuroff *et al.* 1991). This agent would not seem to be significantly superior to placebo, although it does have anticholinergic side-effects, some 19 per cent of patients complaining of a dry mouth (Thuroff *et al.* 1991).

Emepronium bromide is a quaternary ammonium compound with anticholinergic properties. From this description, it should not be surprising that the agent is poorly absorbed from the gastrointestinal tract (Wall 1990). This agent is generally used in a dosage of 800 mg daily, although doses of up to 2000 mg per day may be used in order to obtain maximum benefit (Massey and Abrams 1986). The improvement rates quoted with this agent range between 0 and 79 per cent, which has made its place in clinical practice difficult to elucidate (Andersen *et al.* 1988; Massey and Abrams 1986; Meyhoff and Nordling 1981; Meyhoff *et al.* 1983; Robinson and Brocklehurst 1983; Walter *et al.* 1982). Although minor anticholinergic side-effects occur in 13 per cent of patients, the serious drug-induced side-effect of acute oesophagitis with ulceration at the lower end of the oesophagus led to the withdrawal of emepronium bromide and the re-introduction of the newer agent emepronium carrageenate which appears to be free from this side-effect even in doses of up to 2000 mg per day (Hillman *et al.* 1981; Massey and Abrams 1986).

Flavoxate hydrochloride is a musculotropic agent (direct acting smooth muscle relaxant) which competes with acetylcholine at the neuromuscular junction. The drug is not especially effective, with results giving between 0 and 58 per cent improvement, although there is some evidence that the increased dose of 1200 mg per day may be more effective than the more usual 600 mg per day Chapple *et al.* 1990; Gruneberger 1984; Milani *et al.* 1988). Anti-cholinergic side-effects of dry mouth and blurred vision occur in 21 per cent of patients (Gruneberger 1984).

Oxybutynin was the first truly effective agent in the drug treatment of detrusor instability. It is a tertiary amine with musculotropic, anticholinergic, and local anaesthetic effects. It is convincingly superior to placebo with improvement rates occurring in 57–69 per cent of patients in the usual dose of 15 mg daily, although up to 30 mg daily may be prescribed (Baigrie *et al.* 1988; Holmes *et al.* 1989*a*; Moisey *et al.* 1980; Tapp *et al.* 1990; Thuroff *et al.* 1991). The majority of patients receiving this drug will report side-effects. Nausea and constipation occur in up to 14 per cent of patients, whilst a dry mouth occurs in up to 88 per cent (Baigrie *et al.* 1988; Moore *et al.* 1990; Ouslander *et al.* 1988).

In current clinical practice, oxybutynin is the current first-line agent of choice, the other agents generally being reserved for patients who develop unacceptable side-effects whilst taking oxybutynin (Milani *et al.* 1993; Robinson and Castleden 1994).

Tricyclic antidepressants   These agents are anticholinergic, sympathomimetic, and have a central sedative effect. In dosages of between 75 and 150 mg either daily or purely at night, daytime symptoms or nocturnal bedwetting have been reduced in 74 per cent and 60 per cent of patients, respectively (Castleden *et al.* 1981, 1986). Side-effects include drowsiness (10 per cent) and postural hypotension (20 per cent), whilst the theoretical risk of cardiac conduction disturbances means that these agents are relatively contraindicated in patients with bundle branch block (Wall 1990).

Antiprostaglandins   As antiprostaglandins may cause contraction of bladder muscle in both human and animal experiments, clinical trials of prostaglandin synthetase inhibitors were tried in detrusor instability. However, these drugs were not superior to placebo and caused gastrointestinal side-effects (Cardozo *et al.* 1980).

Antidiuretic hormone analogues   Synthetic vasopressin (DDAVP), given in the form of nasal droplets, can reduce urine production and has been used at night to treat nocturnal enuresis and nocturia. This drug is superior to placebo, but is contraindicated in the presence of ischaemic heart disease, cardiac failure, and hypertension (Hilton and Stanton 1982; Ramsden *et al.* 1982). Although the results of larger studies are not available, and although it cannot, obviously, be used both night and day, it is one of the few useful preparations for adult nocturnal enuresis (Cardozo 1990*a*).

In a review of 12 randomized controlled trials involving the use of DDAVP in the treatment of enuresis, most trials reported a 40–65 per cent reduction in wet nights with few and trivial side-effects (Klauber 1989).

Oestrogens Although there is good evidence for the benefit of oestrogens in treating non-specific lower urinary tract symptoms in post-menopausal women (especially frequency, urgency, and dysuria associated with the urethral syndrome) (Smith 1972), there is no evidence that oestrogen is superior to placebo in reducing incontinence in patients who have an unstable bladder (Cardozo 1990*b*; Wall 1990).

Bladder drill

Bladder drill, also known as bladder retraining, is a simple, but effective, technique for the treatment of idiopathic detrusor instability. The rationale of bladder drill is to make patients aware of the problem and enlist their help in treatment by using behavioural therapy and a structured regime. It is a technique used essentially with idiopathic detrusor instability and an intact nervous system; it is important, therefore, that other pathology has first been excluded. It has been claimed that patients may be equally well treated by out-patient (Frewen 1978) as by in-patient therapy. This is not the author's experience and as the therapy depends to some extent on positive feedback and encouragement from medical and nursing staff, it is to be expected that in-patient therapy will be more successful. Moreover, should out-patient therapy fail, then it is most unlikely that in-patient therapy can be made to succeed.

The patient should understand the rationale of bladder retraining; this requires some explanation as to the nature of detrusor instability as a loss of normal physiological function rather than being a disease. The patient is then instructed to void 'by the clock' choosing a time interval at which it is thought that the patient will succeed. In general, this is in the region of 1.5 hours, and the patient must void, therefore, every 1.5 hours whether she wishes to or not. The patient may not void earlier; incontinence is preferred rather than allowing the patient to void before the allocated time. No specific instruction is given as regards a voiding regime overnight. Following a successful day of reaching the target, the voiding is increased for the following day in half-hourly increments. The patient is encouraged to keep a fluid balance chart during the period of admission. This allows the clinician to assess that the patient's input is neither excessive nor has been curtailed, and it allows the patient to develop a concept of voiding volume and, most importantly, forms part of the 'reward' by recording success (Jarvis and Millar 1980).

The short-term effects of both bladder drill and placebo are illustrated in Table 10.5, from which it can be seen that bladder drill resulted in 90 per cent of patients becoming continent, whilst 23 per cent of patients in the control group also became continent (Jarvis and Millar 1980). Similar success rates have been recorded by other authors (Fantl *et al.* 1981 ; Frewen 1984; Jarvis 1981*b*; Mahady and Begg 1981). However, there is a definite relapse rate

Table 10.5 The effect of bladder drill

Symptoms	Pretreatment		Post-treatment	
	Bladder drill (n = 30)	Control (n = 30)	Bladder drill	Control
Frequency	30	30	5	23
Nocturia	27	25	3	20
Urgency	30	30	4	23
Urge incontinence	30	30	3	23

From Jarvis and Millar (1980)

and up to 40 per cent of patients have relapsed within three years (Holmes *et al.* 1983).

Not all studies have demonstrated this high success rate in achieving continence. A recent study has shown that whilst 87 per cent of patients had a significant reduction in their urinary symptoms after bladder drill, only 12 per cent were actually totally continent (Fantl *et al.* 1991).

Biofeedback

Biofeedback is the technique by which the patient is made aware of an autonomic function using visual or auditory signals in order to demonstrate the strength of that autonomic function. Using this technique, 40 per cent of patients were cured on objective testing, a further 20 per cent improved, and 40 per cent remained unchanged (Cardozo *et al.* 1978). More recent studies have also demonstrated that up to 80 per cent of women with detrusor instability can be symptomatically improved by this technique (Holmes *et al.* 1989*b*). The process is, however, very time-consuming.

Hypnosis

Since it is likely that there is a psychogenic element in the aetiology of this condition, it is not surprising that hypnosis is an effective, but time-consuming, form of treatment. Freeman and Baxby (1982) treated 63 incontinent women with detrusor instability by hypnosis. Each patient received 12 sessions of hypnosis over a one-month period, hence this treatment is very time-consuming. The effects of therapy was to render 58 per cent of patients symptom-free, to improve 28 per cent, whilst 14 per cent remained unchanged. Some 50 per cent of those patients who were followed for two years relapsed.

Acupuncture

Acupuncture has also been used to treat this condition. Philp *et al.* (1988) reported 16 patients with detrusor instability treated by acupuncture, of whom 69 per cent were either cured or improved. Other studies have suggested some benefit, but the detailed scientific assessment of this technique in detrusor instability is yet to be established (Chang 1988).

Surgery

Up to 90 per cent of patients with detrusor instability will be satisfactorily treated with those conservative measures outlined above, therefore, surgical treatment should be reserved for those in whom conservative management has failed. The options are enumerated below:

(1) cystoscopy with or without urethral dilation;

(2) prolonged cystodistension under epidural block;

(3) transvesical phenol injection;

(4) bladder denervation procedures;

(5) augmentation cystoplasty;

(6) urinary diversion.

When assessing the results of surgery from the scientific literature, it is important to distinguish detrusor instability from detrusor hyper-reflexia, and whether or not the procedure is being performed primarily for diurnal symptoms or nocturnal enuresis, for detrusor instability and diurnal symptoms are generally more successfully treated than are detrusor hyper-reflexia or nocturnal enuresis.

Cystoscopy and urethral dilation   Jarvis and Millar (1980) demonstrated that cystoscopy and urethral dilatation (together with reassurance) relieved, both symptomatically and urodynamically, detrusor instability in 23 per cent of patients. It is not clear whether this is a true beneficial effect of treatment or a placebo effect. In the absence of outlet obstruction, it is unlikely that cystoscopy and urethral dilatation will be any more beneficial than cystoscopy alone. Similarly, Farrar *et al.* (1976) reported a series in which 33 per cent of patients with coexisting detrusor instability and bladder outlet obstruction were cured or improved by cystoscopy and urethral dilatation.

Prolonged cystodistension under epidural block   Prolonged hydrostatic bladder distension produces ischaemic nerve damage when the intravesical pressure is maintained midway between systolic and diastolic blood pressure using a fluid column. This technique is based on treatment previously described for carcinoma of the bladder, by prolonged cystodistension, a two-hour period is considered appropriate.

The initial result by Dunn *et al.* (1974) demonstrated that of 20 patients with refractory detrusor instability, 70 per cent became continent following the prolonged cystodistension, a further 25 per cent were improved, and 5 per cent unchanged. The initial improvement was maintained over the longterm.

More recently, Korda *et al.* (1987) reported that 18 months after this procedure, 18 per cent of patients were symptom-free, a further 30 per cent were improved, but 54 per cent were unchanged. The most disappointing results come from Pengelly *et al.* (1978) who reported that only 2 per cent of patients became continent and only 7 per cent showed some improvement following this treatment. An overview of the results has suggested that 50 per cent of patients will show significant improvement following prolonged cystodistension under epidural (Wall 1990).

The procedure carries the complication of bladder rupture in up to 8 per cent of patients (Wall 1990). Fortunately, the bladder rupture tends to be extra-peritoneal and the bladder heals spontaneously after prolonged catheter drainage.

The author finds that the technique of prolonged cystodistension under epidural block significantly improves between one-third and one-half of patients who have not improved with the above treatment regimes. The mode of action of prolonged cystodistension is thought to be hypoxia-induced partial bladder denervation (Wall 1990).

Transvesical phenol injection In the female, the pelvic parasympathetic and sympathetic nerves form a plexus upon the anterolateral aspect of the upper one-third of the vagina. The transvesical injection of 10 ml of 6 per cent aqueous phenol into the trigone, midway between the ureteric orifices and into the perivesical space, should dissipate through this plexus.

The initial results described for this procedure seemed encouraging with 40 per cent of patients improved (Blackford *et al.* 1984). However, more recent studies have suggested that the initial improvement is short-lived with only 11 per cent of patients having a noticeable benefit six months after the procedure and only 2 per cent of patients with any benefit at one year (Chapple *et al.* 1991; Ramsay *et al.* 1992; Rosenbaum *et al.* 1988).

Moreover, there have been reports of a fistula occurring after this procedure related to sloughing of the trigone (Cameron-Strange and Millard 1988).

This procedure is now discredited.

Bladder denervation procedures It is not possible (or? desirable) to denervate the bladder, for the nerve supply is distributed along with the blood supply. It is possible, however, to decentralize the bladder from the central nervous system and spinal cord, leaving only the motor and sensory innervation of the trigone intact, thus, it is argued, significantly reducing involuntary detrusor contractions, yet allowing the patient to be aware of a full bladder and to initiate micturition. As the same motor supply is involved, presumably, for voluntary and involuntary detrusor activity, and as denervation must by its very nature always be incomplete, the scientific basis for these procedures and the success must be limited.

The techniques of sacral or presacral neurectomy are now rarely practised. Ingelman-Sundberg (1959) described a transvaginal operation aimed at dividing a branch of the inferior pelvic plexus via the lateral vaginal formic, where it may be found between the bladder and pubococcygeus muscle. Some 88 per cent of patients were improved or cured. However, the operation has not found widespread favour in current clinical practice.

Bladder transection procedures, performed abdominally, are also designed to denervate the bladder. An incision is made into the bladder wall, full thickness, from just above one ureteric canal and across the posterior wall of the bladder to an area just above the other ureteric canal. Essenhigh and Yeates (1973) treated 15 women with nocturnal enuresis and detrusor instability by this technique. The desire to void was unaffected, diurnal frequency reduced, urgency almost invariably relieved, and 93 per cent of the 15 patients described the improvement in their nocturnal enuresis as 'very good' or 'excellent'. Conversely, Mundy (1988) reported a significant relapse rate following this procedure, such that 74 per cent of patients were cured initially, 65 per cent after two years but only 19 per cent after five years. This high relapse rate, together with the introduction of oxybutynin, has significantly reduced the number of patients who undergo this technique.

Transvaginal endoscopic bladder transection has been described by Parsons *et al.* (1984), who concluded that the symptomatic improvement in over 60 per cent of 30 patients justified the inclusion of this technique as a surgical option.

Augmentation cystoplasty   The description of a successful augmentation cystoplasty has resulted in this becoming the major operative procedure of choice in patients who remain incontinent despite prolonged cystodistension under epidural blockade. The technique of 'clam' augmentation ileocystoplasty was described by Bramble (1982). The technique involves almost complete bisection of the bladder in the coronal plane down as far as the ureters on either side, and then the insertion of an isolated vascular loop of ileum approximately 25 cm in length to restore bladder integrity. Mundy and Stephenson (1985) reported a series of 40 patients treated by this procedure. Some 90 per cent became continent, but only 75 per cent of the patients were able to void spontaneously, 15 per cent of the patients who became continent had so significant a voiding disorder that they needed to rely on longterm clean intermittent self-catheterization.

However, the complications of this procedure are significant, partly because of the need for a bowel anastamosis, and partly because there is some evidence that the mucosa of the ileum which is attached to the bladder may undergo a malignant change associated with the chronic irritation by urine. Until it is known whether or not this is a real risk, patients should be advised to undergo annual cystoscopy (Mundy 1988). There is also the effect of large residual urines with the danger of stasis, infection, and voiding disorders as described above, and contracture of the bladder suture line in order to form a large diverticulum. Despite these problems, the clam cystoplasty is currently the most popular and successful longterm surgical treatment for refractory detrusor instability.

Urinary diversion   The place of urinary diversion will be discussed in the section on longterm incontinence.

In clinical practice, the management of detrusor instability consists of excluding pathology, explaining the nature of the condition to the patient with appropriate reassurances, and offering drug treatment with oxybutynin. Should this fail, other drugs may be tried and if these fail bladder drill is usually offered. Should this fail, prolonged cystodistension under epidural would be offered and should that technique fail, the patient would be counselled about the advantages and disadvantages of a clam ileocystoplasty.

When detrusor instability and genuine stress incontinence coexist

Although 50 per cent of incontinent women complain of both urge incontinence and stress incontinence, only 5 per cent have both detrusor instability and genuine stress incontinence. The advantage of a cystometrogram in this situation is that the diagnosis is not only refined but some assessment as to which condition is of the greater clinical importance may be made and hence, treated initially.

The advantage of treating the detrusor instability before the genuine stress incontinence is that the treatment is generally medical and, if successful, the patient may be so satisfied in her improvement that she no longer wishes surgical intervention for her genuine stress incontinence. The disadvantage of this line of treatment is that detrusor instability may prove difficult to treat, success rates are generally lower than for genuine stress incontinence, and, hence, some surgeons would prefer to treat the genuine stress incontinence in the first instance. In this situation, any residual detrusor instability may be treated during the post-operative period by either drugs or bladder retraining. The disadvantage of this line of management is that detrusor instability is a known complication of surgery for genuine stress incontinence and the surgery may, in fact, make this complication worse post-operatively if it is present pre-operatively.

Should surgery be offered in this situation, it should be performed in the knowledge that the continence rate will be less than that anticipated for the surgical correction of genuine stress incontinence. In this situation, continence rates in the region of 45 per cent may be anticipated (Hilton and Mayne 1991).

Longterm incontinence

Untreatable incontinence is both privately and socially unacceptable, and, hence, help and advice to the patient in whom the other methods of treatment have failed is required, regardless of the cause of the incontinence. The advice of a local Continent Nurse Advisor may be sought (Mandelstam 1990).

Incontinence garments

These include absorbent pants and pads, with the two caveats that those prescribed should not only keep the patient drier but that continuing supplies are readily available either from the hospital or local retailers. No successful urethral female appliance along the lines of the successful male condom appliance has yet been described.

Catheters

In-dwelling catheters are useful for patients with poor mobility and mental state, and are of more use in the presence of a stable bladder than in the presence of an unstable bladder, for leakage around the catheter in the presence of detrusor instability may result. The treatment is not the insertion of a larger catheter if this happens — it is coincidental drug therapy and the use of a smaller retaining balloon to try to reduce the involuntary contraction. Other complications include urinary infection (approaching 100 per cent), catheter blockage by debris (reduced by an increased fluid intake), and care with local hygiene (for example twice or thrice daily washing).

Artificial urinary sphincters

Artificial sphincters may be used in specific circumstances (Scott 1974). The sphincter consists of an inflatable cuff implanted surgically around the bladder neck or proximal urethra. The pressure within the cuff is maintained by a regulating balloon some way away from the cuff and the two are connected by a control pump placed subcutaneously in the labia. When the control pump is pressed, the cuff empties to allow voiding and, after a specific period of time, the cuff reinflates automatically.

Such sphincters are expensive, with problems of cuff erosion, mechanical failure, and infection. They are more useful in the presence of a stable bladder, and they are of particular use in children with congenital or neuropathic damage (Kil and de Vries 1993).

Urinary diversion

A patient with untreatable urinary incontinence may choose to be kept dry and comfortable by diverting the urinary tract, of which the most common technique is the use of an ileal conduit with a collecting bag. Clearly, this is a significant sized operation which should be regarded as a final treatment, in that 'urinary undiversion' should not be undertaken lightly.

Voiding disorders

The term 'voiding disorders' covers a spectrum of urinary dysfunction ranging from a painful episode of acute retention which requires catheterization, through the early phase of chronic retention which is characterized by difficulty in micturition, poor stream, hesitancy, and the feeling of incomplete emptying, to a late phase characterized by chronic retention with overflow incontinence. Stanton *et al.* (1983) has reported that up to 16 per cent of women with urinary incontinence have urodynamic evidence of a voiding disorder. Of those patients who have a urodynamically proven voiding disorder, only 40 per cent admit to any of the classical symptoms, whereas one-third of all women with the classical symptoms of a voiding disorder do not have one. Of those patients who do have a voiding disorder, some 7 per cent have a past history of acute urinary retention which require catheterization. There would, therefore, seem to be difficulties in making the clinical diagnosis, and there is evidence that the condition is underdiagnosed.

Aetiology

(1) neurological;

(2) pharmacological;

(3) acute inflammation;

(4) obstruction;

(5) psychogenic.

Neurological

Neurological causes include both upper and lower motor neurone lesions and autonomic lesions. There may also be a local pain reflex such as that following pelvic surgery, especially to the perianal region. A radiographic evaluation including lumbar myelography and CT scan should be performed (Barone and Berger 1993).

Pharmacological

Pharmacological agents, including the tricyclic antidepressants and anticholinergic agents, may cause voiding difficulties, especially in the older age group in whom detrusor function may already be prejudiced. Epidural analgesia during labour may be associated with poor voiding function either during labour or within the first few hours of delivery.

Acute inflammation

Acute inflammatory conditions affecting the urethra, vulva, vagina, or anus may all result in acute urinary retention.

Obstruction

Bladder outflow obstruction may arise post-operatively, especially following bladder neck surgery for genuine stress incontinence. The mechanism is multi-factorial and includes pain, urethral oedema, and a pre-existing voiding difficulty which may be worsened by those operations associated with a higher incidence of voiding difficulty, for example colposuspension or bladder sling surgery. Distal urethral stenosis is an unusual condition, and a pelvic mass such as a uterine fibroid, ovarian cyst, retroverted gravid uterus or haematocolpos may also cause bladder outlet obstruction.

Psychogenic

Psychogenic causes of urinary retention are not uncommon and should be diagnosed only after the exclusion of other causes.

Investigations

General investigations

Back-pressure influences on the kidneys should be excluded by measuring serum urea and creatinine levels, and assessing the renal anatomy by either ultrasound or intravenous urography.

Urodynamic investigations

The following parameters are generally considered indicative of voiding dysfunction. There should be a peak flow rate which is consistently below 15 ml per second for a voided volume of at least 200 ml; the maximum detrusor pressure during voiding may exceed 70 cm of water although ultimately, as the bladder fails, this pressure may fall to approach zero when the bladder becomes hypotonic; a residual volume of urine, consistently above 200 ml, is also characteristic.

Treatment

(1) prophylactic measures;
(2) drug treatment;
(3) urethral dilatation;
(4) urethrotomy;
(5) clean intermittent self-catheterization.

It is possible that post-operative or post-delivery urinary retention may predispose to longterm urinary dysfunction. Parys et al. (1989) described 36 women who underwent abdominal hysterectomy for benign disease. Five of these women, who were demonstrated pre-operatively to be free of voiding difficulty, developed both evidence of voiding difficulties post-operatively together with evidence of neurological damage based on nerve conduction studies (14 per cent). It is possible that prompt attention to retention may prevent these longterm problems.

Drug therapy is of limited value and may be aimed either at cholinergic therapy, in order to stimulate the detrusor (for example bethanechol, 100 mg per day) or alpha-adrenergic blocking agents (such as phenoxybenzamine, up to 40 mg daily) in order to reduce urethral resting pressure. Diazepam may be useful both as a muscle relaxant and as an anxiolytic, whilst prostaglandins have been shown to be of very limited value.

Urethral dilatation has long been used in clinical practice, but there is very little scientific evidence to justify the procedure. Urethrotomy using the Otis urethrotome may be used if there is either proven evidence of either a bladder neck or proximal urethral stenosis (Stanton 1990).

Clean, intermittent self-catheterization is an effective longterm treatment, but requires a high degree of patient motivation and compliance. Permanent catheter drainage should only be used if all else fails.

Conclusions

Female urinary incontinence is a common problem yet is often incompletely investigated and inappropriately treated. The best person to treat such patients is not necessarily a gynaecologist or a urologist, but someone with an understanding and interest in the underlying problem and the therapeutic options. The ideal drug for detrusor instability and the ideal operation for genuine stress incontinence have probably yet to be described.

References

Allen, R. E., Hosker, G. I., Smith, A. R. B., and Warrell, D. W. (1990). Pelvic floor damage in childbirth. *British Journal of Obstetrics and Gynaecology* **97**, 770–9.

Anderson, J. R., Lose, G., Norgaard, M., Stimpel, H., and Andersen, J. T. (1988). Terodiline, emepronium or placebo for the treatment of female detrusor overactivity. *British Journal of Urology* **61**, 310–13.

Applegate, G. B., Bass, K. M., and Kubick, C. J. (1987). Urethral obstruction as a complication of the Burch colposuspension. *American Journal of Obstetrics and Gynecology* **156**, 445.

Ashken, M. H. (1990). Follow-up results with the Stamey operation for stress incontinence of urine. *British Journal of Urology* **65**, 168–9.

Baigrie, R. J., Kelleher, J. P., Fawcett, D. P., and Pengelly, A. W. (1988). Oxybutynin: is it safe? *British Journal of Urology* **62**, 319–22.

Barone, J. G. and Berger, Y. (1993). Acute urinary tension in females. *International Urogynecology Journal* **4**, 152–6.

Bates, C. P., Whiteside, C. G., and Turner-Warwick, R. T. (1970). Synchronous cine/pressure/flow/cystourethrography with special reference to stress and urge incontinence. *British Journal of Urology* **42**, 714–23.

Beck, R. P. and Hsu, M. (1965). Onset of urinary stress incontinence in 1000 random cases. *American Journal of Obstetrics and Gynecology* **91**, 820–3.

Beck, R. P., McCormick, S., and Nordstrom, L. (1991). 25-year experience with 519 anterior colporrhaphy procedures. *Obstetrics and Gynecology* **78**, 1011-18.

Benness, C. J., Barnick, C. J., and Cardozo, L. (1989). Is there a place for routine videocystourethrography in the assessment of lower urinary tract dysfunction? *Neurosurgery and Urodynamics* **8**, 299-300.

Bergman, A. and Bhatia, N. N. (1985). Uroflowmetry for predicting post-operative voiding difficulties in women with genuine stress incontinence. *British Journal of Obstetrics and Gynaecology* **92**, 835-8.

Bergman, A., Mathews, L., Ballard, C. A., and Roy, S. (1987). Suprapubic versus transurethral bladder drainage after surgery for stress urinary incontinence. *Obstetrics and Gynecology* **69**, 546-9.

Bergman, A., Coonings, P. P., and Ballard, C. A. (1989). Primary stress urinary incontinence and pelvic relaxation: prospective randomized trial comparison of three different operations. *American Journal of Obstetrics and Gynecology* **161**, 97-101.

Bhatia, N. N., Bergman, A., and Karram, M. M. (1989). Effect of estrogen on urethral function in women with urinary incontinence. *American Journal of Obstetrics and Gynecology* **160**, 178-82.

Blackford, H. N., Murray, K., Stephenson, T. P., and Mundy, A. R. (1984). The results of transvesical infiltration of the pelvic plexus with phenol. *British Journal of Urology* **56**, 647-9.

Blaivas, J. G., Labib, K. B., Michalik, S. J., and Zahed, A. A. H. (1980). Cystometric response to propantheline in detrusor hyperreflexia. *Journal of Urology* **124**, 259-62.

Brading, A. F. and Turner, W. F. (1994). The unstable bladder—towards a common mechanism. *British Journal of Urology* **73**, 3-8.

Bramble, F. J. (1982). The treatment of adult enuresis and urge incontinence by enterocystoplasty. *British Journal of Urology* **54**, 593-6.

Brocklehurst, J. C. (1993). Urinary incontinence in the community—analysis of a MORI poll. *British Medical Journal* **306**, 832-4.

Byrne, D. J., Stewart, P. A. H., and Gray, B. K. (1987). The role of urodynamics in female urinary stress incontinence. *British Journal of Urology* **59**, 228-9.

Cameron-Strange, A. and Millard, R. J. (1988). Management of refractory detrusor instability by transvesical phenol injections. *British Journal of Urology* **62**, 323-5.

Cardozo, I. D. (1990*a*). Detrusor instability—medical management. In *Female Urinary Incontinence* (ed. G. J. Jarvis), pp. 59-64. Royal College of Obstetricians and Gynaecologists, London.

Cardozo, L. D. (1990*b*). Detrusor instability—current management. *British Journal of Obstetrics and Gynaecology* **97**, 463-6.

Cardozo, L. D., Abrams, P. H., Stanton, S. L., and Feneley, R. C. L. (1978). Idiopathic detrusor instability treated by biofeedback. *British Journal of Urology* **5031**, 521-3.

Cardozo, L. D., Stanton, S. I., Robinson, H., and Hole, D. (1980). Evaluation of flurbiprofen in detrusor instability. *British Medical Journal* **280**, 281-2.

Carter, P. G., Lewis, P., and Abrams, P. (1991). Urodynamic morbidity and dysuria prophylaxis. *British Journal of Urology* **67**, 4001.

Caspi, E. and Langer, R. (1991). Colpo-needle suspension for the treatment of urinary stress incontinence. *British Journal of Obstetrics and Gynaecology* **98**, 1183-4.

Castleden, C. M., George, C. F., Renwick, A. C., and Asher, M. G. (1981). Imipramine—a possible alternative to current therapy for urinary incontinence in the elderly. *Journal of Urology* **125**, 318-20.

Castleden, C. M., Duffin, C. M., and Gulati, R. S. (1986). Double-blind study of imipramine and placebo for incontinence due to detrusor instability. *Age and Aging* **15**, 299-302.

Chang, P. L. (1988). Urodynamic studies in acupuncture for frequency, urge incontinence, and dysuria. *Journal of Urology* **140**, 563–6.

Chapple, C. R., Helm, C. W., Blease, S., Milroy, E. J. G., Richards, D., and Osborne, J. L. (1989). Asymptomatic bladder neck incompetence in nulliparous females. *British Journal of Urology* **64**, 357–9.

Chapple, C. R., Parkhouse, H., Gardener, C., and Milroy, E. J. G. (1990). Double-blind placebo controlled study of flavoxate in the treatment of idiopathic detrusor instability. *British Journal of Urology* **66**, 491–4.

Chapple, C. R., Hampson, S. J., Turner-Warwick, R. T., and Worth, P. H. L. (1991). Subtrigonal phenol injection — how safe and effective is it? *British Journal of Urology* **68**, 483–6.

Coptcoat, M. J., Reed, C., Cumming, J., Shah, P. J. R., and Worth, P. H. L. (1988). Is antibiotic prophylaxis necessary for routine urodynamic investigations? *British Journal of Urology* **61**, 302–3.

Craggs, M. and Stephenson, J. (1976). The real bladder electromyogram. *British Journal of Urology* **48**, 443–51.

Creighton, S. M., Plevnik, S., and Stanton, S. I. (1991). Distal urethral electrical conductance — a preliminary assessment of its role as a quick screening test for incontinent women. *British Journal of Obstetrics and Gynaecology* **98**, 68–72.

Davila, G. W. (1994). Ambulatory urodynamics in urge incontinence evaluation. *International Urogynecology Journal* **5**, 25–30.

De Lancey, J. O. L. (1986). Correlative study of para-urethral anatomy. *Obstetrics and Gynecology* **68**, 91–7.

Dunn, M., Smith, J. C., and Ardran, G. M. (1974). Prolonged bladder distension as a treatment of urgency and urge incontinence of urine. *British Journal of Urology* **46**, 645–52.

Dwyer, P. L., Lee, E. T. C., and Hay, D. M. (1988). Obesity and urinary incontinence in women. *British Journal of Obstetrics and Gynaecology* **95**, 91–6.

Eardley, I. and Fowler, C. J. (1993). Urethral sphincter electromyography. *International Urogynecology Journal* **4**, 282–6.

Edwards, L. and Malvern, J. (1974). Urethral pressure profile: theoretical considerations and clinical application. *British Journal of Urology* **46**, 325–6.

Elia, G. and Bergman, A. (1993). Pelvic muscle exercises — when do they work? *Obstetrics and Gynecology* **81**, 283–6.

English, P. J. and Fowler, J. W. (1988). Videourodynamic assessment of the Stamey procedure for stress incontinence. *British Journal of Urology* **62**, 550–2.

Eriksen, B. C., Hagen, B., Eik-Nes, S. H., Mone, K., Mjolnerod, O. K., and Romslo, I. (1990). Long-term effectiveness of the Burch colposuspension in female urinary stress incontinence. *Acta Obstetrica et Gynaecologica Scandinavica* **69**, 45–50.

Essenhigh, D. M. and Yeates, W. K. (1973). Transection of the bladder with particular reference to enuresis. *British Journal of Urology* **45**, 299–304.

Fantl, J. A., Hurt, W. G., and Dunn, L. J. (1981). Detrusor instability syndrome. *American Journal of Obstetrics and Gynecology* **140**, 885–90.

Fantl, J. A., Wyman, J. F., McClish, D. K., Hawkins, S. W. Elswick, R. K., Taylor, J. R., *et al.* (1991). Efficacy of bladder training in older women with urinary incontinence. *Journal of the American Medical Association* **265**, 609–13.

Fantl, J. A., Cardozo, L., and McClish, D. K. (1994). Oestrogen therapy in the management of urinary incontinence in post-menopausal women: a meta-analysis. *Obstetrics and Gynecology* **83**, 12–18.

Farrar, D. J., Osborne, J. L., Stephenson, T. P., Whiteside, C. G., Weir, J., Berry, J., *et al.* (1976). A urodynamic view of bladder outflow obstruction in the female. *British Journal of Urology* **47**, 815–22.

Ferguson, K. L., McKey, P., Bishop, K. R., Kloen, P., Verhevl, J. B., and Dougherty, M. C. (1990). Stress urinary incontinence: effect of pelvic muscle exercise. *Obstetrics and Gynecology* **75**, 671–5.

Francis, W. J. A. (1960). The onset of stress incontinence. *Journal of Obstetrics and Gynaecology of the British Empire* **67**, 899–903.

Freeman, R. M. and Baxby, K. (1982). Hypnotherapy for incontinence caused by detrusor instability. *British Medical Journal* **284**, 1831–4.

Frewen, W. K. (1978). An objective assessment of the unstable bladder of psychosomatic origin. *British Journal of Urology* **50**, 246–9.

Frewen, W. K. (1984). The significance of the psychosomatic factor in urge incontinence. *British Journal of Urology* **56**, 330–3.

Galloway, N. T. M., Davis, N., and Stephenson, T. P. (1987). The complications of colposuspension. *British Journal of Urology* **60**, 122–4.

Gilpin, S. A., Gosling, J. A., Smith, A. R. B., and Warrell, D. W. (1989). The pathogenesis of genitourinary prolapse and stress incontinence of urine: a histological and histochemical study. *British Journal of Obstetrics and Gynaecology* **96**, 15–23.

Green, T. H. (1975). Urinary stress incontinence. *American Journal of Obstetrics and Gynecology* **122**, 364–400.

Gruneberger, A. (1984). Treatment of motor urge incontinence with clenbuterol and flavoxate hydrochloride. *British Journal of Obstetrics and Gynaecology* **91**, 275–8.

Hafner, R. J., Stanton, S. I., and Guy, J. (1977). A psychiatric study of women with urgency and urge incontinence. *British Journal of Urology* **49**, 211–14.

Haylen, B. T., Frazer, M. I., and Sutherst, J. R. (1988). Diuretic response to a fluid load in women with urinary incontinence. *British Journal of Obstetrics and Gynaecology* **62**, 331–3.

Haylen, B. T., Sutherst, J. R., and Frazer, M. I. (1989). Is the investigation of most stress incontinence really necessary? *British Journal of Urology* **64**, 147–9.

Henalla, S. M., Kirwan, P., Castleden, C. M., Hutchins, C. J., and Breeson, A. J. (1988). The effect of pelvic floor exercises in the treatment of genuine urinary stress incontinence in women at two hospitals. *British Journal of Obsteterics and Gynaecology* **95**, 602–6.

Henriksson, L. and Ulmsten, U. (1978). A urodynamic evaluation of the effects of vaginal sling urethroplasty in women with stress incontinence. *American Journal of Obstetrics and Gynecology* **131**, 77–82.

Hillmann, L. C., Scobie, B. A., Pomare, E. W., and Austad, W. I. (1981). Acute oesophagitis due to emepronium bromide. *New Zealand Medical Journal* **94**, 4–6.

Hilton, P. (1990). Anatomy and pathophysiology. In *Female urinary incontinence* (ed. G. J. Jarvis), pp. 1–14. Royal College of Obstetricians and Gynaecologists, London.

Hilton, P. and Mayne, C. J. (1991). The Stamey endoscopic bladder neck suspension: a clinical and urodynamic investigation, including actuarial follow-up over four years. *British Journal of Obstetrics and Gynaecology* **98**, 1141–9.

Hilton, P. and Stanton, S. L. (1982). The use of desmopressin in nocturnal urinary frequency in the female. *British Journal of Urology* **54**, 252–5.

Hilton, P. and Stanton, S. L. (1983*a*). Urethral pressure measurement by transducer. *British Journal of Obstetrics and Gynaecology* **90**, 919–33.

Hilton, P. and Stanton, S. L. (1983*b*). The use of intravaginal oestrogen cream in genuine stress incontinence. *British Journal of Obstetrics and Gynaecology* **90**, 940–4.

Hodgkinson, P. (1978). Recurrent stress urinary incontinence. *American Journal of Obstetrics and Gynecology* **132**, 844–60.

Holmes, D. M. Stone, A. R., Barry, P. R., Richards, C. J., and Stephenson, T. P. (1983). Bladder training — three years on. *British Journal of Urology* **55**, 660–4.

Holmes, D. M., Montz, F. J., and Stanton, S. L. (1989a). Oxybutynin versus propantheline in the management of detrusor instability. *British Journal of Obstetrics and Gynaecology* **96**, 607–12.

Holmes, D. M., Plevnik, S., and Stanton, S. L. (1989b). Bladder neck electrical conductance in the treatment of detrusor instability with biofeedback. *British Journal of Obstetrics and Gynaecology* **96**, 821–6.

Ingelman-Sundberg, A. (1959). Partial denervation of the bladder. *Acta Obstetrica et Gynaecologica Scandinavica* **38**, 497–502.

International Continence Society Committee on Standardization of Terminology (1990). The standardization of terminology in lower urinary tract function. *British Journal of Obstetrics and Gynaecology* **97**, Supp. 6, 1–16.

Jarvis, G. J. (1981a). Detrusor muscle instability — a complication of surgery? *American Journal of Obstetrics and Gynecology* **139**, 219.

Jarvis, G. J. (1981b). A control trial of bladder drill and drug therapy in the management of detrusor instability. *British Journal of Urology* **53**, 565–6.

Jarvis, G. J. (1990). The place of urodynamic investigation. In *Female urinary incontinence* (ed. G. J. Jarvis), pp. 15–20. Royal College of Obstetricians and Gynaecologists, London.

Jarvis, G. J. (1993). Urinary incontinence in the community. *British Medical Journal* **306**, 809–10.

Jarvis, G. J. (1994). On the surgery of genuine stress incontinence. *British Journal of Obstetrics and Gynaecology* in press.

Jarvis, G. J. and Fowlie, A. (1985). A clinical and urodynamic assessment of the porcine dermis bladder sling in the treatment of genuine stress incontinence. *British Journal of Obstetrics and Gynaecology* **92**, 1189–91.

Jarvis, G. J. and Millar, D. R. (1980). Control trial of bladder drill for detrusor instability. *British Medical Journal* **281**, 1322–3.

Jarvis, G. J., Hall, S., Stamp, S., Millar, D. R., and Johnson, A. (1980). An assessment of urodynamic examination in incontinent women. *British Journal of Obstetrics and Gynaecology* **87**, 893–6.

Jeffcoate, T. N. A. (1961). Functional disturbances of the female urethra and bladder. *Journal of the Royal College of Surgeons of Edinburgh* **7**, 28–47.

Jones, D. J., Shah, P. J. R., and Worth, P. H. L. (1989). Modified Stamey procedure for bladder neck suspension. *British Journal of Urology* **63**, 157–61.

Karram, M. M., Yeko, T. R., Sauer, M. K., and Bhatia, N. N. (1989). Urodynamic changes following hormone replacement therapy. *Obstetrics and Gynecology* **74**, 208–11.

Kersey, J. (1983). The gauze hammock sling operation in the treatment of stress incontinence. *British Journal of Obstetrics and Gynaecology* **90**, 945–9.

Kil, P. J. M. and de Vries, J. D. M. (1993). The artificial urinary sphincter in the treatment of incontinence in the female patient. *International Urogynecology Journal* **4**, 35–42.

Kinder, R. B. and Mundy, A. R. (1987). Pathophysiology of idiopathic detrusor instability and detrusor hyperreflexia. *British Journal of Urology* **60**, 509–15.

Kirby, R. S. and Whiteway, J. E. (1989). Assessment of the results of Stamey bladder neck suspension. *British Journal of Urology* **63**, 21–3.

Klauber, G. T. (1989). Clinical efficacy and safety of desmopressin in the treatment of nocturnal enuresis. *Journal of Pediatrics* **114**, 719–22.

Kohorn, E. I. (1989). The surgery of stress urinary incontinence. *Obstetrics and Gynecology Clinics of North America* **16**, 841–52.

Korda, A., Kriger, M., and Hunter, P. (1987). The use of prolonged cystodistension in the treatment of intractable urinary incontinence in women with detrusor instability. *Australian and New Zealand Journal of Obstetrics and Gynaecology* **27**, 155–8.

Korda, A., Ferry, J., and Hunter, P. (1989a). Colposuspension for the treatment of female urinary incontinence. *Australian and New Zealand Journal of Obstetrics and Gynaecology* **29**, 146–9.

Korda, A., Peat, B., and Hunter, P. (1989b). Experience with silastic slings for female urinary incontinence. *Australian and New Zealand Journal of Obstetrics and Gynaecology* **29**, 150–4.

Lagro-Janssen, A. L. M., Debruyne, F. M. J., and Van Weel, C. (1991). Value of the patient's case history in diagnosing urinary incontinence in general practice. *British Journal of Urology* **67**, 569–72.

Lockhart, J. C., Ellis, G. F., Helal, M., and Pow-Sang, J. M. (1990). Combined cystourethropexy for the treatment of type III and complicated female urinary incontinence. *Journal of Urology* **143**, 722–5.

Lose, G., Jorgennsen, L., Mortensen, S. O., Molsted-Petersen, L., and Krisensen, J. K. (1987). Voiding difficulties after colposuspension. *Obstetrics and Gynecology* **69**, 33–8.

Macauley, A. J. (1988). Psychiatric aspects. In *The unstable bladder* (ed. R. Freeman and J. Malvern), pp. 38–44. Wright, London.

Mahady, I. W. and Begg, B. M. (1981). Long-term symptomatic and cystometric cure of the urge incontinence syndrome using a technique of bladder re-education. *British Journal of Obstetrics and Gynaecology* **88**, 1038–43.

Mainprize, T. C. and Drutz, H. P. (1988). The Marshall–Marchetti–Krantz procedure: a critical review. *Obstetric and Gynaecological Survey* **43**, 724–9.

Mandelstam, D. (1990). The role of the continence advisor. In *Female urinary incontinence* (ed. G. J. Jarvis), pp. 87–9. Royal College of Obstetricians and Gynaecologists, London.

Massey, J. A. and Abrams, P. (1985). Urodynamics of the lower urinary tract. *Clinics in Obstetrics and Gynaecology* **12**, 319–11.

Massey, J. A. and Abrams, P. (1986). Dose tritration in clinical trials. *British Journal of Urology* **58**, 125–8.

Meyhoff, H. H. and Nordling, J. (1981). Different cystometric types of deficient micturition reflex control in female urinary incontinence with special reference to the effect of parasympatholytic treatment. *British Journal of Urology* **53**, 129–33.

Meyhoff, H. H., Gerstenberg, T. C., and Nordling, J. (1983). Placebo—the drug of choice in female motor urge incontinence. *British Journal of Urology* **55**, 34–7.

Milani, R., Scalambrino, S., Quadri, G., Algeri, M., and Marchesin, R. (1985). Marshall–Marchetti–Krantz procedure and Burch colposuspension in the surgical treatment of female urinary incontinence. *British Journal of Obstetrics and Gynaecology* **92**, 1050–3.

Milani, R., Scalambrino, S., Carrera, S., Pezzoli, P., and Ruffmann, R. (1988). Comparison of flavoxate hydrochloride in daily dosages of 600 versus 1200 mg for the treatment of urgency and urge incontinence. *Journal of International Medical Research* **16**, 244–8.

Milani, R., Scalambrino, S., Milia, R., Sambruni, I., Riva, D., Pulici, L., et al. (1993). Double-blind crossover comparison of flavoxate and oxybutynin in women affected by urinary urge syndrome. *International Urogynecology Journal* **4**, 3–8.

Moisey, C. U., Stephenson, T. P., and Brendler, C. B. (1980). The urodynamic and subjective result of treatment of detrusor instability with oxybutynin chloride. *British Journal of Urology* **52**, 472–5.

Moore, K. H., Hay, D. M., Imrie, A. E., Watson, A., and Goldstein, M. (1990).

Oxybutynin hydrochloride in the treatment of female idiopathic detrusor instability. *British Journal of Urology* **66**, 479–85.

Morgan, J. E., Farrow, G. A., and Stewart, F. E. (1985). The Marlex sling operation in the treatment of recurrent stress urinary incontinence. *American Journal of Obstetrics and Gynecology* **151**, 224–6.

Mouritsen, L. (1994). Pelvic floor exercises for female stress urinary incontinence. *International Urogynecology Journal* **5**, 44–51.

Mundy, A. R. (1988). Detrusor instability. *British Journal of Urology* **62**, 393–7.

Mundy, A. R. and Stephenson, T. P. (1985). Clam ileocytoplasty for the treatment of refractory urge incontinence. *British Journal of Urology* **57**, 641–6.

Norton, P. A., MacDonald, L. D., Sedgewick, P., and Stanton, S. L. (1988). Distress and delay associated with urine incontinence, frequency, and urgency in women. *British Medical Journal* **297**, 1187–9.

Norton, P. A., Peattie, A. S., and Stanton, S. L. (1989). Estimation of residual urine by palpation. *Neurourology and Urodynamics* **8**, 330–1.

O'Brien, J., Austin, M., Sethi, P., and O'Boyle, P. (1991). Urinary incontinence: prevalence, need for treatment, and effectiveness of intervention by nurse. *British Medical Journal* **303**, 1308–12.

Obrink, A., Bunne, G., Ulmsten, U., and Ingleman-Sundberg, A. (1978). Urethral pressure profile before, during, and after pubococcygeal repair for stress incontinence. *Acta Obstetrica et Gynaecologica Scandinavica* **57**, 49–61.

Olah, K. S., Bridges, N., Denning, J., and Farrar, D. J. (1990). The conservative management of patients with symptoms of stress incontinence: a randomized, prospective study comparing weighted vaginal cones and interferential therapy. *American Journal of Obstetrics and Gynecology* **162**, 87–92.

Onuora, C. O., Ardoin, J. A., Dannihoo, D. R., and Otterson, W. N. (1991). Vaginal estrogen therapy in the treatment of urinary tract symptoms in post-menopausal women. *International Urogynecological Journal* **2**, 3–5.

Ouslander, J. G., Blaustein, J., Connor, A., Orzeck, S., and Yong, C. L. (1988). Pharmacokinetics and clinical effects of oxybutynin in geriatric patients. *Journal of Urology* **140**, 47–50.

Parks, A. G., Swash, M., and Urich, H. (1977). Sphincter denervation in ano-rectal incontinence and rectal prolapse. *Gut* **18**, 656–65.

Parsons, K. F., Machin, D. G., Woolfenden, K. A., Walmsley, B., Abercrombie, G. F., and Vinnicombe, J. (1984). Endoscopic bladder resection. *British Journal of Urology* **56**, 625–8.

Parys, B. T., Haylen, B. T., Hutton, J. L., and Parsons, K. F. (1989). The effects of simple hysterectomy on vesicourethral function. *British Journal of Urology* **64**, 594–9.

Peattie, A. B. and Stanton, S. L. (1989). The Stamey operation for correction of genuine stress incontinence in the elderly woman. *British Journal of Obstetrics and Gynaecology* **96**, 983–6.

Peattie, A. B., Plevnik, S., and Stanton, S. L. (1988*a*). Distal urethral electrical conductance: a screening test for female urinary incontinence. *Neurourology and Urodynamics* **7**, 173–4.

Peattie, A. B., Plevnik, S., and Stanton, S. L. (1988*b*). Vaginal cone: a conservative method for treating genuine stress incontinence. *British Journal of Obstetrics and Gynaecology* **95**, 1049–53.

Pengelly, A. W., Stephenson, T. P., Milroy, E. J. G., Whiteside, C. J., and Turner-Warwick, R. T. (1978). Results of prolonged bladder distension as a treatment for detrusor instability. *British Journal of Urology* **50**, 243–5.

Penttinen, J., Kaar, K., and Kauppila, A. (1989). Effective suprapubic operation on urethral closure. *British Journal of Urology* 63, 389–91.

Philp, T., Shah, P. J. R., and Worth, P. H. L. (1988). Acupuncture in the treatment of bladder instability. *British Journal of Urology* 61, 490–3.

Quinn, M. J., Beynon, J., Mortensen, N. J. M., and Smith, P. J. B. (1988). Transvaginal endosonography. *British Journal of Urology* 62, 414–18.

Quinn, M. J., Benyon, J., Mortensen, N. J. M., and Smith, P. J. B. (1989). Vaginal endosonography in the post-operative assessment of colposuspension. *British Journal of Urology* 63, 295–300.

Ramsay, I. N., Clancy, S., and Hilton, P. (1992). Subtrigonal phenol injections in the treatment of idiopathic detrusor instability in the female—a long-term urodynamic follow-up. *British Journal of Urology* 69, 363–5.

Ramsden, P. D., Hindmarsh, J. R., Price, D. A., Yeats, W. K., and Bowditch, J. D. P. (1982). DDAVP for adult enuresis. *British Journal of Urology* 54, 256–8.

Ravichandran, G. (1983). The accuracy of a hand-held real time ultrasound scanner for estimating bladder volume. *British Journal of Urology* 55, 25–7.

Raz, S., Siegel, A. L., Short, J. L., and Synder, J. A. (1989). Vaginal wall sling. *Journal of Urology* 141, 43–6.

Robinson, J. M. and Brocklehurst, J. C. (1983). Emepronium bromide and flavoxate hydrochloride in the treatment of urinary incontinence associated with detrusor instability in elderly women. *British Journal of Urology* 55, 371–6.

Robinson, T. G. and Castleden, C. M. (1994). Drugs in focus—oxybutynin hydrochloride. *Prescriber's Journal* 34, 27–30.

Rosenbaum, T. P., Shah, P. J. R., and Worth, P. H. L. (1988). Transtrigonal phenol—the end of the era. *Neurourology and Urodynamics* 7, 294–5.

Rud, T. (1980). The effects of oestrogen and gestogens on the urethral pressure profile in urinary continent and stress incontinent women. *Acta Obstetrica et Gynaecologica Scandinavica* 59, 265–70.

Sand, P. K., Bowen, L. W., Panganiban, R., and Ostergard, D. R. (1987). The low pressure urethra is a factor in failed retropubic urethropexy. *Obstetrics and Gynecology* 69, 399–402.

Sand, P., Hill, R. C., and Ostergard, D. R. (1988). Incontinence history as a predictor of detrusor instability. *Obstetrics and Gynecology* 71, 257–60.

Scott, F. B., Bradley, W. E., and Timm, G. W. (1974). Treatment of urinary incontinence by an implantable prosthetic urethral sphincter. *Journal of Urology* 112, 75–80.

Shull, B. L. and Baden, W. F. (1989). A six-year experience with paravaginal defect repair for stress urinary incontinence. *American Journal of Obstetrics and Gynecology* 160, 1432–40.

Smith, A. R. B. (1991). The aetiology of genuine stress. *Advances in Obstetrics and Gynaecology* 1, 3–9.

Smith, A. R. B., Hosker, G. L., and Warrell, D. W. (1989a). The role of pudendal nerve damage in the aetiology of genuine stress incontinence in women. *British Journal of Obstetrics and Gynaecology* 96, 29–32.

Smith, A. R. B., Hosker, G. L., and Warrell, D. W. (1989b). The role of partial denervation of the pelvic floor in the aetiology of genitourinary prolapse and stress incontinence of urine: a neurophysiological study. *British Journal of Obstetrics and Gynaecology* 96, 24–8.

Smith, P. (1972). Age changes in the female urethra. *British Journal of Urology* 44, 667–72.

Snooks, S. J., Badnoch, D. F., Tiptaft, R. C., and Swash, M. (1985). Perineal nerve damage and genuine stress incontinence. *British Journal of Urology* 57, 422–6.

Spence-Jones, C., Kamm, M. A., Henry, M. M., and Hudson, C. N. (1994). Bowel dysfunction: a pathogenic factor in utero-vaginal prolapse and urinary stress incontinence. *British Journal of Obstetrics and Gynaecology* 101, 147–52.

Stamey, T. A. (1980). Endoscopic suspension of vesical neck for urinary incontinence in females. *Annals of Surgery* 192, 465–71.

Stamey, T. A., Schaeffer, A. J., and Condy, M. (1975). Clinical and roentgenographic evaluation of endoscopic suspension in the vesical neck for urinary incontinence. *Surgery, Gynecology, and Obstetrics* 140, 355–60.

Stanton, S. L. (1990). Voiding difficulties. In *Female urinary incontinence* (ed. G. J. Jarvis), pp. 73–80. RCOG, London.

Stanton, S. L. and Cardozo, I. D. (1979). Results of the colposuspension operation for incontinence and prolapse. *British Journal of Obstetrics and Gynaecology* 86, 693–7.

Stanton, S. L., Hilton, P., Norton, C., and Cardozo, L. D. (1982). Clinical and urodynamic effects of anterior colporrhaphy and vaginal hysterectomy for prolapse with and without incontinence. *British Journal of Obstetrics and Gynaecology* 89, 459–63.

Stanton, S. L., Ozsoi, C., and Hilton, P. (1983). Voiding difficulties in the female: prevalence, clinics, and urodynamic review. *Obstetrics and Gynecology* 61, 144–7.

Steel, S. A., Cox, C., and Stanton, S. L. (1985). Long-term follow-up of detrusor instability following the colposuspension operation. *British Journal of Urology* 58, 138–42.

Stone, C. B. and Judd, G. E. (1978). Psychogenic aspects of urinary incontinence in women. *Clinical Obstetrics and Gynaecology* 21, 807–15.

Sultan, A. H., Kamm, M. A., and Hudson, C. N. (1994). Pudendal nerve damage during labour. *British Journal of Obstetrics and Gynaecology* 101, 22–8.

Sutherst, J. R. (1979). Sexual dysfunction and urinary incontinence. *British Journal of Obstetrics and Gynaecology* 96, 387–8.

Sutherst, J. R. and Brown, M. C. (1980). Detection of urethral incompetence in women using the fluid bridge test. *British Journal of Urology* 52, 138–42.

Sutherst, J. R., Brown, M. C., and Shawer, M. (1981). Assessing the severity of urinary incontinence in women by weighing perineal pads. *Lancet* i, 1128–30.

Tapp, A. J. S., Cardozo, L. D., Versi, E., Montgomery, J., and Studd, J. (1988). The effect of vaginal delivery on the urethral sphincter. *British Journal of Obstetrics and Gynaecology* 95, 142–6.

Tapp, A. J. S., Hills, B., and Cardozo, L. D. (1989). Randomized study comparing pelvic floor physiotherapy with the Burch colposuspension. *Neurourology and urodynamics* 8, 356–7.

Tapp, A. J. S., Cardozo, L. D., Versi, E., and Cooper, D. (1990). The treatment of detrusor instability in post-menopausal women with oxybutynin chloride: a double-blind controlled study. *British Journal of Obstetrics and Gynaecology* 97, 521–6.

Thomas, T. M., Plymat, K. R., Blannin, J., and Meade, T. W. (1980). Prevalence of urinary incontinence. *British Medical Journal* 281, 1243–5.

Thunedburg, P., Fischer-Rasmussen, W., and Jensen, S. B. (1990). Stress urinary incontinence and posterior bladder suspension defects. *Acta Obstetrica et Gynaecologica Scandinavica* 69, 55–9.

Thuroff, J. W., Bunke, B., Ebner, A., Faber, P., De Geeter, P., Hannappel, J., et al. (1991). Randomized double-blind multicentre trial of treatment of frequency, urgency and incontinence related to detrusor hypersensitivity. *Journal of Urology* 145, 813–17.

Turner-Warwick, R. T. (1979). Observations on the functions and dysfunction of sphincter and detrusor mechanisms. *Urologic Clinics of North America* 6, 13–30.

van Geelen, J. M., Leemans, W. A. J. G., Eskes, T. K. A. B., and Martin, C. B. (1982).

The urethral pressure profile in pregnancy and after delivery in healthy nulliparous women. *American Journal of Obstetrics and Gynecology* **144**, 636–49.

van Geelen, J. N., Theuwes, A. G. M., Eskes, T. K. A. B., and Martin, C. B. (1988). The clinical and urodynamic effects of anterior vaginal wall and Burch colposuspension. *American Journal of Obstetrics and Gynecology* **159**, 137–44.

Varma, J. S., Fides, A., McInnes, A., Smith, A. N., and Chisholm, G. D. (1988). Neurophysiological abnormalities in genuine female stress urinary incontinence. *British Journal of Obstetrics and Gynaecology* **95**, 705–10.

Versi, E. (1990). Discriminent analysis of urethral pressure profilometry data for the diagnosis of genuine stress incontinence. *British Journal of Obstetrics and Gynaecology* **97**, 251–9.

Versi, E., Cardozo, L. D., Studd, J. W. W., Brincat, N., O'Dowd, T. M., and Cooper, D. J. (1986). Internal urinary sphincter maintenance of female continence. *British Medical Journal* **292**, 166–7.

Versi, E., Cardozo, L., Brincat, M., Cooper, D. J., Montgomery, J., and Studd, J. (1988). Correlation of urethral physiology and skin collagen in post-menopausal women. *British Journal of Obstetrics and Gynaecology* **95**, 147–52.

Versi, E., Cardozo, I., Anand, D., and Cooper, D. (1991). Symptom analysis for the diagnosis of genuine stress incontinence. *British Journal of Obstetrics and Gynaecology* **98**, 815–19.

Vordermark, J. S., Brannen, G. E., Wettlaufer, J. N., and Modarelli, R. O. (1979). Suprapubic endoscopic vesical neck suspension. *Journal of Urology* **122**, 165–7.

Wall, L. L. (1990). Urinary incontinence due to detrusor instability. *Obstetric and Gynaecologic Survey* **45**, 1S–47S.

Wall, L. L. and Davidson, T. G. (1992). *Obstetrical and Gynecological Survey* **47**, 322–31.

Walter, S. and Oleson, K. P. (1982). Urinary incontinence and genital prolapse in the female. *British Journal of Obstetrics and Gynaecology* **89**, 393–401.

Walter, S., Hansen, J., Hamsen, L., Maejaard, E., Meyhoff, H. A., and Nordling, J. (1982). Urinary incontinence in old age. *British Journal of Urology* **54**, 249–51.

Warrell, D. W. (1989). In *Pathophysiology of genuine stress incontinence in micturition* (ed. J. O. Drife, P. Hilton, and J. Stanton), pp. 203–8. Springer-Verlag, London.

Weil, A., Rayes, H., Bischoff, P., Rottenberg, R. D., and Krauer, F. (1984). Modifications of the urethral rest and stress profiles after different types of surgery for urinary stress incontinence. *British Journal of Obstetrics and Gynaecology* **91**, 46–55.

Wilson, P. D., Al Samarrai, T., Deakin, M., Colbe, E., and Brown, A. D. G. (1987*a*). An objective assessment of physiotherapy for female genuine stress incontinence. *British Journal of Obstetrics and Gynaecology* **94**, 575–82.

Wilson, P. D., Faragher, B., Butler, B., Bulock, D., Robinson, E. L., and Brown, A. D. G. (1987*b*). Treatment with oral piperazine oestrone sulphate for genuine stress incontinence in post-menopausal women. *British Journal of Obstetrics and Gynaecology* **94**, 568–74.

Wiskind, A. K., Miller, K. F., and Wall, L. L. (1994). One hundred unstable bladders. *Obstetrics and Gynecology* **83**, 108–12.

11 The management of cervical intraepithelial neoplasia

There are over 4000 recorded cases of invasive carcinoma of the cervix, and over 2000 deaths from this disease, in England and Wales every year. In the United States, 7.8 out of every 100 000 white women, and 15.5 out of every 100 000 black women, develop cancer of the cervix. Whilst it cannot be expected that screening will eradicate the disease, the natural history of the progression from a normal cervix through the stages of intraepithelial neoplasia and thence to invasive disease allow an opportunity for this history to be interrupted. The term cervical intraepithelial neoplasia will be used throughout this chapter in preference to the previous terms of dysplasia and carcinoma *in situ*.

Is cervical intraepithelial neoplasia truly premalignant?

There can now be no doubt that some patients with cervical intraepithelial neoplasia (CIN) will develop invasive cancer of the cervix unless the natural history of the condition is interrupted. Some of the evidence for this is circumstantial. For instance, Fidler *et al.* (1962) demonstrated that the mean age for the diagnosis of carcinoma *in situ* was 34 years, for microinvasive disease 34.7 years, for occult carcinoma 48.6 years, and for clinically invasive carcinoma 52 years.

The more important evidence comes from longterm follow-up studies of patients with untreated CIN. Stern and Neely (1964) followed 130 women with atypical smears for between six months and nine years. There was a progression rate into invasive carcinoma of 6.8 per cent per year. However, perhaps the most convincing evidence comes from what has been described as 'an unfortunate experiment' performed in Auckland (McIndoe *et al.* 1984). The background to this study was the belief that carcinoma *in situ* was not believed to be a premalignant lesion. Lee *et al.* (1956) reported a three-year follow-up of 53 women with carcinoma *in situ*, none of whom developed an invasive carcinoma despite the fact that no treatment was offered. Similarly, Green and Donovan (1970) reported 75 women with persistent histological evidence of carcinoma *in situ* despite previous treatment. These women were followed for a mean of 61 months (range 15–141 months) and none developed invasive disease. It was a result of this study that the larger Auckland study took place. Some 948 women with histological evidence of carcinoma *in situ* were followed for between 5 and 28 years. Of 817 patients whose smears reverted to normal (with or without treatment) 1.5 per cent developed invasive carcinoma of the cervix, whilst of 131 patients whose smears continued to be abnormal, 22 per cent developed carcinoma of the cervix. Patients with a continuing cytological abnormality after the diagnosis of carcinoma *in situ*, with or without treatment, were 24.8 times more likely to develop invasive carcinoma than those whose cytology had reverted to normal. Using time–life tables, the authors concluded that a woman with untreated carcinoma *in situ* (CIN III) has an 18 per cent chance of developing carcinoma of the cervix within 10 years and a 36 per cent chance of developing carcinoma of the cervix at 20 years (McIndoe *et al.* 1984).

However, such evidence should not necessarily be taken to mean that every woman with cervical intraepithelial neoplasia warrants treatment. There is good evidence that spontaneous regression of CIN I and CIN II occurs (Fox 1967). He demonstrated that of a cohort of women with CIN I and CIN II, 31 per cent regressed, 9 per cent remained stable, but 60 per cent progressed to CIN III. CIN III did not regress. However, some 33 per cent of those lesions which regressed then recurred.

From the statistics, it would seem that if a woman has CIN I which itself has a 60 per cent chance of progressing to CIN III which then has a 36 per cent chance of progressing to invasive carcinoma, then this patient has a 22 per cent chance of developing invasive carcinoma of the cervix without treatment. Yet, this figure is greater than would be expected from those small series in which patients with CIN I have been followed without treatment (Fletcher *et al.* 1990). In this series of 666 patients, 7 per cent underwent initial treatment because the lesion was thought to be worse than initially anticipated, but the rest of the patients remained untreated for a mean follow-up period of 4.5 years none of whom outside this initial biopsy group developed cervical cancer.

It would, therefore, seem logical to offer treatment to all patients with CIN III and probably with CIN II also. Whether or not all patients with CIN I should be treated requires further scientific evaluation, and the ultimate decision as to whether or not a woman with CIN I should undergo treatment will depend upon both the results of such studies and upon the wishes of the patient. It is considered safe practice that women with mildly dyskaryotic smears could have a smear repeated six months later rather than undergo immediate colposcopy, but be referred for colposcopy if that smear is also atypical. More severely abnormal smears should be followed by immediate colposcopy (Johnson *et al.* 1993; Shafi *et al.* 1992).

Does cervical cytology screening prevent carcinoma?

It is surprisingly difficult to demonstrate the role of cervical cytology screening in the prevention of carcinoma of the cervix since the aim is to prevent cancer and not merely to detect premalignant lesions. Difficulties have included the fact that population screening tends to be incomplete, that controlled trials would not be ethical, that the incidence of invasive disease was falling even before screening commenced, and selective interpretation of the statistics by certain authors.

The first region to make a serious attempt to introduce cohort cervical cytology screening was British Columbia in 1949. Ahluwalia and Doll (1968) reported no significant difference between the rate of fall of the incidence of carcinoma of the cervix in British Columbia and those areas of Canada in which screening was less intensive. They concluded that there were three possible explanations for this. First, screening would not influence the incidence of carcinoma of the cervix; secondly, that insufficient time had been allowed for the benefit of screening to become apparent; or, thirdly, that screening of only 50 per cent of the population was insufficient. However, Fidler *et al.* (1968) was able to show that in every year from 1961 to 1966 the incidence of invasive carcinoma of the cervix was greater in the unscreened population than in the screened population, averaging an incidence of 28.6 per 1000 in the unscreened population compared with 4.8 per 1000 in the screened population. The arguments for and against population cervical cytology screening will now be discussed.

Cervical cytology screening—the case for

There is a large body of circumstantial evidence which suggests that cervical cytology screening of discrete populations has been associated with a fall in the incidence of carcinoma of the cervix. Most of this evidence comes from Canada, Scandinavia, Scotland, and Kentucky.

In 1976, the Walton report was produced for the Canadian Government. This report concluded that screening had shown evidence of a reduction in the mortality of carcinoma of the cervix, the main evidence arising from a comparison between changes in the incidence of carcinoma of the cervix and the screening rate in different provinces. The greatest fall (over 40 per cent) was in British Columbia where the screening rate was the highest, a reduced fall (20–40 per cent) occurred in areas with poorer screening rates, and the lowest fall (less than 20 per cent) occurred in Prince Edward Island, New Brunswick, and Newfoundland where the lowest screening rates existed.

In Iceland, cervical cytology screening commenced in 1964, and by 1969 the incidence of carcinoma of the cervix, which had previously been rising, began to fall. Thus between 1965 and 1969, 54 women died from cancer of the cervix, whereas only 32 died between 1970 and 1974 (Johannesson *et al.* 1978). Walton (1982) reported that in Denmark, Sweden, Iceland, and Finland there was a decreasing incidence of carcinoma of the cervix and increasing widespread screening programmes, whereas in Norway, which had not yet introduced a screening programme, the incidence of carcinoma of the cervix was increasing. There is now evidence to show that in all five Nordic countries (Denmark, Finland, Iceland, Norway, and Sweden) the mortality rates from carcinoma of the cervix have fallen since screening programmes were introduced. Moreover, the size of the fall is greatest in those countries with the widest screening pro-

Table 11.1 Mortality and screening

Country	% Population targeted	% Decline in mortality
Norway	5	10
Denmark	40	25
Sweden	100	34
Finland	100	50
Iceland	100	80

From Hakama and Louhivuori (1988); Laara *et al.* (1987)

Table 11.2 The effect of cervical cytology in Aberdeen

Years	No. of cases of cancer of cervix
1961–3	73
1964–6	52
1967–9	42

From Macgregor *et al.* (1971)

gramme. Thus, in Norway, where 5 per cent of the population were screened, the mortality fell by 10 per cent, whilst in Denmark, where 40 per cent of the population were screened, the mortality has fallen by 25 per cent. These statistics are illustrated in Table 11.1. (Hakama and Louhivuori 1988; Laara *et al.* 1987).

The value of cervical cytology screening in the UK was first reported by Macgregor *et al.* in 1971. In Aberdeen between 1960 and 1969, 97.3 per cent of the women aged 25–60 years were screened. In every triennia between 1946 and 1963, the number of reported cases of carcinoma of the cervix had ranged between 54 and 73. After 1963, there was a progressive fall in the number of cases of cancer of the cervix reported, as shown in Table 11.2. Furthermore, carcinoma of the cervix tended to present at an earlier stage. Thus, between 1951 and 1954, 62 per cent of patients presented with a stage I or stage II lesion, whilst between 1966 and 1969 76 per cent of patients tended to present with a stage I or stage II lesion. In addition, age-specific death rates from carcinoma of the cervix between 1968 and 1976 continued to fall for all women between the ages of 35 and 64 years in England, Scotland, and Wales (Macgregor and Teper 1978). The death rates in Grampian and Tayside, with the most comprehensive screening programmes in Scotland, had the lowest age-specific death rates. Parkin *et al.* (1985) discovered that, despite the increase in incidence of CIN III, there was a fall in the incidence of carcinoma of the cervix in women aged 35–55 years over the 15-year period 1963–1978 in the UK. Similarly, Duguid *et al.* (1985) reported that the incidence of carcinoma of the cervix, rising in the Dundee region prior to the introduction of screening, peaked three years after the introduction of screening, and fell progressively thereafter.

In the United States, Christopherson (1970) found that over 90 per cent of the adult female population of Kentucky had been screened at least once between 1956 and 1968. The overall incidence rate for carcinoma of the cervix had decreased by 38 per cent. When carcinoma of the cervix did arise, it tended to present at an earlier stage, the proportion of cases of stage I increasing from 32 per cent to 57 per cent. Cramer (1974) was able to show that, although the incidence of carcinoma of the cervix was falling in the United States before screening was introduced, there was good correlation between the different levels of screening in different states and the rates of decline of carcinoma of the cervix, the highest decline occurring in those states with the highest incidence of screening.

There is, therefore, good circumstantial evidence that in populations where cervical cytology screening is widely performed, there is a fall in the overall incidence of carcinoma of the cervix together with an earlier presentation of women with the disease.

Cervical cytology screening—the case against

Those who would argue that cervical cytology screening has not had a significant influence upon the incidence of carcinoma of the cervix, in general, are highlighting the deficiencies in the screening process rather than the concept of screening itself. Cervical cytology screening could never, realistically, be expected to result in the prevalence of carcinoma of the cervix approaching zero. In an editorial entitled 'Cancer of the cervix: death by incompetence' (*Lancet* 1985), it was suggested that in the preceding 20 years, 40 million smears had been taken in England and Wales yet 45 000 women had died from carcinoma of the cervix, whilst it was unlikely that more than 1500 had been prevented from this fate. It also needs to be noted that the natural history of cervical intraepithelial neoplasia is such that the majority of lesions would not have progressed and hence the majority of surgical interventions will have been unnecessary.

The following reasons may, to some degree, explain the difficulties with a cervical cytology screening programme:

1. Not all the at-risk population has been screened.
2. Not all cervical cancer is preventable.
3. There is an incidence of false-negative reporting.
4. The sample obtained is unsatisfactory.
5. The screening programme is suboptimal.

There are some women who develop invasive cancer of the cervix who have never had a smear in their lives. The incidence of this observation varies greatly, being reported as 92 per cent (Macgregor 1981), 72 per cent (Walker *et al.* 1983), 61 per cent (Carmichael *et al.* 1984), 29 per cent (Boyce *et al.* 1990), and 8 per cent (Bearman *et al.* 1987).

If the population is to be screened, especially the high-risk population, then screening needs to be offered on a systematic basis rather than an opportunistic one. Ross (1989) discovered that only 80 per cent of 870 women aged 20–64 years had undergone a cervical smear during the previous five years. Standing and Mercer (1984) found that intensive encouragement by the general practitioner would increase the percentage of patients undergoing smears. Thus, of 558 women aged 16–64, 37 per cent had never had a smear. After such intensive encouragement, this figure fell to 4 per cent. Personal invitations to attend for screening have been advocated (*Lancet* 1990), but such encouragement can only work if it reaches the patients at risk. In one series, 47 per cent of 'invitation letters' sent to women by a family practitioner committee were sent to an incorrect address (Beardow *et al.* 1989). It would seem unlikely, therefore, that cervical cytology screening will ever reach 100 per cent of the population.

Not all cervical cancer is preventable. Although much is known of the natural history of cervical cancer, the minimum length of time in which a cervical cancer may develop is clearly not known. It is theoretically possible that some lesions are so aggressive that the cervix progresses from normality to invasive disease in so short a period of time that either there is no opportunity to take a cervical smear or the stages of cervical precancer are not apparent. At the current time, such a view is conceptual, being based upon observation and mathematical models. That this concept is real waits to be proven (Silcocks and Moss 1988).

There is an incidence of false-negative cervical cytology which may be explained by either of the following three situations:

1. The smear was truly abnormal but reported as normal.

2. The technique used to take the cervical smear was unsatisfactory.

3. The lesion did not shed abnormal cells, that is the smear was truly false-negative.

Several authors have reviewed the smear history of women presenting with invasive carcinoma of the cervix. When cervical smears previously reported as negative have been reviewed, a significant percentage were, in fact, abnormal. Again, there is considerable variation in the incidence of this finding which has been reported as occurring in 20 per cent (Walker *et al.* 1983), 36 per cent (Mitchell *et al.* 1990), and 59 per cent (Paterson *et al.* 1984) of smears which were previously reported as being negative.

The technique used to take the cervical smear may be unsatisfactory. It is very difficult to place an accurate scientific estimate upon this, but the spatula used to sample the cervix should sample all 360° of the squamocolumnar junction and should be supplemented by a sample taken from the posterior vaginal fornix (Koss 1989).

Not all abnormal lesions will shed abnormal cells; this occurs in 2–24 per cent of patients with histologically proven CIN (Husain *et al.* 1974; Nyirjesy 1972).

The overall incidence of false-negative reporting may be reduced by both quality control in the laboratory and by alterations in sampling techniques

(Macgregor 1993). It is estimated that an overall false-negative figure of 2 per cent should be achievable (Husain *et al.* 1974). One simple technique which will reduce the incidence of false-negative reporting is the taking of two simultaneous smears which are then sent for independent reporting. Such a technique in smears taken from patients with known CIN reduce the false-negative result from 11 per cent in a single smear to 7 per cent in paired smears (Beilby *et al.* 1982).

A possible explanation for the problem of truly false-negative smears may be the size of the atypical transformation zone, this was found to be statistically significantly smaller in women with CIN and a negative smear when compared with women with CIN and an abnormal smear (Barton *et al.* 1989).

Whilst laboratories tend to reject cervical cytology specimens which they consider to be unsatisfactory, there is nevertheless an incidence of unsatisfactory smears being reported. For instance, Paterson (1984) reported that 19 per cent of cervical smears which were previously reported as negative in women who subsequently developed carcinoma of the cervix were unsatisfactory.

Several techniques have been used in order to assess whether or not a smear is satisfactory. There has been considerable recent interest concerning the presence or absence of endocervical cells in the specimen. Since the atypical transformation zone tends to involve the squamocolumnar junction, the presence of both ectocervical and endocervical cells in a smear has been taken to suggest that the squamocolumnar junction must have been smeared. However, the absence of endocervical cells cannot be taken to conclude that the squamocolumnar junction has not been smeared, and hence assume the smear to be unsatisfactory. In up to 35 per cent of women, endocervical cells cannot be obtained (Beilby *et al.* 1982; Koss 1989). Moreover, the use of different spatulas or of a cytobrush has not been associated with improved sampling techniques as judged by the incidence of abnormalities on cervical smears. Two recent randomized trials compared the use of different spatulas. Both of these trials demonstrated that samples which contained endocervical cells were no more likely to be associated with an abnormality than those which did not (Goorney *et al.* 1989; Woodman *et al.* 1991). For instance, in one of these trials involving women attending a colposcopy clinic, one spatula was associated with an incidence of endocervical cells on 50 per cent of smears, whilst the other was associated with endocervical cells on 24 per cent of smears, but the incidence of dyskaryotic smears was statistically similar with both spatulas (41 and 45 per cent, Woodman *et al.* 1991).

Similarly, the use of a cytobrush to sample the endocervical canal is not an alternative to the use of a spatula, although it may reduce the false-negative rate (Wolfendale 1990). In one series, the rate of detection of a dyskaryotic smear increased from 0.8 to 3 per cent when a cytobrush was used in addition to an Ayre's spatula (Murata *et al.* 1990).

It is now advised that women whose smears are reported as negative but lacking an endocervical component should *not* be rescreened any earlier than women with a negative smear which includes an endocervical component (Mitchell and Medley 1991).

The problem of a suboptimal screening programme is now debated.

Table 11.3 Percentage reduction in the accumulated rates of invasive carcinoma with screening

Frequency of screening	% Fall in invasive cancer
Annual	93.5
Two-yearly	92.5
Three-yearly	90.8
Five-yearly	83.6
Ten-yearly	64.1

From International Agency for Research on Cancer (1986)

What constitutes an optimal screening programme?

There must be guidelines in any screening programme, and these must take into account the age at which screening should commence, the frequency of that screening, and the age at which it should cease.

Even recently, the advice has been to commence screening at the age of 35 years and this is the age at which the UK national 'call programme' commences. The *British Medical Journal* (1980) concluded:

'at present, too much effort is spent in trying to detect cervical cancer in too young an age group where, even with 100% coverage and effectiveness, fewer than 10 out of over 2000 deaths would be prevented.'

However, this view is no longer valid since the registration of cancer of the cervix in women aged 35 years or less has increased from less than 5 per cent to 17 per cent (Adelstein *et al.* 1981; Parliamentary Reply 1986). The only logical age at which to commence cervical cytology screening is at the age of first sexual contact.

The frequency at which cervical screening takes place will influence the degree of protection offered to the woman who has been screened. The frequency at which cervical cytology screening should be offered will depend on two major factors; the incidence of false-negative smears and the natural history of the disease. If the incidence of false-negative smears can be brought down in all laboratories to 2 per cent, then two smears in rapid succession should bring down the false-negative rate to below 2 per cent but above 0.4 per cent, and perhaps, therefore, all women should commence their cytology screening career with two cervical smears a short period apart.

The frequency at which screening should take place thereafter has been studied by the International Agency for Research on Cancer (1986) who have obtained data from 18 screening programmes in eight countries. This data is summarized in Table 11.3. It is clear that the more frequently is the cervix smeared, the greater is the expected fall in the incidence of invasive cancer. The

IARC concluded that the optimal programme screened every three years, yet the figures lend strong support to the concept of an annual screening programme. Screening every two years is probably as protective as annual screening (Shy *et al*. 1989).

The age at which cervical cytology screening should cease is also a matter of some debate (van Wijngaarden and Duncan 1993). Fletcher (1990) reported that, whilst 40 per cent of the deaths from cancer of the cervix occurred in women beyond the age of 65 years, only 4 per cent of all smears taken were from women above the age of 60 years. Thus, older women would appear to be offered a less satisfactory screening programme. Perhaps screening for carcinoma of the cervix should not cease at any age group.

Of these three issues, it is the optimal frequency of screening which has yet to be adequately assessed but this is 'fine tuning', whilst the need to ensure that every woman at risk has even one smear is a greater public health issue. It has been estimated that a woman with even one negative cervical smear has a reduced relative risk of developing cancer of the cervix for up to six years after that smear compared with women who have never had a smear (Macgregor *et al*. 1985).

However, as must be clear from the above, even women with several negative cervical smears are not immune from cancer of the cervix, and, hence, a suspicious history should not be disregarded in the presence of a recent negative smear. In one series of 138 women with carcinoma of the cervix, 13 per cent had one or more negative smears during, the three years prior to diagnosis (Mitchell *et al*. 1990).

Screening after hysterectomy

Although carcinoma of the vagina accounts for less than 4 per cent of all gynaecological malignancies, a premalignant phase of vaginal intraepithelial neoplasia (VAIN) is well recognized. Moreover, there is an association between the occurrence of CIN and the occurrence of VAIN (Ireland and Monaghan 1988). In one recent series of over 4000 women with CIN, 2.5 per cent had a coexisting vaginal epithelial abnormality (Nwabineli and Monaghan 1991). In a series of 177 women treated by hysterectomy for CIN III, 4 per cent developed VAIN whilst 0.6 per cent developed a subsequent invasive carcinoma of the vagina (Burghardt and Holzer 1988). In 97.5 per cent of patients with VAIN, a lesion was present at the vaginal vault (Petrilli *et al*. 1988). It is because of evidence such as this that vault cytology screening is advocated for women with a past history of both CIN and hysterectomy.

However, the evidence that vault cytology screening will prevent vaginal carcinoma is poor. Fawdry (1984) reported 1062 women with CIN III diagnosed at hysterectomy. Of 24 per cent of women who underwent regular vault cytology, invasive carcinoma occurred in the vagina of one (0.4 per cent), whilst a similar lesion developed in the vagina of 0.2 per cent of the 76 per cent who did not undergo regular cytology. Similarly, Gemmell *et al.* (1990) reviewed 341 women who had undergone a hysterectomy in association for CIN III and who had completed ten years of vaginal vault cytology. Abnormal cytology developed in 4 per cent of patients but the smears reverted to normal spontaneously in two-thirds of these. No patient subsequently developed invasive vaginal carcinoma. The authors concluded that this data would support taking three vault smears within the first two years of a hysterectomy in the presence of CIN and then taking vault smears every five years thereafter.

Continuing vault cytology after hysterectomy in patients in whom there has never been a past history of abnormal cervical cytology does not carry scientific support. In patients due to have a hysterectomy and who have a past history of an abnormal smear, preoperative colposcopy of the upper vagina should be considered in case a lesion is present which then becomes sequestrated above the vaginal suture line.

Other benefits of screening

There may be other advantages for screening, over and above that of detecting the presence of invasive carcinoma of the cervix.

Edwards (1974) reported 2656 women undergoing cervical cytology, In addition to the diagnosis of three invasive carcinomata of the cervix at the time of screening, 68 women had a pelvic mass on vaginal examination and, of these, three were ovarian carcinomata. Thomas (1970) reports a series of 3967 women undergoing cervical cytology screening. In addition to the diagnosis of five cervical carcinomata, there were 83 pelvic masses of which 20 were ovarian tumours, although the histology was not stated. It is likely that a vaginal examination at the time of cervical screening will diagnose ovarian cancer in approximately 1 in 900 women.

Endometrial cells may be found in up to 12 per cent of all cervical smears taken from premenopausal women and in 0.6 per cent taken from postmenopausal women (Vooigs *et al.* 1987). There is an association with endocervical carcinoma or hyperplasia, especially in post-menopausal women. Thus, in one series, no premenopausal woman with normal-looking endometrial cells on a cervical smear had a coexisting endometrial carcinoma. Only the presence of atypical endometrial cells was associated with endometrial carcinoma in the premenopausal woman. However, 13.5 per cent of post-menopausal women with apparently normal endometrial cells on the cervical smear had either endometrial hyperplasia or carcinoma. Thus, *any* endometrial cells in the smear of a post-menopausal woman should constitute an indication for further investigation (Yancey *et al.* 1990).

Cytology and histology

Although a cervical smear may give some indication as to the underlying pathology, it cannot replace a histological diagnosis. Ideally, both a colposcopy and a biopsy should be performed. In the presence of CIN alone, there is a close correlation (91 per cent) between the grade of the CIN on colposcopy and on histology (Wetrich 1986). However, a biopsy is required in order to exclude, in as much as is possible, microinvasive or invasive carcinoma of the cervix since up to 16 per cent of patients with a microinvasive or occult invasive cervical cancer have lesions whose colposcopic appearance is not sufficiently distinct to permit an accurate diagnosis to be made (Benedet *et al.* 1985). It is likely that the larger the biopsy specimen, the more representative will it be of the lesion. Hence, a specimen taken by loop excision, cold knife cone biopsy, or laser cone biopsy will be less likely to miss a microinvasive or invasive lesion than will a colposcopically directed punch biopsy (Buxton *et al.* 1991; Howe and Vincenti 1991; McIndoe *et al.* 1989; Skehan *et al.* 1990; Wright *et al.* 1992*a*).

Cervical cytology alone may 'under represent' the severity of CIN. Between 33 per cent and 69 per cent of patients whose smears show mild dyskaryosis have CIN II or CIN III (Giles *et al.* 1989; Walker *et al.* 1986). Moreover, up to 27 per cent of patients with an atypical smear do not have CIN (Giles *et al.* 1989). Any patient with a dyskaryotic smear should, therefore, have the benefit of a colposcopic examination.

The reporting of a smear as showing inflammatory changes may also represent an under-diagnosis. Up to 47 per cent of patients with an inflammatory smear have underlying CIN yet only 29 per cent have evidence of an infective organism (Frisch 1987; Lawley *et al.* 1990; Parsons *et al.* 1993; Walker *et al.* 1986; Wilson *et al.* 1990).

The treatment of cervical intraepithelial neoplasia

Increasing numbers of abnormal cervical smears are being reported, and clearly this carries an implication if these are all to be investigated and treated. Wolfendale *et al.* (1983) analysed smears over the period 1965–1979, and found an increase in the incidence of abnormal smears. In previously unscreened women, the incidence rose from 5.8 to 12.9 per 1000 smears. In previously screened women, the incidence rose from 0.9 to 3.6 per 1000 smears. Although these increases were seen especially in the 20–40 age groups, the increase also occurred in the 40–60 group. This particular problem of younger women was highlighted by Bamford *et al.* (1982) who reported an increasing incidence in the rate of cervical atypia (of 4 per cent) in women attending a family planning clinic. Singer *et al.* (1984) reported that of 379 women with an abnormal smear and histological evidence of CIN, 68 per cent were less than 35 years old and 46 per cent were nulliparous. Such statistics demonstrate the need for effective but conservative methods of treatment.

There is no satisfactory method for determining which patients with CIN will progress and which will persist or regress. However, Yao *et al.* (1981) reported a retrospective study of chromosomal karyotyping of CIN lesions. Of 100 biopsies demonstrating CIN, 34 ultimately regressed to normal, of these, 85 per cent were either euploid or polyploid, and 15 per cent were aneuploid. The CIN persisted in 58 patients, of whom only 5 per cent showed polyploidy and 95 per cent aneuploidy. Invasive carcinoma of the cervix occurred in eight patients, all these biopsies having shown aneuploidy. Thus, of those initial biopsies showing aneuploidy, 81 per cent persisted, 12 per cent became invasive, and only 7 per cent regressed. It may be that such investigations would ultimately define which patients with CIN require treatment and which require follow-up but no treatment.

Hysterectomy is generally only indicated in the presence of another indication, and hence most patients will be treated by a more conservative method. Whichever treatment modality is used, there will be a treatment failure of up to 5 per cent and follow-up is mandatory (Soutter 1991).

The treatment modalities to be discussed are:

(1) cone biopsy;

(2) laser cone;

(3) cold coagulation;

(4) cryosurgery;

(5) electrodiathermy;

(6) laser vaporization;

(7) loop excision.

Cone biopsy

In 1981, a leading article in *The Lancet* concluded that 'cone biopsy remains the standard for simultaneous diagnosis and treatment', but in current practice cone biopsy is now used to treat less than 20 per cent of patients, the majority being treated by some form of local destructive therapy. The advantage of cone biopsy remains the preservation of the abnormal tissue for detailed histological examination, but complications, together with a need for general anaesthesia, have reduced its use.

Haemorrhage has been reported in 13 per cent of patients. Luesley *et al.* (1985) reported primary haemorrhage occurring in 6 per cent of 915 patients undergoing cone biopsy and secondary haemorrhage in 7 per cent. The haemorrhage was sufficient that nine patients were treated by hysterectomy and 30 (3 per cent) by transfusion alone. Statistically, the size of the cone was also relevant, larger cones carrying a minimally greater risk of haemorrhage than smaller cones.

The efficacy of cone biopsy in the treatment of CIN is well documented. Bevan *et al.* (1981) reported a series of 567 patients with CIN treated by cone biopsy, of whom 91 per cent needed no further treatment for their CIN. Of the 9 per cent of patients with subsequent atypia, 7 per cent had an incomplete cone biopsy and 2 per cent subsequently developed atypical smears, again having had normal cytology on initial follow-up. However, this series followed patients for only three years. McIndoe *et al.* (1984) reported 948 patients with CIN III, of whom 86 per cent had negative cytology following treatment but 1.5 per cent developed carcinoma of the cervix, indicating the need for longterm follow-up.

Some authors believe that too many cone biopsies are still being performed. Lopes *et al.* (1989) reported 332 patients who had undergone a cone biopsy (using laser) for abnormal cytology in the presence of an unsatisfactory colposcopy. There was no histological abnormality demonstrated in 34 per cent of these patients. Soutter (1989) reiterated that the indications for cone biopsy were:

(1) squamocolumnar junction not seen in entirety;

(2) CIN in a previously treated cervix;

(3) glandular cells on the smear.

The effect of cone biopsy on subsequent pregnancy will be discussed later in this chapter.

Laser cone

A cone biopsy performed using the laser rather than a cold knife maintains the advantage of cone biopsy in that the complete lesion is available for histological examination, but the procedure may be performed on an out-patient basis under local anaesthesia (Partington *et al.* 1989).

The efficacy of the treatment has been illustrated by Baggish *et al.* (1989) who reported 954 patients who underwent a laser cone, after treatment cytology was negative in 97 per cent.

The major complication of laser cone is haemorrhage which occurs in approximately 14 per cent of patients treated by this technique (Wright *et al.* 1983). In a randomized trial of cold knife versus laser cone, the overall complication rate for haemorrhage, cervical stenosis, and dysmenorrhoea was similar in both groups (Kristensen *et al.* 1990).

Cold coagulation

This is a misnomer, for temperatures of between 100–120 °C are reached using this technique which can destroy tissue to a depth of approximately 4 mm without the need for anaesthesia. The efficacy of the procedure equates with other techniques and the complications are minimal.

Byrne *et al.* (1988) reported a series of 1005 patients with CIN treated by cold coagulation, of whom 97 per cent had initially normal cervical cytology and 93 per cent remained normal after seven years. Gordon and Duncan (1991) treated

1628 women with CIN III by cold coagulation. Overall, 95 per cent were successfully treated, but 0.25 per cent ultimately developed malignant cervical disease (Loobuyck and Duncan 1993).

Cryosurgery

This initially promising technique is now rarely used for the treatment of CIN as there appears to be difficulty in achieving an appropriate depth of tissue destruction. Charles and Savage (1980) reviewed the literature concerning the cryosurgical treatment of 2888 patients with CIN, they demonstrated initial cure rates varying from 27 to 96 per cent. Richart *et al.* (1980) reported a multicentre study of 2839 women treated for CIN using crysosurgery. This study was remarkable in that over 99 per cent of patients appeared to be treated successfully. After ten years, only 0.4 per cent of patients had a recurrence of an atypical smear.

However, the technique fell into disrepute following a report of eight patients who developed carcinoma of the cervix after having had prior treatment by cryosurgery (Sevin *et al.* 1979). There was criticism of the management of these patients over and above the occurrence of invasive disease, in that four of the eight patients did not have a pretreatment biopsy and three did not have a pretreatment colposcopy. Although enthusiasm for this technique has been reduced and other out-patient techniques have been developed, cryosurgery is still in use as an economical out-patient method of treatment of CIN (Benedet *et al.* 1992; Draeby-Kristiansen *et al.* 1991).

Electrodiathermy

This technique is able to destroy epithelium to a depth of 10 mm, however, it almost always requires a general anaesthetic. The success of this technique, as judged by the finding of follow-up negative smears, lies between 94 and 97 per cent (Chanen and Rome 1983; Giles *et al.* 1987).

The main complication relates to secondary infection with or without secondary haemorrhage. This complication occurs in up to 3 per cent of patients (Giles *et al.* 1987; Woodman *et al.* 1985).

Laser vaporization

The treatment of CIN using a carbon dioxide laser has the advantage of efficacy combined with out-patient treatment, but laser vaporization has the disadvantage that the specimen is destroyed.

It is this ability to achieve a superior depth of destruction which underlies the current popularity of the technique. Anderson and Hartley (1980) examined 343 cone specimens specifically to assess the depth of crypt involvement by intraepithelial neoplasia. They reported that a mean destruction to 3 mm would eradicate 95 per cent of CIN, but destruction must reach 4 mm in order to eradicate 99.7 per cent of CIN.

The efficacy of laser vaporization is well known. Most series have demonstrated that some 93 per cent of patients were successfully treated after a single vaporization and, if the treatment was repeated where necessary, up to 96 per cent of patients had a negative smear one year after treatment (Ali *et al.* 1986; Baggish *et al.* 1989; Benedet *et al.* 1992; Evans and Monaghan 1983; Jordan *et al.* 1985; Paraskevaidis *et al.* 1991).

Out-patient therapy without general anaesthetic is possible in 93 per cent of patients, the remaining patients being admitted either because of bleeding, pain, or an assessment that they were unsuitable for such therapy (Jordan *et al.* 1985). The complications of the procedure include the need for suturing because of bleeding (1.3 per cent), cervical stenosis (1.1 per cent), and sepsis (0.05 per cent) (Baggish *et al.* 1989). Approximately 0.1 per cent of patients treated by laser vaporization will ultimately present with a cervical carcinoma (Ali *et al.* 1986; Jordan *et al.* 1985).

Loop excision

Loop excision of the transformation zone has also in gained recent popularity, in that a specimen is preserved for histological examination and the apparatus is significantly less expensive than a carbon dioxide laser. The finding of an unsuspected microinvasive carcinoma of the cervix following loop excision has been reported in 1 per cent of patients so treated (Prendiville *et al.* 1989).

The technique appears to be successful, in terms of returning cervical cytology to normal, in between 90 and 98 per cent of patients (Luesley *et al.* 1990; Mor-Yosef *et al.* 1990; Prendiville 1989; Wright *et al.* 1991*b*).

It is likely that this technique will increase in popularity since, like a laser cone, it provides the whole of the abnormal area for histological examination, however, the longterm results have yet to be assessed, whilst thermal artefacts at the excision margin may make interpretation difficult (Krebs *et al.* 1993; Montz *et al.* 1993).

The failure of local destructive techniques

It has already been demonstrated that a small percentage of patients will have an unsuspected microinvasive carcinoma of the cervix discovered when the full transformation zone is subject to histological examination, even though microinvasive disease was 'excluded' by previous colposcopy and/or colposcopically directed biopsy. Pearson *et al.* (1989) reported 3738 women who had undergone previous laser ablation for CIN. At a follow-up of between six months and six years, nine patients (0.24 per cent, or 1 patient in 415) developed cancer of the cervix, in equal proportions of either invasive or microinvasive. If the risk of malignant disease following local destructive treatment of any type is to be minimized, then certain criteria should be satisfied before a patient is so treated. Townsend *et al.* (1981) reported that when the case records of patients who developed invasive disease following local destruction were scrutinized, it was not uncommon to find that such criteria had not been satisfied.

A series of criteria were proposed by Jordan (1981) and are enumerated below:

1. The patient must be assessed by an experienced colposcopist before treatment is commenced.

2. The entire lesion must be seen as should the squamocolumnar junction.

3. Invasive carcinoma must be excluded by a colposcopically directed biopsy.

4. Destructive therapy must be performed under colposcopic control by an experienced colposcopist.

5. There must be adequate follow-up by cytology and/or colposcopy.

Should the upper limit of CIN extend into the endocervical canal beyond the limits of colposcopic vision, as happens in approximately 20 per cent of patients, and more often in post-menopausal patients than in premenopausal patients, then several methods of assessment are possible in order to see the entire extent of the lesion and thus avoid a large cone biopsy. Such techniques include the use of an endocervical curette (Soisson *et al.* 1988), a micro-colpohysteroscope (Soutter *et al.* 1984), ethinyl oestradiol (Prendiville *et al.* 1986), and Lamicel (Johnson *et al.* 1990).

Any patient who has undergone treatment for CIN requires follow-up, by some form of combination of cytology and colposcopy (Mahadevan and Horwell 1993), for three reasons. First, as has been illustrated above, treatment may be incomplete. Secondly, up to 2.5 per cent of women will have a recurrence of CIN (Paraskevaidis *et al.* 1991). Thirdly, up to 0.25 per cent of patients will develop a microinvasive or invasive carcinoma (Anderson 1993; Gordon and Duncan 1991; Pearson *et al.* 1989). The technique by which the patient is followed up is of importance. The evidence suggests that a combination of colposcopy and cervical cytology will detect recurrence earlier than either technique alone, and, hence, all women should be offered at least one colposcopic examination in addition to cervical cytology (Paraskevaidis *et al.* 1991; Soutter 1991). In view of the false-negative cytology rate, as a minimum regime two negative smears should be obtained initially after treatment with annual cytology for the first three years thereafter (Paraskevaidis *et al.* 1991).

Treatment and future pregnancy

Theoretically, there are four ways in which treatment for cervical intraepithelial neoplasia may affect future pregnancy. Cervical damage, either in the form of stenosis with or without amenorrhoea, or cervical incompetence may occur. This is a particular problem related to cone biopsy either by cold knife or laser. The taller is the cone, the more likely cervical stenosis to occur (Luesley *et al.* 1985). These authors reported that symptomatic cervical stenosis occurred in 8 per cent of patients and in 1.3 per cent of patients amenorrhoea coexisted. Hysterectomy was ultimately performed in 3 per cent. This complication may be associated with labour exceeding 12 hours in 20 per cent of patients compared with 10 per cent of controls (Jones *et al.* 1979).

Preterm labour, or late spontaneous abortion, is a known complication of cone biopsy. Following this technique, up to 11 per cent of pregnancies were preterm (compared with 5 per cent of controls) and late spontaneous abortion occurred in 5 per cent of pregnancies (compared with 3.5 per cent of controls) (Larsson *et al.* 1982). When the criteria for local destructive treatment rather than cone biopsy allow, it is preferable that these techniques should be used in women who may wish to have more children. There is no evidence for an increased incidence of cervical stenosis or preterm labour following labour vaporization, cryosurgery, cold coagulation, or loop excision of the transformation zone (Bigrigg *et al.* 1991; Gordon and Duncan 1991; Haffenden *et al.* 1993; Hagen and Skjeldestad 1993; Hammond and Edmonds 1990; Prendiville *et al.* 1989).

The incidence of infection sufficient to interfere with future fertility is not known. It had also been proposed that there was a theoretical risk that laser vaporization may alter cervical glands such that mucus excretion became abnormal with resulting subfertility, but there is no evidence to substantiate this view (Hammond and Edmonds 1990).

Adenocarcinoma *in situ*

Whilst most activity is directed towards the precursors of squamous cancer, a specific and difficult clinical problem is created by the condition of adenocarcinoma *in situ* of the cervix. This was once considered unusual, but it is now being diagnosed in up to 1 per cent of patients following the use of excision techniques for the management of cervical intraepithelial neoplasia (Howe and Vincenti 1991).

In up to 58 per cent of patients dysplastic squamous epithelium coexists (Bertrand *et al.* 1987; Luesley *et al.* 1987). The lesion is only predicted by an atypical smear in 50–72 per cent of patients, being an unsuspected diagnosis on cervical histology in the rest (Hopkins *et al.* 1988; Jaworski *et al.* 1988; Luesley *et al.* 1987) . The precise risk for subsequent development of adenocarcinoma of the cervix in women with adenocarcinoma *in situ* is not known but is presumed to occur (Bousfield *et al.* 1980; Hopkins *et al.* 1988). Colposcopic diagnosis is unhelpful in up to 80 per cent of lesions (Teshima *et al.* 1985).

The treatment of this condition is determined by the observation that a limited biopsy may be insufficient to exclude coexisting malignant disease, and, hence, a significant portion of the transformation zone needs to be excised for histological purposes (Ostor *et al.* 1984). Moreover, some authors believe that the whole of the transformation zone is at risk of malignant disease in adenocarcinoma *in situ* and argue that the minimum acceptable treatment for this treatment is excision of the whole transformation zone. Bertrand *et al.* (1987) reported that adenocarcinoma *in situ* generally affected both the surface of the cervix and the deeper glands, covered a wide area, and extended up the endocervical canal. They argued that a cone biopsy (or presumably loop excision) must include all of the transformation zone and at least 25 mm up the endocervical canal. Whilst some authors believe that such conservative methods of treatment are satisfactory for patients with adenocarcinoma *in situ* who wish to have more children (Luesley *et al.* 1987), others argue that only hysterectomy is an appropriate treatment (Hopkins *et al.* 1988). Which of these two management strategies is the more appropriate will have to await the analysis of those prospective studies currently in progress.

Conclusions

There can no longer be any doubt that cervical cytology screening will prevent some patients developing invasive cancer of the cervix. Exactly what percentage of patients destined to develop cancer of the cervix is preventable is not known, but there is no doubt that if cervical cytology screening is to have a useful place the process must be one which is specifically organized and is not opportunistic (Chomet and Chomet 1990). Although the major details of such a programme, such as frequency screening, have to be scientifically assessed, this seems slightly academic whilst there are still some women in the population who are sexually active yet have never had a cervical smear. In one UK series, only 89 per cent of women eligible for a cervical smear had had one in the five-year period of study (Reid *et al.* 1991).

The technique of smear taking also requires further evaluation if the incidence of false-negative smears is to be reduced. The treatment of CIN also requires further refinement. The argument between destructive techniques and techniques which preserve tissue for histology will continue, and there should soon be an answer to the question of the need to treat patients with CIN I.

It is possible that future strategies for cervical screening will involve the use of cervicography. In this technique, the cervix is stained with 5 per cent acetic acid and photographed. The photograph may then be 'read' at a later date and patients with an abnormality referred for colposcopy. When this technique is compared with screening by cervical cytology, it will detect more abnormalities than will cervical cytology but it is also less specific, increasing the false-positive rate. In one series involving over 3000 screens, there were 39 atypical smears and 301 suspicious cervicographs. Some 14 patients with atypical smears had CIN on colposcopy as did 72 women with suspicious cervicographs (Tawa *et al.* 1988). There would appear to be a significant incidence of observer variability in the interpretation of these cervicographs (Sellors *et al.* 1990).

Although this may become a screening test, it is more likely to be used as a second-line screen following an abnormal smear when colposcopy is not immediately available. Digital imaging of the colposcopic image may also enhance the histological prediction at colposcopy (Shafi *et al.* 1994).

References

Adelstein, A. M., Husain, O. A. N., and Spriggs, A. I. (1981). Cancer of the cervix and screening. *British Medical Journal* **282**, 564.

Ahluwalia, H. S. and Doll, R. (1968). Mortality from cancer of cervix uteri in British Columbia. *British Journal of Preventative and Social Medicine* **22**, 161-4.

Ali, S. W., Evans, A. S., and Monaghan, J. M. (1986). Results of carbon dioxide laser cylinder vaporization of cervical intraepithelial disease in 1234 patients. An analysis of failure. *British Journal of Obstetrics and Gynaecology* **93**, 75-8.

Anderson, M. C. (1993). Invasive carcinoma of the cervix following local destructive treatment for cervical intra-epithelial neoplasia. *British Journal of Obstetrics and Gynaecology* **100**, 657-63.

Anderson, M. C. and Hartley, J. (1980). Cervical crypt involvement by intraepithelial neoplasia. *Obstetrics and Gynecology* **55**, 546-50.

Baggish, M. S., Dorsey, J. H., and Adelson, M. (1989). A 10 year experience treating cervical intraepithelial neoplasia with a carbon dioxide laser. *American Journal of Obstetrics and Gynecology* **161**, 60-8.

Bamford, P. N., Barber, M., and Beilby, J. O. W. (1982). Changing pattern of cervical intraepithelial neoplasia seen in a family planning clinic. *Lancet* **i**, 747.

Barton, S. E., Jenkins, D., Hollingsworth, A., Cuzick, J., and Singer, A. (1989). An explanation for the problem of false-negative smears. *British Journal of Obstetrics and Gynaecology* **96**, 482-5.

Beardow, R., Oerton, J., and Victor, C. (1989). Evaluation of the cervical cytology screening programme in an inner city health district. *British Medical Journal* **299**, 98-100.

Bearman, D. M., MacMillan, J. P., and Creasman, W. T. (1987). Papanicolaou smear history of patients developing cervical cancer. *Obstetrics and Gynecology* **69**, 151-5.

Beilby, J. O. W., Bourne, R., Guillebaud, J., and Steele, S. T. (1982). Paired cervical smears. *Obstetrics and Gynecology* **60**, 46-8.

Benedet, J. L., Anderson, G. H., and Boyers, D. A. (1985). Colposcopic accuracy in the diagnosis of microinvasive and occult invasive carcinoma of the cervix. *Obstetrics and Gynecology* **65**, 557-62.

Benedet, J. L., Miller, D. M., and Nickerson, K. G. (1992). Results of conservative management of CIN. *Obstetrics and Gynecology* **79**, 105-10.

Bertrand, M., Lickrish, G. M., and Colgan, T. J. (1987). The anatomic distribution of cervical adenocarcinoma—*in situ*. *American Journal of Obstetrics and Gynecology* **157**, 21-5.

Bevan, J. R., Attwood, M. E., Jordan, J. A., Lucas, A., and Newton, J. R. (1981). Treatment of pre-invasive disease of the cervix by cone biopsy. *British Journal of Obstetrics and Gynaecology* **88**, 1140-4.

Bigrigg, M. A., Codling, B. W., Pearson, P., Read, M. D., and Swingler, G. R. (1991). Pregnancy after cervical loop diathermy. *Lancet* **337**, 119.

Bousfield, L., Pacey, F., Young, Q., Krumins, I., and Osborne, R. (1980). Expanded cytologic criteria for the diagnosis of adenocarcinoma—*in situ* of the cervix. *Acta Cytologica* **24**, 283-96.

Boyce, J. G., Fruchter, R. G., Romanzi, L., Sillman, F. H., and Mainman, M. (1990). The fallacy of the screening interval for cervical smears. *Obstetrics and Gynecology* **76**, 627-32.

British Medical Journal (1980). High-risk groups and cervical cancer. *British Medical Journal* **261**, 629-30.

Burghardt, E. and Holzer, E. (1980). Treatment of carcinoma *in situ*: evaluation of 1609 cases. *Obstetrics and Gynecology* **55**, 539–45.

Buxton, E. J., Luesley, D. M., Shafi, M. I., and Rollason, M. (1991). Colposcopically directed punch biopsy: a potentially misleading investigation. *British Journal of Obstetrics and Gynaecology* **98**, 1273–6.

Byrne, P., Nava, G., and Woodman, G. B. J. (1988). Premalignant lesions of the lower genital tract. In *Progress in Obstetrics and Gynaecology* (ed. J. Studd), Vol. 6, pp. 365–84. Churchill Livingstone, Edinburgh.

Carmichael, J. A., Jeffrey, J. F., Steele, H. D., and Ohlke, I. D. (1984). The cytological history of 245 patients developing invasive cervical cancer. *American Journal of Obstetrics and Gynecology* **148**, 685–90.

Chanen, W. and Rome, R. M. (1983). Electrocoagulation diathermy for cervical dysplasia and carcinoma *in situ*. *Obstetrics and Gynecology* **61**, 673–9.

Charles, E. H. and Savage, E. W. (1980). Cryosurgical treatment of cervical intra-epithelial neoplasia. *Obstetrics and Gynecological Survey* **35**, 539–48.

Chomet, J. and Chomet, J. (1990). Cervical screening in general practice. *British Medical Journal* **300**, 1504–6.

Christopherson, W. M. (1970). Screening for breast and gynaecological lesions. *Lancet* **ii**, 874.

Cramer, D. W. (1974). The role of cervical cytology in declining morbidity and mortality of cervical cancer. *Cancer* **34**, 2018–27.

Draeby-Kristiansen, J., Garsaae, M., Bruun, M., and Hansen, K. (1991). Ten years after cryosurgical treatment of cervical intraepithelial neoplasia. *American Journal of Obstetrics and Gynecology* **165**, 43–5.

Duguid, H. L. D., Duncan, I. D., and Currie, J. (1985). Screening for intraepithelial neoplasia in Dundee and Angus 1962–81 and its relation to invasive cervical cancer. *Lancet* **ii**, 1053–6.

Edwards, D. (1974). Gynaecological abnormalities found at a cytology clinic. *British Medical Journal* **4**, 218–21.

Evans, A. S. and Monaghan, J. (1983). Treatment of cervical intraepithelial neoplasia using the carbon dioxide laser. *British Journal of Obstetrics and Gynaecology* **90**, 553–6.

Fawdry, R. D. S. (1984). Carcinoma *in situ* of the cervix: is post-hysterectomy cytology worthwhile? *British Journal of Obstetrics and Gynaecology* **91**, 67–72.

Fidler, H. K., Boyes, D. A., Lock, D. R., and Aversperg, N. (1962). The cytology programme in British Columbia. *Canadian Medical Association Journal* **86**, 823–30.

Fidler, H. K., Boyes, D. A., and Worth, A. J. (1968). Cervical cancer detection in British Columbia. *Journal of Obstetrics and Gynaecology of the British Commonwealth* **75**, 392–404.

Fletcher, A. (1990). Screening for cancer of the cervix in elderly women. *Lancet* **335**, 97–9.

Fletcher, A., Metaxas, N., Grubb, C., and Chamberlain, J. (1990). Four-and-a-half year follow-up of women with dyskaryotic cervical smears. *British Medical Journal* **31**, 641–4.

Fox, C. H. (1967). Biological behavior of dysplasia and carcinoma *in situ*. *American Journal of Obstetrics and Gynecology* **99**, 960–72.

Frisch, L. E. (1987). Inflammatory atypia. *Acta Cytologica* **31**, 869–72.

Gemmell, J., Holmes, D. M., and Duncan, I. D. (1990). How frequently need vaginal smears be taken after hysterectomy for cervical intraepithelial neoplasia? *British Journal of Obstetrics and Gynaecology* **97**, 58–61.

Giles, J. A., Walker, P. G., and Chalk, P. A. (1987). Treatment of cervical intraepithelial neoplasia by radical electrocoagulation diathermy: 5 years' experience. *British Journal of Obstetrics and Gynaecology* **94**, 1089–93.

Giles, J. A., Deery, A., Crow, J., and Walker, P. (1989). The accuracy of repeat cytology in women with mildly dyskaryotic smears. *British Journal of Obstetrics and Gynaecology* **96**, 1067–70.

Goorney, B. P., Lacey, C. J. N., and Sutton, J. (1989). Ayre's versus Aylesbury cervical spatulas. *Genitourinary Medicine* **65**, 161–2.

Gordon, H. K. and Duncan, I. D. (1991). Effective destruction of CIN III at 100 °C using the Semm cold coagulator: 14 years' experience. *British Journal of Obstetrics and Gynaecology* **98**, 14–20.

Green, G. H. and Donovan, J. W. (1970). The natural history of cervical carcinoma *in situ*. *Journal of Obstetrics and Gynaecology of the British Commonwealth* **77**, 1–9.

Haffenden, D. K., Bigrigg, A., Codling, B. W., and Read, M. D. (1993). Pregnancy following large loop excision of the transformation zone. *British Journal of Obstetrics and Gynaecology* **100**, 1059–60.

Hagen, B. and Skjeldestad, S. E. (1993). The outcome of pregnancy after carbon dioxide laser conisation of the cervix. *British Journal of Obstetrics and Gynaecology* **100**, 717–20.

Hakama, M. and Louhivuori, K. (1988). A screening programme for cervical cancer that worked. *Cancer Surveys* **7**, 403–16.

Hammond, R. H. and Edmonds, D. K. (1990). Does treatment for CIN affect fertility and pregnancy? *British Medical Journal* **301**, 1344–5.

Hopkins, M. P., Roberts, J. A., and Schmidt, R. W. (1988). Cervical adenocarcinoma – *in situ*. *Obstetrics and Gynecology* **71**, 842–4.

Howe, D. T. and Vincenti, A. C. (1991). Is large loop excision of the transformation zone more accurate than colposcopically directed punch biopsy in the diagnosis of CIN? *British Journal of Obstetrics and Gynaecology* **98**, 588–91.

Husain, O. A. N., Butler, E. B., Evans, D. M. B., Macgregor, J. E., and Yule, R. (1974). Quality control in cervical cytology. *Journal of Clinical Pathology* **27**, 935–44.

International Agency for Research on Cancer (1986). Screening for squamous cell cancer: duration of low-risk after negative results of cervical cytology and its implication for screening policies. *British Medical Journal* **293**, 659–64.

Ireland, D. and Monaghan, J. M. (1988). The management of the patient with abnormal vaginal cytology after hysterectomy. *British Journal of Obstetrics and Gynaecology* **95**, 973–5.

Jaworski, R. C., Pacey, N. F., Greenberg, M. L., and Osborn, R. A. (1988). The histologic diagnosis of adnocarcinoma – *in situ* and related lesions of the cervix uteri. *Cancer* **619**, 1171–81.

Johannesson, G., Geirsson, G., and Day, N. (1978). The effect of mass screening in Iceland. *International Journal of Cancer* **21**, 418–25.

Johnson, N., Crompton, A. C., Wyatt, J., Buchan, P. C., and Jarvis, G. J. (1990). Use of Lamicel to expose high cervical lesions during colposcopic examination. *British Journal of Obstetrics and Gynaecology* **97**, 46–52.

Johnson, N., Sutton, J., Thornton, J. G., Lilford, R. J., Johnson, V. A., and Peel, K. R. (1993). Decision analysis for best management of mildly dyskaryotic smear. *Lancet* **342**, 91–6.

Jones, G. M., Sweetham, P., and Hibbard, E. M. (1979). The outcome of pregnancy after cone biopsy of the cervix. *British Journal of Obstetrics and Gynaecology* **869**, 913–16.

Jordan, J. A. (1981). Treatment of cervical intraepithelial neoplasia by destruction. In *Preclinical neoplasia of the cervix* (ed. J. A. Jordan, F. Sharp, and A. Singer), pp. 185–6. Royal College of Obstetricians and Gynaecologists, London.

Jordan, J. A., Woodman, C. B. J., Mylotte, M. J., Emens, J. M., Williams, D. R., Macalary, M., *et al.* (1985). The treatment of cervical intraepithelial neoplasia by laser vaporization. *British Journal of Obstetrics and Gynaecology* **92**, 394–8.

Koss, L. G. (1989). The Pap test for cervical cancer detection. *Journal of the American Medical Association* **261**, 737–43.

Krebs, H. B., Pastore, L., and Helmkamp, B. F. (1993). Loop electrosurgical excision procedures for cervical dysplasia. *American Journal of Obstetrics and Gynecology* **169**, 288–95.

Kristensen, G. B., Jensen, L.K., and Holund, B. (1990). A randomized trial comparing two methods of cold knife cone with laser conization. *Obstetrics and Gynecology* **76**, 1009–13.

Laara, E., Day, N. E., and Hakama, M. (1981). Trends in mortality from cervical cancer in the Nordic countries. *Lancet* **i**, 1247–9.

Lancet (1981). Cone biopsy of the cervix. *Lancet* **i**, 400–2.

Lancet (1985). Cancer of the cervix: death by incompetence. *Lancet* **ii**, 363–4.

Lancet (1990). Cervical screening. *Lancet* **i**, 466–7.

Larsson, G., Grundsell, H., Gullberg, B., and Svennerud, S. (1982). Outcome of pregnancy after conization. *Acta Obstetrica et Gynaecologica Scandinavica* **61**, 461–6.

Lawley, T. B., Lee, R. B., and Kapela, R. (1990). The significance of moderate and severe inflammation on Papanicolaou smears. *Obstetrics and Gynecology* **76**, 997–9.

Lee, L. E., Melnick, P. J., and Walsh, H. M. (1956). Carcinoma *in situ* of the uterine cervix. *Surgery, Gynecology, and Obstetrics* **102**, 677–82.

Loobuyck, H. A. and Duncan, I. D. (1993). Destruction of CIN I and II with a Semm cold coagulator. *British Journal of Obstetrics and Gynaecology* **100**, 465–8.

Lopes, A., Pearson, S. E., Mor-Yosef, S., Ireland, D., and Monaghan, J. M. (1989). Is it time for a reconsideration of the criteria for cone biopsy? *British Journal of Obstetrics and Gynaecology* **96**, 1345–7.

Luesley, D. M., McCrum, A., Terry, P. B., Wade-Evans, T., Nicholson, H. O., Mylotte, M., *et al.* (1985). Complications of cone biopsy related to the dimension of the cone and the influence of prior colposcopic assessment. *British Journal of Obstetrics and Gynaecology* **92**, 158–64.

Luesley, D. M., Jordan, J. A., Woodman, C. B. J., Watson, N., Williams, D. R., and Wadell, C. (1987). A retrospective review of adenocarcinoma—*in situ* and glandular atypia of the uterine cervix. *British Journal of Obstetrics and Gynaecology* **94**, 699–703.

Luesley, D. M., Cullimore, J., Redman, C. W. E., Lawton, F. G., Emens, J. M., Rollason, T. P., *et al.* (1990). Loop diathermy excision of the cervical transformation zone in patients with abnormal cervical smears. *British Medical Journal* **300**, 1690–3.

Macgregor, J. E. (1981). Screening for preclinical cervical cancer. In *Preclinical neoplasia of the cervix* (ed. J. A. Jordan, F. Sharp, and A. Singer), pp. 95–107. Royal College of Obstetricians and Gynaecologists, London.

Macgregor, J. E. (1993). False-negative cervical smears. *British Journal of Obstetrics and Gynaecology* **100**, 801–2.

Macgregor, J. E. and Teper, S. (1978). Mortality from cancer of cervix uteri in Britain. *Lancet* **ii**, 744–6.

Macgregor, J. E., Fraser, M. E., and Mann, E. M. F. (1971). Improved prognosis of cervical cancer due to comprehensive screening. *Lancet* **i**, 74–6.

Macgregor, J., Moss, S. M., Parkin, D. M., and Day, N. E. (1985). A case-controlled study of cervical cancer screening in N.E. Scotland. *British Medical Journal* **290**, 1543–6.

McIndoe, W. A., McLean, M. R., Jones, R. W., and Mullins, P. R., (1984). The invasive protection of carcinoma—*in situ* of the cervix. *Obstetrics and Gynecology* **64**, 451–8.

McIndoe, G. A. J., Robson, M. S., Tidy, J. A., Mason, P., and Anderson, M. C. (1989). Laser excision rather than vaporization: the treatment of choice for cervical intraepithelial neoplasia. *Obstetrics and Gynecology* **74**, 165–8.

Mahadevan, N. and Horwell, D. H. (1993). The value of cytology and colposcopy in the follow-up of cervical intra-epithelial neoplasia after treatment by laser excision. *British Journal of Obstetrics and Gynaecology* **100**, 563–6.

Mitchell, H. and Medley, G. (1991). Longitudinal study of women with negative cervical smears according to endocervical status. *Lancet* **337**, 265–7.

Mitchell, H., Medley, G., and Giles, G. (1990). Cervical cancers diagnosed after negative reports on cervical cytology. *British Medical Journal* **300**, 1622–6.

Montz, F. J., Holschneider, C. H., and Thompson, L. B. R. (1993). Large loop excision of the transformation zone. *Obstetrics and Gynecology* **81**, 976–82.

Mor-Yosef, S., Lopes, A., Pearson, S., and Monaghan, J. M. (1990). Loop diathermy cone biopsy. *Obstetrics and Gynecology* **75**, 884–6.

Murata, P. J., Johnson, R. A., and McNicholl, K. E. (1990). Controlled evaluation of implementing the cytobrush technique to improve Papanicolaou smear quality. *Obstetrics and Gynecology* **75**, 690–5.

Nwabineli, N. J. and Monaghan, J. M. (1991). Vaginal epithelial abnormalities in patients with CIN: clinical and pathological features and management. *British Journal of Obstetrics and Gynaecology* **98**, 25–9.

Nyirjesy, 1. (1972). Atypical or suspicious cervical smears. *Journal of the American Medical Association* **222**, 691–3.

Ostor, A. G., Pagano, R., Davonen, R. A. M., Fortune, D. W., Chanen, W., and Rome, R. (1984). Adenocarcinoma—*in situ* of the cervix. *International Journal of Gynaecological Pathology* **3**, 179–90.

Paraskevaidis, E., Jandial, L., Mann, E. M. F., Fisher, P. M., and Kitchener, H. C. (1991). Pattern of treatment failure following laser for CIN. *Obstetrics and Gynecology* **78**, 80–3.

Parkin, D. M., Nguyen-Dinh, Z., and Day, N. E. (1985). The impact of cervical screening on the incidence of cervical cancer in England and Wales. *British Journal of Obstetrics and Gynaecology* **92**, 150–7.

Parliamentary Reply (1986). Cervical smear. *Hansard* **101**, 146.

Parsons, W. L., Godwin, M., Robins, C., and Butler, R. (1993). Prevalence of cervical pathogens in women with and without inflammatory changes on smear testing. *British Medical Journal* **306**, 1173–4.

Partington, C. K., Turner, M. J., Soutter, W. P., Griffiths, S. M., and Kraus, Z. T. (1989). Laser vaporization versus laser excision conization in the treatment of CIN. *Obstetrics and Gynecology* **73**, 775–9.

Paterson, M. E. L., Peel, K. R., and Joslin, C. A. F. (1984). Cervical smear histories of 500 women with invasive cervical cancer in Yorkshire. *British Medical Journal* **289**, 896–8.

Pearson, S. E., Whittaker, J., Ireland, D., and Monaghan, J. M. (1989). Invasive cancer of the cervix after laser treatment. *British Journal of Obstetrics and Gynaecology* **96**, 486–8.

Petrilli, E. S., Townsend, D. E., Morrow, C. P., and Nakao, C. Y. (1980). Vaginal intraepithelial neoplasia, *American Journal of Obstetrics and Gynecology* **138**, 321–8.

Prendiville, W. J., Davis, W. A. R., Davis, J. O., and Shepherd, A. M. (1986). Medical dilatation of the non-pregnant cervix: the effect of ethinyl oestradiol on the visibility of the transformation zone. *British Journal of Obstetrics and Gynaecology* **93**, 508–11.

Prendiville, W., Cullimore, J., and Norman, S. (1989). Large loop excision of the transformation zone. *British Journal of Obstetrics and Gynaecology* **96**, 1054–60.

Reid, G. S., Robertson, A. J., Bassett, C., Smith, J., Waugh, N., and Halkerston, R. (1991). Cervical screening in Perth and Kinross since introduction of the new contract. *British Medical Journal* **303**, 447–50.

Richart, R. M., Townsend, D., Crisp, W., De Petrillo, A., Ferenczy, A., Johnson, G., *et al.* (1980). An analysis of long-term follow-up results in patients with cervical intraepithelial neoplasia treated by cryosurgery. *American Journal of Obstetrics and Gynecology* **137**, 823–6.

Ross, S. K. (1989). Cervical cytology screening and government policy. *British Medical Journal* **299**, 101–4.

Sellors, J. W., Nieminen, P., Vesterinen, E., and Paavonen, J. (1990). Observer variability in the scoring of colpophotographs. *Obstetrics and Gynecology* **76**, 1006–8.

Sevin, B. U., Ford, J. H., Girtanner, R. D., Hoskins, W. J., Ng, A. B. P., Nordqvist, S. R. B., *et al.* (1979). Invasive cancer of the cervix after cryosurgery. *Obstetrics and Gynecology* **53**, 465–71.

Shafi, M. I., Luesley, D. M., and Jordan, J. A. (1992). Mal-cervical cytological abnormalities. *British Medical Journal* **305**, 1040–1.

Shafi, M. I., Dunn, J. A., Chenoy, R., Buxton, E.J., Williams, C., and Luesley, D.M. (1994). Digital imaging colposcopy, image analysis, and quantification of the colposcopic image. *British Journal of Obstetrics and Gynaecology* **101**, 234–8.

Shy, K., Chu, J., Mandelson, M., Greer, B., and Figge, D. (1989). Pap smear screening interval and risk of cervical cancer. *Obstetrics and Gynecology* **74**, 838–43.

Silcocks, P. B. S. and Moss, S. M. (1988). Rapidly progressive cervical cancer: is it a real problem? *British Journal of Obstetrics and Gynaecology* **95**, 1111–16.

Singer, A., Walker, P., Tay, S. K., and Dyson, J. (1984). Impact of introduction of colposcopy to a district general hospital. *British Medical Journal* **289**, 1049–51.

Skehan, M., Soutter, W. P., Lim, K., Kraus, Z. T., and Pryce-Davies, J. (1990). Reliability of colposcopy and directed punch biopsy. *British Journal of Obstetrics and Gynaecology* **97**, 811–16.

Soisson, A. P., Molina, C. Y., and Benson, W. L. (1988). Endocervical curettage in the evaluation of cervical disease in patients with adequate colposcopy. *Obstetrics and Gynecology* **71**, 109–11.

Soutter, W. P. (1989). A practical approach to colposcopy. In *Progress in obstetrics and gynaecology* (ed. J. Studd), Vol. 7, pp. 355–7. Churchill Livingstone, Edinburgh.

Soutter, W. P. (1991). Criteria for standards of management of women with an abnormal smear. *British Journal of Obstetrics and Gynaecology* **98**, 1069–72.

Soutter, W. P., Fenton, D. W., Gudgeon, P., and Sharp, F. (1984). Quantitative microcolpohysteroscopic assessment of the extent of an endocervical involvement by cervical intraepithelial neoplasia. *British Journal of Obstetrics and Gynaecology* **91**, 712–15.

Standing, P. and Mercer, S. (1984). Quinquennial cervical smears: every woman's right and every general practitioner's responsibility. *British Medical Journal* **289**, 883–6.

Stern, E. and Neely, P. M. (1964). Dysplasia of the uterine cervix. *Cancer* **17**, 508–12.

Tawa, K., Forsythe, A., Cove, K., Salz, A., Peters, H. W., and Watring, W. G. (1988). A comparison of the Papanicolaou smear and the cervigram. *Obstetrics and Gynecology* **71**, 229–35.

Teshima, S., Shimosato, U., Kishi, K., Kasamatsu, T., Ohmi, K., and Vei, Y. (1985). Early stage adenocarcinoma of the Uterine cervix. *Cancer* **56**, 167–72.

Thomas, B. A. (1970). Screening for breast and gynaecological lesions. *Lancet* **ii**, 409–12.

Townsend, D. E., Richart, R. M., Marks, E., and Neilsen, J. (1981). Invasive cancer following out-patient evaluation and therapy for cervical disease. *Obstetrics and Gynecology* **57**, 145-9.

Van Wijngaarden, W. J. and Duncan, I. D. (1993). Rationale for stopping cervical screening in women over 50. *British Medical Journal* **306**, 967-71.

Vooigs, G. P., van der Graaf, Y., and Vooigs, M. A. (1987). The presence of endometrial cells in relation to the day of the menstrual cycle. *Acta Cytologica Scandinavica* **31**, 427-33.

Walker, E. M., Hare, M. J., and Cooper, P. (1983). A retrospective review of cervical cytology in women developing invasive squamous cell cancer. *British Journal of Obstetrics and Gynaecology* **90**, 1087-91.

Walker, E. M., Dodgson, J., and Duncan, I. D. (1986). Does mild atypia on a cervical smear warrant further investigation? *Lancet* **ii**, 672-3.

Walton, R. J. (1982). Cervical cancer screening programmes. *Canadian Medical Association Journal* **127**, 581-9.

Walton, R. J., Blanchet, M., Boyes, D. A., Carmichael, J., Marshall, K. C., Miller, A. D., *et al.* (1976). Cervical cancer screening programmes. *Canadian Medical Association Journal* **114**, 1003-33.

Wetrich, D. W. (1986). An analysis of the factors involved in the colposcopic evaluation of 2194 patients with abnormal Pap smears. *American Journal of Obstetrics and Gynecology* **154**, 1333-49.

Wilson, J. D., Robinson, A. J., Kinghorn, S. A., and Hicks, D. A. (1990). Implications of inflammatory changes on cervical cytology. *British Medical Journal* **300**, 638-40.

Wolfendale, M. (1990). Cervical samplers. *British Medical Journal* **302**, 1554-5.

Wolfendale, M. R., King, S., and Usherwood, M. McD. (1983). Abnormal cervical smears: are we in for an epidemic? *British Medical Journal* **287**, 526-8.

Woodman, C. B. J., Jordan, J. A., Mylotte, M., Gustafson, R., and Wade-Evans, T. (1985). The management of cervical intraepithelial neoplasia by coagulation electrodiathermy. *British Journal of Obstetrics and Gynaecology* **92**, 751-5.

Woodman, C. B. J., Yates, M., Williams, D. R., Ward, K., Jordan, J., and Luesley, D. (1991). A randomized controlled trial of two cervical spatulas. *British Journal of Obstetrics and Gynaecology* **98**, 21-4.

Wright, T. C., Davies, E., and Riopelle, M. A. (1983). Laser surgery for cervical intraqpithelial neoplasia: principles and results. *American Journal of Obstetrics and Gynecology* **145**, 181-4.

Wright, T. C., Richart, R. M., Ferenczy, A., and Koulos, J. (1992a). Comparison of specimens removed by CO_2 laser conization and the loop electrosurgical excision procedures. *Obstetrics and Gynecology* **79**, 147-53.

Wright, T. C., Gagnon, S., Richart, R. M., and Ferenczy, A. (1992b). Treatment of CIN using the loop electrosurgical excision procedure. *Obstetrics and Gynecology* **79**, 173-8.

Yancey, M., Mangelsson, D., Damaurez. A., and Lee, R. B. (1990). Classification of endocervical cells on cervical cytology. *Obstetrics and Gynecology* **76**, 1000-5.

Yao, S. F., Reagan, J. W., and Richart, R. M. (1981). Definition of precursors. *Gynecologic Oncology* **12**, S2230-1.

12 The management of carcinoma of the cervix

Carcinoma of the cervix results in approximately 2200 deaths in England and Wales every year, compared to 1200 deaths from carcinoma of the body of the uterus, 3500 deaths from cancer of the ovary, and 11 000 from carcinoma of the breast. This chapter is concerned with the aetiology of carcinoma of the cervix and the management of FIGO stages I and IIa.

The aetiology of carcinoma of the cervix

No single aetiological agent for cancer of the cervix has been identified and, indeed, there is no reason why only one should be present. There may be an interplay between different aetiological agents which may act either to induce the carcinoma or to facilitate that induction.

The possible aetiological factors in carcinoma of the cervix are well documented and may be divided into social, biological, and male factors.

Social factors

(1) sexual behaviour;
(2) socio-economic status;
(3) racial;
(4) choice of male partner.

Sexual behaviour

It is frequently quoted that virgins are immune to carcinoma of the cervix whilst prostitutes are at high risk (Skegg *et al*. 1982). Whilst the latter may be true, the former is not. Gagnon (1950) reported three cases of carcinoma of the cervix in nuns, and a recent review of the literature has suggested that the risk of carcinoma of the cervix to nuns is little different from that amongst the general female population (Griffiths 1991). However, it has long been accepted that carcinoma of the cervix occurs up to four times more commonly in prostitutes than amongst the rest of the population (Rojel 1953).

Probably the most important feature of sexual behaviour as a risk factor for carcinoma of the cervix is the age at first intercourse. Rotkin (1973) reported that 51 per cent of patients with carcinoma of the cervix had commenced intercourse before the age of 17 as compared with 28 per cent of the rest of the female population. This association has been confirmed by other authors

Table 12.1 Carcinoma of the cervix, rate per 100 000 of population

Puerto Rican, New York City	105.7
Negro, New York City	49.6
Non-Jewish White, New York City	15.0
Jew, New York City	4.1
Jew, Israel	4.8

From Steward *et al.* (1966)

(Wright and Riopelle 1982). The frequency of coitus is not a risk factor but multiple partners are (Skegg *et al.* 1982; Wright and Riopelle 1982). There is no convincing evidence that patients with carcinoma of the cervix have had more pregnancies than other patients matched for age, race, and social class (Terris and Oalmann 1960).

Socio-economic status

Beral (1974) analysed mortality rates from carcinoma of the cervix by the occupation of the husband or consort. There was a gradient such that Social Class 1 women had a crude mortality rate of 35 per cent that of the mean, whilst women of Social Class 5 had a crude mortality rate of 101 per cent when compared with the mean. Wakefield *et al.* (1973) analysed the husband's occupation of almost 300 000 women with abnormal cervices, showing the lowest prevalence in professional classes and the highest in labourers, miners, and construction workers.

Racial

It is often difficult to separate true racial factors from behavioural ones and this may be particularly relevant in this disease. Kessler (1974) reported that the mortality rate from carcinoma of the cervix in the United States for non-whites was twice that for whites in almost all age categories. Steward *et al.* (1966) compared the rates of carcinoma of the cervix per 100 000 head of population amongst different racial and religious groups, and illustrated the sparing effect of carcinoma of the cervix in Jewish women. The authors believed that the major factors in the explanation of this sparing effect were lack of uncircumcized partners and a delayed age at first coitus, although the exact explanation for this phenomenon is not totally clear. These results can be seen in Table 12.1.

Choice of male partner

The apparent reduction in the incidence of carcinoma of the cervix in women whose male consorts have been circumcized is discussed under 'male factors' (p. 334). Kessler (1976) reported that the previous and subsequent partners of men who have had one wife with carcinoma of the cervix were more likely to develop carcinoma of the cervix than were other women matched for age and social class.

Biological factors

(1) cigarette smoking;

(2) use of oral contraception;

(3) microorganisms.

Cigarette smoking

That cigarette smoking is a risk factor in its own right for carcinoma of the cervix is now accepted, the only debate is the size of that risk. Even when allowance has been made for other known risk factors, including sexual behaviour, some case-controlled studies have reported that the relative risk of carcinoma of the cervix in women who smoked was as high as seven times that of non-smokers (Buckley *et al*. 1981). A review of 33 epidemiological studies which have addressed the relationship between smoking and cervical cancer suggested that smoking was a causal agent in its own right and a meta-analysis suggested an overall relative risk in the region of 2.0 (Winklestein 1990). There is also evidence for a dose-response effect such that the risk is increased with the number of years of smoking (Brinton *et al*. 1986; Winklestein 1990). There is also some evidence that the dose-response is so crucial that there is no increased risk for women who smoke less than 15 cigarettes per day, whilst those who smoke in excess of this may have a relative risk of 3.5 for invasive disease (Greenberg *et al*. 1985).

The mechanism by which smoking may induce cervical cancer is not clear, but it may act either as a cofactor in the oncogenic process or cause direct DNA damage (Barton *et al*. 1988; Phillips *et al*. 1990; Simons *et al*. 1993).

Use of oral contraception

The World Health Organization Study (1985) showed that the relative risk for cervical cancer in oral contraceptive users was 1.2 that of non-users and that the relative risk increased to 1.5 after five years of use. Even when correction was made for other known risk factors, there was a four-fold risk of cervical cancer in women who took the pill for ten years compared with never-users (Beral *et al*. 1988). Vessey *et al*. (1989) reported a 20-year follow-up of over 17 000 women in the Oxford–FPA study and confirmed the increased risk of cervical cancer in oral contraceptive users. In IUCD users, the mortality rate from cervical cancer was 0.9 per 100 000 women-years whereas in oral contraceptive takers it was 4.4.

However, there is some difficulty in attempting to quantify the relative risk for cervical cancer in oral contraceptive users since numerous sources of bias (for example cervical screening frequency, recall of information, numbers of partners) are rarely controlled for in the literature. All that can really be observed is that the range of relative risks quoted in the literature range from 0.6 to 4.7, with most series quoting a relative risk of between 1.2 and 1.7 (Swan and Petitti 1982). The need to advise women taking oral contraceptives to enter a cervical screening programme is clear.

Microorganisms

The mechanism by which a normal cervical cell may transform into a malignant one was proposed by Coppleson and Reid (1968) who initially considered that sperm DNA was the oncogene. They proposed that the immature metaplastic cervical cell, found especially in young women and during a first pregnancy, was able to take up nucleic acid which might then be mutagenic, allowing uncontrolled cellular proliferation. Using tissue culture techniques, post-parturient cervix showed both histological evidence of metaplasia and genetic material from sperm DNA existing in close proximity to cervical cell DNA. Reid *et al.* (1978) suggested that basic sperm protein may be the aetiological factor rather than DNA. Two basic proteins exist in sperm: histone and protamine. The lower the social class of the male, the greater the proportion of basic proteins in sperm, especially protamine. The hypothesis was made that cervical cells were able to take up sperm head protein and mutate to become malignant. Although there is no direct evidence to suggest that some chemical portion of sperm is the aetiological factor, a similar hypothesis may be proposed for any relevant protein, including microorganism nucleic acid.

So far, *Chlamydia trachomatis*, cytomegalovirus (CMV), HSV, and papillomavirus have all been serious contenders as the aetiological agent in carcinogenesis and have been studied along similar lines. However, no organism has (or probably can) satisfy the Koch postulates.

Chlamydia   Naib (1970) examined the cervical smears of 54 mothers of infants affected by TRIC organisms for the presence of inclusion-bearing cells. There were clusters of intracytoplasmic inclusions in the cervical cells of 33 (61 per cent) mothers similar to those seen in the conjunctival cells, whilst 22 (40 per cent) had some degree of squamous atypia, but in only one patient was a cervical biopsy taken and this showed CIN II. Schachter *et al.* (1975) reported a TRIC recovery rate from cervical scrapings (on yolk sac inoculation) of 4.1 per cent in women with cervical dysplasia as compared to 0.8 per cent in a 'well-woman clinic'. However, they found a similar agent in 5.4 per cent of pregnant women and 7.8 per cent of all women attending their gynaecological clinic, but without any correlation with cervical atypia. Paavonen *et al.* (1979) found *Chlamydia* in 16 of the genital tracts of 177 women with cervical atypia.

It would seem that Chlamydia is simply a disease of sexually active women and there is no reason to accept it as an aetiological factor in carcinoma of the cervix.

Cytomegalovirus (CMV)   Lang and Kummer (1972) demonstrated CMV in the semen of an asymptomatic male, whilst Willmott (1975) isolated CMV from 6.6 per cent of women attending a venereal disease clinic, although he also found herpes hominis in 5.3 per cent. Some 25 per cent of those patients with CMV also had genital warts. Pasca *et al.* (1975) found antibodies to CMV in 61 per cent of 151 women with either CIN or invasive carcinoma as compared to 33 per cent of controls, however this was not as discrepant as the findings in herpes (see below). Melnick *et al.* (1978) were able to isolate CMV from cell cultures of 2 out of 10 biopsies taken from squamous cell carcinoma of the cervix.

The above evidence could be interpreted as CMV being merely a coincidental infection in sexually active women.

HSV The rise and fall of herpes simplex virus type-2 as the aetiological agent for cancer of the cervix may be traced through the following pieces of evidence:

1. Cervical biopsies were taken from 32 women whose smears showed cellular material characteristics for herpes simplex infection. CIN was found in 10 patients, non-specific inflammatory changes in 11, changes compatible with herpes infection in 5, and no abnormality in 6 (Naib *et al.* 1966).

2. One hundred and sixty-seven women with CIN III or carcinoma of the cervix were assessed for the presence of antibodies to HSV-2 in cervical mucus. HSV-2 antibodies were found in 83 per cent of women with carcinoma of the cervix, but in only 35 per cent of controls; in 70 per cent of women with CIN III, but only 24 per cent of controls; and 56 per cent of women with CIN I or II, but only 18 per cent of controls. Antibodies to HSV-1 were less common in the mucus from patients with cervical atypia than in controls (Nahmias *et al.* 1970).

3. Blood taken during pregnancy from 15 000 women was analysed for the presence of HSV-2 antibodies. Some 45 of these women subsequently developed CIN III and 35.7 per cent of these had antibodies, whereas only 7.1 per cent of 90 matched controls, who did not develop CIN at any stage, had serological evidence of antibodies to HSV-2 (Catalono and Johnson 1971).

4. In a complement fixation test designed to detect a tumour-specific HSV-2 antigen, antibodies were detected in the sera of 35 per cent of 20 women with CIN I or II, 73 per cent of 22 women with CIN III, and 89 per cent of 27 women with squamous cell carcinoma of the cervix. Although non-specific antibodies to HSV-2 were detected in 56 per cent of age-matched controls, only 5 per cent of these controls contained the tumour-specific antigen AG-4 as assessed by the complement fixation test. It is believed that AG-4 is a tumour antigen induced by HSV-2 infection (Aurelian *et al.* 1973).

5. The oncogenic potential of HSV (albeit HSV-1) was demonstrated in hamster embryo fibroblasts. Tumours were induced in 47 per cent of newborn hamster inoculated with HSV-1 infected embryo fibroblasts, and HSV specific antigen was found in the tumour cells (Duff and Rapp 1973).

6. A prospective study of 673 women with genital herpes showed CIN in 14 per cent and invasive neoplasia of the cervix in 1.6 per cent of these women (Nahmias *et al.* 1974).

7. Further serological studies of HSV-2 antibodies revealed their presence in 17 per cent of controls, 73 per cent of 60 women with CIN III, but in only 51.4 per cent of women with cancer of the cervix (Pasca *et al.* 1975).

8. Using indirect immunofluorescence, HSV-specific antigen was found in 9 per cent of samples from healthy cervical epithelium, 61 per cent of biopsies of CIN, and 94 per cent of 38 biopsies taken from women with carcinoma of the cervix (Pasca *et al.* 1976).

9. Tumours induced in rat embryo cells inoculated with HSV were shown to express HSV-specific antigens (Macnab and Timbury 1976).

10. HSV-2 RNA was identified in 60 per cent of 41 biopsies taken from areas of CIN, but was not identified in any of the five biopsies taken from carcinoma of the cervix. It was also identified in 5 per cent of 75 biopsies taken from apparently normal cervices (McDougall *et al.* 1980).

11. HSV-2 specific DNA-binding antigen was expressed in 38 per cent of 106 biopsies taken from areas of CIN III or carcinoma, but in only 3 per cent of biopsies from CIN I, 4 per cent with squamous metaplasia, and none from normal cervix (Dreesman *et al.* 1980).

12. Using genetic probes and recombination, HSV-2 DNA was reclaimed from the genome of HSV-2 transformed rat embryo cells in a form indistinguishable from the original DNA (Park *et al.* 1980).

13. On cervical biopsy, HSV-specific RNA was detected in 60 per cent of 35 biopsies from squamous cell carcinoma of the cervix, 72 per cent of 43 biopsies from CIN, 72 per cent of 56 biopsies from benign cervices, and 9 per cent of 11 biopsies from adenocarcinoma of the cervix. These researchers repeated these results in a second series and were totally unable to find HSV-specific RNA in internally paired benign epithelia from normal areas of the cervix of the same individuals (Eglin *et al.* 1981, 1984).

14. Although HSV had been shown to transform cells to a malignant potential, there was no consistent set of viral genes either retained or expressed in the transformed cells or in human cervical tumours, and, hence, it was proposed that the virus was either not needed to maintain the transformed phenotype, that is it was a 'hit and run' effect or perhaps it was not truly oncogenic (Galloway and McDougall 1983).

15. Rat embryo fibroblasts inoculated with HSV-2 could be transformed into tumorigenic clones, but there was no evidence of the HSV genome in the tumour cells (Darai *et al.* 1977).

16. Tissue culture of 50 cancers of the cervix resulted in several different cell lines, but none expressed HSV-DNA (Kitchener 1988).

17. It has been proposed that HSV does not cause cervical cancer but initiates a change in the cervical cells, acting as a cofactor for the oncogenic agent (Hausen 1982).

From the above evidence, it may be seen that there is a close relationship between HSV infection and carcinoma of the cervix. Furthermore, although HSV is oncogenic in animal models, there is no evidence to demonstrate that it is able to induce carcinoma of the cervix in human cells, nor can the HSV genome be obtained consistently from the chromosomes of malignant cells. Although a 'hit and run' hypothesis may help to explain some of the discrepancies, the evidence may be better interpreted by a high incidence of coincidental herpetic infection in women who develop carcinoma of the cervix. Koch's postulates are not satisfied.

Papillomavirus   Numerous different papillomaviruses have been identified, but types 6, 11, 16, and 18 appear to have a particular association with infections of the genital tract, and it may be that the association between papillomavirus and carcinoma of the cervix has run a similar course to that described for herpes simplex. The evidence associating papillomavirus with carcinoma of the cervix is summarized below:

1. Meisels *et al.* (1977) drew attention to the confusion between, and frequent coexistence of, condylomatous lesions of the cervix and cervical atypia. The smears of 726 women with condylomatous lesions of the cervix were examined and reported as showing 'mild dyskaryosis' in 152 (20.9 per cent). Following colposcopy and biopsy, CIN was reported in only 4 per cent. Condylomatous lesions of the crevix were found in 1 per cent of 1000 cervices examined, but found in 5 per cent of 1000 cervices of 'young women'. In this series, the prevalence of CIN I or II was 5.1 per 1000 smears, CIN III 0.8 per 1000 smears, and carcinoma 0.7 per 1000 smears.

2. The prevalence of genital wart infection is increasing in both men and women in England and Wales, and is twice as common in men as in women. In 1971, genital warts affected 20.32 per 100 000 of the female population, but in 1978 this figure had risen to 34.58 per 100 000, making genital wart infection 50 times more common than herpes. Although there was evidence of papillomavirus infection of the cervix in 1.3 per cent of all cervical smears, 53.3 per cent of these smears were in women below the age of 25 years. On follow-up, 68 per cent of these cervical lesions spontaneously regressed, however, 10 per cent of these women developed CIN (Meisels *et al.* 1982).

3. Walker *et al.* (1983*a*) performed colposcopy on 50 women with vulval warts. Some 50 per cent of these patients had evidence of cervical wart virus infection, 36 per cent had CIN I, and in 18 per cent both CIN I and wart virus infection coexisted.

4. The presence of HPV-11-DNA was demonstrated in 50 per cent of 14 papillomata of the larynx, 100 per cent of 5 cervical condylomata, 21 per cent of 63 vulval condylomata, and 8 per cent of 13 carcinomata of the cervix. HPV-6-DNA was found in 65 per cent of 63 vulval condylomata (Gissmann *et al.* 1983).

5. HPV-16-DNA was discovered in 61.1 per cent of 18 biopsies of invasive carcinoma of the cervix, but in only 22.2 per cent of 9 CIN III lesions, and 10 per cent of 20 CIN I lesions. HPV-16-DNA was also found in 28.6 per cent of 7 vulval carcinomata (Durst *et al.* 1983).

6. HPV-6-DNA was discovered in 59 per cent of biopsies taken from CIN lesions (McCance *et al.* 1983).

7. Papillomavirus protein was found in 43 per cent of 152 lesions of CIN I, 15 per cent of 82 lesions of CIN II, 17 per cent of 47 lesions of 'severe dysplasia', and 10 per cent of 41 lesions with CIN III. However, the cells containing papillomavirus protein were not necessarily within the histological lesion but often only in the transitional zone generally (Kurman *et al.* 1983).

8. In 200 women with an atypical smear who underwent colposcopy, evidence of wart virus was found on colposcopic appearance in 29 per cent of cervices, and evidence of wart virus was shown on histological examination of 30 per cent of cervical biopsies from these patients. However, there was poor correlation between the colposcopic appearances and the histology, both the colposcopic appearances of wart virus infection coinciding only in 83 per cent of the patients in each group. Colposcopic lesions thought to be due to wart virus infection should, therefore, be biopsied in order to confirm or refute the presence of CIN (Walker *et al.* 1983*b*).

9. Using immune histochemical techniques, HPV antigen was found in 8.0 per cent of 25 totally benign cervices, 14.3 per cent of lesions of CIN I, 25.0 per cent of CIN II, 17.2 per cent of CIN III, but was not found in any biopsy taken from squamous cell carcinoma of the cervix. In patients with colposcopic and histological evidence of wart virus infection, HPV antigen was discovered in 57.1 per cent of specimens (Walker *et al.* 1983*c*).

10. Serum assayed for IgG antibody to a group-specific papillomavirus antigen was not present in either children or in 108 adult controls, but was discovered in 95 per cent of 60 patients with anogenital warts, 60 per cent of 92 patients with CIN, and 93 per cent of 46 patients with squamous cell carcinoma of the cervix (Baird 1983).

11. Cervical warts were analysed for HPV-DNA by hybridization techniques. Of 23 cervical warts analysed, 10 had abnormal mitotic figures and of these, 7 contained HPV-16-DNA. Of 13 lesions which did not have abnormal mitotic figures, only one contained HPV-16-DNA and seven contained various other forms of HPV-DNA. In seven of the 23 lesions there was no evidence of HPV-DNA content (Crum *et al.* 1984).

12. Some 19 of 25 women (76 per cent) who were sexual consorts of men with penile warts had similar lesions in their lower genital tracts, and 32 per cent had CIN on colposcopy. Biopsy of the cervical lesions demonstrated similar HPV-DNA to that found in biopsies of the penile lesions, expecially the presence of HPV-16 (Campion *et al.* 1985).

13. HPV-16-DNA was found in 62 per cent of 78 lesions of CIN and in 90 per cent of 13 lesions of invasive cell carcinoma, whereas HPV-6-DNA was not found in any of the invasive lesions but was found in 28 per cent of the CIN lesions. However, in the CIN lesions the viral DNA was free in the

cells, whereas it was generally bonded to the cell chromosomal DNA in invasive lesions (McCance *et al.* 1985).

14. HPV-DNA was found in 68 per cent of 82 cytologically abnormal cervices and in 2.2 per cent of 229 cytologically normal cervices (Schneider *et al.* 1985).

15. In tissue cultures of benign cervical cells incubated with papillomavirus taken from condylomata acuminata, HPV-6 and HPV-11, but not HPV-16, could be demonstrated in those previously normal cervical cells which had transformed into cells indistinguishable histologically from dysplastic cervical cells (Kreider *et al.* 1985).

16. Some 51 women with histological features of cervical warty atypia, but no CIN, were followed for 12 months. The lesion resolved in 47 per cent, was unchanged in 37 per cent, and had progressed to either CIN or microinvasive disease in 16 per cent (Evans and Monaghan 1985).

17. Some 343 women with histological evidence of papillomavirus infection of the cervix were followed for a mean of 18.7 months using colposcopy, cytology, and punch biopsy. Regression occurred in 25 per cent, the lesion persisted in 61 per cent, and had progressed into CIN (but not invasive disease) in 14 per cent (Syrjanen *et al.* 1985).

18. Some 846 women with cytological evidence of papillomavirus of the cervix, but no CIN, were followed for a mean of six years. Whereas the expected number of patients who should develop CIN was 1.9, some 30 patients (3.5 per cent) developed CIN III, demonstrating a relative risk for HPV of 15.6. If only women below the age of 25 were considered then the relative risk became 38.7 (Mitchell *et al.* 1986).

19. Although HPV-16-DNA was found in 84 per cent of 25 squamous cell carcinomata of the cervix or vulva, it was also found in 73 per cent of 11 clinically and histologically normal control tissues up to 5 cm away from the tumour site in these patients (Macnab *et al.* 1986).

20. There was evidence of the presence of HPV-DNA in 66 per cent of 47 biopsies taken from patients with invasive carcinoma of the cervix, however, the viral genome was only integrated with the DNA of the whole cell in 15 per cent. HPV-DNA was discovered in 35 per cent of 26 biopsies from normal cervical tissue, but there was no integration of HPV-16-DNA into the host cell DNA in any of these. There was also a close association between the presence or absence of HPV-16-DNA and age, papillomavirus being found only in women below the age of 40 years. Once the above results were adjusted for age, there was no significant difference between cases and controls as to HPV-16-DNA presence, suggesting that this may be an age effect and not an oncogene (Meanwell *et al.* 1987).

21. De Villiers *et al.* (1987) examined 9295 cervical smears for HPV-6, -11, -16, and -18. Of the 94 per cent of normal smears, evidence of HPV infection was found in 10 per cent of women below the menopause and less than 5

per cent of women above the menopause. Of 6 per cent with CIN, evidence of HPV infection was found in almost 40 per cent and 'almost all' of these women were premenopausal.

22. Murdoch (1988) found HPV-16-DNA in 60 per cent of biopsies taken from normal areas of the transformation zone in women who also showed evidence of CIN. It is not known whether any of these areas underwent dysplastic change at a later date.

23. Using immunochemical techniques, HPV antigen was found in 72 per cent of biopsies from CIN with histological evidence of HPV infection in 71 per cent. However, using paired biopsies from apparently normal areas of cervix, there was histological evidence of HPV in 39 per cent and immunochemical evidence of HPV antigen in 4.2 per cent of the normal biopsies, even in biopsies taken from normal cervix outside the transformation zone (Cassidy 1988).

As with herpes simplex virus infection, there is good evidence to show a correlation between the presence of infection and the presence of CIN or invasive disease, and papillomavirus DNA may be found in cervical tumours. However, further evidence is required, including follow-up studies on apparently normal cervical tissue which also contains the papillomavirus genome, in order to assess whether papillomavirus is merely another coexisting sexually transmitted disease in women with CIN and cervical neoplasia. It is unlikely to be an aetiological agent in its own right but may be a cofactor, facilitating the development of malignant transformation of cervical cells (Wright and Richart 1990).

We still do not know the cause of carcinoma of the cervix.

Male factors

(1) smegma;

(2) sperm DNA and proteins:

(3) microorganisms.

In that some aspect of coitus is clearly the aetiological factor in carcinoma of the cervix, means that the male must be involved. Evidence of the variation in sperm basic protein together with the observation that subsequent partners of men who have had one wife with carcinoma of the cervix were more likely to develop carcinoma of the cervix than were other women has led to the concept of the 'high-risk male'.

It has been suggested that having a male partner who is circumcized may reduce the risk of carcinoma of the cervix.

Steward *et al.* (1966) reported a lower prevalence of carcinoma of the cervix in Jewish women compared with that in non-Jewish women. Handley (1936) also drew attention to the apparently protective effect of circumcision. He had observed that the incidence of carcinoma of the cervix in Amsterdam in non-Jewish inhabitants was 10 per 100 000, whereas it was four per 100 000 for Jewish women. He visited Fiji in 1927 where the larger Fijian population practised circumcision but the smaller Indian population did not. During an 8-year period, three Fijians were diagnosed as having carcinoma of the cervix compared with 26 Indians. Such studies were not controlled for sexual behaviour and it may be that this is the factor, rather than the practice of circumcision, which acts as an aetiological factor. To explain non-circumcision as a factor, smegma has been implicated as the aetiological agent even though there is no evidence that it is carcinogenic.

The other male factors have already been discussed.

Microinvasive carcinoma of the cervix

The literature concerning microinvasive carcinoma of the cervix is complicated by a changing definition of what constitutes the histological picture of microinvasion. Currently, for microinvasive disease to be diagnosed, the depth of invasion should not exceed 1 mm to be defined as stage Ia1, or should not exceed 5 mm and the largest diameter of the lesion should not exceed 7 mm to be diagnosed as stage Ia2 (Shepherd 1989). It is likely that microinvasive carcinoma of the cervix represents a spectrum extending between CIN III and occult invasive carcinoma of the cervix.

Clinically, the peak age of microinvasive carcinoma of the cervix occurs between 44 and 48 years, some two-thirds of patients are free of all symptoms whilst one-third complain of intermenstrual bleeding, post-coital bleeding or post-menopausal bleeding. Naked eye appearances may vary from normality to red or white patches on the cervix, and colposcopic examination reveals bizarre vessel branching over raised acetowhite areas.

Suggested treatments have included cone biopsy, hysterectomy, radical hysterectomy, radical hysterectomy with pelvic lymphadenectomy, and radical radiotherapy. The five-year survival should approach 100 per cent. The survival rate in this condition will be less if the lesion appears to be invading capillary-like spaces (either lymphatic or vascular) or if pelvic lymph nodes contain metastases. Pelvic lymph node metastases occur in 1.5 per cent of such patients (Sedlis *et al.* 1979).

The likelihood of pelvic lymph node metastases will be a major factor in deciding upon the appropriate treatment for patients with microinvasive carcinoma of the cervix. There is good evidence to suggest that the depth of invasion within the cervix is closely related to the risk of pelvic lymph node metastasis. For instance, Hasumi *et al.* (1980) reported that only 0.9 per cent of patients with a depth of stromal invasion of less than 3 mm had positive pelvic lymph nodes, whereas 14 per cent of patients with a depth of invasion greater than 3 mm had evidence of pelvic node metastases. Other authors have confirmed the virtual absence of positive pelvic lymph nodes when the depth of invasion in the cervix was less than 3 mm (Simon *et al.* 1986; Van Nagell *et al.* 1983). It would seem that patients with a lesion showing a depth of invasion of less than 3 mm may safely be treated by either cone biopsy (especially if future fertility was desired) or by simple hysterectomy (Burghardt *et al.* 1991). Following such treatment, lymph node involvement or local recurrence did not occur (Creasman *et al.* 1985).

When stromal invasion to a depth of greater than 3 mm, but less than 5 mm, occurs there is an appreciable incidence of pelvic lymph node metastases, with quoted incidences in the literature varying from 2 to 14 per cent (Creasman *et al.* 1985; Hasumi *et al.* 1980; Simon *et al.* 1986; Van Nagell *et al.* 1983). Such patients even have an appreciable mortality (5 per cent, Creasman *et al.* 1985). It would seem logical that should the depth of invasion of the initial lesion in microinvasive carcinoma of the cervix exceed 3 mm, the patient should be treated in the same way as a stage Ib squamous cell carcinoma of the cervix (Burghardt *et al.* 1991; Morgan *et al.* 1993).

The management of stage Ib carcinoma of the cervix

Over the past 25 years it has been noted that patients with carcinoma of the cervix tend to present earlier. Boyce *et al.* (1981) reported that in New York between 1961 and 1965, only 27 per cent of carcinoma of the cervix were stage I, whereas between 1971 and 1975, 43 per stage were stage I. However, there has been very little, if any, improvement in the 5- and 10-year survival rates of stage Ib carcinoma of the cervix over this time, these figures being 86 per cent and 84 per cent, respectively.

The FIGO definition of a stage Ib carcinoma of the cervix is an occult or overt lesion, strictly confined to the cervix, invading to a depth of greater than 5 mm or a width of greater than 7 mm. Any involvement of the corpus uteri is disregarded (Shepherd 1989).

Prognostic factors in stage Ib

The following prognostic factors should be taken into account:

(1) lymph node involvement;

(2) tumour volume;

(3) histological differentiation;

(4) lymphovascular invasion;

(5) age of patient.

Lymph node involvement

Most authors report that between 10 and 15 per cent of patients with stage Ib carcinoma of the cervix have metastases in pelvic lymph nodes (La Polla *et al.* 1986; Larson *et al.* 1987). However, once pelvic lymph node involvement has occurred, the disease is potentially a systemic one, with spread outside of the pelvis. Thus, there is an incidence of between 2–6 per cent positive para-aortic lymph node involvement in stage Ib (Averette *et al.* 1987; La Polla *et al.* 1986). In patients who have para-aortic node involvement, there is a 7 per cent incidence of scalene lymph node involvement, demonstrating the potential for even early disease to be widespread (Stehman *et al.* 1987).

In order to identify such patients with lymph node involvement beyond the pelvis, various techniques have been advocated. Surgical staging has been used in order that a more individualized treatment can be planned for those patients with extrapelvic spread, but there is no good evidence that surgical staging will improve the survival of the patient, partly because the treatment options for distant spread (surgery, radiotherapy, or chemotherapy) have limitations and the operation of surgical staging itself will carry a morbidity and mortality risk. La Polla *et al.* (1986) reported one post-operative death from pulmonary embolus in 96 patients undergoing surgical staging. Imaging of the lymph nodes by either CT scan or the use of lymphograms are also of limited value. To be visible on a CT scan, a lymph node needs to be greater than 1 cm in size. In one study, CT scans correctly predicted the presence of positive para-aortic node involvement in 75 per cent of patients with such involvement, but failed to diagnose lymph node metastases in 25 per cent. Similarly, the technique falsely predicted positive lymph nodes in 9.4 per cent of patients with histologically negative nodes. Even fine needle aspiration of the nodes, based on CT findings, did not significantly improve the diagnostic accuracy (Ballon *et al.* 1981).

The importance of lymph node involvement is in the prediction of both recurrence and survival. The recurrence rate following treatment for a stage Ib cervical carcinoma is 7 per cent when lymph nodes are negative, but 34 per cent when they are positive (Burke *et al.* 1987; Larson *et al.* 1987). Moreover, the five-year survival rate in the presence of negative lymph nodes is between 90 and 93 per cent, whilst the five-year survival in the presence of positive lymph nodes is between 55 and 63 per cent (Fuller *et al.* 1989; Rampone *et al.* 1973).

Tumour volume

The positive relationship between tumour volume, incidence of lymph node metastases, and survival has been documented by many authors (Baltzer *et al.* 1982; Chung *et al.* 1980; Dareng *et al.* 1985). For instance, Fuller *et al.* (1989) found that a tumour of less than 4 cm in diameter was associated with a 13 per cent incidence of positive lymph nodes and an 84 per cent five-year survival, whereas a tumour of greater than 4 cm in diameter was associated with a 31 per cent incidence of lymph node involvement and a 65 per cent five-year survival. Similarly, Hopkins and Morley (1991) reported that the five-year survival for stage Ib tumours was 76 per cent if tumour diameter was greater than 3 cm, but 91 per cent if it was less than 3 cm, whilst Peipert *et al.* (1993) reported 79 per cent and 92 per cent respectively.

Histological differentiation

The degree of differentiation is the single most important histological feature which correlates with recurrence and survival (Smiley *et al.* 1991). Moreover,

Table 12.2 Actual (or predicted) death rate by age per 100 000 women

	Age (years) 20–24	30–34	35–39	50–54
1950–54	0.1	2.9	5.4	21.1
1960–64	0.1	2.0	7.0	18.5
1970–74	0.3	7.3	3.7	19.8
1980–83	0.4	4.3	5.6	11.2
1990–94*	0.4	7.7	10.6	13.0
2000–04*	0.4	7.7	12.8	20.0

* = prediction; From Beral and Booth (1986)

the more dedifferentiated was the tumour, the more bulky was the lesion, the higher was the incidence of lymph node metastases, and the lower was the disease-free survival (Chung *et al*. 1981). For instance, Prempree *et al*. (1983) analysed 561 patients with carcinoma of the cervix, subdivided by Broder's grade. The five-year survival for stage Ib with a Broder's grade I was 79 per cent, whereas the corresponding figure for Broder's grade III (poorly differentiated) was 43 per cent. Similarly, Hopkins and Morley (1991) reported that the five-year survival for stage Ib was 82 per cent for poorly differentiated tumours and 95 per cent for well-differentiated tumours.

Lymphovascular invasion

The presence or absence of lymphovascular invasion by the tumour shows a positive correlation with lymph node involvement and a negative correlation with survival. Hoskins (1988) accumulated six series of over 1000 patients. If the original lesion failed to show lymphovascular invasion, the incidence of positive pelvic lymph nodes was 15 per cent, whereas if the initial lesion did show lymphovascular invasion, the corresponding figure for pelvic lymph nodes was 50 per cent. Similarly, the recurrence rate was 8 per cent in the absence of lymphovascular invasion and 46 per cent in its presence, whilst the five-year survival was 93 per cent in the absence of lymphovascular invasion and 62 per cent in its presence.

However, Fuller *et al*. (1989) stratified results for different prognostic features and found that, once the presence or absence of lymph node involvement was considered, the presence or absence of lymphovascular invasion was no longer related to survival and was, therefore, not an independent factor in its own right.

Age of patient

It is frequently stated that patients below the age of 35 years have a lower five-year survival rate, stage for stage, than do patients above this age (Beral and Booth 1986; Yule 1978). Beral and Booth (1986) predicted (as can be seen from Table 12.2) that there was an increased mortality from carcinoma of the cervix in all women and that the increase would work throughout the population such that the decreased survival currently seen in younger women would become a characteristic of all age groups. Other authors have drawn attention to the possibly more aggressive nature of cervical cancer in the younger age group with the suggestion that, stage for stage, women below the age of 40 years had a higher incidence of positive lymph nodes and poor differentiation than did women above this age group (Buckley *et al*. 1988; Prempree *et al*. 1983; Stanhope *et al*. 1980).

However, the majority of authors have been unable to find any disadvantage for survival in younger women with survival cancer (Baltzer *et al*. 1982; Burke 1987; Junor *et al*. 1989).

The largest study of the influence of age upon survival was reported by Meanwell *et al*. (1988). In a series of 10 022 patients with carcinoma of the cervix, the overall five-year survival was, in fact, greater in women below the age of 40 years, being 69 per cent in this group compared with 45 per cent for those above this age. After a regression analysis for other known variables, younger age was still a weak but favourable prognostic factor. Similarly, other authors have confirmed that younger age is, at worst, a neutral factor in survival, and may, in fact, be a favourable factor in survival since younger women tend to present at an earlier stage, or with a smaller volume tumour, than do older women (Peel *et al*. 1991; Russell *et al*. 1987; Sigurdsson *et al*. 1991; Smale *et al*. 1987).

It should no longer be considered that younger age is an adverse factor in survival, but rather that it is either a neutral or even a favourable prognostic factor.

The treatment of carcinoma of the cervix

This discussion is designed to deal primarily with stages Ib and IIa, where the controversy between surgery or radiotherapy as a primary form of treatment is still not resolved. This debate could perhaps have been solved had prospective randomized controlled trials been performed. The results of survival for patients treated by either radical surgery or radiotherapy have to be compared with caution since patient selection may have played a role, in that younger fitter patients with smaller tumours may be more likely to have been treated by surgery than by radiotherapy (Iversen *et al*. 1982). However, several series have suggested that the five-year survival for stages Ib and IIa in patients treated by radical radiotherapy alone varies between 70 and 86 per cent (Brady 1979; Einhorn *et al*. 1985; Iversen *et al*. 1982; Martimbeau *et al*. 1978; Morley and Seski 1976; Peel *et al*. 1991; Perez *et al*. 1988). The overall survival rate for patients with stage IIa treated by radiotherapy alone is in the region of 67 per cent (Perez *et al*. 1988).

The use of radical surgery alone is an option for patients with stage Ib disease, and, to a lesser extent, for patients with stage IIa. The overall five-year survival rate for patients with stage Ib treated with radical surgery alone ranges between 77 and 90 per cent (Benedet *et al.* 1980; Brady 1979; Burghardt *et al.* 1987; Morley and Seski 1976; Webb and Symmonds 1979). The five-year survival rate is greater if pelvic lymph nodes are negative (81.4 per cent) than if they are positive (61.5 per cent) (Benedet *et al.* 1980). The overall five-year survival rate following surgery alone is significantly lower in patients with stage II disease, being 69 per cent (Webb and Symmonds 1979).

A further treatment option, and one, which is currently popular, is primary surgical treatment but offering radical pelvic radiotherapy to those patients who have positive pelvic lymph nodes. This regime may be especially beneficial in premenopausal women who may have one or both ovaries preserved and then only irradiated should there be histological evidence of pelvic lymph node metastasis. Since between 9 and 15 per cent of patients will have lymph node metastases, the vast majority of patients will be treated by surgery alone and ovarian function will continue (Falk *et al.* 1982; Peel *et al.* 1991). Only 0.5 per cent of women with stage Ib squamous cell carcinoma of the cervix will have an ovarian metastasis (Sutton *et al.* 1992). Using such a regime, the overall five-year survival rate for patients with stage Ib and IIa disease was 81.9 per cent (Peel *et al.* 1991) or up to 91.5 per cent for patients with stage Ib disease only (Falk *et al.* 1982). The logic behind post-operative radiotherapy to the pelvis, when pelvic lymph nodes have been removed but demonstrated to be histologically involved with tumour, is the observation that surgical lymphadenectomy is complete only in a minority of patients (26 per cent) in whom the technique was attempted (Kjorstad and Bond 1984).

Perhaps the earliest regime for the treatment of carcinoma of the cervix related to pre-operative irradiation followed, generally six weeks later, by radical hysterectomy with pelvic lymphadenectomy (Meigs 1951; Wertheim 1912). The overall five-year survival rate in patients with stage Ib disease treated by this regime ranged between 84 and 88 per cent (Burch and Chalfont 1970; Churches *et al.* 1974; Currie 1971; Iversen *et al.* 1982; Rampone *et al.* 1973). However, the major problem with such a regime is that the complication rate is greater following surgery and radiotherapy than after surgery alone. In one series of patients, the incidence of fistula was 5 per cent following irradiation alone but 15 per cent following a combination of radiation and surgery (Rotman *et al.* 1979), whereas another series reported that the overall major complication rates following surgery alone was 6 per cent, but following surgery and radiotherapy this figure rose to 12 per cent (Morrow 1980). Peel *et al.* (1991) reported that 1.6 per cent of patients treated by surgery alone developed a fistula as compared with 2.1 per cent of patients treated with surgery following radiotherapy. However, in this series the highest incidence of serious morbidity followed radiotherapy alone when 3.8 per cent of patients developed a stricture of either the small or large bowel. Similarly, Morley and Seski (1976) attempted to treat alternate patients by surgery or radiotherapy alone. The five-year survival was similar in both groups, but the overall complication rates were greater during and following radiotherapy (24 per cent) than during or following surgery (20 per cent).

In an attempt to assess optimal figures for surgery and radiotherapy, Brady (1979) conducted a survey of USA institutions with regard to their treatment for stage Ib disease. His results may be shown as follows:

1. Of 93 institutions favouring primary surgery, 6815 patients had an 81 per cent five-year survival, whereas 6446 patients were treated by radiotherapy with a 70 per cent five-year disease-free survival.
2. Of 26 institutions favouring radiotherapy, 3430 patients had a 75 per cent five-year disease-free survival.

The same surveys carried out for stage IIa showed that:

1. Of 76 institutions favouring primary surgery, 4506 patients had a 62 per cent five-year disease-free survival, whereas 9564 patients treated by radiotherapy had a 48 per cent five-year disease-free survival.
2. Of 43 institutions favouring radiotherapy, 10 152 patients had a 56 per cent disease-free five-year survival.

All these results have been summarized in Table 12.3, from which it can be seen that there is a trend towards better results from surgery alone compared with radiotherapy alone, but that the best results probably arise when surgery has been augmented by post-operative radiotherapy should pelvic lymph nodes have been involved. Whilst the need for further series, perhaps even in the form of randomized trials, concerning these observations is clear, on present-day evidence the optimal treatment for a younger woman with stage Ib disease must be primary surgery with conservation of an ovary followed by radiotherapy should the lymph nodes have been involved. There is an additional major benefit from such a regime in that there are less problems with sexual dysfunction after surgery than after radiotherapy. For instance, Abitbol and Davenport (1974) reported that 78.6 per cent of 28 patients with carcinoma of the cervix treated by radiotherapy alone had a shortened vagina which interfered with sexual function, whereas only 6.3 per cent of 32 patients treated with surgery alone had this complication. Similarly, Siebel *et al.* (1980) reported a statistically significant decrease in both sexual enjoyment and frequency of intercourse in women who had been treated by radiotherapy compared with those treated surgically.

The significant longterm mortality, whichever treatment modality is chosen, demonstrates that, for a significant percentage of patients with stage Ib lesions, the disease is systemic and cannot be cured by local treatment. Some 40 per cent of patients have a recurrence outside the pelvis, yet none of the treatments described so far could have influenced this statistic (Hacker 1988). Because of this, alterations in treatment have been made in order to include either para-aortic lymph node irradiation or systemic chemotherapy.

Enlarging the field of treatment to include the para-aortic nodes does not seem to be sufficient to combat this spread of disease. Haie *et al.* (1988) reported the results of the randomized European Collaborative Study which compared pelvic irradiation with pelvic and para-aortic nodes irradiation for

Table 12.3 Five-year survival rates for stages Ib

Radiotherapy alone			Surgery alone			Pre-operative irradiation			Post-operative irradiation		
Reference	No.	%	Reference	No.	%	Reference	No.	%	Reference	No.	%
Brady (1979)	6646	70.0	Benedet et al. (1980)	76	77.6	Burch and Chalfont (1970)	511	85.5	Falk et al. (1982)	141	91.5
	3430	75.0									
Einhorn et al. (1985)	113	81.0	Brady (1979)	6815	81.0	Churches et al. (1974)	577	72.4	Peel et al. (1991)	181	81.9
Iversen et al. (1982)	147	71.0	Burghardt et al. (1987)	112	82.2	Currie (1971)	189	86.3			
Martimbeau et al. (1978)	75	73.6	Morley and Seski (1976)	100	89.0	Iversen et al. (1982)	542	84.0			
Morley and Seski (1976)	100	86.0	Webb and Symmonds (1979)	144	90.0	Rampone et al. (1973)	537	88.3			
Peel et al. (1991)	132	73.1									
Perez et al. (1988)	353	85.0									

stage I and stage II disease. There was no significant difference in four-year disease-free survival whether or not the para-aortic nodes were irradiated, but irradiation of the para-aortic nodes resulted in severe bowel damage in 5 per cent of patients, whereas irradiation of the pelvic nodes alone resulted in severe bowel damage in 4 per cent. Furthermore, death occurred from bowel complications in 3 per cent of 201 patients in the pelvic and para-aortic treated group compared with 2 per cent of 215 patients in the pelvic irradiated group alone. The authors concluded that routine para-aortic irradiation was unlikely to be beneficial.

The role of chemotherapy, either before or after surgery, may have a role in preventing recurrence and increasing survival, and, hence, warrants consideration. Kim *et al*. (1988) have advocated chemotherapy before radical surgery treatment for patients with stage Ib or stage II disease. The response was judged by the histology of the surgical specimen, and an overall response was noted in 89 per cent of 35 patients so treated. There was a complete remission in 16 (46 per cent) and partial remission in 15 (43 per cent). No nodal metastases were found in the complete remission group, whilst metastases were found in the partial remission and no treatment group. It is possible that pre-operative chemotherapy may, in the future, have some role to play in reducing tumour volume and lymph node metastases. Other small series have shown some benefit from pre-operative chemotherapy, especially in the presence of a bulky cancer of the cervix, and this treatment modality warrants further study (Dottino *et al*. 1991).

The role of adjuvant chemotherapy following surgery has also been studied (Lai *et al*. 1989; Remy *et al*. 1990) and the early results suggest that this technique deserves further evaluation. In one series, the three-year disease-free interval following surgery with post-operative chemotherapy (cisplatin, vincristine, and bleomycin) for patients with stage I and IIb disease was 75 per cent compared with 47 per cent for those who were not treated with adjuvant chemotherapy.

It may be that such chemotherapy, especially given post-operatively to patients with positive lymph nodes, will become a standard treatment modality but the need for further information is apparent.

Chemotherapy has been used in the treatment of later stages or following recurrence. Thigpen *et al*. (1981) treated 34 patients with advanced or recurrent squamous cell carcinoma using *cis*-platinum. In 22 patients who had had no previous chemotherapy, there was a 50 per cent response rate with three complete responses and eight partial responses. In 12 patients who had had prior radiotherapy, the response rate was only 17 per cent and those were all partial. The mean duration of response was six months and the mean survival for responders was nine months compared to a mean survival of less than six months for non-responders. Friedlander *et al*. (1983) evaluated 33 women after treatment with *cis*-platinum, vinblastine, and bleomycin. Two-thirds of the patients showed some degree of response, with one-third of the patients showing complete remission. Survival was longer in responders than non-responders, but toxicity included nausea, vomiting, and alopecia. It is not yet known whether triple therapy has any increased benefits over single agent therapy, although a recent trial of the latter found a 23 per cent partial response rate but a zero complete response rate (Rabinovich *et al*. 1991). The use of bromocriptine has been suggested because of some value in the treatment of prostatic cancer, but this drug has not been shown to cause even partial remission in patients with cervical cancer (Ruge *et al*. 1985).

Adenocarcinoma of the cervix

Adenocarcinoma of the cervix accounts for between 10 and 20 per cent of cases of invasive carcinoma of the cervix, with a median age at diagnosis of 47 years (Brand *et al*. 1988; Shingleton *et al*. 1981). When matched for age, race, stage, and treatment with patients with squamous cell carcinoma of the cervix, there were no differences in the rate of recurrence, survival, metastases, or radioresistance (Ireland *et al*. 1985; Shingleton *et al*. 1981). There is, therefore, no good reason to treat adenocarcinoma of the cervix any differently from squamous cell carcinoma of the cervix (Brand *et al*. 1988). In young women undergoing radical surgery for adenocarcinoma of the cervix, ovarian conservation can be considered since an ovarian metastasis is found in only 1.7 per cent of patients with a stage Ib adenocarcinoma of the cervix (Sutton *et al*. 1992).

Conclusions

Although there have been some modifications in the detail of treatment of patients with carcinoma of the cervix in the recent past, there has been no improvement in the survival rate from this disease. Moreover, there is good epidemiological evidence to believe that, despite cervical screening, the disease is going to increase in incidence over the next two decades. Survival rates are good for those patients with early disease, without nodal metastases, and morbidity may be reduced by treatment with surgery alone. It is not clear how best to treat the patients who do have pelvic node involvement, and it may be that survival in these patients, and in those patients with later stages, may be improved by advances in chemotherapy. The psychosexual implications of gynaecological cancer and the need for this to be discussed with patients are becoming apparent (Crowther *et al*. 1994).

References

Abitbol, M. M. and Davenport, J. H. (1974). Sexual dysfunction after therapy for cervical carcinoma. *American Journal of Obstetrics and Gynecology* **119**, 181–9.

Aurelian, L., Davis, H. J., and Julian, C. G. (1973). Herpes virus type 2 induced tumour specific antigens in cervical cancer. *American Journal of Epidemiology* **98**, 1–9.

Averette, H. E., Donato, D. M., Lovecchio, J. L., and Sevin, B. (1987). Surgical staging of gynaecological malignancies. *Cancer* **60**, 2010–20.

Baird, P. J. (1983). Serological evidence for the association of papillomavirus and cervical neoplasia. *Lancet* **ii**, 17–18.

Ballon, S. C., Berman, M. L., Lagasse, L. D., and Petrelli, E. S. (1981). Survival after extra-peritoneal pelvic and para-aortic lymphadenectomy and radiation therapy in cervical cancer. *Obstetrics and Gynecology* **57**, 90–5.

Baltzer, J., Keopcke, W., Lohe, K. J., Ober, K. G., and Zander, J. (1982). Age and five-year survival rates in patients with carcinoma of the cervix. *Gynecologic Oncology* **14**, 220–4.

Barton, J. E., Maddox, P. H., Jenkins, D., Edwards, R., Cuzick, J., and Singer, A. (1988). Effect of cigarette smoking on cervical epithelial immunity. *Lancet* **ii**, 652–4.

Benedet, J. L., Turko, M., Boyes, D. A., Nickerson, K. G., and Bienkowska, B. T. (1980). Radical hysterectomy in the treatment of cervical cancer. *American Journal of Obstetrics and Gynecology* **137**, 254–62.

Beral, V. (1974). Cancer of the cervix: a sexually transmitted disease? *Lancet* **i**, 1037–40.

Beral, V. and Booth, M. (1986). Predicting cervical cancer incidence and mortality in England and Wales. *Lancet* **i**, 495.

Beral, V., Hannaford, P., and Kay, C. (1988). Oral contraceptive use and malignancies of the genital tract. *Lancet* **ii**, 1331–4.

Boyce, J. G., Fruchter, R. G., and Nicastri, A. F. (1981). Prognostic factors in stage I cancer of the cervix. *Gynecologic Oncology* **12**, 154–65.

Brady, L. W. (1979). Surgery or radiotherapy for stage I and IIa carcinoma of the cervix. *International Journal of Radiation, Oncology, Biology, and Physics* **5**, 1877–9.

Brand, E., Berek, J., and Hacker, N. (1988). Controversies in the management of cervical adenocarcinoma. *Obstetrics and Gynecology* **71**, 261–9.

Brinton, L. A., Schairer, C., Haenszel, W., Stolley, P., Lehman, H. F., Levine, R., *et al.* (1986). Cigarette smoking and invasive cervical cancer. *Journal of the American Medical Association* **255**, 3265–9.

Buckley, J. D., Harris, R. C. W., Doll, R., Vessey, M. P., and Williams, D. (1981). Case controlled study of husbands of women with carcinoma of cervix uteri. *Lancet* **ii**, 1010–14.

Buckley, C. H., Beards, C. S., and Fox, H. (1988). Pathological prognostic indicators in cervical cancer with particular reference to patients under the age of 40 years. *British Journal of Obstetrics and Gynaecology* **95**, 47–56.

Burch, J. C. and Chalfont, R. L. (1970). Pre-operative radium irradiation and radical hysterectomy in the treatment of carcinoma of the cervix. *American Journal of Obstetrics and Gynecology* **106**, 1054–64.

Burghardt, E., Pickel, H., Haas, J., and Lahousen, M. (1987). Prognostic factors and operative treatment of stages Ib and IIb cervical cancer. *American Journal of Obstetrics and Gynecology* **157**, 988–96.

Burghardt, E., Girardi, F., Lahousen, M., Pickel, H., and Tamussino, K. (1991). Microinvasive carcinoma of the uterine cervix. *Cancer* **67**, 1037–45.

Burke, T. W., Hoskins, W. J., and Heller, P. B. (1987). Prognostic factors associated with radical hysterectomy failure. *Gynecologic Oncology* **26**, 153–9.

Campion, M. J., Singer, A., Clarkson, P. K., and McCance, D. J. (1985). Increased risk of cervical neoplasia in consorts of men with penile condylomata accuminata. *Lancet* **i**, 943–6.

Cassidy, L. J. (1988). Human papillomavirus in paired normal and abnormal cervical biopsies. *British Journal of Obstetrics and Gynaecology* **95**, 1092–5.

Catalano, L. W. and Johnson, L. D. (1971). Herpes virus antibody and carcinoma-*in-situ* of the cervix. *Journal of the American Medical Association* **217**, 447–50.

Chung, C. K., Nahhas, W. A., Stryker, J. A., Curry, S. L., and Mortel, R. (1980). Analysis of factors contributing towards treatment failures in stages Ib and IIa carcinoma of cervix. *American Journal of Obstetrics and Gynecology* **138**, 550–6.

Chung, C. K., Stryker, J. A., Ward, S. P., Nahhas, W. A., and Mortel, R. (1981). Histological grade and prognosis of carcinoma of the cervix. *Obstetrics and Gynecology* **57**, 636–42.

Churches, C. K., Kurrie, G. R., and Johnson, B. (1974). Treatment of carcinoma of the cervix by combination of irradiation and operation. *American Journal of Obstetrics and Gynecology* **118**, 1033–40.

Coppleson, M. and Reid, B. (1968). The aetiology of squamous carcinoma of the cervix. *Obstetrics and Gynecology* **32**, 432–6.

Creasman, W. T., Fetter, B. F., Clarke-Pearson, D. L., Kaufman, L., and Parker, R. T. (1985). Management of stage Ia carcinoma of the cervix. *American Journal of Obstetrics and Gynecology* **153**, 164–72.

Crowther, M. E., Corney, R. H., and Shepherd, J. H. (1994). Psychosexual implications of gynaecological cancer. *British Medical Journal* **308**, 869–70.

Crum, C. P., Idenberg, H., Richard, R. M., and Gissman, L. (1984). Human papillomavirus type-16 and early cervical neoplasia. *New England Journal of Medicine* **310**, 880–3.

Currie, D. W. (1971). Operative treatment of carcinoma of the cervix. *Journal of Obstetrics and Gynaecology of the British Commonwealth* **78**, 385–405.

Darai, G., Braun, R., Flugel, R. M., and Munk, K. (1977). Malignant transformation of rat embryo fibroblasts by herpes simplex virus. *Nature* **265**, 744–5.

Dareng, D., Frobert, J. L., and Beau, G. (1985). Tumour volume in the assessment of cervical cancer prognosis. *Gynecologic Oncology* **22**, 12–22.

De Villiers, A., Wagner, D., Schneider, A., Wesch, H., Miklaw, H., Wahrendorf, J., *et al.* (1987). Human papillomavirus infection in women with and without abnormal cervical cytology, *Lancet* **ii**, 703–5.

Dottino, D. R., Plaxe, S. C., Beddoe, A. M., Johnson, C., and Cohen, C. J. (1991). Induction chemotherapy followed by radical surgery in cervical cancer. *Gynecologic Oncology* **40**, 7–11.

Dreesman, G. R., Burek, J., Adam, A., Kaufman, R. H., Melnick, J. L., Powell, K. L., *et al.* (1980). Expression of herpes virus induced antigens in human cervical cancer. *Nature* **283**, 591–3.

Duff, R. and Rapp, F. (1973). Oncogenic transformation of hamster embryo cells after exposure to herpes simplex virus type I. *Journal of Virology* **12**, 209–17.

Durst, M., Gissmann, L., Ikenberg, H., and Hausen, H. (1983). A papillomavirus DNA from a cervical carcinoma. *Proceedings of the National Academy of Science USA* **80**, 3812–15.

Eglin, R. P., Sharp, F., MacLean, A. B., Macnab, J. C. M., Clements, J. B., and Wilkie, N. M. (1981). Detection of RNA complimentary to HSV-DNA in human cervical cell neoplasms. *Cancer Research* **41**, 3597–603.

Eglin, R. P., Kitchener, H. C., MacLean, A. B., Denholm, R. B., Cordiner, J. F., and Sharp, F. (1984). The presence of RNA complimentary to HSV-2 DNA in cervical intraepithelial neoplasia after laser therapy. *British Journal of Obstetrics and Gynaecology* **91**, 265–9.

Einhorn, N., Patek, E., and Sjoberg, B. (1985). Outcome of different treatment modalities in cervical carcinoma stages Ib and IIa. *Cancer* **55**, 949–55.

Evans, A. S. and Monaghan, J. M. (1985). Spontaneous resolution of cervical warty atypia. *British Journal of Obstetrics and Gynaecology* 92, 165–9.

Falk, V., Lundgren, N., Wuarfordt, L., and Arstrom, K. (1982). Primary surgical treatment of carcinoma stage I of uterine cervix. *Acta Obstetrica et Gynaecologica Scandinavica* 61, 481–6.

Friedlander, M., Kaye, S. B., Sullivan, A., Atkinson, K., Elliott, P., Coppleson, M., *et al.* (1983). Cervical carcinoma: a drug responsive tumour. *Gynaecologic Oncology* 16, 275–81.

Fuller, A. F., Elliott, N., Kosloff, C., and Lewis, J. L. (1989). Determinants of increased risk for recurrence in patients undergoing radical surgery for stage Ib and IIa cervical cancer. *Gynaecological Oncology* 33, 34–9.

Gagnon, F. (1950). Contribution to the study of aetiology of cancer of the cervix. *American Journal of Obstetrics and Gynecology* 60, 516–22.

Galloway, D. A. and McDougall, J. K. (1983). The oncogenic potential of herpes simplex viruses. *Nature* 302, 21–4.

Gissmann, L., Wolnick, L., Ikenberg, H., Koldovsky, O., Schmurch, H. G., and Hausen, H. (1983). Human papilloma-virus types 6 and 11 DNA sequences in genital and laryngeal papillomas and cervical smears. *Proceedings of the National Academy of Science USA* 80, 560–8.

Greenberg, E. R., Vessey, M., McPherson, K., and Yeates, D. (1985). Cigarette smoking and cancer of the uterine cervix. *British Journal of Cancer* 51, 139–41.

Griffiths, M. (1991). 'Nuns, virgins, and spinsters'. Rigoni–Stern and cervical cancer revisited. *British Journal of Obstetrics and Gynaecology* 98, 797–802.

Hacker, N. F. (1988). Clinical and operative staging of cervical cancer. *Ballière's Clinical Obstetrics and Gynaecology* 2, 747–59.

Haie, C., Pejovic, M. H., Gerbaulet, A., Hariot, J. C., Pourquier, H., Delouche, J. *et al.* (1988). Is prophylactic para-aortic irradiation worthwhile in the treatment of advanced cervical carcinoma? *Radiotherapy and Oncology* 11, 101–12.

Handley, W. S. (1936). The prevention of cancer. *Lancet* i, 987–91.

Hasumi, K., Sakamoto, A., and Sugano, H. (1980). Microinvasive carcinoma of the uterine cervix. *Cancer* 45, 928–31.

Hausen, H. Z. (1982). Human genetic cancer. *Lancet* ii, 1370–2.

Hopkins, M. P. and Morley, G. W. (1991). Stage Ib squamous cell carcinoma of the cervix: clinicopathological features related to survival. *American Journal of Obstetrics and Gynecology* 164 1520–9.

Hoskins, W. J. (1988). Prognostic factors for risk of recurrence in stages Ib and IIa cervical cancer. *Ballière's Clinical Obstetrics and Gynaecology* 2, 817–28.

Ireland, D., Hardiman, P., and Monaghan, J. M. (1985). Adenocarcinoma of the uterine cervix. *Obstetrics and Gynecology* 65, 82–5.

Iversen, T., Kjorstad, K. E., and Martimbeau, P. W. (1982). Treatment results in carcinoma of the cervix stage Ib in a total population. *Gynaecologic Oncology* 14, 1–5.

Junor, E. J., Symonds, R. P., Watson, E. R., and Lamont, D. W. (1989). Survival of younger cervical cancer patients treated by radical radiotherapy in the west of Scotland, 1964–84. *British Journal of Obstetrics and Gynaecology* 96, 522–8.

Kessler, I. I. (1974). Perspectives on the epidemiology of carcinoma of the cervix. *Cancer Research* 34, 1091–110.

Kessler, I. I. (1976). Human cervical cancer as a venereal disease. *Cancer Research* 36, 783–91.

Kim, D., Moon, H., Hwang, Y., and Cho, S. (1988). Pre-operative adjuvant chemotherapy in the treatment of cervical cancer stage Ib, IIa, and IIb with bulky tumour. *Gynaecologic Oncology* 29, 321–32.

Kitchener, H. C. (1988). Genital virus infections and cervical neoplasia. *British Journal of Obstetrics and Gynaecology* **95**, 182–91.

Kjorstad, K. E. and Bond, B. (1984). Stage Ib adenocarcinoma of the cervix. *American Journal of Obstetrics and Gynecology* **150**, 297–9.

Kreider, J. W., Howett, W. K., Wolfe, S. A., Bartlett, G. L., Zianu, R. J., Sedlacek, T. V., *et al.* (1985). Morphological transformation *in vivo* of human uterine cervix with papillomavirus. *Nature* **317**, 639–41.

Kurman, R. J., Jenson, A. B., and Lancaster, W. D. (1983). Papillomavirus infection of the cervix. *American Journal of Surgical Pathology* **7**, 39–52.

Lai, C. H., Lin, T. S., Solng, Y. K., and Chen, H. F. (1989). Adjuvant chemotherapy after radical hysterectomy for cervical cancer. *Gynecologic Oncology* **35**, 193–8.

Lang, D. J. and Kummer, J. F. (1972). Demonstration of cytomegalovirus in semen. *New England Journal of Medicine* **387**, 756–8.

La Polla, J. P., Schlaerth, J. B., Baddis, O., and Morrow, C. P. (1986). The influence of surgical staging on the evaluation and treatment of patients with cervical carcinoma. *Gynaecologic Oncology* **24**, 194–206.

Larson, D. M., Stringer, C. A., Copeland, L. J., Gershenson, D. M., Malone, J. M., and Rutledge, F. N. (1987). Stage Ib cervical carcinoma treated with radical hysterectomy and pelvic lymphadenectomy: role of adjuvant radiotherapy. *Obstetrics and Gynecology* **69**, 378–81.

McCance, D. J., Walker, P. G., Dyson, S. L., Coleman, D. V., and Singer, A. (1983). Presence of human papillovirus DNA sequences in cervical intraepithelial neoplasia. *British Medical Journal* **287**, 784–8.

McCance, D. J., Campion, M. J., Clarkson, P. K., Chesters, P. M., Jenkins, D., and Singer, A. (1985). Prevalence of human papillovirus type-16 DNA sequences in cervical intraepithelial neoplasia and invasive cancer of the cervix. *British Journal of Obstetrics and Gynaecology* **92**, 1101–5.

McDougall, J. K., Galloway, D. A., and Fenoglio, C. M. (1980). Cervical carcinoma. *International Journal of Cancer* **25**, 1–8.

Macnab, J. C. M. and Timbury, M. C. (1976). Combination of ts-mutants by a herpes simplex virus ts-transformed cell line. *Nature* **261**, 233–5.

Macnab, J. C. M., Walkinshaw, S. A., Cordiner, J. W., and Clements, J. B. (1986). Human papillomavirus in clinically and histologically normal tissue of patients with genital carcinoma. *New England Journal of Medicine* **315**, 1052–8.

Martimbeau, P. W., Kjorstad, K. E., and Iversen, T. (1978). Stage Ib carcinoma of the cervix, the Norwegian Radium Hospital. *American Journal of Obstetrics and Gynecology* **131**, 389–94.

Meanwell, C. A., Cox, M. F., Blackledge, B., and Maitland, N. J. (1987). Human papillomavirus 16 DNA in normal and malignant cervical epithelium. *Lancet* i, 703–7.

Meanwell, C. A., Kelly, K. A., Wilson, S., Roginski, C., Woodman, C., Griffiths, R., *et al.* (1988). Young age as a prognostic factor in cervical cancer. *British Medical Journal* **296**, 386–91.

Meigs, J. B. (1951). Radical hysterectomy with bilateral pelvic lymph node dissections. *American Journal of Obstetrics and Gynecology* **62**, 854–65.

Meisels, A., Fortin, R., and Roy, M. (1977). Condylomatous lesions of the cervix. *Acta Cytologica* **61**, 379–90.

Meisels, A., Morin, C., and Casas-Cordero, M. (1982). Human papillomavirus infection of the uterine cervix. *International Journal of Gynaecological Pathology* **1**, 75–94.

Melnick, J. L., Lewis, R., Wimberley, I., Kaufman, R. H., and Adam, E. (1978). Association of cytomegalovirus infection with cervical cancer. *Intervirology* **10**, 115–19.

Mitchell, H., Draker, M., and Medley, G. (1986). Prospective evaluation of risk of cervical cancer and the cytological evidence of human papillovirus infection. *Lancet* i, 573–5.

Morgan, P. R., Anderson, M. C., Buckley, C. H., Murdoch, J. B., Lopes, A., Duncan, I. D., *et al.* (1993). The Royal College of Obstetricians and Gynaecologists microinvasive carcinoma of the cervix study. *British Journal of Obstetrics and Gynaecology* **100**, 664–8.

Morley, G. W. and Seski, J. C. (1976). Radical pelvic surgery versus radiation therapy for stage I carcinoma of the cervix. *American Journal of Obstetrics and Gynecology* **126**, 785–98.

Morrow, C. O. (1980). Is pelvic irradiation beneficial in the post-operative management of stage Ib carcinoma of the cervix with pelvic lymph node metastases treated by radical hysterectomy and pelvic lymphadenectomy? *Gynaecologic Oncology* **10**, 105–10.

Murdoch, J. B. (1988). Histological and cytological evidence of viral infection in human papillomavirus type-16 DNA sequences in cervical intraepithelial neoplasia and normal tissue. *British Medical Journal* **296**, 318–25.

Nahmias, A. J., Jocey, W. E., Naib, J. M., Luce, C. F., and Guest, B. A. (1970). Antibodies to herpes virus hominis types I and II in human. *American Journal of Epidemiology* **91**, 547–52.

Nahmias, A. J., Naib, Z. M., and Josey, W. (1974). Epidemiological studies relating genital herpes infection to cancer of the cervix. *Cancer Research* **34**, 1111–17.

Naib, Z. M. (1970). Cytology of TRIC agent infection of the eyes of newborn infants. *Acta Cytologica* **14**, 390–5.

Naib, Z. M., Nahmias, A. J., and Jocey, W. E. (1966). Cytology and histopathology of cervical herpes simplex infection. *Cancer* **19**, 1026–30.

Paavonen, J., Vesterinen, E., Mayer, B., Saikku, P., Suni, J., Purola, E., *et al.* (1979). Genital chlamydia infections in patients with cervical atypia. *Obstetrics and Gynecology* **54**, 589–91.

Park, M., Lonsdale, D. M., Timbury, M. C., Subak-Sharpe, J. H., and Macnab, J. C. M. (1980). Genetic retrieval of viral genome sequences from herpes simplex virus transformed cells. *Nature* **285**, 412–15.

Pasca, A. S., Kummerlander, L., Pejtsik, B., and Pali, K. (1975). Herpes virus antibodies and antigens in patients with cervical anaplasia and controls. *Journal of the National Cancer Institute* **55**, 775–81.

Pasca, A. S., Kummerlander, L., Pejtsik, B., Krammer, K., and Pali, K. (1976). Herpes simplex virus specific antigens in exfoliated cervical cells from women with and without cervical anaplasia. *Cancer Research* **36**, 2130–2.

Peel, K. R., Khoury, G. G., Joslin, C. A. F., O'Donovan, P. J., Mgaya, H., Keates, G., *et al.* (1991). Cancer of the cervix in women under 40 years of age, a regional survey. *British Journal of Obstetrics and Gynaecology* **98**, 993–1000.

Perez, C. A., Kuske, R. R., Camel, H. M., Galakatos, A. E., Henderman, M. A., Kao, M. S., *et al.* (1988). Analysis of pelvic tumour control and impact on survival in cancer of the uterine cervix treated with radiation alone. *International Journal of Radiation, Oncology, Biology and Physics* **14**, 613–21.

Phillips, D. H., Hewer, A., Malcolm, A. D. B., Ward, W., and Coleman, D V. (1990). Smoking and DNA damage in cervical cells. *Lancet* **335**, 417.

Pipert, J. F., Wells, C. J., Schwartz, P. E., and Feinstein, A. R. (1993). The importance of symptoms and comorbidity on prognosis in stage IB cervical cancer. *American Journal of Obstetrics and Gynecology* **169**, 598–604.

Prempree, T., Patanaphan, V., Sewchand, W., and Scott, R. M. (1983). The influence of patient's age and tumour grade on the prognosis of carcinoma of the cervix. *Cancer* **51**, 1764–71.

Rabinovich, M. G., Focaccia, G., Ferreyra, R., Elem, R., Elem, Y., Leone, B. A., *et al.* (1991). Neoadjuvant chemotherapy for cervical carcinoma. *Obstetrics and Gynecology* **78**, 685–8.

Rampone, J. F., Klem, V., and Kjolstad, P. (1973). Combined treatment of stage Ib carcinoma of the cervix. *Obstetrics and Gynecology* **41**, 163–7.

Reid, B., French, P. W., Singer, A., Hogan, B. E., and Coppleson, M. (1978). Sperm basic proteins in cervical carcinoma. *Lancet* ii, 60–2.

Remy, J. C., Maio, T. D., Fruchter, R. G., Sedlis, A., Boyce, J. G., Sohn, C. K., *et al.* (1990). Adjunctive radiation after radical hysterectomy in stage Ib squamous cell carcinoma of the cervix. *Gynecologic Oncology* **38**, 161–5.

Rojel, J. (1953). Uterine cancer and syphilis. *Acta Pathologica et Microbiologica Scandinavica* **Supp. 97**, 46–58.

Rotkin, I. D. (1973). A comparison and review of key epidemiological factors in cancer of the cervix. *Cancer Research* **33**, 1353–67.

Rotman, M., John, M. J., Moon, S. H., Choi, K. N., Stowe, S. M., Abitbol, A., *et al.* (1979). Limitations of adjunctive surgery in carcinoma of the cervix. *International Journal of Radiation Oncology, Biology, and Physics* **5**, 327–32.

Ruge, S., Pagel, J., and Hording, U. (1985). Bromocriptine in the treatment of carcinoma of the cervix. *Gynecologic Oncology* **21**, 356–8.

Russell, J. M., Blair, V., and Hunter, R. D. (1987). Cervical carcinoma: prognosis in younger patients. *British Medical Journal* **295**, 300–3.

Schachter, J., Hill, E. C., King, E. B., Coleman, V. R., Jones, P., and Mayer, K. F. (1975). Chlamydial infection in women with cervical dysplasia. *American Journal of Obstetrics and Gynecology* **123**, 753–7.

Schneider, A., Kraus, H., Schuhmann, R., and Gissmann, L. (1985). Papillomavirus infection of the lower genital tract. *International Journal of Cancer* **35**, 443–8.

Sedlis, A., Fall, S., Tsukada, Y., Park, R., Mungan, C., Shingleton, L. I., *et al.* (1979). Microinvasive carcinoma of the uterine cervix—a clinicopathological study. *American Journal of Obstetrics and Gynecology* **137**, 64–74.

Siebel, M. M., Freeman, M. G., and Graves, W. L. (1980). Carcinoma of the cervix and sexual function. *Obstetrics and Gynecology* **55**, 484–7.

Shepherd, J. H. (1989). Revised FIGO staging for gynaecological cancer. *British Journal of Obstetrics and Gynaecology* **96**, 889–92.

Shingleton, H. M., Gore, H., Bradley, D.H., and Soong, S. J. (1981). Adenocarcinoma of the cervix. *American Journal of Obstetrics and Gynecology* **139**, 799–813.

Sigurdsson, K., Hrafnkelsson, J., Geirsson, G., Gudmundsson, J., and Salvarsdottir, A. (1991). Screening as a prognostic factor in cervical cancer. *Gynecologic Oncology* **43**, 64–70.

Simon, N. L., Gore, H., Shingleton, H. M., Soong, S. J., Orr, J., and Hatch, K. D. (1986). Study of superficially invasive carcinoma of the cervix. *Obstetrics and Gynecology* **68**, 19–23.

Simons, A. M., Phillips, D. H., and Coleman, D. V. (1993). Damage to DNA in cervical epithelium related to tobacco smoking. *British Medical Journal* **306**, 1444–8.

Skegg, D. C. G., Corwin, P. A., Paul, C., and Doll, R. (1982). Importance of the male factor in cancer of the cervix. *Lancet* ii, 581–3.

Smale, S. E., Perry, C. M., Ashby, M. A., and Baker, J. W. (1987). Influence of age on prognosis in carcinoma of the cervix. *British Journal of Obstetrics and Gynaecology* **94**, 784–7.

Smiley, L. M., Burke, T. W., Silva, E. G., Morris, M., Gerschenson, D. M., and

Wharton, J. T. (1991). Prognostic factors in stage Ib squamous cell carcinoma patients. *Obstetrics and Gynecology* **77**, 271-5.

Stanhope, C. R., Smith, J. P., Wharton, J. T., Rutledge, F. N., Fletcher, G. H., and Gallagher, H. S. (1980). Carcinoma of the cervix: effect of age on survival. *Gynaecologic Oncology* **10**, 188-93.

Stehman, F. B., Bundy, B. N., Hanjani, P., Fowler, W. C., Abdulhay, G., and Whitney, C. W. (1987). Biopsy of the scalene fat pad in carcinoma of the cervix uteri. *Surgery, Gynaecology, and Obstetrics* **165**, 503-6.

Steward, H. L., Dunham, L. J., Casper, J., Dorn, H. F., Thomas, L. B., Edgecomb, J. H., *et al.* (1966). Epidemiologies of cancers of uterine cervix and corpus, breast, and ovary in Israel and New York City. *Journal of the National Cancer Institute* **37**, 1-95.

Sutton, G. P., Bundy, D. N., Delgardo, G., Sevin, B. U., Creasman, W. T., Major, F. J., *et al.* (1992). Ovarian metastases and carcinoma of the cervix. *American Journal of Obstetrics and Gynecology* **166**, 50-3.

Swann, S. H. and Petitti, D. B. (1982). A review of problems of bias and confounding in epidemiologic studies of cervical neoplasia and contraceptive use. *American Journal of Epidemiology* **115**, 10-18.

Syrjanen, K., Vayrynen, M., Saarikoski, R., Mantyiari, R., Parkkinen, S., Hippelainen, M., *et al.* (1985). Natural history of cervical human papillomavirus infection based on prospective follow-up. *British Journal of Obstetrics and Gynaecology* **92**, 1086-92.

Terris, M. and Oalmann, M. C. (1960). Carcinoma of the cervix. *Journal of the American Medical Association* **174**, 1847-51.

Thigpen, T., Shingleton, H., Homesley, H., Lagasse, L., and Blessing, J. (1981). *Cis*platinum in treatment of advanced or recurrent squamous cell carcinoma of the cervix. *Cancer* **48**, 899-903.

Van Nagell, J. R., Greenwell, N., Powell, D. F., Donaldson, E. S., Hanson, M. B., and Gay, E. C. (1983). Microinvasive carcinoma of the cervix. *American Journal of Obstetrics and Gynecology* **145**, 981-91.

Vessey, M. P., Villard-Mackintosh, L., McPherson, A., and Yeates, D. (1989). Mortality amongst oral contraceptive users. *British Medical Journal* **299**, 1487-91.

Wakefield, J., Yule, R., Smith, A., and Adelstein, A. M. (1973). Carcinoma cervix uteri related to husband's occupation. *British Medical Journal* **2**, 142-3.

Walker, P. G., Colley, N. V., Grubb, C., Tejerin, A., and Oriel, J. D. (1983*a*). Abnormalities of the uterine cervix in women with vulval warts. *British Journal of Venereal Diseases* **59**, 120-3.

Walker, P. G., Singer, A., Dyson, J. L., Shah, K. V., Wilten, J., and Coleman, D. V. (1983*b*). Colposcopy in the diagnosis of papillomavirus infection of the cervix. *British Journal of Obstetrics and Gynaecology* **90**, 1082-6.

Walker, P. G., Singer, A., Dyson, J. L., Shah, K. V., To, A., and Coleman, D. V. (1983*c*). The prevalence of human papillomavirus antigens in patients with cervical intraepithelial neoplasia. *British Journal of Cancer* **48**, 99-101.

Webb, M. J. and Symmonds, R. E. (1979). Wertheim hysterectomy—a reappraisal. *Obstetrics and Gynecology* **54**, 140-5.

Wertheim, E. (1912). Extended abdominal operation for carcinoma uteri (based on 500 operative cases). *American Journal of Obstetrics and Gynecology* **66**, 196-232.

Willmott, F. E. (1975). C. M. V. in female patients. *British Journal of Venereal Diseases* **51**, 278-80.

Winklestein, W. (1990). Smoking and cervical cancer—current status: a review. *American Journal of Epidemiology* **131**, 945-57.

World Health Organization Collaborative Study of Neoplasia and Steroid Contraception

(1985). Invasive cervical cancer and combined oral conraception. *British Medical Journal* **290**, 961–5.

Wright, T. C. and Richart, R. M. (1990). Role of human papillomavirus in the pathogenesis of genital tract warts and cancer. *Gynecologic Oncology* **37**, 151–64.

Wright, V. C. and Riopelle, M. A. (1982). Age at time of first intercourse versus chronological age as a basis for Pap smear screening. *Canadian Medical Association Journal* **127**, 127–31.

Yule, R. (1978). Mortality from carcinoma of the cervix. *Lancet* **i**, 1031–2.

13 The management of carcinoma of the ovary

Approximately 4500 new cases of ovarian cancer are diagnosed every year in England and Wales and 3800 women per year die, the highest mortality for any gynaecological malignancy. One woman in 70 (1.4 per cent) will develop ovarian cancer during her life and 1 in 100 will die from it. Ovarian cancer is the fifth commonest malignancy in women, following breast, skin, lung, and colon, and results in more deaths in England and Wales than all other gynaecological malignancies combined. This data is illustrated in Table 13.1 (Office of Population, Census, and Surveys 1985).

The disease occurs more frequently in highly industrialized countries, with an age-adjusted annual incidence of between 11 and 15 per 100 000 women in Sweden, USA, New Zealand, West Germany, Canada, and the UK. In Japan, however, the age-adjusted annual incidence is only 3 per 100 000. There is other evidence of racial variation, with an incidence of 9.3 per 100 000 for black American women and 14.2 per 100 000 for white women. When Japanese women emigrate to the United States, the prevalence of carcinoma of the ovary in their daughters is closer to that of the white American population than to that of their counterparts in Japan.

The prevalence of the disease is age-related, with an increased risk after 45 years and a peak between 60 and 75 years. Thus, the annual incidence between the ages 20 and 29 is 2 per 100 000, whilst it is 55 per 100 000 at age 70. Although the age range at presentation is wide, 80 per cent of women present between the ages of 40 and 70 years, whilst 13 per cent are below the age of 40 years and 7 per cent are above the age of 70 years (Smith and Day 1979).

The survival figures for women with carcinoma of the ovary are particularly gloomy. As can be seen from Table 13.2, only 25 per cent of women present with stage I disease and although the five-year survival figure is 95 per cent for FIGO stage Ia, the overall five-year survival for all cases of stage I carcinoma of the ovary is only 70 per cent (Oram and Jacobs 1987; Smith and Day 1979).

The majority of patients with ovarian cancer have an epithelial carcinoma, although other histological types occur, especially at the extremes of age. Epithelial carcinoma accounts for 89 per cent of tumours (please see Table 13.3) (Smith and Day 1979).

Table 13.1 Cancer in females

Site	Registrations	Deaths
All	99 032	66 021
Breast	22 064	13 454
Skin (excluding melanoma)	10 746	198
Trachea, bronchus, and lung	9771	9789
Colon	7953	6362
Ovary	4406	3831
Cervix uteri	3970	1956
Corpus uteri	3386	1014

From Office of Population, Census, and Surveys (1985)

Table 13.2 Five-year survival figures

Stage at presentation	% Of patients	% Five-year survival
I	25.2	69.7
II	17.6	45.0
III	39.5	13.3
IV	17.7	4.1
All	100	30.6

From Oram and Jacobs (1987); Smith and Day (1979)

The aetiology of ovarian cancer

(1) family history;

(2) reproductive age span;

(3) pregnancy;

(4) oral contraception;

(5) hormone replacement therapy;

(6) viral infections;

(7) talc and asbestos;

(8) diet;

(9) blood group.

Family history

There are numerous reports which suggest a hereditary factor in the aetiology of ovarian cancer. Cramer *et al.* (1983) compared 215 women with ovarian

Table 13.3 Histology of ovarian malignancy

Tumour histology	% Of patients
Epithelial carcinoma	89.1
Germ cell tumour	2.6
Granulosa cell tumour	2.5
Teratoma	1.9
Endodermal sinus tumour	1.4
Sarcoma	1.2
Other	1.3

From Smith and Day (1979)

cancer with 215 female controls matched by age, race, and residence. There was a zero incidence of a family history of ovarian cancer in the controls compared with 1.9 per cent in the index group. Many other series have confirmed the increased risk of carcinoma of the ovary in the presence of a positive family history, quoting a relative risk of between 2 and 10 when a sibling or mother has this disease (Lynch *et al.* 1991; Parazzini *et al.* 1991).

Although it is not generally accepted that epithelial ovarian cancer has a premalignant stage, Gusberg and Deligdisch (1984) reported that the normal identical twin sisters of three women who developed an epithelial ovarian cancer after the menopause were subjected to prophylactic bilateral oophorectomy. Although the ovaries appeared macroscopically normal, they showed histological changes comparable to the dysplasia seen in other epithelial sites within the genital tract.

Reproductive age span

It has been suggested in some epidemiological studies that an early menarche and a late menopause are predisposing factors for ovarian cancer. There is very little evidence for the former. Although some studies have found an increased risk of ovarian cancer in women whose menarche occurred before the age of 11 years (Franceschi *et al.* 1982), most studies have not confirmed an early menarche to be a separate aetiological factor (Booth *et al.* 1989; Cramer *et al.* 1983; Parazzini *et al.* 1991).

However, the number of ovulations which occur during a woman's life, and a late menopause are both aetiological factors for the development of cancer of the ovary (Booth *et al.* 1989; Franceschi *et al.* 1982; Parazzini *et al.* 1991), and this lends weight to the theory of incessant ovulations. This theory, supported by the epidemiological evidence of the influence of parity and contraception also, would suggest that women with more than 30 years of ovulation have a relative risk of 1.6 of developing carcinoma of the ovary when compared with women with less than 30 years of ovulation (Whittemore *et al.* 1992; Wu *et al.* 1988). It is proposed that repeated ovulation induces trauma in the epithelial surface of the ovary which then predisposes to the development of ovarian cancer (Casagrande *et al.* 1979; Khoo 1986).

Pregnancy

The protective effect of pregnancy against the development of ovarian cancer is now well documented. For instance, Cramer *et al.* (1983), in a comparison of 215 white women from Boston compared with 215 controls matched by age, race, and residence, demonstrated that 36.3 per cent of the patients with ovarian cancer were nulliparous as compared to 18.1 per cent of the controls. Giving nulliparity a relative risk of one, the relative risk following one or two pregnancies was 0.51, after three or four pregnancies 0.32, and after five or more pregnancies 0.26. The age at the first pregnancy was not relevant. Other authors have produced similar relative risks (Booth *et al.* 1989; Franceschi *et al.* 1982).

   In order to reduce the risk of ovarian cancer, a pregnancy does not have to have been completed. Even miscarriages produce a decrease in the risk of cancer comparable to that from a term pregnancy (Parazzini *et al.* 1991). The age at first pregnancy is no longer considered to be a significant aetiological factor so long as that pregnancy occurred before the age of 35 years (Booth *et al.* 1989; Parazzini *et al.* 1991).

Oral contraception

There would appear to be a significant protective effect from the use of oral contraception over and above other methods of contraception, and this would be expected from the theory of incessant ovulation (Khoo 1986; Villard-Mackintosh *et al.* 1989).

   Vessey *et al.* (1989) reported the results of the Oxford Family Planning Group statistics. When standardized for age, parity, and social class, they found:

(1) never-users: 9.2 deaths from ovarian cancer per 100 000 women-years of observation;

(2) users for less than 48 months: 12.1 deaths from ovarian cancer per 100 000 women-years of observation;

(3) users for between 48 and 95 months: 1.8 deaths from ovarian cancer per 100 000 women-years of observation;

(4) users for more than 96 months: 1.5 deaths from ovarian cancer per 100 000 women-years of observation.

   The conclusion from this study is that longterm users of oral contraception have a relative risk of 0.16 for the development of ovarian cancer compared with never-users.

   The Cancer and Steroid Hormone Study Group in the USA (1987) came to similar but less dramatic conclusions. They compared 548 women with epithelial ovarian cancer with 4228 controls. Ever-users of oral contraception had a relative risk of 0.6 compared with never-users. This protective effect appeared to start within three months of commencement of oral contraception and lasted until 15 years after cessation of use. The results were independent of the formulation of the oral contraceptive.

From a review of the literature, the range of relative risks quoted for the development of ovarian cancer in women who used oral contraceptives ranged between 0.16 and 1.8, with most studies quoting a very significant benefit with a relative risk in the region of 0.4–0.6 (Parazzini *et al.* 1991). Translated into clinical terms, women who use oral contraceptives have, potentially, a 60 per cent reduction in the incidence of this disease. Women who are at high risk of cancer of the ovary should perhaps be encouraged to use oral contraception and hence reduce their risk (Gross and Schlesselman 1994).

Hormone replacement therapy

The effect of hormone replacement therapy upon the prevalence of ovarian cancer is not yet clear. Although it is tempting to equate hormone replacement therapy with oral contraception, this is not valid and such extrapolation should not take place. Cramer *et al.* (1982) has suggested that hormone replacement is associated with an increased relative risk of 1.56 for the development of ovarian cancer compared with women who do not take hormone replacement therapy. Other studies have also suggested an increase in the risk of ovarian cancer in women taking hormone replacement therapy. For instance, Booth *et al.* (1989) quote a relative risk of 1.2. However, this is an area of controversy since other authors have suggested a decreased relative risk of 0.8 (La Vecchia *et al.* 1982). A review of the data has suggested either a neutral risk (Booth *et al.* 1989), except for a possible increased risk in the development of endometroid ovarian cancer (Weiss *et al.* 1982) and perhaps an improved survival rate (Eeles *et al.* 1991).

Viral infections

Viral infections are not an important aetiological feature in the development of ovarian cancer but require discussion since many of the earlier epidemiological studies have assessed this factor with conflicting results. Newhouse *et al.* (1977) observed that a past history of mumps appeared to exert a protective effect as regards carcinoma of the ovary, whilst there was a smaller, but nevertheless statistically significant, protective effect from a past history of measles, rubella, and chickenpox. Cramer *et al.* (1983) concluded from their data that a past history of mumps depleted the oocyte, reduced the reproductive span, and hence increased the risk of cancer of the ovary despite the fact that a greater percentage of controls (62 per cent) gave a past history of mumps compared with age-matched women with epithelial ovarian cancer (50 per cent). These authors concluded that subclinical mumps occurred to a greater extent in those patients with ovarian cancer since there was an excess of parotitis in patients with ovarian cancer.

No recent study has provided satisfactory epidemiological data and it is unlikely that a past history of viral infections exert either a protective or a deleterious effect.

Talc and asbestos

Talc is found in powders, soaps, and contraceptive diaphragms and is able to reach the ovary by transvaginal migration as demonstrated by Venter (1981), he was able to show migration of a particulate radioactive tracer attached to talc ([^{99m}Tc]HAM) from the vagina to the peritoneal cavity and the ovaries in 67 per cent of 24 subjects, whilst Henderson *et al.* (1971) found talc particles in ovarian tumours and in normal ovaries, but also found evidence of talc particles in other gynaecological tumours, including cervical tumours.

Epidemiological studies have shown that the use of talc in the genital areas increases the risk of ovarian cancer. For instance, Cramer and Welch (1983) reported that 43 per cent of women with carcinoma of the ovary regularly used talc, either as a dusting powder on the perineum or on their sanitary towels, as compared with 28 per cent of controls. The relative risk for any talc use, adjusted for parity, was 1.9, but in those women who regularly used talc on both sides, the relative risk increased to 3.3. Other studies have confirmed that regular (daily or weekly) use of talc in the genital areas may increase the relative risk of ovarian cancer and perhaps women should be discouraged from this practice (Booth *et al.* 1989; Whittemore *et al.* 1988).

Asbestos has been studied, partly because of the implication of asbestos in the genesis of peritoneal mesotheliomata and, partly because one type of asbestos (anthophyllite) is converted naturally to talc, female workers in the asbestos industry have a small increase in risk for the development of ovarian cancer (Acheson *et al.* 1982; Newhouse *et al.* 1985).

Diet

The evidence that diet may be an aetiological factor in carcinoma of the ovary is difficult to assess for the results are often contradictory, may not be controlled for other factors, and those dietary factors studied often represent random observation. For instance, it is not clear whether the low incidence in Japanese women whilst in Japan, relates to diet or to other environmental factors.

However, there is consistent evidence that coffee drinking represents an aetiological factor, perhaps even showing a dose-response effect (La Vecchia *et al.* 1984). These workers demonstrated that, allowing for other risk factors, and giving non-coffee drinkers a relative risk of 1.0, the relative risk of developing ovarian cancer for drinkers of two, three, or four or more cups of coffee per day was 1.3, 1.7, and 1.8, respectively. There was no increased risk for tea intake or cigarette smoking (La Vecchia *et al.* 1984; Whittemore *et al.* 1988). When the evidence from epidemiological studies was pooled, the relative risk for coffee drinkers compared with non-coffee drinkers was 1.3 (Parazzini *et al.* 1991).

Blood group

Women of blood group A have an increased risk of developing ovarian cancer. In one study, blood group A was identified in 39 per cent of blood donors, but in 44 per cent of women with malignant ovarian disease. When compared to women of blood group O, the relative risk to blood group A women of developing epithelial ovarian cancer was 1.4 (Osborne and De George 1963). This association has been confirmed by other authors (Bjorkolm 1984; Mori *et al.* 1988). It is unlikely that blood group antigens themselves exert any influence on the development of ovarian cancer. It is more likely that this forms part of a more widespread genetic predisposition.

Screening for ovarian tumours

Since prevention would appear to be possible for only a minority of patients, various techniques for screening asymptomatic women in an attempt to diagnose ovarian cancer at a surgically treatable stage have been the subject of recent studies. The screening techniques involved include:

(1) cervical cytology;

(2) pelvic examination;

(3) ultrasound screening;

(4) serological tests.

Cervical cytology

Although a close association would not be expected between cervical cytology and ovarian tumours, Shapiro and Nunez (1983) reported that psommoma bodies may be seen in 10–30 per cent of smears taken from women with adenocarcinoma of the ovary. However, they have also been reported in association with mesothelioma of the peritoneum, adenocarcinoma of the Fallopian tube, and in women wearing an IUCD, and hence cervical cytology does not represent a practical screening option for this disease.

Pelvic examination

The incidence of ovarian tumours being diagnosed at the time of vaginal examination when taking a cervical smear was discussed in the Chapter 11 (Cervical intraepithelial neoplasia). Probably the largest series in the literature

(MacFarlane *et al.* 1955) reported 18 753 vaginal examinations over a 15-year period in women aged 30–80 years. Some 17 pelvic cancers were diagnosed of which six were ovarian. It is unlikely that routine vaginal examination will have a significant impact on the diagnosis of carcinoma of the ovary at an earlier stage.

Ultrasound screening

There is evidence that ultrasound screening of the pelvis will be more accurate than vaginal examination in the diagnosis of asymptomatic ovarian tumours. Andolf *et al.* (1986) performed transabdominal ultrasound and bimanual pelvic examinations in 805 women. In the 39 women with an ultrasonically detected ovarian swelling, only 11 had been detected on bimanual examination and all 4 malignant lesions had been missed. Ultrasound screening is, therefore, superior to bimanual pelvic examination in the detection of ovarian cancer.

Campbell *et al.* (1989 and 1990) screened, with transabdominal ultrasound, 5479 self-referred asymptomatic women aged 18–78 years. Some 5.9 per cent of women had an abnormal scan. The odds that an abnormal scan would indicate the presence of a benign ovarian tumour, any ovarian cancer, or primary ovarian cancer were 1 in 2, 1 in 26, and 1 in 50, respectively. No malignant ovarian tumour was believed to have been missed, and hence the technique would detect a malignant ovarian tumour in 0.2 per cent of all examinations.

The use of transvaginal colour-flow imaging may help to distinguish between malignant and benign pelvic masses in that the new vessel formation associated with malignant tumours is detectable as an area of increased vascularity (Bourne *et al.* 1989; Kawai *et al.* 1992; Kurjack *et al.* 1989). However, the value of this technique in cohort screening is yet to be proven.

Serological tests

It is well recognized that ovarian tumours containing trophoblastic elements may produce hCG, whilst endodermal sinus elements may produce AFP, the former common in germ cell tumours and the latter in yolk sac tumours (Jacobs *et al.* 1993*a*). In terms of screening, the most interesting tumour marker would appear to be CA125. This is a high molecular weight glycoprotein expressed in coelomic epithelium during embryonic development, and defined by radio-immunoassay using murine monoclonal antibodies raised against a serous ovarian cancer cell-line. Bast *et al.* (1983) found evidence of CA125 in the serum of 1 per cent of 888 healthy people, in 6 per cent of 143 in-patients with non-malignant, non-gynaecological disease, but in 82 per cent of 101 patients with known ovarian cancer. Other authors have found raised circulating levels of CA125 in a similar percentage of patients with ovarian cancer (Heinonen *et al.* 1985), but the marker may also be found in women with other conditions including benign ovarian tumours, endometriosis, chronic pelvic inflammatory disease, a fibroid uterus, and pregnancy (Barbieri *et al.* 1986; Heinonen *et al.* 1985; Jacobs *et al.* 1988*a*).

Table 13.4 Screening tests

	No. of patients	No. with any ovarian tumour	No. with malignant ovarian tumour
CA125 +ve and VE +ve	1	1	1
CA125 +ve and VE −ve	30	0	0
CA125 −ve and VE +ve	27	8	0
CA125 −ve and VE −ve	925	0	0

* Vaginal examination
From Jacobs *et al.* (1988*b*)

Table 13.5 Screening tests

	% Specificity
CA125 alone	97.0
VE alone	97.3
CA125 and VE	100
VE and ultrasound	99.0
CA125 and ultrasound	99.8
All three	100

From Jacobs *et al.* (1988 *b*)

The place of CA125 in ovarian cancer screening of asymptomatic women has been studied by Jacobs *et al.* (1988*b* and 1993*b*). These workers recruited 1010 post-menopausal women (age range 45–83 years) to an ovarian cancer screening programme. On the basis of an initial assay and a vaginal examination, the women were divided into four groups and offered ultrasound examination should either the CA125 level have been raised or vaginal examination abnormal. The results of this study, shown in Tables 13.4 and 13.5, suggested a place for whole population screening. In the presence of a normal vaginal examination, it has been estimated that CA125 screening would produce 50 false-positive screening tests for each cancer detected, whilst the combination of both an abnormality on vaginal examination and a raised CA125 assay would be highly suggestive of ovarian cancer (Jacobs *et al.* 1988*b*; Westhoff and Randall 1991).

The place of CA125 screening and ultrasound screening, either together or singly, requires assessment before such tests are offered to the asymptomatic population in general. In the interim, perhaps women considered to be at an increased risk of ovarian cancer (especially those with a strong family history) should currently be offered one or other screening tests on an annual basis (Bourne *et al.* 1991; Sparks and Varner 1991). In a recent review on ovarian cancer screening, the authors argued that the number of lives which could be saved by screening would represent only a proportion of those which would be saved by the more widespread use of oral contraceptives (Creasman and DiSaia 1991). The multimodality to cervical cancer screening is stressed (Karlan *et al.* 1993; Webb 1993).

The place of prophylactic oophorectomy

There is diverse opinion, both amongst doctors and patients, about prophylactic oophorectomy which, in general, is only an option at the time of abdominal hysterectomy for benign pathology.

There have been numerous studies which have estimated the percentage of women who present with ovarian cancer who have previously undergone surgery for benign pelvic pathology (generally abdominal hysterectomy) and therefore who had an opportunity for prophylactic oophorectomy. By performing prophylactic oophorectomy at the time of hysterectomy in women below the age of the menopause, these studies have suggested that somewhere between 4–14 per cent of subsequent cases of ovarian carcinoma would have been prevented (Counseller *et al.* 1955; McGowan 1987; Parazzini *et al.* 1993; Sightler *et al.* 1991). Jacobs and Oram (1988) gathered ten series of 4106 patients with ovarian cancer, of whom 5.6 per cent had undergone a previous abdominal hysterectomy for benign disease. The place of prophylactic oophorectomy at the time of hysterectomy for benign disease should probably be discussed with patients who can be informed of the pros and cons of prophylactic oophorectomy together with the pros and cons of longterm hormone replacement therapy.

It has been suggested that the prevalence of ovarian cancer in patients who have had their ovaries conserved at the time of abdominal hysterectomy will be significantly less than the prevalence in the overall population, since the ovaries will have been inspected. Should this be so, then the above argument would not hold, or at least the figure of 5.6 per cent would have to be revised (Booth *et al.* 1989). However, the evidence does not support this view. Oram and Jacobs (1987) accumulated 12 series which represented 30 555 women who had both ovaries conserved at hysterectomy and, of these, 0.2 per cent ultimately developed cancer of the ovary. Based upon the annual prevalence of 15 cases per 100 000, the expected incidence would have been 0.16 per cent, and, therefore, there would seem no reason to believe that women who have had their ovaries conserved at the time of hysterectomy will have a lower than expected chance of developing ovarian cancer.

Prophylactic oophorectomy at the time of abdominal hysterectomy for benign disease should, therefore, be considered and debated. Unfortunately, prophylactic oophorectomy does not completely remove the risk of development of epithelial ovarian cancer. The germinal epithelium of the ovary is continuous with the peritoneum and it has been reported that high-risk women who have undergone prophylactic oophorectomy have subsequently developed an ovarian-type malignancy arising from the abdominal or pelvic peritoneum (Tobacman *et al.* 1982).

Treatment of ovarian cancer

The optimal surgery in early (stage I) ovarian cancer is total abdominal hysterectomy with bilateral salpingo-oophorectomy and infracolic omentectomy. That omentectomy is indicated is evidenced by the observation that microscopic metastases will be found in an omentum which was macroscopically normal in between 8.9–11 per cent of patients with stage I ovarian cancer (Buchsbaum and Lifshitz 1984; Young *et al.* 1983). The five-year survival following this combination of surgical procedures may be as high as 98 per cent or as low as 70 per cent (Dembo *et al.* 1990; Finn *et al.* 1992).

It is clear, therefore, that one of the reasons why patients with stage I cancer of the ovary have such a bad five-year prognosis is that the disease has often spread beyond the pelvis, even though the surgeon on initial laparotomy may consider that it has not. Young *et al.* (1983) also reported that 9 per cent of patients with stage I and 12 per cent of patients with stage II disease had positive para-aortic nodes, whilst 10 per cent had positive pelvic lymph nodes. On a review of 100 consecutive patients thought to have either stage I or stage II disease by the initial surgeon, some 23 per cent had stage III ovarian cancer. The importance of thorough abdominal examination may be demonstrated by the observation that 10 per cent of patients thought to be stage I, and 20 per cent of patients thought to be stage II, had diaphragmatic involvement. Some surgeons suggest direct visualization of the undersurface of the diaphragm using a fibre-optic light source (Wijnen and Rosenheln 1980). Whilst it may be argued whether or not all cases of ovarian cancer should be dealt with by specialized gynaecological units, it seems inappropriate that up to 25 per cent of all patients with ovarian cancer have their primary operation performed by a general surgeon and not by a gynaecologist (Wijnen and Rosenheln 1980).

Conserving one ovary

When bilateral macroscopic disease is present, the patient is approaching the menopause, or the patient is post-menopausal, removal of both ovaries seems appropriate. However, in younger women who only have macroscopic evidence of unilateral disease, should one ovary be preserved?

There is no evidence that bilateral ovarian removal offers additional survival if the tumour is of borderline malignancy, although it would be wise surgical practice to bisect the contralateral ovary before a decision on its rejection is made (Carter *et al.* 1993; Conrad and Woodruff 1972; Hart and Norris 1973).

The situation with unilateral frankly invasive disease is not as acceptable. Munnell (1969) reported 144 women with unilateral ovarian cancer who underwent total abdominal hysterectomy and bilateral salpingo-oophorectomy, and 46 in whom the other appendage was conserved (and generally the uterus also). This series was not random and the five-year survival for the bilateral salpingo-oophorectomy group was 79 per cent and for the unilateral salpingo-oophorectomy group 74 per cent, but these differences were not statistically significant. However, a microscopic focus of invasive cancer was found in 5 per cent of the 144 patients in whom a clinically normal contralateral ovary was removed. Similarly, Williams and Dockerty (1976) reported 65 women in whom the surgeon found cystic ovarian cancer. In 17 per cent, neoplasia was suspected and confirmed in the other ovary. In 9 per cent, it was not suspected, yet microscopic invasive cancer was found on histological examination of the apparently normal ovary. In apparent stage I disease, whether or not conservative surgery is contemplated, a thorough staging laparotomy should be undertaken. This would involve biopsies of the contralateral ovary, omentum, abdominal and pelvic peritoneal surfaces including diaphragmatic cytology, and retroperitoneal lymph nodes. It is likely that preservations of the contralateral ovary in the presence of an epithelial ovarian cancer is contraindicated unless the tumour is of borderline malignancy.

The role of adjuvant therapy in stage I

In view of the unsatisfactory five-year survival even in stage I disease, adjuvant therapy, either by radiotherapy or cytotoxic therapy, has been considered. This debate still remains controversial.

Most series which consider the role of adjuvant radiotherapy are retrospective and consist of selected patients. Fuks (1975) assessed the results of eight series which compared surgery with surgery and external irradiation for stage I disease. The survival seemed to be improved by irradiation in two series and made worse in six. He also assessed seven series which compared surgery with surgery and external irradiation for stage II disease. Survival was improved by irradiation in all seven. It would seem that adjuvant radiotherapy may be beneficial in stage II disease, but not for stage I.

There have been several randomized trials in which patients who have undergone optimal surgery for stage I disease were randomized to receive no further treatment, or adjuvant therapy either in the form of external irradiation or chemotherapy involving melphalan or *cis*-platinum (Drouin 1979; Redman *et al.* 1987; Young *et al.* 1990). None of these trials showed any statistically significant benefit in survival following adjuvant therapy, either with radiotherapy or chemotherapy, as opposed to no further treatment. However, one randomized trial did demonstrate a decreased rate for recurrences following chemotherapy compared with either no treatment or radiotherapy (Hreshchyshyn *et al.* 1980). In this trial, in which 86 women with stage I ovarian cancer treated surgically were subsequently randomized to no further treatment, external beam radiotherapy, or chemotherapy with melphalan, the recurrence rate at a median of 36 months was 17 per cent, 30 per cent, and 6 per cent, respectively.

Current practice tends, therefore, to favour the view that adjuvant chemotherapy following surgery for stage I disease is not of benefit, but the

Table 13.6 Residual tumour and prognosis

Size of maximum deposit (cm)	No.	Mean survival time (months)
0	29	39
0–0.5	28	29
0.6–1.5	16	18
>1.5	29	11

From Griffiths (1975)

controversy will not be resolved without the results from further larger studies.

It has been suggested that peritoneal cytology may be of help in the management of ovarian malignancy in that peritoneal washings from the pouch of Douglas in a patient with stage I ovarian cancer might indicate the need for chemotherapy should the cytology of the washings be positive but not if they are negative (Keettel *et al.* 1974). There is some evidence that patients with positive washings on cytological examination have an increased survival after adjuvant chemotherapy (Dembo *et al.* 1990; Finn *et al.* 1992) and again, this specific point needs to be the subject of further randomized trials.

Cytoreductive surgery

When the complete removal of all macroscopic tumour at the time of initial surgery is not possible, there is an abundance of evidence that the efficacy of any further therapy, which in general will be chemotherapy or radiotherapy, will be inversely proportional to the size of any residual tumour deposits following primary surgery. Griffiths (1975) reported 102 women with stage II and Ill epithelial ovarian cancer in whom the major determinants of survival were the histological grade of the tumour and the size of the largest residual deposit after primary surgery. In general, poorly differentiated tumours carried a poor prognosis. Similarly, the larger was the size of tumour deposits following cytoreductive surgery, the poorer was the survival, as illustrated in Table 13.6. Similarly, other authors have demonstrated that the smaller is the residual disease after debulking, the longer is the survival following chemotherapy (Delgardo *et al.* 1984; Greco *et al.* 1981; Hacker *et al.* 1983). For instance, Hacker *et al.* reported that the median survival in 31 patients with optimal cytoreduction (no tumour mass larger than 1.5 cm diameter) was 18 months compared with six months for 16 patients in whom this could not be achieved, whilst Delgardo *et al.* reported that the mean survival was 45 months in patients who had been optimally debulked compared with 16 months in those who have not.

So energetically was cytoreductive therapy performed during the last 20 years, that up to 10 per cent of patients underwent bowel resection as part of a cytoreductive regime (Castaldo *et al.* 1981), or underwent partial cystectomy, or even urinary diversion (Berek *et al.* 1982; Carter *et al.* 1991).

However, the view that debulking is of longterm benefit to the patient is now being questioned. For instance, Potter *et al.* (1991) could find no survival benefit between those patients with residual disease after primary surgery and those with residual disease who underwent radical attempts at debulking, including bowel resection. The ability to debulk may, like survival, depend upon the biological characteristics of the tumour such that debulking is only possible in the less aggressive tumours.

A recent review of the evidence concerning the proposed benefit of maximum cytoreductive surgery has suggested that maximum cytoreductive surgery is associated with only a small improvement in median survival time (Hunter *et al.* 1992). These authors performed a meta-analysis of 58 studies which included 6962 patients with advanced ovarian cancer. Using the technique of multiple linear regression to analyse the effects on median survival time, each 10 per cent increase in the number of patients who underwent optimal cytoreductive surgery was associated with a 4 per cent increase in median survival time. This increase in median survival time became relatively unimportant when compared with the observation from the same study that the use of platinum-containing chemotherapy improved the median survival time by 53 per cent.

The only randomized trial of debulking surgery in advanced epithelial ovarian cancer has failed to show a benefit for further debulking surgery, compared with chemotherapy without debulking surgery in patients with bulky residual disease after primary surgery (Redman *et al.* 1994).

Radiotherapy

The place of pelvic radiotherapy in stage I and stage II disease has already been discussed. Hacker *et al.* (1985) reported the place of whole abdominal irradiation in 32 women with residual epithelial ovarian cancer deposits in the abdomen despite cytoreductive surgery and chemotherapy (stage III). Some 47 per cent of patients completed treatment without interruption, 23 per cent completed treatment with interruptions (generally because of myelosuppression), and 30 per cent did not complete treatment (because of either myelosuppression or rapidly progressive disease). Significant myelosuppression, therefore, occurred in 34 per cent of the patients, whilst 30 per cent of the patients required a laparotomy because of small bowel intestinal obstruction.

Similar studies have suggested that irradiation to treat residual abdominal disease is unlikely to be successful (Kjorstad *et al.* 1977; Kucera *et al.* 1990), whilst the complications of irradiation, especially inflammatory bowel disease or intestinal obstruction, remain high (Bolis *et al.* 1990).

Chemotherapy

Since approximately 70 per cent of patients with ovarian cancer present with stage III and IV disease, and since approximately 30 per cent of patients with stage I and II disease relapse, chemotherapy has an important role in the management of ovarian cancer. Overall, the complications of chemotherapy are less than those of radiotherapy in this situation, and, hence, chemotherapy is the treatment option in current practice (Bruzzone *et al.* 1990).

Before discussing the results and complications which may be anticipated in clinical practice, it is perhaps appropriate to trace the development of chemotherapy in ovarian cancer.

Initially, single alkylating agents were used. In an assessment of the results of over 1000 patients treated with melphalan, chlorambucil, or cylcophosphamide, the response rates were up to 65 per cent, with the median survival for responders being between 17 and 20 months, whilst the median survival for non-responders was between six and 13 months. The overall five-year survival was, however, only 7 per cent, suggesting that whilst chemotherapy may prolong survival in a significant number of patients, it cannot really be considered as a curative measure in late disease (Ozols and Young 1984).

Following the limited success of single alkylating agent treatment, combination therapy became popular, and although some series showed an increased survival with combination therapy compared with single therapy, they also demonstrated an increased toxicity (Young *et al.* 1978).

In the 1970s, platinum-containing compounds became available for clinical use, with *cis*-platinum (*cis*-diammine-dichlorplatinum) and its analogues, especially carboplatin, becoming the commonest cytotoxic agents used against ovarian cancer in the UK. Wiltshaw and Kroner (1976) reported 34 women with advanced ovarian cancer resistant to 'conventional chemotherapy'. Some 27 per cent of these patients showed a therapeutic response, one patient having a complete response and eight having partial responses. The mean duration of response was six months with a mean survival time for responders being 12 months after the commencement of therapy as compared with six months in non-responders. Decker (1982) reported a prospective randomized trial of cyclophosphamide in 21 patients with cyclophosphamide and *cis*-platinum in another 21 patients. These patients had advanced ovarian cancer after initial cytoreductive surgery and were reassessed by second-look laparotomy. At the end of two years, there was no progression of tumour in 9.5 per cent of the cyclophosphamide alone group, with a two-year survival of 19 per cent. For the combination group, there was no progression of tumour after two years in 52 per cent with a survival of 62 per cent, suggesting the benefit of *cis*-platinum over alkylating agents (see also p. 000).

There has since been a trend towards the use of the cytotoxic agent carboplatin rather than *cis*-platinum since these drugs seem to be equally effective, both are myelosuppressive, but carboplatin has a lower incidence of nephrotoxicity, ototoxicity, and peripheral neuropathy (Pecorelli *et al.* 1988; Wiltshaw

Table 13.7 Platinum agents

	cis-Platinum (n = 21)		Carboplatin (n = 18)	
Overall response	11	52%	9	50%
Complete response	3	14.3%	3	16.7%
Nephrotoxicity (%)	71		12	
Ototoxicity (%)	65		0	
Peripheral neuropathy (%)	19		0	
Transfusion (%)	38		18	

From Wilshaw *et al.* (1983)

et al. 1983). The results from a randomized comparison of these two agents are shown in Table 13.7. Several authors demonstrated that platinum-containing regimes, in randomized trials, gave superior survival rates and improved clinical response compared with non-platinum regimes. For instance, one randomized trial demonstrated that the *cis*-platinum-containing regime gave a complete clinical response in 63 per cent of patients with a median survival of 19 months compared with a complete clinical response of 38 per cent with a median survival of 12 months in the non-platinum-containing regime (Lambert and Berry 1985). It is possible that the newer platinum analogue CHIP (*cis*-dichloro-*trans*-dihydro-bis-isopropylamine-platinum) is currently under investigation, but no real clinical studies are as yet available.

There is no clear evidence as to the optimal number of courses of platinum-containing compounds, with advice varying between 4–12 cycles, although the rate of response may decline after five courses. It has also been suggested that courses some 21 days apart gave a reasonable balance between side-effects, drug dosage intensity, and performance (Levin and Hryniuk 1987; Thigpen *et al.* 1984).

In order that conclusions may be drawn from chemotherapy trials, the technique of meta-analysis is required since any one trial must be relatively small. There have been several such meta-analyses reported recently and these have allowed certain conclusions to be drawn.

In an analysis of 33 randomized trials of chemotherapy for ovarian carcinoma, Levin and Hryniuk (1987) concluded that multiple agent regimes were associated with a distinct survival advantage over single alkylating agent regimes, and that multi-agent regimes containing *cis*-platinum had particular advantage.

In a second meta-analysis, Peto and Easton (1989) came to the following conclusions:

1. From an analysis of 17 trials comprising 3081 patients, they concluded that non-platinum combinations were probably not significantly superior to non-platinum single agent regimes.

2. From 16 trials comprising 2058 patients, they concluded that *cis*-platinum regimes were statistically significantly superior to non-*cis*-platinum regimes.

3. From four trials comprising 670 patients, they concluded that *cis*-platinum in multi-agent regimes was statistically significantly superior to *cis*-platinum alone.

The most recent meta-analysis assessed 45 randomized trials involving 8139 patients (Advanced Ovarian Cancer Trialists Group 1991). They came to the following conclusions:

1. Despite the wealth of literature currently available, *no firm conclusions* can be reached, and, hence, the rest of the conclusions are no stronger than suggestions.

2. Single platinum based regimes were as effective as non-platinum combinations, but no more so.

3. Platinum-containing combinations were superior to non-platinum-containing combinations.

4. Platinum-containing combinations were superior to single platinum regimes.

5. *Cis*-platinum and carboplatin were equally effective.

6. Survival tended to be in the region of 15–20 per cent at five years.

These meta-analyses have allowed several conclusions to be drawn, Perhaps the four most important conclusions are that platinum-containing combinations are currently the most effective form of chemotherapy available, that carboplatin is the agent of choice, that new drugs or drug-containing regimes need to be assessed in large multicentre randomized trials, and that survival is still very limited, but that the median survival time may be increased by 53 per cent (Hunter *et al.* 1992).

A rational approach to the choice of chemotherapeutic agent has been suggested by *in vitro* drug sensitivity testing, but this will be of limited value because only 40–50 per cent of tumour cells grow under laboratory conditions, and the response *in vitro* is not necessarily the same as the response *in vivo* (Ozols and Young 1984). However, Hunter *et al.* (1987) grew ovarian tumour cells in culture with cytotoxic agents with and without danazol and with danazol alone, danazol being known to affect protein synthesis adversely via an inhibitory effect on enzyme systems and the RNA synthesis. Of 33 cultured tumours (out of 40 attempted) danazol alone had no effect, whereas danazol had a statistically significant enhancing effect on the inhibition of cell growth when combined with *cis*-platinum, adriamycin, bleomycin, and chlorambucil as compared to the cytotoxic agent alone, but did not improve the inhibitory effect of thiotepa. This has not yet been tested in clinical practice.

There is no doubt that the side-effects of cytotoxic therapy often limit their use, both in terms of dosage and duration. However, recent developments have enabled significant reductions to be made in the severity of the commonest important complications of platinum therapy, namely nephrotoxicity, nausea and vomiting, neurotoxicity, and bone marrow depression.

Platinum-containing compounds are nephrotoxic, probably having a direct toxic effect on both the renal glomerular apparatus and the renal tubules (Meijer *et al.* 1983). There is biochemical evidence of nephrotoxicity in the majority of patients given *cis*-platinum but in only 12 per cent of those given carboplatin (Wiltshaw *et al.* 1983). This complication may be reduced to an almost negligible incidence by an excessive intravenous hydration with forced diuresis at the time of administration of the agent (Ozols *et al.* 1984).

Nausea with vomiting is a common and unpleasant side-effect of platinum-containing compounds and, without prophylaxis, occurs in 100 per cent of patients (Cubeddu *et al.* 1990; Gralla *et al.* 1988). Non-specific antiemetic therapy, such as chlorpromazine and metoclopramide, is of benefit, albeit limited, in reducing the number of episodes of vomiting in patients receiving such therapy (Cunningham *et al.* 1985; Gralla *et al.* 1981). The observation that 5-hydroxytryptamine (serotonin or 5-HT) selective antagonists ameliorates the vomiting has allowed for the development of more specific and powerful agents (Cunningham *et al.* 1987). Recent studies have demonstrated that the 5-HT_3 antagonist ondansetron (in a dosage of 4 mg given by intravenous injection 30 minutes before commencing cytotoxic therapy) reduced the mean number of episodes of vomiting by up to 83 per cent, whilst 46 per cent of patients experienced neither nausea nor vomiting (Cubeddu *et al.* 1990; *Drug and Therapeutics Bulletin* 1992; Jones *et al.* 1991; Marty *et al.* 1990). Side-effects from ondansetron are relatively unusual, but headache may occur (Cubeddu *et al.* 1990: Marty *et al.* 1990). Dexamethasone (8 mg intravenously before chemotherapy and orally in a reducing dose thereafter) is equally as effective as ondansetron in the prevention of cytotoxic therapy induced vomiting, and may even reduce the incidence of vomiting further when given in combination with ondansetron (Jones *et al.* 1991; *Lancet* 1991). The mechanism of action of dexamethasone, and the optimal treatment regime, have yet to be elucidated.

Peripheral sensory neuropathy may develop in up to 45 per cent of patients receiving platinum therapy, especially when increased dosage is considered (Mollman 1990; Ozols *et al.* 1985). Randomized studies have demonstrated that using a neurotrophic peptide ACTH analogue not only reduced the incidence of neurotoxicity (from 43 per cent to 8 per cent), but allowed for higher doses of *cis*-platinum to be used before neurotoxicity occurred. There were no side-effects for ACTH which is believed to facilitate neural repair (van der Hoop *et al.* 1990). If larger studies confirm the value of this agent in the prevention of neurotoxicity, the prognosis for selected patients with cancer who may be able to receive higher doses of platinum-containing compounds may be dramatically improved (Mollman 1990).

Bone marrow depression is a potentially lethal complication of cytotoxic therapy resulting in aplastic anaemia and infection, distressing morbidity may also occur, such that in one series 63 per cent of patients receiving *cis*-platinum required blood transfusion for their symptomatic anaemia (Wiltshaw *et al.*

1986). When bone marrow recovery is slow or absent, the individual cell lines may be stimulated by individual growth factors, although at the current time no single growth factor has been identified which will stimulate all cell lines. Thus, red-cell lines can be stimulated with erythropoeitin, white-cell lines by specific recombinant growth factors (such as granulocyte colony-stimulating factor), and platelet cell-lines by interleukin 6 (Brandt *et al.* 1988; Khwaja and Goldstone 1991; Sheridan *et al.* 1989). The ultimate clinical place for these growth factors has yet to be determined by controlled clinical trials with specific end-points.

It may be seen that the side-effects of cytotoxic therapy, which currently limit their value, may well be controllable and at a minimal level this would improve the quality of life of these patients, but controlling the side-effects potentially has important implications for survival if it allows for more effective chemotherapy to be given.

It may be that higher concentrations of drugs can be administered with fewer side-effects when direct intraperitoneal administration takes place. This is particularly attractive in the control of ascites. Myers (1984) reviewed nine series consisting of 44 patients who underwent intraperitoneal drug treatment involving adriamycin, methotrexate, or 5-fluorouracil. Of these 44 patients, six showed a complete response and eight a partial response, suggesting no obvious benefit over systemic administration. However, the clinical evidence upon which to make any judgement is still very limited.

Radioisotopes

The use of intraperitoneal radioactive compounds, initially zinc and then gold, have been superseded by radioactive phosphorus (^{32}P). This isotope is administered in a colloidal suspension of chromic phosphate, via an intraperitoneal catheter, and emits electrons into the peritoneum.

Although this has yet to be confirmed in larger studies, there is some evidence that adjuvant therapy using intraperitoneal ^{32}P-labelled compounds may improve survival compared with surgery alone (Piver *et al.* 1978). However, the major indication for intraperitoneal radioisotopes relates to the treatment of residual disease, there is evidence that this therapy is as effective as single agent alkylating agents but no evidence to show that it is as effective as platinum-containing combination regimes (Young 1987; Young *et al.* 1990). The complications from this treatment include abdominal pain in 25 per cent of patients and a chemical peritonitis in 1.5 per cent (Young *et al.* 1990).

More recently, intraperitoneal radioimmunotherapy has been attempted using radioisotope-labelled monoclonal antibodies (Stewart *et al.* 1989) with some success in small tumour deposits, but the technique currently remains experimental.

Hormonal therapy

Progestogen therapy has been assessed as an alternative to chemotherapy for advanced ovarian cancer. Ward (1972) reported 23 women with advanced ovarian cancer treated with high-dose hydroxyprogesterone caproate, of whom 35 per cent showed no response and 65 per cent some response. However, the mean duration of response was only 3.5 months. Trope *et al.* (1982) reported 25 women with stage III or stage IV ovarian cancer treated with medroxy-progesterone acetate. No patient showed a complete response, one patient had a partial response for three months and survived for four months. Thigpen *et al.* (1984) accumulated 176 women from 10 reports involving progestogen therapy. Some 12 per cent of these patients showed a significant response, especially in well-differentiated serous or endometroid tumours. The authors describe this result as 'modest at best'.

Schwartz *et al.* (1982) reported that the antioestrogen tamoxifen induced a partial response in 7.7 per cent of 13 women. These results would suggest a very limited role for hormonal therapy in ovarian cancer.

Immunotherapy

Stimulation of the patient's own macrophage system within the peritoneal cavity has been attempted in ovarian cancer. Berek *et al.* (1985) reported 21 patients with progressive epithelial ovarian cancer at second-look laparotomy despite previous surgery and chemotherapy. These patients received *Corynebacterium parvum*, via a peritoneal dialysis catheter, every two weeks for up to four courses. The rationale behind this treatment is that *Corynebacterium* spp. activate natural cytotoxic lymphocyte activity within the peritoneal cavity. The results were assessed by a third-look procedure. Some 9.5 per cent of patients had a complete response, with a mean survival of 35 months after immuno-therapy, but ultimately died from ovarian cancer. Some 19 per cent of patients had a partial response and 71.5 per cent of patients were either unchanged or had progressive disease. Toxicity was common, with 78 per cent of patients experiencing abdominal pain and/or fever, 40 per cent nausea, and 22 per cent vomiting.

Interferon exhibits much of the activity of lymphocyte-derived macrophage activating factor, and might, therefore, have an effect on host–tumour function. Abdulhay *et al.* (1985) gave intramuscular human lymphoblastoid interferon to 28 patients with residual ovarian disease after previous treatment had failed. Some 7 per cent of patients had a complete response, 11 per cent had a partial response, 50 per cent had stable disease, and 32 per cent progressive disease. The side-effects included fatigue, leukopenia, and thrombocytopenia.

The place of this therapy in current practice is yet to become clear, but it may be that its most useful role will be in the maintenance of response following multi-agent cytotoxic regimes.

Monitoring the response to treatment

Judging the response of residual disease to treatment may be made in several different ways, including clinical response, imaging techniques, or second-look laparoscopy or laparotomy. The place of second-look procedures will be discussed below. Perhaps the widest used assessment technique is biochemical and involves the serial measurement of tumour markers in the patient's circulation. Bast et al. (1983) reported that rising or falling serum levels of CA125 correlated with the course of the disease in 93 per cent of patients with ovarian cancer. Other workers have demonstrated that a fall in serum CA125 levels post-operatively correlates with clinically non-progressive disease (Brand and Lidor 1993; Brioschi et al. 1987; Heinonen et al. 1985).

The rate of fall in circulating levels with CA125 is the best prognostic feature. Van de Burg et al. (1988) reported that the pretreatment level of CA125 had no prognostic value, but there was a close association between the half-life of CA125 and the prognosis in 37 patients after treatment. If the half-life was greater than 20 days, the chance of a patient having progressive disease was 3.2 times that of patients whose circulating levels of CA125 had a half-life of less than 20 days. Similarly, Hawkins et al. (1989) reported an actuarial two-year survival of 76 per cent in patients with a CA125 half-life of less than 20 days compared with a 48 per cent actuarial two-year survival for those with a CA125 half-life of between 20 and 40 days, and a zero two-year survival in patients with a CA125 half-life of greater than 40 days.

Although this technique cannot replace imaging, it allows a simple, relatively non-invasive technique which may be readily repeated between each course of treatment, whilst formal imaging techniques may be used less frequently but as a more definitive method of assessment.

Second-look procedures

The advocates of second-look surgery, either by laparotomy or laparoscopy, in patients following cytoreductive surgery and cytotoxic therapy have argued that it would allow:

(1) a continuation of chemotherapy in patients with clinically undetectable but remaining tumour;

(2) cessation of chemotherapy in patients who are disease-free;

(3) a second attempt at cytoreductive surgery.

There is no doubt that a second-look laparotomy is a more accurate method of assessing whether or not residual disease is present than is CT scan, but it is associated with all the usual surgical complications (Brenner et al. 1985; Goldhirsch et al. 1983).

Laparoscopy could not fulfil all the proposed advantages of the second-look procedure. Berek *et al.* (1981) reported 119 laparoscopies in 57 patients with ovarian cancer. The procedure was only technically successful on 73 per cent of occasions, the commonest reason for failure being adhesions, probably related to the previous omentectomy, which obscured the view of the pelvis. Complications, especially perforation of the transverse colon, occurred in 10 per cent of procedures, with 6.7 per cent of procedures resulting in laparotomy. Furthermore, laparoscopy clearly does not allow any further cytoreductive surgery.

The enthusiasm for second-look laparotomy followed reports such as that by Smith *et al.* (1976) in which patients who had a partial response to cytotoxic therapy following previous incomplete surgery were then able to undergo further surgery and have complete surgical removal of macroscopic residual tumour. Microscopic disease could also be diagnosed using cytological washing which would also allow for further therapy to be given (Copeland *et al.* 1985).

However, two prospective trials of second-look laparotomy as a planned procedure have failed to demonstrate any survival benefit to patients undergoing this technique.

Wiltshaw *et al.* (1985) reported that a planned second-look laparotomy in 53 women some five to seven months after starting an apparently successful course of chemotherapy showed no survival benefit when compared with 56 patients with the same chemotherapeutic regime and no second-look procedure. Luesley *et al.* (1988) reported a prospective randomized trial of second-look laparotomy in 166 patients who had undergone optimal cytoreductive surgery followed by treatment with *cis*-platinum. The patients were then randomly allocated to three groups, group A (53 patients) who had a second-look procedure followed by chlorambucil, group B (56 patients) who underwent a second-look procedure followed by abdominopelvic irradiation, and group C (57 patients) who received chlorambucil but *no* second-look laparotomy. No differences in survival were noted between the three groups.

A large randomized trial of second-look laparotomy versus no second-look surgery in women with an apparent complete clinical remission is probably the next phase in this line of management (Friedman and Weiss 1990).

Since there is no survival benefit from second-look laparotomy in patients with residual disease, it is unlikely that third-look laparotomy will be of value (Copeland *et al.* 1983).

Conclusions

Ovarian cancer is the major gynaecological lethal disease. It is likely that there will be two major groups of advances over the next decade. The first relates to screening procedures, such that asymptomatic patients with stage I disease may be diagnosed and treated. The second group of advances will probably relate to the way cytotoxic therapy is administered. Toxicity has already been reduced in the platinum-containing compounds and hence higher dosages or different agents may become available in clinical practice.

References

Abdulhay, G., DiSaia, F. J., Blessing, J., and Creasman, W. T. (1985). Human lymphoblastoid interferon in the treatment of advanced epithelial ovarian tumours. *American Journal of Obstetrics and Gynecology* **152**, 418–23.

Acheson, E. D., Gardner, M. J., Pipparo, E. C., and Grime, L. P. (1982). Mortality of two groups of women who manufactured gas masks. *British Journal of Industrial Medicine* **39**, 344–8.

Advanced Ovarian Cancer Trialists Group (1991). Chemotherapy in advanced ovarian cancer: an overview of randomized clinical trials. *British Medical Journal* **303**, 884–93.

Andolf, E., Svalenius, E., and Astedt, B. (1986). Ultrasonography for early detection of ovarian carcinoma. *British Journal of Obstetrics and Gynaecology* **93**, 1286–9.

Barbieri, R. L., Niloff, J. M., Bast, R. C., Schaetzl, E., Kistner, R. W., and Knapp, R. C. (1986). Elevated serum concentrations of CA125 in patients with advanced endometriosis. *Fertility Sterility* **45**, 630–4.

Bast, R. C., Klug, T. C., St. John, E., Jenison, E., Niloff, J. M., Lazarus, H., *et al.* (1983). A radioimmunoassay using a monoclonal antibody to monitor the course of epithelial ovarian cancer. *New England Journal of Medicine* **309**, 883–7.

Berek, J. S., Griffiths, C. T., and Leventhal, J. N. (1981). Laparoscopy for second-look evaluation of ovarian cancer. *Obstetrics and Gynecology* **58**, 192–8.

Berek, J. S., Hacker, N. F., Lagasse, L. D., and Luchter, R. S. (1982). Lower urinary tract resection as part of cytoreductive surgery for ovarian cancer. *Gynecologic Oncology* **13**, 87–92.

Berek, J. S., Knapp, R. C., Hackers, N. F., Lichtenstein, A., Jung, T., Spina, A., *et al.* (1985). Intraperitoneal immunotherapy of epithelial ovarian carcinoma with *Corynebacterium parvum*. *American Journal of Obstetrics and Gynecology* **152**, 1003–10.

Bjorkolm, E. (1984). Blood group distribution in women with ovarian cancer. *International Journal of Epidemiology* **13**, 15–17.

Bolis, G., Zanaboni, F., Vanoli, P., Russo, A., Franchi, M., Scarfone, G., *et al.* (1990). The impact of whole abdominal radiotherapy on survival in advanced ovarian cancer. *Gynecologic Oncology* **39**, 150–4.

Booth, M., Beral, V., and Smith, P. (1989). Risk factors for ovarian cancer. *British Journal of Cancer* **60**, 592–8.

Bourne, T., Campbell, S., Steer, C., Whitehead, M. I., and Collins, W. P. (1989). Transvaginal colour flow imaging: a possible new screening technique for ovarian cancer. *British Medical Journal* **299**, 1367–70.

Bourne, T., Whitehead, M. I., Campbell, S., Royston, P., Bhan, V., and Collins, W. P. (1991). Ultrasound screening for familial ovarian cancer. *Gynecologic Oncology* **43**, 92–7.

Brand, E. and Lidor, Y. (1993). The decline of CA125 level after surgery reflects the size of residual ovarian cancer. *Obstetrics and Gynecology* **81**, 29–32.

Brandt, S. J., Peters, W. P., Atwater, S. K., Kurtzberg, J., Borowitz, M. J., Jones, R. B., *et al.* (1988). Effect of recombinant human granulocyte–macrophage colony-stimulating factor in haemopoietic reconstitution after high-dose chemotherapy. *New England Journal of Medicine* **318**, 869–76.

Brenner, D. E., Shaff, M. F., Jones, H. W., Grosh, W. W., Greco, F. A., and Burnett, L. S. (1985). Abdominopelvic computerised tomography. *Obstetrics and Gynecology* **65**, 715–19.

Brioschi, P. A., Irion, O., Bishof, P., Bader, N., Forni, N., and Krauer, F. (1987).

Serum CA125 in patients with ovarian cancer. *British Journal of Obstetrics and Gynaecology* **94**, 196–201.

Bruzzone, M., Repetto, L., Chiara, S., Campara, E., Conte, P. F., Orsatti, M., *et al.* (1990). Chemotherapy versus radiotherapy in the management of ovarian cancer patients. *Gynecologic Oncology* **38**, 392–5.

Buchsbaum, H. J. and Lifshitz, S. (1984). Staging and surgical evaluation of ovarian cancer. *Seminars in Oncology* **11**, 227–37.

Campbell, S., Bakn, V., Royston, P., Whitehead, M. I., and Collins, W. P. (1989). Transabdominal ultrasound screening for early ovarian cancer. *British Medical Journal* **299**, 1363–7.

Campbell, S., Royston, P., Bhan, V. Whitehead, M. I., and Collins, W. P. (1990). Novel screening strategies for early ovarian cancer by transabdominal ultrasound. *British Journal of Obstetrics and Gynaecology* **97**, 304–11.

Cancer and Steroid Hormone Study Group (1987). The reduction in risk of ovarian cancer associated with oral contraceptive use. *New England Journal of Medicine* **316**, 650–5.

Carter, J. C., Ramirez, C., Waugh, R., Atkinson, K., Coppleson, M., Elliott, P., *et al.* (1991). Percutaneous urinary diversion in gynecologic oncology. *Gynecologic Oncology* **40**, 248–52.

Carter, J., Fowler, J., Karlson, J., Karlson, L., and Twiggs, L. B. (1993). Borderline and invasive epithelial ovarian tumour in young women. *Obstetrics and Gynecology* **82**, 752–6.

Casagrande, J. T., Lovie, E. W., Pike, M. C., Roy, S., Ross, R. K., and Henderson, B. E. (1979). Incessant ovulation and ovarian cancer. *Lancet* ii, 170–3.

Castaldo, T. W., Petrilli, E. S., Ballon, S. C., and Lagasse, L. D. (1981). Intestinal operations in patients with ovarian carcinoma. *American Journal of Obstetrics and Gynecology* **139**, 80–4.

Conrad, G. J. and Woodruff, J. D. (1972). The biologic behavior of low grade papillary serous carcinoma of the ovary. *Obstetrics and Gynecology* **40**, 460–7.

Copeland, L. J., Wharton, J. T., Rutledge, F. N., Gershenson, D. M., Seski, J. C., and Henson, J. (1983). The role of third-look laparotomy in the guidance of ovarian cancer treatment. *Gynecologic Oncology* **15**, 145–9.

Copeland, L. J., Gershenson, D. M., Wharton, J. T., Atkinson, E. N., Sneige, N., Edwards, C. L., *et al.* (1985). Microscopic disease at second-look laparotomy in advanced ovarian cancer. *Cancer* **55**, 472–8.

Counseller, V. S., Hunt, W., and Haigler, F. H. (1955). Carcinoma of the ovary following hysterectomy. *American Journal of Obstetrics and Gynecology* **69**, 538–46.

Cramer, D. W. and Welch, W. R. (1983). Determinance of ovarian cancer risk. *Journal of the National Cancer Institute* **71**, 717–21.

Cramer, D. W., Hutchinson, G. B., Welch, W. R., Scully, R. E., and Knapp, R. C. (1982). Factors affecting the association of oral contraception and ovarian cancer. *New England Journal of Medicine* **307**, 1047–51.

Cramer, D. W., Hutchinson, G. B., Welch, W. R., Scully, R. E., and Ryon, K. J. (1983). Determinance of ovarian cancer risk. *Journal of the National Cancer Institute* **71**, 711–16.

Creasman, W. T. and DiSaia, P. J. (1991). Screening in ovarian cancer. *American Journal of Obstetrics and Gynecology* **165**, 7–10.

Cubeddu, L. X., Hoffmann, I. S., Fuenmayor, N. T., and Finn, A. L. (1990). Efficacy of ondansetron and the role of serotonin in *cis*-platin-induced nausea and vomiting. *New England Journal of Medicine* **322**, 810–16.

Cunningham, D., Soukop, M., Gilchrist, N., Forrest, G. J., Hepplestone, A., Calder,

I. T., *et al.* (1985). Randomized trial of intravenous high-dose metoclopramide and intramuscular chlorpromazine in controlling nausea and vomiting induced by cytotoxic agents. *British Medical Journal* **295**, 604–5.

Cunningham, D., Hawthorn, J., Pople, A., Gazet, J. C., Ford, H. T., Challoner, T., *et al.* (1987). Prevention of emesis in patients receiving cytotoxic drugs by a selective 5-HT₃ receptor antagonist. *Lancet* i, 1461–2.

Decker, D. G. (1982). Cyclophosphamide plus *cis*-platin in combination. *Obstetrics and Gynecology* **60**, 481–7.

Delgardo, G., Oram, D. H., and Petrilli, E. J. (1984). Stage III epithelial ovarian cancer: role of maximal surgical reduction. *Gynecologic Oncology* **18**, 293–8.

Dembo, J., Davy, N., Stenwig, A. E., Berle, E. J., Bush, R. J., and Kjorstad, K. (1990). Prognostic factors in patients with stage I epithelial ovarian carcinoma. *Obstetrics and Gynecology* **75**, 263–73.

Drouin, P. (1979). Comparison of external radiotherapy and chemotherapy in ovarian cancer. *Annals of the Royal College of Physicians and Surgeons of Canada* **12**, 61–7.

Drug and Therapeutics Bulletin (1992). Ondansetron to prevent chemotherapy-induced vomiting. *Drug and Therapeutics Bulletin* **30**, 21–3.

Eeles, R. A., Tan, S., Fryatt, I., A'Hern, R. P., Shepherd, J. H., Harmer, C. L., *et al.* (1991). Hormone replacement therapy and survival after surgery for ovarian cancer. *British Medical Journal* **302**, 259–62.

Finn, C. B., Luesley, D. M., Buxton, E. J., Blackledge, J. R., Kelly, K., Dunn, J. A., *et al.* Is stage I epithelial ovarian cancer overtreated both surgically and systemically? *British Journal of Obstetrics and Gynaecology* **99**, 54–8.

Franceschi, S., La Vecchia, C., Helmrich, S. P., Mangioni, C., and Tognoni, G. (1982). Risk factors for epithelial ovarian cancer in Italy. *American Journal of Epidemiology* **115**, 714–19.

Friedman, J. B. and Weiss, N. S. (1990). Second thoughts about second-look laparotomy in advanced ovarian cancer. *New England Journal of Medicine* **322**, 1079–82.

Fuks, Z. (1975). External radiotherapy of ovarian cancer. *Seminars in Oncology* **2**, 253–66.

Goldhirsch, A., Triller, J. K., Greiner, R., Dreker, E., and Davis, B. W. (1983). Computerised tomography prior to second-look laparotomy in advanced ovarian cancer. *Obstetrics and Gynecology* **62**, 630–4.

Gralla, R. J., Itri, L. M., Pisco, S. E., Squillante, A. E., Kelsen, D. P., Braun, D. W., *et al.* (1981). Antiemetic efficacy of high-dose metoclopramide: randomized trials. *New England Journal of Medicine* **305**, 905–9.

Greco, F. A., Julian, C. G., Richardson, R. L., Burnett, L., Hande, K. R., and Oldham, R. K. (1981). Advanced ovarian cancer: brief intensive combination chemotherapy and second-look operation. *Obstetrics and Gynecology* **58**, 199–205.

Griffiths, C. T. (1975). Surgical resection of tumour bulk in the primary treatment of ovarian carcinoma. *National Cancer Insitute Monogram* **42**, 101–4.

Gross, T. P. and Schlesselman, J. J. (1994). The estimated effect of oral contraceptive use on the cumulative risk of epithelial ovarian cancer. *Obstetrics and Gynecology* **83**, 419–24.

Gusberg, S. B. and Deligdisch, L. (1984). Ovarian dysplasia. *Cancer* **54**, 1–4.

Hacker, N. F., Berek, J. S., Lagasse, L. D., Nieberg, R. K., and Elashoff, R. M. (1983). Primary cytoreductive surgery for epithelial ovarian cancer. *Obstetrics and Gynecology* **61**, 413–20.

Hacker, N. F., Berek, J. S., Burnison, C. M., Heintz, P. N., Juillard, G. J. F., and Lagasse, L. D. (1985). Whole abdominal radiation as salvage treatment for epithelial ovarian cancer. *Obstetrics and Gynecology* **65**, 60–6.

Hart, W. R. and Norris, H. J. (1983). Border-line or malignant mucinous tumours of the ovary. *Cancer* **31**, 1031–45.

Hawkins, R. E., Roberts, K., Wiltshaw, E., Mundy, J., Fryatt, I. J., and McCready, V. R. (1989). The prognostic significance of the half-life of serum CA125 in patients responding to chemotherapy for epithelial ovarian carcinoma. *British Journal of Obstetrics and Gynaecology* **96**, 1395–9.

Heinonen, P. K., Tontti, K., Koivula, T., and Pystynen, P. (1985). Tumour-associated antigen CA125 in patients with ovarian cancer. *British Journal of Obstetrics and Gynaecology* **92**, 528–31.

Henderson, W. J., Joslin, C. A. F., Turnbull, A. C., and Griffiths, K. (1971). Talc and carcinoma of the ovary and cervix. *Journal of Obstetrics and Gynaecology of the British Commonwealth* **78**, 266–72.

Hreshchyshyn, M. M., Parc, R. C., Blessing, J. A., Norris, H. J., Levy, D., Lagasse, L. D., and Creasman, W. T. (1980). The role of adjuvant therapy in stage I ovarian cancer. *American Journal of Obstetrics and Gynecology* **138**, 139–45.

Hunter, G., Ashton, K. J., and Merry, B. (1987). *In vitro* sensitivity of human ovarian tumours to chemotherapeutic agents with adjuvant danazol. *Obstetrics and Gynecology* **69**, 233–6.

Hunter, R. W., Alexander, N. D. E., and Soutter, W. P. (1992). Meta-analysis of surgery in advanced ovarian carcinoma. Is maximum cytoreductive surgery an independent determinant of prognosis? *American Journal of Obstetrics and Gynecology* **166**, 504–11.

Jacobs, I. J. and Oram, D. H. (1988). Oophorectomy and prevention of ovarian cancer. In *Contemporary obstetrics and gynaecology* (ed. G. Chamberlain), pp. 397–408. Butterworths, London.

Jacobs, I. J., Fay, T. N., Stabile, I., Bridges, J. E., Oram, D. H., and Grudzinskas, J. G. (1988*a*). The distribution of FCA125 in the reproductive tract of pregnant and non-pregnant women. *British Journal of Obstetrics and Gynaecology* **95**, 1190–4.

Jacobs, I. J., Stabile, I., Bridges, J. E., Kemsley, P., Reynolds, S., Grudzinskas, J. G., *et al.* (1988*b*). Multimodal approach to screening for ovarian carcinoma. *Lancet* **i**, 268–71.

Jacobs, I. J., Rivera, H., Oram, D. H., and Bast, R. C. (1993*a*). Differential diagnosis of ovarian cancer with tumour markers. *British Journal of Obstetrics and Gynaecology* **100**, 1120–4.

Jacobs, I., Davies, A. P., Bridges, J., Stabile, I., Fay, T., Lower, A., *et al.* (1993*b*). Prevalence screening for ovarian cancer in post-menopausal women by CA125 measurement and ultrasonography. *British Medical Journal* **306**, 1030–4.

Jones, A. L., Hill, A. S., Soukop, M., Hutcheon, A. W., Cassidy, J., Kaye, S. B., *et al.* (1991). Comparison of dexamethasone and ondansetron in the prophylaxis of emesis induced by moderately emetogenic chemotherapy. *Lancet* **338**, 483–7.

Karlan, B. Y., Raffel, L. J., Crvenkovic, G., Smart, C., Chen, M. D., Lozez, E., *et al.* (1993). A multi-disciplinary approach to the early detection of ovarian cancer. *American Journal of Obstetrics and Gynecology* **169**, 494–501.

Kawai, M., Kano, T., Kikkawa, F., Maeda, O., Oguchi, H., and Tumoda, Y. (1992). Transvaginal Doppler ultrasound with colour-flow imaging in the diagnosis of ovarian cancer. *Obstetrics and Gynecology* **79**, 163–7.

Keettel, W. C., Pixley, E. E., and Buchsbaum, H. J. (1974). Experience with peritoneal cytology in the management of gynecological malignancies. *American Journal of Obstetrics and Gynecology* **120**, 174–282.

Khoo, S. K. (1986). Cancer risks and the contraceptive pill. *Medical Journal of Australia* **144**, 185–90.

Khwaja, A. and Goldstone, A. H. (1991). Haemopoietic growth factors. *British Medical Journal* **302**, 1164–5.

Kjorstad, K. E., Welander, C., and Kolstad, P. (1977). Pre-operative irradiation in stage III carcinoma of the ovary. *Acta Obstetrica et Gynaecologica Scandinavica* **56**, 449–52.

Kucera, P. R., Berman, M. L., Treadwell, P., Sheets, E. E., Micha, J. P., Rettenmaier, M. A., *et al.* (1990). Whole-abdominal radiotherapy for patients with minimal residual epithelial ovarian cancer. *Gynecologic Oncology* **36**, 338–42.

Kurják, A., Zalud, I., Jurkovic, D., Alfirevia, Z., and Miljan, M. (1989). Transvaginal colour Doppler for the assessment of pelvic circulation. *Acta Obstetrica et Gynaecologica Scandinavica* **68**, 131–5.

La Vecchia, C., Liberati, A., and Franceschi, S. (1982). Non-contraceptive oestrogen use and the occurrence of ovarian cancer. *Journal of the National Cancer Institute* **69**, 1207.

La Vecchia, C., Franceschi, S., Decoli, A., Gentile, A., Liati, P., Rigallo, N., *et al.* (1984). Coffee drinking and the risk of epithelial ovarian cancer. *International Journal of Cancer* **33**, 559–62.

Lambert, H. E. and Berry, R. J. (1985). High-dose *cis*-platinum compared with high-dose cyclophosphamide in the management of advanced epithelial ovarian cancer. *British Medical Journal* **290**, 879–93.

Lancet (1991). Ondansetron versus dexamethasone for chemotherapy-induced emesis. *Lancet* **338**, 478–9.

Levin, L. and Hryniuk, W. M. (1987). Dose intensity analysis of chemotherapy regimes in ovarian carcinoma. *Journal of Clinical Oncology* **5**, 756–67.

Luesley, D., Lauton, F., Blackledge, G., Hilton, C., Kelly, K., Rollason, T., *et al.* (1988). Failure of second-look laparotomy to influence survival in epithelial ovarian cancer. *Lancet* **ii**, 599–603.

Lynch, H. T., Watson, P., Bewtra, C., Conway, T. A., Read, H. C., Kaur, P., *et al.* (1991). Hereditary ovarian cancer. *Cancer* **67**, 1460–6.

MacFarlane, C., Sturgis, M. C., and Fetterman, F. S. (1955). Results of an experiment in the control of the female genital organs. *American Journal of Obstetrics and Gynecology* **69**, 294–8.

McGowan, L. (1987). Ovarian cancer after hysterectomy. Obstetrics and Gynecology **69**, 386–8.

Marty, M., Pouillart, P., Scholl, S., Droz, J. P., Azab, M., Brion, N., *et al.* (1990). Comparison of the 5-hydroxytryptamine antagonist odansetron with high-dose metoclopramide in the control of *cis*-platinum-induced emesis. *New England Journal of Medicine* **322**, 816–21.

Meijer, S., Sleijfer, D. T., Mulder, N. H., Sluiter, W. J., Marrink, J., Koops, H. S., *et al.* (1983). Some effects of combination chemotherapy with *cis*-platinum on renal function. *Cancer* **51**, 2035–40.

Mollman, J. E. (1990). *Cis*-platin neurotoxicity. *New England Journal of Medicine* **322**, 126–7.

Mori, M., Harabuchi, I., Miyake, H., Casagrande, J. T., Henderson, B. E., and Ross, R. K. (1988). Reproduction, genetics, and dietary risk factors for ovarian cancer. *American Journal of Epidemiology* **128**, 771–7.

Munnell, E. W. (1969). Is conservative therapy ever justified in stage I cancer of the ovary? *American Journal of Obstetrics and Gynecology* **103**, 641–53.

Myers, C. (1984). The use of intraperitoneal chemotherapy in the treatment of ovarian cancer. *Seminars in Oncology* **11**, 275–84.

Newhouse, M. L., Pearson, R. N., Fullerton, J. M., Boesen, E. A. N., and Shannon,

H. S. (1977). A case-controlled study of carcinoma of the ovary. *British Journal of Preventative and Social Medicine* **31**, 148–53.

Newhouse, M. L., Berry, G., and Wagner, J. C. (1985). Morbidity of factory workers in East London. *British Journal of Industrial Medicine* **42**, 4–11.

Office of Population, Census and Surveys (1985). *Cancer Statistics.* no. 18. MBI. Her Majesty's Stationery Office, London.

Oram, D. and Jacobs, I. (1987). Improving the prognosis in ovarian cancer. In *Progress in obstetrics and gynaecology* Vol. 6, (ed. J. Studd), pp. 399–432. Churchill Livingstone, Edinburgh.

Osborne, R. H. and De George, F. V. (1963). The ABO blood groups in neoplastic disease of the ovary. *American Journal of Human Genetics* **15**, 380–8.

Ozols, R. F. and Young, R. C. (1984). Chemotherapy of ovarian carcinoma. *Seminars in Oncology* **11**, 251–63.

Ozols, R. F., Corden, B. J., Jacob, J., Wesley, M. N., Ostchego, Y., and Young, R. C. (1984). High-dose *cis*-platin in hypertonic saline. *Annals of Internal Medicine* **100**, 19–24.

Ozols, R. F., Ostchego, Y., Myers, C. E., and Young, R. C. (1985). High-dose *cis*-platin in hypertonic saline in refractory ovarian cancer. *Journal of Clinical Oncology* **3**, 1246–50.

Parazzini, F., Franceschi, S., La Vecchia, C., and Fasoli, M. (1991). The epidemiology of ovarian cancer. *Gynecologic Oncology* **43**, 9–23.

Parazzini, F., Negri, E., La Vecchia, C., Luchini, L., and Mezzopane, R. (1993). Hysterectomy, oophorectomy and subsequent ovarian cancer risk. *Obstetrics and Gynecology* **81**, 363–6.

Pecorelli, S., Bolis, G., and Vassena, L. (1988). Randomized comparison of *cis*-platin and carboplatin in advanced ovarian cancer. *Proceedings of the American Society of Clinical Oncology* **7**, 136.

Peto, J. and Easton, D. (1989). Cancer treatment trials *Cancer Surveys* **8**, 511–33.

Piver, N. S., Barlow, J. J., and Lele, S. B. (1978). Incidence of subclinical metastasis in stage I and II ovarian cancer. *Obstetrics and Gynecology* **52**, 100–4.

Potter, M. E., Partridge, E. E., Hatch, K. D., Soong, S. J., Austin, M., and Shingleton, H. M. (1991). Primary surgical therapy of ovarian cancer: how much and when? *Gynecologic Oncology* **40**, 195–200.

Redman, C. W. E., Lawton, F. D., Luesley, D., Hilton, C., Mould, J., Latief, T., et al. (1987). Randomized trial comparing abdomino-pelvic radiotherapy with *cis*-platin in patients with ovarian cancer with no macroscopic disease after primary surgery. *British Journal of Cancer* **56**, 216–17.

Redman, C. W. E., Warwick, J., Luesley, D. M., Varma, R., Lawton, F. G., and Blackledge, G. R. P. (1994). Intervention debulking surgery in advanced epithelial ovarian cancer. *British Journal of Obstetrics and Gynaecology* **101**, 142–6.

Schwartz, P. E., Keating, G., MacLusky, N., Natfolin, F., and Eisenfeld, A. (1982). Tamoxifen therapy for advanced ovarian carcinoma. *Obstetrics and Gynecology* **59**, 583–8.

Shapiro, S. P. and Nunez, C. (1983). Psammoma bodies in the cervicovaginal smear in association with papillary tumours of the peritoneum. *Obstetrics and Gynecology* **61**, 130–4.

Sheridan, W. P., Morstyn, G., Wolf, M., Dodds, A., Lusk, J., Maher, D., et al. (1989). Granulocyte colony-stimulating factor and neutrophil recovery after high-dose chemotherapy. *Lancet* **ii**, 891–5.

Sightler, S. E., Boike, G. M., Estarpe, R. E., and Averette, H. E. (1991). Ovarian cancer in women with prior hysterectomy. *Obstetrics and Gynecology* **78**, 681–4.

Smith, J. P. and Day, J. (1979). Review of ovarian cancer at the University of Texas. *American Journal of Obstetrics and Gynecology* **135**, 984–93.

Smith, J. P., Delgado, G., and Rutledge, F. (1976). Second-look operations in ovarian cancer. *Cancer* **38**, 1438–42.

Sparks, J. M. and Varner, R. E. (1991). Ovarian cancer screening. *Obstetrics and Gynecology* **77**, 787–92.

Stewart, J. S. W., Hird, V., Sullivan, M., Snook, D., and Epenetos, A. A. (1989). Intraperitoneal radioimmunotherapy for ovarian cancer. *British Journal of Obstetrics and Gynaecology* **96**, 529–36.

Thigpen, J. T., Vance, R. B., Balducci, L., and Khansur, T. (1984). New drugs and experimental approaches in ovarian cancer treatment. *Seminars in Oncology* **11**, 314–26.

Tobacman, J. K., Tucker, M. A., Kasa, R., Greene, M. H., Costa, J., and Fraumeni, J. F. (1982). Intra-abdominal carcinomatosis after prophylactic oophorectomy in ovarian cancer prone families. *Lancet* **ii**, 795–7.

Trope, C., Johnssen, J. E., Sigurdsson, K., and Simonsen, E. (1982). High-dose medroxyprogesterone acetate for the treatment of advanced ovarian carcinoma. *Cancer Treatment Reports* **60**, 1441–3.

Van de Burg, M. E. L., Lammes, F. B., Van Putten, W. L. J., and Stoker, G. (1988). Ovarian cancer: the prognostic value of the serum half-life of CA125 during induction chemotherapy. *Gynecologic Oncology* **30**, 307–10.

van der Hoop, R. J., Vecht, C. J., Van de Burg, M. E. L., Elderson, A., Booger, D. W., Vries, E. P., *et al.* (1990). Prevention of *cis*-platin neuretoxicity with an ACTH analogue in patients with ovarian cancer. *New England Journal of Medicine* **322**, 89–94.

Venter, P. F. (1981). Ovarian epithelial cancer and chemical carcinogenesis. *Gynecologic Oncology* **12**, 281–5.

Vessey, M. P., Villard-Mackintosh, L., McPherson, K., and Yeates, D. (1989). Mortality among oral contraceptive users: 20-year follow-up. *British Medical Journal* **299**, 1487–91.

Villard-Mackintosh, L., Vessey, M. P., and Jones, L. (1989). The effects of oral contraceptives and parity on ovarian cancer trends in women under 55 years of age. *British Journal of Obstetrics and Gynaecology* **96**, 783–8.

Ward, H. W. C. (1972). Progesterone treatment for ovarian carcinoma. *Journal of Obstetrics and Gynaecology of the British Commonwealth* **79**, 555–9.

Webb, M. J. (1993). Screening for ovarian cancer. *British Medical Journal* **306**, 1015–16.

Weiss, N. S., Lyon, J. L., Krishnamurthy, S., Dietert, S., Liff, J. N., and Daling, J. R. (1982). Non-contraceptive oestrogen use and the occurrence of epithelial ovarian cancer. *Journal of the National Cancer Institute* **68**, 95–8.

Westhoff, C. and Randall, M. C. (1991). Ovarian cancer screening. *American Journal of Obstetrics and Gynecology* **165**, 502–5.

Whittemore, A. S., Wu, M. L., Paffenbarger, R. S., Sarles, D.L., Kampert, J. B., Grosser, S., *et al.* (1988). Personal and environmental characteristics related to epithelial ovarian cancer. *American Journal of Epidemiology* **128**, 1228–40.

Whittemore, A. S., Harris, R., and Itnyre, J. (1992). Risk factors for ovarian cancer. *American Journal of Epidemiology* **126**, 1212–20.

Wijnen, J. A. and Rosenheln, N. B. (1980). Surgery in ovarian cancer. *Archives of Surgery* **115**, 863–8.

Williams, T. J. and Dockerty, N. B. (1976). Study of the contralateral ovary in encapsulated low grade malignant tumours of the ovary. *Surgery, Gynaecology, Obstetrics* **143**, 763–6.

Wiltshaw, E. and Kroner, R. T. (1976). Phase II study of *cis*-platinum in advanced adenocarcinoma of the ovary. *Cancer Treatment Report* **60**, 55–60.

Wiltshaw, E., Evans, B. D., Jones, A. C., Baker, J. W., and Calvert, H. (1983). JM8, successor to *cis*-platinum in advanced ovarian carcinoma? *Lancet* **i**, 587.

Wiltshaw, E. Raju, K. S., and Dawson, J. (1985). The role of cytoreductive surgery in advanced carcinoma of the ovary. *British Journal of Obstetrics and Gynaecology* **92**, 522–7.

Wiltshaw, E., Evans, B., Rustin, G., Gilby, E., Baker, J., and Barker, G. (1986). A retrospective randomized trial comparing high-dose *cis*-platin and low-dose *cis*-platin and chlorambucil in advanced ovarian cancer. *Journal of Clinical Oncology* **4**, 722–9.

Wu, M. L., Whittemore, A. S., Paffenbarger, R. S., Sarles, D. L., Kampert, J. B., Grosser, S., *et al.* (1988). Personal and environmental characteristics related to epithelial ovarian cancer. *American Journal of Epidemiology* **128**, 1216–27.

Young, R. C. (1987). Initial therapy for early ovarian cancer. *Cancer* **60**, 2042–9.

Young, R. C., Chabner, B. A., Hubbard, S. P., Fusher, R. I., Bender, R. A., Anderson, T., *et al.* (1978). Prospective trial of melphalan versus combination chemotherapy in ovarian adenocarcinoma. *New England Journal of Medicine* **299**, 1261–6.

Young, R. C., Decker, D. G., Wharton, J. T., Piver, S., Sindelar, W., Edwards, B. K., *et al.* (1983). Staging laparotomy in early ovarian cancer. *Journal of the American Medical Association* **250**, 3072–6.

Young, R. C., Walton, L. A., Ellenberg, S. S., Homesley, H. D., Wilbanks, G. D., Decker, D. G., *et al.* (1990). Adjuvant therapy in stage I and stage II epithelial ovarian cancer. *New England Journal of Medicine* **322**, 1021–7.

14   Surgical practice

This chapter will debate the following topics:

(1) the prevention of thromboembolic disease;

(2) the prevention of infection following gynaecological surgery;

(3) abdominal wound closure;

(4) the increasing incidence of Caesarean section;

(5) Caesarian section scar dehiscence;

(6) the prevention of infection following Caesarean section.

The prevention of thromboembolic disease

Patients undergoing abdominal or pelvic surgery are at specific risk of pulmonary embolus, this being either the main cause of death or a contributory factor in 0.8 per cent of all such patients operated upon, without prophylaxis, for general surgical, urological, or gynaecological problems (Bergqvist and Lindbland 1985). Patients undergoing surgery for malignant disease are at a greater risk of fatal pulmonary embolus, this being recorded in up to 9 per cent of patients undergoing surgery for ovarian cancer (Walsh *et al*. 1974). Non-fatal pulmonary embolus occurs in a higher percentage of patients, often unrecognized clinically. It has been estimated that this complication occurs in up to 2 per cent of patients undergoing hysterectomy (either abdominal or vaginal) for benign disease, but in 8–13.5 per cent of patients undergoing gynaecological surgery for malignant disease (Clarke-Pearson *et al*. 1983*a*; Clarke-Pearson *et al*. 1990; Walsh *et al*. 1974). A deep venous thrombosis is also present more commonly than is clinically recognized, occuring in approximately 7 per cent of patients undergoing vaginal hysterectomy for benign disease and in 12 per cent undergoing abdominal hysterectomy for benign disease (Walsh *et al*. 1974). As with pulmonary embolus, a deep venous thrombosis occurs more commonly following surgery for malignant disease, with evidence of this complication in up to 26 per cent of patients undergoing a Wertheim's hysterectomy and in 45 per cent undergoing surgery for either ovarian or vulval cancer (Clarke-Pearson *et al*. 1990; Walsh *et al*. 1974). The importance of the use of prophylactic agents against deep venous thrombosis and pulmonary embolus may be evidenced by the observation that half of the cases of fatal pulmonary embolus are massive, acute, and without previous clinical suspicion (Sevitts and Gallagher 1959). If these complications are to be avoided, then it is appropriate to examine the evidence for the use of prophylactic agents.

There are two major problems when interpreting these studies, however. First, most studies define a deep venous thrombosis as being one that is detected by radioactive fibrinogen uptake studies rather than by a clinical diagnosis, and, hence, the figures quoted may initially seem excessive to the clinician. Secondly, most of the comparative studies which can be performed at one centre are too small in that in order to demonstrate a beneficial effect from any form of treatment at a statistical level, a series should consist ideally of at least 500 patients, should deep venous thrombosis be the end-point, 5000 patients if a reduction in the incidence of pulmonary embolus is to be tested, or 20 000 patients if death from pulmonary embolus is to be assessed. Very few series reach this size (Collins *et al.* 1988).

Numerous trials have now addressed the question of prophylaxis using subcutaneous heparin. All the evidence would suggest that subcutaneous heparin reduces the incidence of both deep venous thrombosis and pulmonary embolus, but that the dosage required as prophylaxis in the presence of benign disease is not necessarily an adequate dose for the prevention in the presence of malignant disease.

The benefit of prophylactic heparin in the presence of benign gynaecological disease has been assessed in several studies. Ballard *et al.* (1973) demonstrated that subcutaneous heparin, given in a dosage of 5000 IU two hours preoperatively and 12-hourly thereafter for seven days, reduced the incidence of deep venous thrombosis as detected by radioactive fibrinogen estimation, from 29 per cent in a control group to 3.6 per cent in a treatment group. Similarly, the Groote Schuur group (1979) reported that the incidence of deep venous thrombosis was 12 per cent in heparin-treated patients compared with 27 per cent of controls.

In order that the effect of subcutaneous heparin in the prevention of pulmonary embolus, both fatal and non-fatal may be assessed, the evidence from large multicentre trials or from a meta-analysis of the available smaller trials is required. The International Multicentre Trial first reported in 1975 but then re-reported in 1977 in view of 'inconsistencies in the data from one of the centres'. This centre (Grubber *et al.* 1977) then reported separately. The International Multicentre Trial consisted of 4121 patients, aged 40 years and over who underwent a range of major surgical procedures and who were randomly allocated into no drug prophylactics or to receive calcium heparin 5000 units subcutaneously two hours pre-operatively and every eight hours there-after for seven days. This data, shown in Table 14.1, demonstrated that heparin reduced the incidence of deep venous thrombosis from 24 per cent to 6 per cent, the incidence of non-fatal pulmonary embolus from 6 per cent to 3 per cent, and the incidence of fatal pulmonary embolus from 0.3 per cent to zero. The study from Grubber *et al.* (1977) gave similar results. Collins *et al.* (1988) reported an overview of 84 randomized prospective trials throughout surgical specialities. As can be seen from Table 14.2, the incidence of deep venous thrombosis was reduced from 15 per cent to 7 per cent, the incidence of non-fatal pulmonary embolus from 2 per cent to 1.3 per cent, and the incidence of

Table 14.1 Thromboembolic disease

	No. of patients	No. of deaths	DVT at post-mortem (%)	Fatal PE (%)	Non-fatal PE at post-mortem (%)
Heparin	1998	76	6	0	3
Controls	2033	94	24	0.3	6

From International Multicentre Trial (1977)

Table 14.2 Thromboembolic disease

	No. of patients	DVT	Non-fatal PE	Bleeding (non-fatal)	Fatal PE	Fatal haemorrhage
Heparin	8112	524 (7%)	105 (1.3%)	419 (5.2%)	19 (0.2%)	8 (0.1%)
Controls	7486	1077 (15%)	147 (2.0%)	244 (3.3%)	55 (0.7%)	6 (0.08%)

From Collins *et al.* (1988)

fatal pulmonary embolus from 0.7 per cent to 0.2 per cent. This meta-analysis demonstrated that not only was subcutaneous heparin effective, but that for benign disease there was no advantage in using heparin every 8 hours instead of every 12 hours.

The major anxiety with subcutaneous heparin is the risk of bleeding either during the operation or in the immediate post-operative period. Major haemorrhage, defined as the need for a blood transfusion, is no more likely when heparin is given than when it is not (Collins *et al.* 1988; International Multicentre Trial 1977). However, there is a trend towards a statistically non-significant increase in the incidence of wound haematoma in the heparin-treated group (International Multicentre Trial 1977). It is possible that the newer low molecular weight heparins will increase in popularity, since they can be administered once daily and may be more efficacious for the prophylaxis against venous thrombosis, yet give a lower incidence of unwanted haemorrhage because of a smaller disruptive effect on platelet function (Kakkar *et al.* 1993; Leizorovicz *et al.* 1992).

When performing major gynaecological surgery for benign disease, surgeons should not be afraid to give their patients subcutaneous heparin two hours pre-operatively and every 12 hours thereafter, and we may be reaching the time when it will be considered negligent not to do so.

What evidence there is suggests that a greater dose of heparin is needed for prophylaxis against deep venous thrombosis in the presence of malignant disease. Low-dose heparin, defined as 5000 units 2 hours pre-operatively and every 12 hours thereafter, was not superior to 'no treatment' in the prevention of deep venous thrombosis in surgery for malignant gynaecological disease (Clarke-Pearson *et al.* 1983*a*). However, when heparin 5000 IU two hours pre-operatively was followed by the same dose every eight hours for seven days, the incidence of fibrinogen-proven deep venous thrombosis was halved, from 18 per cent to 9 per cent, without any increase in the risk of life-threatening haemorrhage (Clarke-Pearson *et al.* 1990). In view of the high incidence of pulmonary embolus in patients undergoing major gynaecological surgery for malignant disease, such a heparin regime should be instituted.

Oral anticoagulation has been used prophylactically and although it is as effective as heparin, it suffers from the inconvenience that therapy needs to commence some five days pre-operatively and continue into the second post-operative week. Moreover, the patient may be vomiting in the initial post-operative period and warfarin is more difficult to reverse than is heparin.

Taberner *et al.* (1978) randomly allocated a group of 145 patients, aged 40 or over, undergoing major abdominal surgery to receive either oral anticoagulation, subcutaneous low-dose calcium heparin, or subcutaneous saline. The incidence of fibrinogen-detected DVT in each group was 6 per cent, 6 per cent, and 23 per cent, respectively, whilst the incidence of wound haematoma or the need for transfusion was 6 per cent, 2 per cent, and zero, respectively.

The use of high molecular weight Dextran was assessed by Bonnar and Walsh (1972), who compared the use of one litre of Dextran 70, given from the time of induction of anaesthesia, with a control group who received clear intravenous fluids only. There were no significant differences between blood loss or blood transfusion requirements between the groups, but the Dextran groups for both abdominal hysterectomy and vaginal hysterectomy had statistically significantly lower incidences of deep venous thrombosis. However, subcutaneous heparin is a more effective prophylaxis against deep venous thrombosis than is high molecular weight Dextran. In one comparison of these agents, deep venous thrombosis occurred in 13 per cent of patients undergoing major surgery and receiving subcutaneous heparin but in 22 per cent of patients receiving Dextran (Grubber *et al.* 1977).

The value of venous calf compression, either continuously or intermittently, has been advocated for the prevention of deep venous thrombosis. The use of graduated stockings will reduce the incidence of deep venous thrombosis following surgery for benign gynaecological disease, although not as effectively as heparin, but it does not seem to reduce the incidence following gynaecological surgery for malignant disease (Clarke-Pearson *et al.* 1983*b*; Colditz *et al.* 1986; *Drug and Therapeutics Bulletin* 1992). The value of intra-operative intermittent venous calf compression was demonstrated by Rosenberg *et al.* (1975) in a randomized prospective controlled trial of patients undergoing major abdominal surgery, patients being allocated to undergo intermittent calf stimulation, subcutaneous calcium heparin (5000 IU eight-hourly for six days), or no specific prophylaxis, and subdivided for both benign and malignant disease. As can be seen from Table 14.3, the low-dose heparin was effective as a prophylaxis in all patients, whilst calf stimulation appeared to help only those with benign disease. The beneficial effect of heparin was statistically greater than that of calf compression in patients with benign disease. Since malignant disease is itself a known risk factor for thromboembolism, pre-

Table 14.3 Thromboembolic disease

	Laparotomy for benign disease			Laparotomy for malignant disease		
	No.	All DVT (%)	DVT above knee (%)	No.	All DVT (%)	DVT above knee (%)
Calf compression	37	16.2	0	13	61.5	15.4
Heparin	34	8.8	0	21	4.8	0
No specific prophylaxis	57	35.1	12.3	32	59.4	12.5

From Rosenberg *et al.* (1975)

sumably prophylaxis needs to be extended into the post-operative period, whereas calf compression ceases when the patient leaves the operating theatre. However, it is clear from this study that heparin is superior to calf compression, although more recent studies have suggested that intermittent calf compression is as effective as low dose heparin even in the presence of malignant disease (Clarke-Pearson *et al.* 1993).

Although the above evidence has been used to suggest that all patients undergoing major gynaecological surgery should receive subcutaneous heparin prophylaxis, it is clear that some patients are at a greater risk than others. The increased risk associated with malignant disease has already been stressed and there is an increased risk in women above the age of 40 years (Bergqvist and Lindbland 1985). In women below the age of 40 years it is possible to be more selective, and, instead of offering subcutaneous heparin to all, it is possible by means of two simple laboratory blood tests (euglobulin lysis time and serum fibrinogen antigen concentration) to identify those patients who are at increased risk of deep venous thrombosis. However, since these tests are not totally specific and sensitive, they are not in widespread use (Crandon *et al.* 1980).

The prevention of infection following gynaecological surgery

Over and above the usual aseptic precautions, the risk of infection after gynaecological surgery in general, and hysterectomy in particular, may be reduced by cleansing the vagina pre-operatively and by the use of prophylactic antibiotics. Walker *et al.* (1982) claimed that the use of povidone iodine is the most effective vaginal cleansing agent, but did not quote specific evidence to support this. Blackmore *et al.* (1981), however, considered that cleansing the vagina with chlorhexidine at the start of surgery was as equally effective as using povidone iodine pessaries every eight hours for at least four applications pre-operatively. In a randomized prospective trial involving patients undergoing both abdominal and vaginal hysterectomy, the incidence of vault infection in those patients who had been treated with iodine was 41 per cent, whilst it was 23 per cent for those treated with chlorhexidine. This difference was not statistically significant, and the diagnosis of infection was based on positive bacteriological growth rather than pyrexia.

There is no convincing evidence that any particular antiseptic used to paint the skin prior to incision is more effective than any other in the prevention of wound infection (Graham *et al.* 1991; Magnann *et al.* 1993).

Without antibiotic prophylaxis, infection of wound, urine, or pelvis will occur in between 21 and 26 per cent of patients undergoing abdominal hysterectomy and in between 21–71 per cent of patients undergoing vaginal hysterectomy (Grossman 1979; Polk *et al.* 1980). The commonly held view that infection is commoner after vaginal than abdominal hysterectomy is only true whilst urinary tract infections are included, otherwise the rates of infections are comparable or perhaps even increased following abdominal hysterectomy (Shapiro *et al.* 1982).

All the evidence suggests that the use of prophylactic antibiotics will reduce this incidence of infection, although the percentage reduction is greater after vaginal hysterectomy than after abdominal hysterectomy. Perhaps this is to be expected since antiseptic skin preparation is the only prophylaxis against abdominal wound infection and clearly there is no abdominal wound following vaginal hysterectomy. The infecting organisms in pelvic infection after hysterectomy tend to be bacteroides, anaerobic streptococci, and, to a lesser degree, *Escherichia coli* (Grossman 1979; Polk *et al.* 1980).

Following abdominal hysterectomy, prophylactic antibiotics will reduce the incidence of febrile morbidity by approximately one-third (Mittendorf *et al.* 1993). Thus, Polk *et al.* (1980) reported an incidence of infection of 14 per cent of 206 women who received an antibiotic at the time of abdominal hysterectomy compared with 21 per cent in 223 who received a placebo. Similarly, antibiotic prophylaxis reduced the incidence of post-operative febrile morbidity from 24 per cent to 14 per cent in a recent randomized trial of antibiotics against placebo at the time of abdominal hysterectomy (Munck and Jensen 1989). There was no evidence from these studies that the use of prophylactic antibiotics will reduce the patients' stay in hospital.

Following vaginal hysterectomy, a more significant reduction in febrile morbidity will occur following the use of prophylactic antibiotics. Thus, in one series, 71 per cent of 24 patients who received a placebo had an infection compared with 18 per cent of 28 patients who received a cephaloridine and 19 per cent of 26 patients who received a penicillin (Grossman 1979). Similarly, when 44 patients received antibiotic prophylaxis at the time of vaginal hysterectomy and were compared with 42 patients who did not, the incidence of febrile morbidity was lower (14 per cent compared with 31 per cent), there was less pelvic infection (2 per cent compared with 21 per cent), and there was a shorter stay in hospital (eight days compared with nine days) (Polk *et al.* 1980).

There is a small price to pay for this prophylaxis in that a rash occurred in 3.6 per cent of patients receiving an antibiotic and diarrhoea in 0.8 per cent

Table 14.4 The timing of antibiotic prophylaxis

Hours relative to incision (incision at '0' hours)	No. of patients	% Wound infection
> − 2	369	3.8
−2 to 0	1708	0.6
0 to +3	282	1.4
> + 3	488	3.3
All	2847	1.5

From Classen *et al.* (1992)

compared with 2.3 per cent and 0.4 per cent, respectively after placebo (Polk *et al.* 1980). The cost of the antibiotics is more than compensated for by the reduction in hospital stay in those patients receiving prophylactic antibiotics at the time of vaginal hysterectomy (Davey *et al.* 1988).

In the UK, metronidazole is popularly used as part of a prophylactic regime, whereas it tends to be omitted in the USA. Metronidazole given in the form of suppositories immediately pre-operatively is as effective in the reduction of infection, and significantly cheaper, than when given intravenously (McLean *et al.* 1983). In a double-blind trial of 100 women undergoing abdominal hysterectomy, the incidence of post-operative pyrexia was 28 per cent in the women who received metronidazole but 33 per cent in those who received a placebo (Walker *et al.* 1982).

There is no real evidence to favour any one logically chosen antibiotic over any other (Berkeley *et al.* 1988; Davey *et al.* 1988; Gordon 1988; Multicentre Study Group 1989). Similarly, a single injection of an appropriate antibiotic agent at the time of surgery is as effective as multiple dose regimes in the prevention of post-operative infection (Berkeley *et al.* 1988; Gordon 1988; Orr *et al.* 1988; Orr *et al.* 1990*a*). The single agent may be as effectively given either intramuscularly one hour pre-operatively as intra-venously intra-operatively (Hemsell *et al.* 1990).

There is good evidence that the timing of antibiotic prophylactic administration is critical to the risk of surgically-induced wound infection. In a non-randomized study of 2847 'clean surgical procedures', the lowest wound infection rate occurred if antibiotics had been administered within the two hours immediately prior to the incision, whilst higher rates occurred if administration was greater than two hours pre-incision or if prophylaxis occurred following the incision. These results are shown in Table 14.4 (Classen *et al.* 1992).

The surgeon may confidently use a single dose of either a third-generation cephaloridine or ampicillin intramuscularly one hour pre-operatively as an effective agent in the prophylaxis against infection following hysterectomy.

Particular attention has been given to the prevention of urinary tract infections. Ireland *et al.* (1982) was able to demonstrate, in a randomized trial, a reduction in post-operative urinary tract infection following abdominal hysterectomy, from 50 per cent to 4 per cent, when a single intramuscular injection of co-trimoxazole was given immediately pre-operatively. If post-operative catheter drainage is used, antiseptic irrigation is unhelpful in preventing infection, but intermittent drainage into a closed system will result in a lower infection rate than will continuous drainage (Pollock 1988). Moreover, the use of a suprapubic catheter will be associated with an approximate reduction of 50 per cent in the infection rate compared with a urethral catheter (Sethia *et al.* 1987).

Abdominal wound closure

Abdominal gynaecological procedures will be performed using either a low transverse (Pfannensteil) incision, a midline incision, or a paramedian incision. The lowest incidence of wound dehiscence post-operatively will occur after the use of a low transverse incision. Mowat and Bonnar (1971) reported 2175 women delivered by Caesarean section and found that the incidence of wound dehiscence following a vertical incision was 3 per cent, whereas the incidence of wound dehiscence following the low transverse incision was only 0.4 per cent. The incidence of abdominal dehiscence following different types of vertical abdominal incisions has been reported by Guillou *et al.* (1980) who also described the newer lateral paramedian incision. The lateral paramedian incision is made at least two-thirds of the width of the rectus sheath away from the midline. In a randomized trial of 207 laparotomy incisions, the incidence of burst abdomen was zero after either a midline incision or a lateral paramedian incision, but was 1.5 per cent following the medial paramedian incision. It would seem that a midline or a lateral paramedian incision are preferable to the classical medial paramedian incision.

Whichever incision is chosen, the technique of wound closure is important in the avoidance of both abdominal dehiscence and of an incisional hernia. Ellis (1984) advised that wide bites of tissue are taken, involving a minimum of 1 cm of tissue from the wound edge, and that the sutures are placed at intervals of 1 cm, or less, apart, not too tight in order to allow for post-operative abdominal distension, thus the length of suture used will measure approximately four times that of the length of the original wound.

Although it was probably beneficial to close the abdominal wall in layers when catgut was the only available material, there is increasing evidence that this is no longer a valid concept. Ellis and Heddle (1977) argued that closure of the peritoneum is not necessary. This hypothesis has been tested for laparotomy incisions. In a non-randomized trial of closure of laparotomy incisions, with or without peritoneal suturing, followed by interval laparoscopy, there were no differences in wound healing or in the incidence of intra-abdominal adhesions between the groups (Tulandi *et al.* 1988). In a recent randomized study of closure of the peritoneum or not at the time of lower section Caesarean section, there were no demonstrable adverse effects on post-operative recovery in those patients in whom the visceral and parietal peritoneum was not closed (Hull and Varner 1991).

With the advent of the newer, synthetic, slowly absorbable suture materials as an alternative to catgut, mass closure of a vertical abdominal incision is again being considered. Mass closure is the technique in which peritoneum, muscle, and sheath are closed using the same suture, a separate suture being used for the skin (and fat layer if this is to be closed). The newer synthetic materials (vicryl or polyglactin, dexon or polyglycolic acid, and PDS or polydioxone) have been advocated for abdominal closure because of their delayed absorption, retention of tensile strength (especially in the presence of infection), and lower levels of tissue reaction (Aronson and Lee 1990). In one prospective study of 1129 major laparotomy wounds, the incidence of abdominal dehiscence was 1 per cent when mass closure was employed using either a newer synthetic material or nylon, whereas abdominal dehiscence occurred in 3 per cent of patients when the abdominal wall was closed conventionally in layers (Bucknall *et al.* 1982). In a more recent study of 285 patients undergoing gynaecological surgery (60 per cent for malignant disease) only one dehiscence occurred (0.4 per cent) after mass closure using polyglycolic acid, suggesting that this is a safe and effective method of abdominal closure (Gallup *et al.* 1990). Other recent randomized studies support this view (Orr *et al.* 1990*b*).

Since it is the abdominal incision which the patient sees, the good cosmetic appearance of this scar is important. The use of skin staples is significantly faster than the use of conventional sutures, and while some trials have demonstrated that a skin incision closed with staples is as cosmetic as one closed with interrupted nylon (Meiring *et al.* 1982) other studies have demonstrated that up to 14 per cent of wounds closed with a stapler have some degree of skin inversion and hence a reduction in cosmetic appearance (Stockley and Elson 1987). Moreover, 6 per cent of patients complained that suture removal is painful compared with 21 per cent of patients who complain of pain on removal of the staples (Stockley and Elson 1987).

There is an increasing trend towards the use of subcuticular wound closure, especially using prolene. This is considered to give a good cosmetic appearance, to be safe even in the presence of infection, and to be more comfortable than interrupted skin sutures (Cassie *et al.* 1988; Vipond and Higgins 1991).

The type of suture material used for the closure of the vaginal vault is itself a potential cause of morbidity due to the occurrence of granulation tissue. Thus, in a randomized trial of vicryl against chromic catgut, vault granulation occurred in 21 per cent of patients in the former group but in 45 per cent of the latter, suggesting that vicryl, or the chemically similar dexon, is preferable to catgut for vaginal vault closure (Manyonda *et al.* 1990).

Table 14.5 Indications for Caesarean section

Indication	%
In labour	60.5
Dystocia	24.7
Fetal distress	20.6
Breech	6.1
Others	9.1
Not in labour	39.5
Breech	12.5
Hypertension	10.6
APH	4.2
Other	12.2
Total	100.0

From Yudkin and Redman (1986)

The increasing incidence of Caesarean section

There is no doubt that the incidence of Caesarean section is increasing. In 1965, Caesarean section rates of 3.5 per cent and 4.5 per cent were quoted for England and Wales and the USA, respectively, whereas current levels in the UK are in the region of 14 per cent and one area in the USA quotes a current Caesarean section rate of 31.8 per cent (Goyert *et al*. 1989). There is no single fact which accounts for this increase, and suggested factors have included a change in the incidence of various obstetric complications, the increase in incidence of previous Caesarean sections, changes in maternal age distribution, changes in paediatric services, the influence of malpractice litigation, the influence of continuous electronic monitoring, the wishes of the patient, and the style of the doctor (Chamberlain 1993; Stafford *et al*. 1993).

The major indications for Caesarean section have been reported by Yudkin and Redman (1986). Some 30.3 per cent of all Caesarean sections were performed because of a previous Caesarean section and the primary indications for the remainder are shown in Table 14.5. It should be noted that 60.5 per cent of Caesarean sections were performed during labour and 39.5 per cent electively. It has been reported that the incidences of some of the commonest indications for Caesarean section (dystocia, fetal distress, and breech presentation) are increasing (Anderson and Lomas 1985; Bottoms *et al*. 1980). Once a patient has had a Caesarean section, there is a likelihood of between 45–61 per cent that she will have a repeat Caesarean section, with two-thirds of these being performed electively and one-third being performed during labour (Paterson and Saunders 1991; Paul *et al*. 1985; Rosen and Dickinson 1990; Yudkin and Redman 1986).

The relationship between Caesarean section rates and continuous fetal heart rate monitoring is discussed in Chapter 18 (The management of labour).

There is evidence that the introduction of a neonatal intensive care service is associated with an increase in Caesarean section, although this may relate in some degree to *in utero* transfers and not just to a change in attitude. Gleicher *et al.* (1985) reported that the Caesarean section rate before the introduction of neonatal intensive care was 14.3 per cent but in the following year it had risen to 18.5 per cent. There is, however, only a poor correlation between the increasing Caesarean section rate and decreasing perinatal mortality rates, whether the whole population is considered or just the very low birthweight population (Bergsjo *et al.* 1983; De Mott and Sandmire 1990; Olshan *et al.* 1984). These authors reported that variations in the Caesarean section rate were associated with only a small inverse correlation in the perinatal mortality rate and accounted for only a small amount of the differences in perinatal mortality rates between different populations.

Whilst one would have expected an increased Caesarean section rate in 'clinic patients, (free treatment) rather than private patients since it is likely that the former are, overall, of a lower socio-economic group than the latter, this is not so. De Regt *et al.* (1986) reviewed over 65 000 deliveries and found that the relative risk for Caesarean section in private patients was 1.3 that of clinic patients. The overall incidence of Caesarean section was 21 per cent in private patients and 17 per cent in clinic patients. Other authors have reported a higher incidence of Caesarean section in the higher socio-economic group of patients (Gould *et al.* 1989). Manning *et al.* (1984) reported that the incidence of Caesarean section in patients who were privately insured on an item for service basis was 28 per cent, higher than the incidence of Caesarean sections in patients who were privately insured in a prepaid scheme.

There is also evidence that the incidence of Caesarean section relates, in some degree, to the 'style of practice' of the physician concerned. Recent US studies of Caesarean section rates have demonstrated a wide variation in Caesarean section rates within the same population, ranging between 5.6 and 19.7 per cent in one population, 10.9 and 17.3 per cent in another, and 9.2 and 31.8 per cent in a third (De Mott and Sandmire 1990; Gould *et al.* 1989; Goyert *et al.* 1989). Some 3 per cent of obstetricians would agree to perform a Caesarean section should the patient wish it in the absence of any specific medical indication (Johnson *et al.* 1986).

It is not clear whether the fear of litigation has influenced Caesarean section rates. Some authors have claimed that this fear has increased Caesarean section rates (De Mott and Sandmire 1990; Ennis *et al.* 1991; Gould *et al.* 1989), whereas others have argued that there is no relationship between the fear of litigation and the Caesarean section rate (Banfield *et al.* 1991; Belizan *et al.* 1991). No doubt obstetricians, patients, and lawyers will watch closely for any relationship in the next few years.

From the above, it would seem that the current Caesarean section rates could be reduced without any significant detriment in fetal or neonatal safety. There is evidence that Caesarean section rates may now have reached a plateau (Macfarlane and Chamberlain 1993; Notzon *et al*. 1994) and could be encouraged to fall by a combination of careful assessment of clinical indications and genuine intent (Socol *et al*. 1993; Treffers and Pel 1993).

Caesarean section scar dehiscence

One of the factors in repeat Caesarean section is the avoidance of scar dehiscence. This complication probably occurs in a significant number of patients without identification, and should be distinguished from a true rupture of the uterus (Finley and Gibbs 1986). Current series generally make this distinction and hence quote statistics which differ from those reported by Dewhurst in 1957. Dewhurst reported 1530 patients with a previous lower segment Caesarean section from six previously published series, together with 762 patients with a classical Caesarean section from six previously published series. For the lower segment group, the incidence of scar rupture was 0.5 per cent for all patients, 0.8 per cent for those in labour, and 1.2 per cent of those delivering vaginally. For the classical Caesarean section group, the incidence of scar rupture was 2.2 per cent for all patients, 4.7 per cent for those in labour, and 8.9 per cent for those delivering vaginally. The need to avoid vaginal delivery in patients with a previous classical section was clear.

More recent series have suggested that some degree of scar dehiscence may be detected at repeat Caesarean section in up to 4 per cent of patients, although a true rupture of the uterus following a lower segment Caesarean section occurs in less than 0.5 per cent of patients (Finley and Gibbs 1986; Paul *et al*. 1985).

Perhaps it is the relative infrequency with which obstetricians now see a ruptured uterus which has led some authors to consider whether or not a classical Caesarean section should be performed more often, especially as it might be more gentle for the delivery of the preterm infant (Westgren and Paul 1985). However, it would seem likely that this would increase the maternal risks, and it has been suggested that such a trend should not be introduced into clinical practice without a well-monitored randomized trial (Halperin *et al*. 1988).

The prevention of infection following Caesarean section

The incidence of febrile morbidity following Caesarean section is surprisingly high, even after elective Caesarean section. One study of 1546 women delivered by Caesarean section demonstrated a wound infection rate following emergency Caesarean section of 12 per cent and following elective Caesarean section of 8 per cent (Webster 1988). The incidence of wound infection was related to the length of time of membrane rupture such that the longer were the membranes ruptured, the higher was the incidence of both wound infection and endometritis. Cunningham *et al*. (1978) reported that in patients whose membranes were intact at the time of Caesarean section, the incidence of wound infection was zero and the incidence of endometritis was 29 per cent, but when the membranes had been ruptured for up to six hours before Caesarean section, the incidence of wound infection was 4 per cent and endometritis 67 per cent, whilst the incidence of wound infection was 24 per cent and endometritis 85 per cent if the membranes had been ruptured for longer than six hours. Because of such observations, there have been numerous trials which have assessed the efficacy of prophylactic antibiotics in the prevention of such sepsis.

There is now no doubt that prophylactic antibiotics reduce the incidence of both wound infection and endometritis following both emergency and elective Caesarean section (Smaill 1992). There have been several overviews of the literature which have enabled such conclusions to be reached. Duff (1987) assessed 25 prospective randomized controlled trials and concluded that prophylactic antibiotics would reduce the overall incidence of sepsis by 60 per cent. Mungford *et al.* (1989) assessed the results of 58 prospective controlled trials comprising 7777 women in whom prophylactic antibiotics were compared with either a placebo or no treatment. When an antibiotic was given, the overall risk of wound infection was 35 per cent that found without an antibiotic and the overall risk of endometritis was 25 per cent of that found without an antibiotic. Enkin *et al.* (1989) reported a meta-analysis of 44 placebo-controlled randomized trials of antibiotic prophylaxis for Caesarean section. There was a 65 per cent reduction in the incidence of wound infection and 75 per cent for endometritis following emergency Caesarean section. There was a similar reduction in the incidence of endometritis when antibiotics were given at the time of elective Caesarean section, but the wound infection rate fell by 90 per cent.

Whilst there is no doubt that antibiotic prophylaxis at the time of Caesarean section will reduce infection, the existing evidence supports the view that a broad-spectrum antibiotic, such as ampicillin, is as effective as a third-generation cephalosporin and that a single dose of antibiotic is as effective as a multiple dose regime (Duff 1987; Enkin *et al.* 1989; Faro *et al.* 1990; Mungford *et al.* 1989; Stein 1991). In one randomized trial involving 1580 patients delivered by Caesarean section who were allocated to receive one of seven different antibiotics in ten different regimes, ampicillin, 2 g in a single dose given intravenously at the moment that the cord was clamped, was as good as any other regime in the reduction of post-operative infection (13 per cent) (Faro *et al.* 1990). Not only is a single dose of antibiotic as good as a multiple dose, short-acting single antibiotics are as effective as long-acting antibiotics in single dose (Carlson and Duff 1990).

There is only limited evidence concerning the place of metronidazole as a prophylactic agent at the time of Caesarean section. In one trial involving 100 women undergoing Caesarean section, metronidazole, 1 g, given intravenously immediately after cord clamping, but without any other antibiotic, was associated with an incidence of post-operative wound infection of 2 per cent and endometritis of 14 per cent, whereas the relative figures following placebo were 8 per cent and 30 per cent (Moreno *et al.* 1991). The randomized trial which compares the use of either a broad-spectrum antibiotic or a third-generation cephaloridine with metronidazole has not been performed.

With our current state of knowledge, all patients undergoing Caesarean section, emergency or elective, should receive a single injection of an antibiotic when the cord is clamped.

Conclusions

There is no doubt that attention to surgical technique will reduce the complications following gynaecological or obstetric surgery. However, the use of peri-operative agents is also a major factor in the reduction of morbidity. There can now be no doubt that the use of prophylactic anticoagulants, especially in patients over the age of 40 years or with malignant disease, will reduce the thromboembolic complications of major gynaecological surgery. In addition, there is no doubt that a single antibiotic given during surgery will reduce the incidence of post-operative sepsis.

There is still scope for a further examination of the type of incision used and the way in which that incision is closed. As new suture materials are developed, this process of examination will continue.

Acknowledgement

The author wishes to thank Mr N. J. St G. Saunders for his advice on this chapter.

References

Anderson, G. M. and Lomas, J. (1985). Explaining variations in Caesarean section rates. *Canadian Medical Association Journal* **132**, 253–9.

Aronson, M. P. and Lee, R. A. (1990). Chromic catgut should be abandoned for fascial closure of the anterior abdominal wall in favour of newer stronger delayed absorbable suture material. *Journal of Gynecological Surgery* **6**, 59–61.

Ballard, R. M., Bradley-Watson, P. J., Johnstone, F. D., Kenney, A., McCarthy, T. G., Campbell, S., *et al.* (1973). Low doses of subcutaneous heparin in the prevention of deep venous thrombosis after gynaecological surgery. *Journal of Obstetrics and Gynaecology of the British Commonwealth* **80**, 469–72.

Banfield, P., O'Hanlon, M. Chapple, J., and Mugford, M. (1991). Obstetric practice and the fear of litigation. *Lancet* **338**, 1019.

Belizan, J. M., Quaranta, P., Paquez, E., and Villar, J. (1991). Caesarean section and fear of litigation. *Lancet* **338**, 1462.

Bergqvist, D. and Lindbland, B. (1985). A 30-year survey of pulmonary embolism verified at autopsy. *British Journal of Surgery* **72**, 105–8.

Bergsjo, P., Schmidt, E., and Pusch, D. (1983). Differences in reported frequencies of some obstetrical intervention in Europe. *British Journal of Obstetrics and Gynaecology* **90**, 628–32.

Berkeley, A. S., Freedman, K. S., Ledger, W. J., Orr, J. W., Benigno, B. B., Gordon, S. F., *et al.* (1988). Comparison of cefotetan and cefoxitin prophylaxis for abdominal and vaginal hysterectomy. *American Journal of Obstetrics and Gynecology* **158**, 706–9.

Blackmore, M. A., Turner, G. M., Adams, M. R., and Speller, D. C. E. (1981). The effect of pre-operative povidone iodine vaginal pessaries on vault infection after hysterectomy. *British Journal of Obstetrics and Gynaecology* **88**, 308–13.

Bonnar, J. and Walsh, J. J. (1972). Prevention of thrombosis after pelvic surgery by Dextran 70. *Lancet* **i**, 614–16.

Bottoms, S. F., Rosen, M. G., and Sokol, R. J. (1980). The increase in Caesarean birth rate. *New England Journal of Medicine* **302**, 559–63.

Bucknall, T. E., Cox, P. J., and Ellis, H. (1982). Burst abdomen and incisional hernia. *British Medical Journal* **284**, 931–3.

Carlson, C. and Duff, P. (1990). Antibiotic prophylaxis for Caesarean delivery. *Obstetrics and Gynecology* **76**, 343–6.

Cassie, A. B., Chatterjee, A. K., Mehta, S., and Haworth, J. M. (1988). Pain and wound healing. *Annals of the Royal College of Surgeons of England* **70**, 339–42.

Chamberlain, G. (1993). What is the correct Caesarean section rate? *British Journal of Obstetrics and Gynaecology* **100**, 403–4.

Clarke-Pearson, D. L., Coleman, R. E., Synan, I. S., Hinshaw, W., and Creasman, W. T. (1983*a*). Venous thrombosis prophylaxis in gynaecological oncology. *American Journal of Obstetrics and Gynecology* **145**, 606–13.

Clarke-Pearson, D. L., Jelovsek, F. R., and Creasman, W. T. (1983*b*). Thromboembolism complicating surgery for cervical and uterine malignancy. *Obstetrics and Gynecology* **61**, 87–94.

Clarke-Pearson, D. L., De Long, E., Synan, I. S., Soper, J. T., Creasman, W. T., and Coleman, R. E. (1990). A controlled trial of two low-dose heparin regimens for the prevention of post-operative deep venous thrombosis. *Obstetrics and Gynecology* **75**, 684–9.

Clarke-Pearson, D. L., Synan, I. S., Dodge, R., Soper, J. T., Berchuck, A., and Coleman, R. E. (1993). A randomized trial of low dose heparin and intermittent calf compression for the prevention of deep venous thromboses. *American Journal of Obstetrics and Gynecology* **168**, 1146–54.

Classen, D. C., Evans, R. S., Pestotnik, S. L., Horn, S. D., Menlove, R. L., and Burke, J. P. (1992). The timing of prophylactic administration of antibiotics and the risk of surgical wound infection. *New England Journal of Medicine* **326**, 281–6.

Colditz, G. A., Tuden, R. L., and Oster, G. (1986). Rates of venous thrombosis after general surgery. *Lancet* **ii**, 143–6.

Collins, R., Scrimgeour, A., Yasuf, S., and Peto, R. (1988). Reduction in fetal pulmonary embolus and venous thrombosis by perioperative administration of subcutaneous heparin. *New England Journal of Medicine* **318**, 1162–73.

Crandon, A. J., Peel, K. R., Anderson, J. A., Thompson, V., and McNicol, G. P. (1980). Post-operative deep venous thrombosis: identification of high-risk pregnancies. *British Medical Journal* **281**, 343–5.

Cunningham, F. G., Hauth, A. C., Strong, J. D., and Kappus, S. S. (1978). Infectious morbidity following Caesarean section. *Obstetrics and Gynecology* **52**, 656–61.

Davey, P. G., Duncan, I. D., Edward, D., and Scott, A. C. (1988). Cost–benefit analysis of cephradine and mezlocillin prophylaxis for abdominal and vaginal hysterectomy. *British Journal of Obstetrics and Gynaecology* **95**, 1170–7.

De Mott, R. K. and Sandmire, H. F. (1990). The Green Bay Caesarean Section Study. *American Journal of Obstetrics and Gynecology* **162**, 1593–602.

De Regt, R., Minkoff, H. L., Feldman, J., and Schwartz, R. H. (1986). Relation of private or clinic care to the Caesarean birth rate. *New England Journal of Medicine* **315**, 619–24.

Dewhurst, C. H. (1957). The ruptured Caesarean section scar. *Journal of Obstetrics and Gynaecology of the British Empire* **64**, 113–18.

Drug and Therapeutics Bulletin (1992). Preventing and treating deep venous thrombosis. *Drug and Therapeutics Bulletin* **30**, 9–12.

Duff, P. Prophylactic antibiotics for Caesarean delivery (1987). *American Journal of Obstetrics and Gynecology* **157**, 794–8.

Ellis, H. (1984). Midline abdominal incisions. *British Journal of Obstetrics and Gynaecology* **91**, 1–2.

Ellis, H. and Heddle, R. (1977). Does the peritoneum need to be closed at laparoscopy? *British Journal of Surgery* **64**, 733–6.

Enkin, M., Enkin, E., Chalmers, I., and Hemminki, E. (1989). Prophylactic antibiotics in association with Caesarean section. In *Effective care in pregnancy and childbirth* (ed. I. Chalmers, M. Enkin, and M. J. N. C. Keirse), pp. 1246–69. Oxford University Press, Oxford.

Ennis, M., Clark, A., and Grudzinskas, J. G. (1991). Change in obstetric practice in response to fear of litigation in the British Isles. *Lancet* **338**, 616–18.

Faro, S., Martens, M. G., Hammill, H. A., Riddle, G., and Tortolero, G. (1990). Antibiotic prophylaxis—is there a difference? *American Journal of Obstetrics and Gynecology* **162**, 900–9.

Finley, B. E. and Gibbs, C. E. (1986). Emergent Caesarean delivery in patients undergoing a trial of labour with a transverse lower segment scar. *American Journal of Obstetrics and Gynecology* **155**, 936–9.

Gallup, D. G., Nolan, T. E., and Smith, R. P. (1990). Primary mass closure of midline incision with a continuous polyglyconate monofilament absorbable suture. *Obstetrics and Gynecology* **76**, 872–5.

Gleicher, N., Vermesh, M., Rotmesch, Z., Thornton, J., and Elrad, H. (1985). Caesarean section patterns—the influence of a perinatology service. *Mount Sinai Journal of Medicine* **52**, 100–5.

Gordon, S. F. (1988). Results of a single centre study of cefotetan prophylaxis in abdominal and vaginal hysterectomy. *American Journal of Obstetrics and Gynecology* **158**, 710–14.

Gould, J. B., Davey, B., and Stafford, R. S. (1989). Socio-economic differences in the rates of Caesarean section. *New England Journal of Medicine* **321**, 233–9.

Goyert, G. L., Bottoms, S. F., Treadwell, M. C., and Nehra, P. C. (1989). The physician factor in Caesarean birth rates. *New England Journal of Medicine* **320**, 706–9.

Graham, G. P., Dent, C. M., and Fairclough, J. A. (1991). Preparation of skin for surgery. *Journal of the Royal College of Surgeons of Edinburgh* **36**, 264–6.

Groote Schuur Hospital Thromboembolism Study Group (1979). Failure of low-dose heparin to prevent significant thrombo-embolic complications. *British Medical Journal* **1**, 1447–50.

Grossman, J. H. (1979). Prophylactic antibiotics in gynaecological surgery. *Obstetrics and Gynecology* **53**, 537–44.

Grubber, U. F., Duckert, F., Friedrich, R., Torhurst, J., and Rem, J. (1977). Prevention of post-operative thromboembolism by Dextran 40, low doses of heparin, or xantinol nicotinate. *Lancet* **i**, 207–10.

Guillou, P. J., Hall, T. J., Donaldson, D. R., Broughton, A. C., and Brennan, T. J. (1980). Vertical abdominal incisions—a choice? *British Journal of Surgery* **67**, 395–9.

Halperin, M. E., Moore, D. C., and Hannah, W. J. (1988). Classical versus lower segment transverse incision for preterm Caesarean section. *British Journal of Obstetrics and Gynaecology* **95**, 990-6.

Hemsell, D. L., Johnson, E. R., Hemsell, P. G., Nobles, B.J., and Heard, M. C. (1990). Cefazolin for hysterectomy prophylaxis. *Obstetrics and Gynecology* **76**, 603-6.

Hull, D. B. and Varner, M. W., (1991). A randomized study of closure of the peritoneum at Caesarean delivery. *Obstetrics and Gynecology* **77**, 818-21.

International Multicentre Trial (1975). Prevention of fatal post-operative pulmonary embolus by low doses of heparin. *Lancet* **ii**, 45-51.

International Multicentre Trial (1977). Prevention of fatal post-operative pulmonary embolus by low doses of heparin. *Lancet* **i**, 567-9.

Ireland, D., Tacchi, D., and Bint, A. J. (1982). Effect of single-dose prophylactic co-trimoxazole on the incidence of gynaecological post-operative urinary tract infection. *British Journal of Obstetrics and Gynaecology* **89**, 578-80.

Johnson, S. R., Elkins, T. E., Strong, C., and Phelam, J. P. (1986). Obstetrics decision-making. *Obstetrics and Gynecology* **67**, 847-50.

Kakkar, V. V., Cohen, A. T., Edmondson, R. A., Phillips, M. J., Cooper, D. J., Das, S. K., *et al.* (1993). Low molecular weight versus standard heparin for the prevention of venous thromboembolism after major abdominal surgery. *Lancet* **341**, 259-65.

Leizorovicz, A., Hough, M. C., Chapuis, F. R., Samama, M. M., and Boissel, J. P. (1992). Low molecular weight heparin in prevention of peri-operative thrombosis. *British Medical Journal* **305**, 913-20.

Macfarlane, A. and Chamberlain, G. (1993). What is happening to Caesarean section rates? *Lancet* **342**, 1005-6.

McLean, A., Ioannides-Demos, L., Somogyi, A., Tong, N., and Spicer, J. (1983). Successful substitution of rectal metronidazole administration for intravenous use. *Lancet* **i**, 41-2.

Magnann, E. F., Dodson, M. K., Ray, M. A., Harris, R. L., Martin, J. N., and Morrison, J. C. (1993). Pre-operative skin preparation and intra-operative pelvic irrigation. *Obstetrics and Gynecology* **81**, 922-5.

Manning, W. G., Leibowitz, A., Goldberg, G. A., Rogers, W. H., and Newhouse, J. P. (1984). A controlled trial of the effect of a prepaid group practice on use of services. *New England Journal of Medicine* **310**, 1505-10.

Manyonda, I., Welch, C. R., McWhinney, N. A., and Ross, L. D. (1990). The influence of suture material on vaginal vault granulation following abdominal hysterectomy. *British Journal of Obstetrics and Gynaecology* **97**, 608-12.

Meiring, L., Silliers, K., Barry, R., and Nel, C. H. C. (1982). A comparison of a disposable skin stapler and nylon sutures for wound closure. *South African Medical Journal* **62**, 371-2.

Mittendorf, R., Aronson, M. P., Berry, R. E., Williams, M. A., Kupelnick, B., Klickstein, A., *et al.* (1993). Avoiding serious infection associated with abdominal hysterectomy. *American Journal of Obstetrics and Gynecology* **169**, 1119-21.

Moreno, R., Garcia-Rojas, J. M., and Leon, J. D. L. (1991). Prevention of post-Caesarean infectious morbidity with a single dose of intravenous metronidazole. *International Journal of Gynecology and Obstetrics* **34**, 217-20.

Mowat, J. and Bonnar, J. (1971). Abdominal wound dehiscence after Caesarean section. *British Medical Journal* **2**, 256-7.

Multicentre Study Group (1989). Single dose prophylaxis in patients undergoing vaginal hysterectomy. *American Journal of Obstetrics and Gynecology* **160**, 1198-201.

Munck, A. M. and Jensen, H. K. (1989). Pre-operatively clindomycin treatment and vaginal drainage in hysterectomy. *Acta Obstetrica et Gynaecologica Scandinavica* **68**, 241–5.

Mungford, M., Kingston, J., and Chalmers, I. (1989). Reducing the incidence of infection after Caesarean section. *British Medical Journal* **299**, 1003–6.

Notzon, F. C., Cnattingius, S., Cole, S., Taffel, S., Irgens, L., and Daltveit, A. K. (1994). Caesarean section delivery in the 1990s. *American Journal of Obstetrics and Gynecology* **170**, 495–504.

Olshan, A. F., Shy, K. K., Luthy, D., Hickok, D., Weiss, N. S., and Daling, J. R. (1984). Caesarean birth and neonatal morbidity in very low birthweight infants. *Obstetrics and Gynecology* **64**, 267–70.

Orr, J. W., Sisson, P. F., Barrett, J. M., Ellington, J. R., Jennings, R. H., and Taylor, D. L. (1988). Single centre study results of cefotetan and cefoxitin prophylaxis for abdominal or vaginal hysterectomy. *American Journal of Obstetrics and Gynecology* **158**, 714–16.

Orr, J. W., Sisson, P. F., Patsner, B., Barrett, J. M., Ellington, J. R., Jennings, R. H., *et al.* (1990*a*). A single-dose antibiotic prophylaxis for patients undergoing extended pelvic surgery for gynecologic malignancy. *American Journal of Obstetrics and Gynecology* **162**, 718–21.

Orr, J. W., Orr, P. F., Barrett, J. M., Ellington, J. R., Jennings, R. H., Paredes, K. B., *et al.* (1990*b*). Continuous or interrupted fascial closure: a prospective evaluation. *American Journal of Obstetrics and Gynecology* **163**, 1485–9.

Paterson, C. M. and Saunders, N. J. S. G. (1991). Mode of delivery after one Caesarean section. *British Medical Journal* **303**, 818–21.

Paul, R. H., Phelan, J. P., and Yeh, S. (1985). Trial of labour in the patient with a prior Caesarean birth. *American Journal of Obstetrics and Gynecology* **151**, 297–304.

Polk, B. F., Tager, I. B., Shapiro, M., Goren-White, B., Goldstein, P., and Schoenbaum, S. C. (1980). Randomized trial of perioperative cefozilin in preventing infection after hysterectomy. *Lancet* **i**, 437–40.

Pollock, A. V. (1988). Surgical prophylaxis. *Lancet* **i**, 225–9.

Rosen, M. G. and Dickinson, J. C. (1990). Vaginal birth after Caesarean section: a meta-analysis of indicators for success. *Obstetrics and Gynecology* **76**, 865–9.

Rosenberg, I. L., Evans, M., and Pollock, A. V. (1975). Prophylaxis of post-operative leg venous thrombosis by low-dose subcutaneous heparin or pre-operative calf stimulation. *British medical Journal* **1**, 649–51.

Sethia, K. K., Selkon, J. B., Berry, A. V., Turner, C. M., Kettlewell, M. G., and Gough, G. H. (1987). Prospective controlled trial of urethral versus suprapubic catheterisation. *British Journal of Surgery,* **74**, 624–5.

Sevitts, S. and Gallagher, N. G. (1959). Prevention of venous thrombosis and pulmonary embolism in injured patients. *Lancet* **ii**, 981–9.

Shapiro, M., Munoz, A., Tager, I. B., Schoenbaum, S. C., and Polk, B. F. (1982). Risk factors for infection at the operative site after abdominal or vaginal hysterectomy. *New England Journal of Medicine* **307**, 1661–6.

Smaill, F. (1992). Antibiotic prophylaxis in Caesarean section. *British Journal of Obstetrics and Gynaecology* **99**, 789–90.

Socol, M. L., Garcia, P. M., Peaceman, A. M., and Dooley, S. L. (1993). Reducing Caesarean births at a primarily private university hospital. *American Journal of Obstetrics and Gynecology* **168**, 1748–58.

Stafford, R. S., Sullivan, S. D., and Gardner, L. B. (1993). Trends in Caesarean section use in California. *American Journal of Obstetrics and Gynecology* **168**, 1293–302.

Stein, G. E. (1991). Patient costs for prophylaxis and treatment of obstetric and gynecologic surgical infections. *American Journal of Obstetrics and Gynecology* **154**, 1377–80.

Stockley, I. and Elson, R. (1987). Skin closure using staples or nylon sutures. *Annals of the Royal College of Surgeons of England* **69**, 76–8.

Taberner, D. A., Poller, L., Burslem, R. W., and Jones, J. B. (1978). Oral anticoagulants controlled by the British comparative thromboplastin ratio versus low-dose heparin in prophylaxis of deep venous thrombosis. *British Medical Journal* **1**, 272–6.

Treffers, P. E. and Pel, M. (1993). The rising trend for Caesarean birth. *British Medical Journal* **307**, 1017–18.

Tulandi, T., Hum, H. S., and Gelfand, M. M. (1988). Closure of laparotomy incision with or without peritoneal suturing. *American Journal of Obstetrics and Gynecology* **158**, 536–7.

Vipond, M. N. and Higgins, A. F. (1991). Subcuticular prolene or PDS for skin closure? *Journal of the Royal College of Surgeons of Edinburgh* **36**, 97–102.

Walker, E. M., Gordon, A. J., Warren, R. E., and Hare, M. J. (1982). Prophylactic single-dose metronidazole before abdominal hysterectomy. *British Journal of Obstetrics and Gynaecology* **89**, 957–61.

Walsh, J. J., Bonnar, J., and Wright, J. W. (1974). A study of pulmonary embolus and deep leg venous thrombosis after major gynaecological surgery. *Journal of Obstetrics and Gynaecology of the British Commonwealth* **81**, 311–16.

Webster, J. (1988). Post-Caesarean wound infection. *Australian and New Zealand Journal of Obstetrics and Gynaecology* **28**, 201–7.

Westgren, M. and Paul, R. (1985). Delivery of the low birthweight infant by Caesarean section. *Clinical Obstetrics and Gynecology* **28**, 752–62.

Yudkin, P. I. and Redman, C. W. G. (1986). Caesarean section dissected 1978–1983. *British Journal of Obstetrics and Gynaecology* **93**, 135–44.

15 Routine antenatal care

It is arbitrarily and traditionally taught that pregnant women should seek medical advice early in their pregnancies in order to initiate antenatal care which, at a minimal level, will consist of a visit to a doctor or a midwife every four weeks until the twenty-eighth week of pregnancy, every second week until the thirty-sixth week of pregnancy, and then weekly until delivery. Taking England and Wales as an example, there are currently approximately 700 000 maternities per year, and if the average patient first attended at the eighth week and delivered at the fortieth week, there would be 9 100 000 antenatal visits per year. This huge commitment of the time of doctors, midwives, and patients requires a closer analysis.

This chapter will deal specifically with the causes of perinatal mortality, the changing style of antenatal care, and the value of certain selected areas of advice given to pregnant women. Specific discussions concerning specific conditions, such as intrauterine growth retardation or pre-eclampsia, will be debated in the appropriate chapters.

Perinatal mortality

The perinatal mortality rate has been used traditionally as a 'measure' of the quality of perinatal care, yet there is little reason to continue with this statistic unless it is modified. There are two major reasons for this. The first concerns the deficiencies in the statistic itself, whilst the second concerns the quality of the conclusions drawn from these statistics.

The perinatal mortality rate only concerns itself with death after the 28th week of pregnancy and before the end of the first week of life. The improvements in neonatal survival, especially of preterm infants, have prevented many deaths but have deferred others to the post-perinatal period. There is a need to consider not only the perinatal mortality rate, but the late neonatal mortality rate and the post-neonatal mortality rate (*Lancet* 1991*a*) The current definition of a perinatal death excludes death *in utero* before the 28th week of pregnancy, yet there is some argument in favour of reducing this gestational age to include infants dying *in utero* during the late second trimester since these may have a similar cause to those in the third trimester.

There is much to recommend the use of 'weight-related' statistics rather than merely gestational statistics which would include all infants, for instance, of birthweight in excess of 500 g whether live or stillborn. Currently, liveborn infants of any gestation are included in perinatal mortality statistics should they die within seven days of birth, yet a fetus of the same weight and gestation

Table 15.1 Perinatal mortality rate and antenatal visits

Number of antenatal visits	Percentage of pregnant population	Mortality ratio
0	0.6	502
1	0.4	409
2	0.8	378
3–4	3.4	315
5–9	28.6	126
10–14	40.2	67
15–19	16.5	58
20–24	5.3	58
25–29	1.6	78
>30	1.0	122
Unknown	1.6	199

From Perinatal Mortality Survey (Butler and Bonham 1963)

which dies *in utero* is excluded. In the European Study of Pregnancy Outcome involving 1644 deaths between the 22nd and 28th week of gestation, 55 per cent of babies were liveborn and would be included in a perinatal mortality statistic, whereas 45 per cent were stillborn and would have been excluded (Working Party on the Very Low Birthweight Infant 1990). There is much to be said for quoting figures corrected for lethal fetal abnormality since this is a major but largely unpreventable cause of death (see below).

Many of the factors involved in perinatal loss were described in the Perinatal Mortality Survey (Butler and Bonham 1963). This survey analysed data from 16 994 pregnancies during a particular month in 1958 in England and Wales. Whilst much valuable information came from this study, it has sometimes been misused as evidence that there is some relationship between the number of antenatal visits and the perinatal mortality rates such that, within reason, the more visits the lower the perinatal mortality. This survey made use of the 'mortality ratio' which is the relative risk of a perinatal mortality for that group in particular compared with the cohort study. The relationship between the mortality ratio and the number of antenatal visits is shown in Table 15.1.

There is no doubt that the triad of age, parity, and social class are major determinants of perinatal mortality rates yet cannot be influenced by obstetric care (Balarajan and Botting 1989; Chamberlain 1978; Cnattingius *et al.* 1993). From Tables 15.2, 15.3, and 15.4. it can be seen that the lowest perinatal mortality will occur in a patient aged between 25 and 29 years, having her second baby, and belonging to social class I. It is also possible to construct tables (Tables 15.5 and 15.6) which relate perinatal mortality rate to birthweight of the overall population, and of the population corrected for singleton or multiple births (Alberman 1989; Balarajan and Botting 1989).

Table 15.2 Perinatal mortality rate and maternal age

Maternal age	Perinatal mortality rate
All ages	10
<20 yrs	13
20–24	10
25–29	9
30–34	10
35–39	12
40 +	17

From Balarajan and Botting (1989)

Table 15.3 Perinatal mortality rate and parity

Parity	Perinatal mortality rate
All parities	10
P_0	10
P_1	8
P_2	9
P_3 or more	12

From Balarajan and Botting (1989)

Table 15.4 Perinatal mortality rate and social class

Social class	Perinatal mortality rate
All classes (legitimate)	9.5
All classes (illegitimate)	12.7
I	7.2
II	7.8
IIIN	8.4
IIIM	9.2
IV	10.6
V	12.0

From Balarajan and Botting (1989)

There is a further complication in drawing conclusions from all the above data, in that pregnant women of social class V, young pregnant women, and pregnant women who were para four or more were more likely to attend later in pregnancy for their first antenatal visit than were pregnant women in general. Thus 18 per cent of women of social class V attend for their first antenatal visit after the 20th week of pregnancy compared with 9 per cent of women of social classes I and II. Some 19 per cent of pregnant women below the age of 20 years

Table 15.5 Perinatal mortality rate and birthweight

Birthweight (g)	Perinatal mortality rate
All	10
<2500	94
2500–2999	7
3000–3499	3
3500–3999	2
4000 +	3

From Balarajan and Botting (1989)

Table 15.6 Perinatal mortality rate and birthweight

Birthweight (g)	Perinatal mortality rate	
	Singleton	Multiple
1500	360.0	302.3
1500–1999	107.3	43.2
2000–2499	30.8	12.2
2500–2999	7.1	10.0
3000–3499	2.7	7.6
3500–3999	1.8	4.0
4000 +	3.1	—
Total	9.1	47.7

From Alberman (1989)

attended their first antenatal visit beyond the 20th week compared with 9 per cent of all other age groups, whilst 33 per cent of women who were para four or more attended for their first antenatal visit beyond the 20th week of pregnancy compared with 9 per cent of women who were para three or less (O'Brien and Smith 1981).

Numerous studies now exist which add detail to the bland perinatal mortality rate statistic. MacFarlane *et al.* (1986), using data from Scotland, showed that the stillbirth rate was 5.4 per 1000 total births, perinatal mortality rate 9.8, and neonatal mortality 5.4 per 1000 total births. It is likely that the quality of antenatal care will only affect perinatal deaths due to asphyxia, trauma, or immaturity (Clarke *et al.* 1993).

Congenital abnormality accounted for 10 per cent of stillbirths, 18 per cent of perinatal deaths, and 31.5 per cent of neonatal deaths. The relative importance of the major causes of perinatal death have also been widely reported. For instance, Bucknell and Wood (1985) reported a survey of 335 perinatal deaths occurring in the Wessex region of England in 1982 and representing a perinatal mortality rate of 10.1 per 1000 births; lethal fetal abnormality accounted for 24 per cent of these. Of the normally formed infants, 49 per cent died before labour, 13 per cent during labour, and 38 per cent after delivery. Some 25 per cent of the deaths in normally formed infants were related to intrauterine growth retardation and 23.2 per cent to prematurity. Similarly, Alberman (1989) showed that the major causes of stillbirth before labour were unknown (73 per cent) and asphyxia (21 per cent), whilst the major causes of death during labour were asphyxia (61 per cent) and congenital malformation (24 per cent). The major causes of early neonatal death were immaturity (42 per cent), congenital malformation (31 per cent), and asphyxia 15 per cent).

The gestational age at which death *in utero* occurs was surveyed by McIlwaine *et al*. (1979) who reported 1150 perinatal deaths in Scotland. This survey showed that 20 per cent of all stillbirths occurred between the 28th and 31st weeks of pregnancy, 39 per cent between the 32nd and 36th week, 28 per cent between the 37th and 39th weeks, 11 per cent between the 40th and 41st weeks, and 2 per cent beyond the 42nd week of pregnancy.

An analysis of such statistics may allow the obstetrician to tailor the antenatal care to the risk factors which are either present when the patient presents at the beginning of pregnancy, or become apparent during the pregnancy. They also demonstrate those areas where investigation, preventative medicine, and research require direction. It is clearly inappropriate to offer the same antenatal care to all patients.

The pattern of antenatal care

How antenatal care is offered depends not only upon the clinical requirements of the recipient (and their views) but also upon the perceptions of the roles of the specialist, general practitioner, and midwife. This inter-relationship is seen in different ways in different countries, often with widely divergent regimes even within the same country (Blondel *et al*. 1985; Heringa and Huisjes 1988). An assessment of the overall value of antenatal care in general has not, and never can be, tested for a randomly allocated trial of care versus no care; this would ethically unacceptable. However, trials of individual aspects of care should be performed and these will be debated either in this chapter, or in other specific chapters, as appropriate. It is, however, of some interest to assess the obstetric outcome in groups who do not accept antenatal care. Kaunitz *et al*. (1984) reported 344 pregnancies between 1975 and 1982 in the Faith Assembly, a religious group in Indiana comprising approximately 2000 members who received no antenatal care and delivered at home without, trained attendance. Their fertility is also greater than average. The 344 pregnancies included 21 perinatal deaths (without any lethal fetal abnormalities) and six maternal deaths (four due to haemorrhage and two due to infection) giving a perinatal mortality rate of 61 per 1000 and a maternal mortality rate of 1744.2 per 100 000. Compared to the rest of Indiana, the perinatal mortality rate was increased by a factor of 2.7 and a maternal mortality rate by a factor of 92.

In a detailed review of clinical trials designed to assess different methods of provision of antenatal care in hospitals or in the community, by medical specialists, midwives, and additional supporters, no real benefits could be identified from any one style of care (Bryce 1990). However, two major trends currently exist within the provision of antenatal care. The first is a trend to increase the volume of care in the community with a corresponding decrease in that which is hospital based, but with shared responsibility between both groups (Anderson 1993; Dunlop 1993). Of the more recent studies, there is evidence to show that such a style increased patient satisfaction but without any evidence as to tangible clinical benefits or detriments (Hepburn 1990; Marsh 1985). In such a situation, good communication between providers is invaluable (Elbourne *et al.* 1987; Thomas *et al.* 1983). Street *et al.* (1991) reported a community study in which 30 per cent of the entire antenatal population received all their antenatal care from general practitioners and midwives without any apparent detriment. What appears to be required is cooperation rather than competition (Keirse 1989).

The second trend relates to the provision of day care in obstetric practice. The use of maternal and fetal assessment units for high-risk patients who might have otherwise become in-patients is being increasingly advocated. The value of this style of treatment in the management of patients with such problems as decreased fetal movements, pregnancy-induced hypertension and intrauterine growth retardation has been recently assessed (Soothill *et al.* 1991; Tuffnell *et al.* 1992). Such units would appear to have the advantages of keeping patients at home other than for their hospital visits, with a corresponding reduction in hospital costs without any obvious detriment. They are destined to play a greater role in antenatal care.

The first real audit of antenatal care was reported by Hall *et. al.* (1980) who stressed that it was the quality rather than the quantity of antenatal care which required reassessment. They performed a retrospective study of the case records of 1907 women delivering in Aberdeen in 1975; this accounted for 1907 booking visits and 19 451 return visits by the patient to either the hospital or the general practitioner. In this series, only 44 per cent of all patients with intrauterine growth retardation (IUGR) were diagnosed antenatally and there were 2.5 false-positive diagnoses for every case accurately diagnosed. The incidence of detection of IUGR for the first time at any one antenatal visit ranged between 0.2 and 0.7 per cent depending upon gestational age. Some 88 per cent of 58 breech presentations at delivery were detected antenatally, the incidence of diagnosis at any one antenatal visit ranging between 0.1 and 0.9 per cent. Of 1884 women with a singleton pregnancy, 259 (13.7 per cent) had evidence of elevated blood pressure and of these, 183 (9.7 per cent) were evident antenatally. The incidence of elevated blood pressure at any antenatal visit only exceeded the 1 per cent level after the 34th week of pregnancy and only exceeded 2 per cent after the 38th week. The incidence of patients with raised blood pressure was 3.2 per cent of visits at the 38th and 39th week and 4.0 per cent at the 40th week or above in primigravidae; for multiparous patients, the incidence was always equal to or less than 0.7 per cent per antenatal visit until the patients were beyond 40 weeks when the level was 1.4 per cent. They concluded that the maximum number of abnormalities that could be diagnosed at any one antenatal visit should they have all arisen at the same time, and before the 40th week, was 4.8 per cent.

The same unit (Chng *et al.* 1980) also assessed the quality of the information obtained at the first (booking) hospital antenatal visit. In a retrospective survey of 1907 case records they found that, in up to 50 per cent of cases, the doctor had failed to identify, or to take note of, such features as previous perinatal death, intrauterine growth retardation, or retained placenta when planning the style of antenatal care or agreeing upon the place of delivery. Whilst the identification of risk factors at the booking visit should influence the style of antenatal care given, it has to be recalled that even in this study 50 per cent of the perinatal deaths occurred to won without identifiable risk factors at booking. More recent studies have demonstrated the low detection rates for small for gestation age (14 per cent), breech presentation (69 per cent), and twin pregnancies (94 per cent) (Backe and Nakling 1993).

Perhaps not all patients require the traditional level of antenatal surveillance, especially multiparous women, and perhaps each antenatal visit, particularly when it is made to a hospital, should be made with a particular reason for surveillance in mind. Evidence from this and subsequent chapters may be used to suggest that a 'low-risk patient' need visit the hospital on only three occasions, the first occasion at between the 16th and 18th weeks of pregnancy for an ultrasound examination to exclude fetal abnormality and multiple pregnancy, a second visit at between the 30th and 34th weeks of pregnancy in order to have a clinical and ultrasound assessment of fetal growth, and a third visit at the 41st week of pregnancy for a clinical reassessment. The style of antenatal care needs to be flexible, being influenced by previous events and responding to events during the current pregnancy, whilst accepting that no one schedule of care has superior scientific justification (Hall 1990; Steer 1993).

The classification of a patient as either 'low risk' or 'high risk' is generally clinical, but there is some evidence that refinement of antenatal care may be based upon the degree of risk as established by a risk score rather than clinical perception. Many risk scores have been proposed, some being generalized (Hobel 1973; Knox *et al.* 1993), whilst others aim to predict the risk of a specific problem, for example intrauterine growth retardation (Adelstein and Fedrick 1978) and preterm labour (Lumley 1988). Thus Hobel proposed a score based on 51 antenatal factors, 40 intrapartum factors, and 35 neonatal factors. On a prospective assessment of 738 pregnancies, Hobel found that 340 were 'low risk' both for the antenatal and intrapartum period, 135 were 'high risk' antenatally but 'low risk' for labour, 144 were 'low risk' antenatally but 'high risk' for labour, and 119 were 'high risk' for both the antenatal and intrapartum period. The perinatal mortality rate for each of these four groups is shown in Table 15.7. Such formal scoring systems have failed to find popular support. Lilford and Chard (1983) argued that traditional risk scoring systems probably

Table 15.7 Antenatal risk factors

	Number of patients	%	Antenatal	Intrapartum	Perinatal mortality rate
	340	46	low	low	3
	135	18	high	low	22
	144	20	low	high	35
	119	16	high	high	145
Total	738	100	all	all	34

From Hobel (1973)

have no advantage over clinical practice, as too many factors, both known and unknown, combine in order to dictate outcome and, hence, make a precise prediction impossible.

Prepregnancy care

The overall effect of prepregnancy counselling may be aimed at influencing attitudes rather than events, although there are specific situations where the benefits of prepregnancy counselling may clearly be shown. These situations include the avoidance of potentially hazardous drugs, the optimal care of diabetes mellitus, advice concerning the need for early care in a forthcoming pregnancy following a previous tubal pregnancy, and an opportunity to plan the management in the presence of an increased risk of a genetically abnormal fetus. There is an opportunity for balanced advice concerning smoking and alcohol consumption, both of which will be discussed later in this chapter. Two areas should be discussed in greater detail, however, and relate to the assessment of rubella status and the place of prepregnancy vitamin supplementation in the presence of a previous neural tubal defect.

Kudesia *et al.* (1985) reported that 67 per cent of schoolgirls in the UK already have natural immunity to rubella and, following, rubella vaccination, 98 per cent of those vaccinated will show levels of immunity based on serological testing. Rabo and Taranger (1984) argue that although some 10–15 per cent of those previously seroconverted with vaccine will show a decline in immunity, they will have an antibody response after a booster revaccination. Moreover, the use of rubella vaccine at the time of immunization against mumps and measles in infants will reduce the susceptible population and may, therefore, reduce the pool of subjects available to the virus in order to continue its existence. The importance of rubella immunity prior to the first pregnancy was demonstrated by Peckham (1978) who reported that 41 per cent of 430 children born with congenital rubella were firstborns.

O'Shea *et al.* (1984), in a study of 93 previously vaccinated and seroconverted women, showed that antibody levels persisted for at least eight years in 58 per cent of subjects and could be demonstrated in some subjects vaccinated up to 18 years previously. Overall, however, there was a decline in immunity in 10 per cent of subjects after a mean of eight years. Previous vaccination with a history of serconversion should not, therefore, be taken as evidence of continuing immunity and should perhaps be checked in, or ideally before, each pregnancy.

The risk of rubella vaccination to a fetus, should it be given within three months prior to conception or even inadvertently during pregnancy, is probably small but is best avoided outside of an epidemic. Banatvala (1985) reported that the infection rate of such fetuses is only 1.7 per cent should vaccination be given inadvertently during early pregnancy, and that the risk to a fetus conceived within three months after rubella vaccination is 'so small as to be negligible'.

Neural tube defects may be found in approximately five in every 1000 fetuses in the UK, but will be found in one in twenty fetuses in women who have already had one fetus with a neural tube defect. The possible benefit of periconceptual vitamin supplementation was reported by Smithells *et al.* (1980). Women who had given birth to one or more infants with a neural tube defect were admitted to a prospective controlled trial of periconceptual vitamin supplementation using Pregnavite Forte F for at least 28 days prior to conception and until the eighth week of pregnancy, whilst a control group of such women received no medication. Some 13 of 260 infants or fetuses delivered to unsupplemented mothers had a neural tube defect (5.0 per cent), in contrast to only one of 178 (0.6 per cent) infants or fetuses delivered to fully supplemented mothers. This trial was criticized because it was not randomly allocated and it was, therefore, repeated (Smithells *et al.* 1983). A second cohort of 254 mothers were given periconceptual vitamin supplementation and there were two neural tube defect recurrences (0.9 per cent) as compared with 11 in 215 infants or fetuses born to unsupplemented mothers (5.1 per cent) over the same period of time. When these results were combined, the overall recurrence rate was 0.7 per cent for 454 supplemented mothers as opposed to 4.7 per cent for 518 unsupplemented mothers. The recurrence rates in unsupplemented mothers after one previous neural tube defect was 4.2 per cent and after two, 9.6 per cent. A small double-blind randomized control trial of folic acid demonstrated similar results in the prevention of a recurrent neural tube defect (Laurence *et al.* 1981).

The Medical Research Council randomized double-blind trial of periconceptual folic acid supplementation was reported in 1991. Each participant, who had a previous conceptus with a neural tube defect, was assigned randomly to one of four groups, 4 mg folic acid per day, a multivitamin preparation and folic acid, a multivitamin preparation alone, or a placebo and treated from the day of randomization until the 12th week of pregnancy. The results, shown in Table 15.8, were such that the trial ceased prematurely because of the strength of the effect once 1195 pregnancies of known outcome were analysed. This trial demonstrated a reduction in risk of recurrence of 78 per cent, giving a relative risk of the recurrence of a neural tube defect of 0.28 in folic acid takers com-

Table 15.8 The effect of folic acid supplementation

Group	No.	No. with recurrence
Folic acid	298	2
Multivitamin and folic acid	295	4
Multivitamin alone	302	8
Placebo	300	13

From Medical Research Council (1991)

pared with non-takers. This represented a 1 per cent risk of recurrence in folic acid takers compared with 3.5 per cent in non-takers. Although not all authors have demonstrated a reduction in risk of neural tube defect with folic acid supplementation (Mills *et al.* 1989), there is now little doubt that women with a history of a neural tube defect in a previous pregnancy should receive periconceptual folic acid supplementation (Acheson and Poole 1991; Centres for Disease Control 1991; *Lancet* 1991*b*).

What is not known is the minimum dose of folic acid which is required for this prevention, or the minimum length of time for which preconceptual supplementation must be given. Although the MRC trial advocated folic acid 4 mg per day from as soon as the pregnancy is planned until the end of the 12th week of gestation, no such preparation is currently available. The nearest available dose to this is 5 mg. It would also be prudent to advise such women to eat food rich in folic acid, such as lettuce, raw or lightly cooked green vegetables, bread, potatoes, and nuts. Although liver is rich in folic acid, it is not advised during pregnancy since it may contain excessive levels of vitamin A (see below). Primary prevention is discussed under 'Folic acid'.

The value of dietary supplementation

Extremes of diet clearly have adverse effects on pregnancy, the famine of the Second World War and the Dutch famine being associated with increased prematurity and perinatal mortality rates (Malhotra and Sawers 1986), whilst obesity is associated with an increased incidence of pre-eclampsia, operative and difficult delivery, and overweight babies (Tracy and Miller 1969). However, other than in these extreme circumstances, there is little evidence to suggest that dietary supplementation during pregnancy would have a beneficial effect on outcome, including low birthweight. In a randomized trial involving a poor black urban population in New York, Rush *et al.* (1980) were unable to detect any significant increase in birthweight in the offspring of women who received protein supplementation antenatally.

Iron

The use of routine iron prophylaxis during pregnancy is no longer indicated but rather reserved for high-risk groups, a haemodilutional anaemia of pregnancy being normal and related to the presence of an increase in the total red cell mass being eclipsed by a greater rise in plasma volume. Paintin *et al.* (1966) reported that, although 80 per cent of women will increase their haemoglobin with routine iron supplementation, it seems unreasonable to assume that this means that 80 per cent of women were iron-deficient. In a prospective trial, they gave placebo or low-dose iron (4 mg Fe) and high-dose iron (35 mg Fe) three times daily to 57, 60, and 56 primigravidae, respectively, the incidence of a late pregnancy haemoglobin of less than 10 g/dl being 30 per cent, 30 per cent and 7 per cent in each group, but patients were equally likely to feel tired in all groups. Although the numbers were small, there were no differences between the three groups for the incidence of preterm labour, antepartum haemorrhage, pre-eclampsia, or any other obstetric complication.

Taylor and Lind (1976) showed a reduced haemoglobin during the second trimester whether iron supplementation was given or not, whilst some patients taking iron supplementation developed macrocytosis, suggesting a possible 'over-sufficiency' of iron. Routine iron supplementation should only be given to women with microcytosis in the absence of thalassaemia, or for the treatment of iron deficiency anaemia, and should not be given to all antenatal patients regardless of other factors (*Drug and Therapeutics Bulletin* 1994; Terry 1990).

Folic acid and pyridoxine

Likewise, there is no proven haematological benefit for the administration of routine folic acid, with or without iron, in the absence of folate deficiency or high risk of folate deficiency. Fletcher *et al.* (1971), in a double-blind trial of folic acid supplementation with iron (322 patients), compared with iron alone (321 patients), could find no differences in the incidence of anaemia, infection, pre-eclampsia, antepartum haemorrhage, low birthweight, or preterm labour. Hemminki and Starfield (1978) reviewed 17 controlled clinical trials, from the scientific literature, related to the routine administration of iron and vitamins during pregnancy. No study reported an improvement in the incidences of anaemia, low birthweight, preterm labour, infant morbidity or mortality, or serious maternal morbidity. One trial showed that the administration of vitamin B_6 produced less dental caries in pregnant women, and one trial associated multivitamin administration with a reduced incidence of pre-eclampsia. No other benefits could be found.

Since it has already been demonstrated that folic acid supplementation periconceptually will reduce the recurrence of a neural tube defect in a fetus, it has been extrapolated that folic acid supplementation may be of use in primary prevention. Interestingly enough, pregnant women were urged to take periconceptual folic acid supplementation for primary prevention even in the absence of any scientific evidence to support this view (Report from an Expert Advisory Group 1992). Such primary prevention would take the form of folic acid 0.4 mg daily (obtainable over the counter from pharmacies and health food stores) or by the enrichment of foods, especially cereals. Such advice has been reinforced without providing additional evidence (Wald and Bower 1994). There is, however, now a single randomized trial which would support this advice (Czeizel 1993). In this Hungarian trial, women were randomized to receive folic acid 0.8 mg daily or trace element supplements for at least one month before conception and for at least two months after conception. Neural tube defects were not seen in any of 2104 folate supplemented pregnancies but were seen in six of 2052 trace element supplemented pregnancies. It would seem likely that primary prevention with folic acid is a real option when pregnancy is planned but there is clearly a need for a confirmatory trial.

Calcium and vitamin D

The case for calcium or vitamin D supplementation in selected groups carries more weight. Raman *et al.* (1978) randomly allocated 87 pregnant women of low socio-economic status to receive either no supplementation (*n* = 38), 300 mg of calcium supplementation per day (*n* = 24). Although the infants were of the same mean birthweights in each group, infant bone densities (ulna, radius, tibia, and fibula) were greater in the supplemented than the unsupplemented group. Such studies may be of relevance to the Asian population of the UK in whom osteomalacia is a well-recognised complication of pregnancy. Brooke *et al.* (1980) reported a double-blind trial of vitamin D (1000 IU/day) administration to 59 pregnant Asian women and a placebo to 67 controls, during the last trimester of pregnancy. The pretreatment maternal serum 25-hydroxyvitamin D concentrations were equally low in both groups, but the treatment group showed a better maternal weight gain with both mothers and babies having normal plasma 25-HVD levels, whilst in the placebo group, mothers and infants showed continuing low plasma concentrations of 25-HVD. Some five of these infants (7.5 per cent) developed symptomatic hypocalcaemia with hyperirritability. Although the incidence of IUGR was 29 per cent in the placebo group and 15 per cent in the treatment group, these figures approached but did not reach statistical significance. Brooke *et al.* (1981*a*) followed these infants during their first year. Those who had received antenatal vitamin D had a greater weight gain and growth in length (but not in head circumference) than did those who received placebo. Brooke *et al.*, therefore, advocated vitamin D supplementation to Asian women during the last trimester of pregnancy. It has, therefore, been advised that pregnant women who have either an inadequate dietary intake of calcium or vitamin D during pregnancy (1200 mg and 400 IU per day, respectively), or who are at high risk of an inadequate intake (economically deprived communities, Asian immigrant in temperate regions during winter, and those living at high altitude) should have supplements prescribed during pregnancy (Brooke *et al.* 1981*b*; Misra and Anderson, 1990; Terry 1990).

Zinc

Zinc is of current interest, and is required for cell division. The danger when assessing the possible association between complications of pregnancy and the circulating maternal level of a given substance is that the normal level during pregnancy may be lower than the normal level in the non-pregnant state, and this is true for zinc. There is a pathological condition termed acrodermatitis enteropathica in which a severe zinc deficiency occurs because of poor intestinal absorption, and this is associated with abnormalities of the fetus including achondroplasia (Epstein and Vedder 1960) and anencephaly (Neldner and Hambidge 1975), but this does not necessarily equate with pregnancy in the absence of this disease.

Possible zinc deficiency, based on leukocyte zinc content, has been implicated as a cause of IUGR. Meadows *et al.* (1981) showed a statistically significant association between decreased maternal leukocyte zinc content and babies with IUGR when compared with either normal weight or preterm babies. Solton and Jenkins (1982) showed that plasma zinc concentrations were lower in the maternal blood of 54 women giving birth to babies with a wide variety of congenital abnormalities (including neural tube defects and Potter syndrome) when compared with 56 controls; the cord serum zinc concentrations in 20 congenitally abnormal babies were also lower than in 20 normal controls. Buamah *et al.* (1984) reported a statistically significant lower maternal serum zinc level in nine women with anencephalic fetuses when compared with 244 pregnant controls.

However, Campbell-Brown *et al.* (1985) were unable to find any association between any measure of zinc during pregnancy and birthweight, whilst Ghosh *et al.* (1985) was unable to find any statistically significant correlation between maternal serum or hair zinc levels and the incidence of miscarriage or fetal abnormality. In a double-blind randomized control trial of zinc supplementation during 494 pregnancies, Mahomed *et al.* (1989) could find no difference between the two groups in the incidences of low birthweight or congenital abnormality.

There is, therefore, no good evidence to suggest that the general pregnant population suffer as a result of zinc deficiency, nor do they require supplementation (Hytten 1985).

Vitamin A hazards

In addition to unnecessary dietary supplementation, there may be hazards. There have been a small but steady number of reports which have associated excessive vitamin A intake with fetal abnormality (including urinary tract abnormalities, microcephaly, and facial deformity), but the size of this risk is not known (*Lancet* 1985). Although the scientific information available on vitamin A toxicity is not sufficient to define a specific minimum threshold level for teratogenic effects, patients are now advised to avoid excessive vitamin A intake during pregnancy. In practical terms, an intake in excess of 25 000 IU per day is considered to be 'excessive', and supplements, either dietary (especially liver) or in the form of multivitamin preparations should be avoided (Hathcock *et al.* 1990). The advice to avoid liver in excessive quantities during pregnancy relates to the observation that vitamin A accumulates in liver, and, hence, this may represent a particularly rich source of this substance.

The effect of smoking

There is good evidence that smoking, especially during the second half of pregnancy, may be associated with a decrease in the potential birthweight of the fetus. In 1959, Lowe compared the mean birthweight of the fetuses of 2042 pregnant women in relation to their smoking habits. The mean birthweight of fetuses of mothers who never smoked during pregnancy was 7.33 kg ($n = 1155$), of women who smoked during early pregnancy and then ceased 7.36 kg ($n = 181$), of women who smoked during early pregnancy, ceased, and then restarted 7.11 kg ($n = 38$), and women who smoked throughout pregnancy 6.93 kg ($n = 668$). The mean reduction in birthweight associated with smoking throughout pregnancy compared with never-smoking was 400 g or 5.5 per cent. Andrews and McGarry (1972) reported a retrospective study from Wales analysing 18 631 maternities subdivided into smokers, ex-smokers and non-smokers. The following results were found:

1. The patients' estimates of their smoking was inconsistent.
2. The average weight reduction of babies born to women who smoked, corrected from social class was 170 g.
3. There was no evidence of an increased incidence of either preterm labour or preterm rupture of the membranes in smokers when compared with non-smokers.
4. The perinatal mortality rate in smokers was 31 per 1000 compared with 25 per 1000 in non-smokers. This increase in smokers was comparable to that reported by Butler and Bonham (1963) who reported a perinatal mortality rate in smokers of 44.8 and non-smokers 32.4.
5. There was no statistical differences in the incidence of congenital abnormalities in the babies born to smokers or non-smokers.
6. For all social classes, hypertension, mild or moderate pre-eclampsia, and proteinuric hypertension were less common in smokers than non-smokers (see Table 15.9).
7. The incidence of placental abruption was commoner in smokers than non-smokers for all parities (see Table 15.10).

Other authors have found a mean birthweight reduction of approximately 300–450 g (Murphy *et al.* 1980; Wen *et al.* 1990).

Table 15.9 Smoking and raised blood pressure

	Hypertension (%)	Mild or moderate pre-eclampsia (%)	Proteinuric hypertension (%)	All (%)
Non-smokers	14.6	5.8	0.7	21.1
Smokers	9.6	4.1	0.3	10.04

From Andrews and McGarry (1972)

Table 15.10 Smoking and placental abruption

	Para 0	Para 1–3	Para 4 or more	All
Non-smokers	2.04	1.61	1.67	5.32
Smokers	2.88	2.4	3.16	8.44

From Andrews and McGarry (1972)

Table 15.11 Smoking during pregnancy

Risk	Relative risks	
	smokes < 20/day	smokes > 20/day
Birthweight less than 2.5 kg (any cause)	1.52	2.30
Preterm labour	1.2	1.5
Perinatal mortality rate	1.2	1.35
Placental abruption	1.24	1.68

From Meyer *et al.* (1976)

Even when corrected for other known risk factors, smoking still exerts an effect in its own right. Meyer *et al.* (1976), using a multiple regression analysis, analysed 50 000 births, which included 1300 perinatal deaths, in order to assess any effect of smoking during pregnancy. After adjustments were made for socio-economic status, maternal height, prepregnancy weight, sex of child, past obstetric history, maternal age, and parity, the authors reported that smokers, when compared with non-smokers, had an increased risk of low birthweight babies, preterm babies, perinatal mortality, and placental abruption, and that these risks were to some degree related to the number of cigarettes smoked (Table 15.11). Lumley *et al.* (1985) analysed the cigarette consumption and alcohol intake of mothers in almost 15 000 pregnancies, and found that the percentage of mothers who smoked during pregnancy increased as the social class declined (social class I, 13.9 per cent; social class V, 45.5 per cent). When corrected for differences in drinking habits, there was an increase in the incidence of low birthweight babies in all socio-economic groups, and in all parity groups in smokers compared with non-smokers, and an increased percen-

Table 15.12 Smoking, drinking, and abortion

Relative risks of second trimester abortion

Cigarettes per day	Alcoholic drinks per day		
	0	1	>1
0	1.0	1.05	3.18
0 – 30	1.05	1.27	2.24
30 +	1.13	2.00	3.29

From Evans et al. (1979)

tage in heavy smokers (10.0 per cent) compared to light smokers (5.7 per cent) compared with non-smokers (3.3 per cent). The mean reduction of birthweight in fetuses born to mothers who were in the heavy smoking group was 200 g.

There is evidence that the earlier in pregnancy that a woman stops smoking, the less is the depression of birthweight. Thus, the mean birthweight of infants of women who stopped smoking before the sixth week of pregnancy was 3404 g (similar to non-smokers), whilst the mean birthweight in women who stopped smoking at some stage beyond the 16th week of pregnancy was 3324 g. The mean birthweight in women who persisted with smoking throughout pregnancy was 3140 g (McArthur and Knox 1988).

There may also be an increased risk of spontaneous abortion in smokers. Himmelberger (1978) surveyed 27 686 women doctors, nurses, and operative theatre assistants who had 12 918 pregnancies resulting in 10 523 live births. After correcting for age, exposure to anaesthetic gases, and past obstetric history, there was a relative risk of spontaneous abortion in smokers of 1.7 when compared with non-smokers. There was also an age-dependent relative risk of congenital abnormality in the infants, varying from 1.1 at a maternal age of less than 25 years to 2.2 at a maternal age of 40 years. Harlap and Shiono (1980) analysed 32 019 pregnancies using a regression analysis, and found that both smoking and drinking were risk factors for spontaneous abortion, drinking being a greater risk factor than smoking. Similarly, Evans et al. (1979) reported a series of 67 609 singleton births in which the risk of congenital abnormality was identical in smokers and non-smokers (2.8 per cent), but that both smoking and alcohol consumption were risk factors for spontaneous abortion, especially in the second trimester (Table 15.12).

The possible association between maternal cigarette smoking during pregnancy and childhood cancer is unclear, contradictory, and complicated by any effects of post-delivery passive smoking. Stjernfeld et al. (1986), in a Swedish case-controlled study of 305 children with cancer and 340 children with insulin-dependent diabetes (used as controls), reported that the cancer risk in the children of mothers who smoked during pregnancy was increased by 50 per cent when compared with controls, and the major risks appeared to lie with non-Hodgkin lymphoma, acute lymphoblastic leukaemia, and Wilm's tumour.

Table 15.13 The effect of advice

	Control	Intervention advice
Number	473	463
Ceased smoking by 36th week	20.0%	43.0%
Stillbirths	2.4%	2.0%
Birthweight < 2.5 kg	8.9%	6.8%
Birthweight < 1.5 kg	1.1%	1.9%
Mean gestational age (weeks)	39.7	39.7

From Sexton and Hebel (1984)

Buckley *et al.* (1986) reported a case-controlled study consisting of 1814 cases of childhood cancer compared with 720 normal control children, and were unable to find any increased risk of either childhood cancers overall or any of the three particular malignancies reported in the Swedish study.

There is evidence that pregnant women respond in some measure to advice to stop smoking during pregnancy. Donovan (1977) randomized 1274 pregnant smokers to receive either no advice or intensive antismoking advice. This series did not show any apparent effect on birthweight following antismoking advice, but no separation of results was shown for those who were advised and continued smoking and those who were advised and ceased smoking. Sexton and Hebel (1984) reported a controlled prospective randomized trial of 936 pregnant smokers, dividing them into two well-matched groups, one receiving no specific advice on smoking. The benefits associated with this advice are shown in Table 15.13. The style of the antismoking intervention may influence its efficacy. Windsor *et al.* (1985) randomly allocated 309 pregnant smokers either to receive no advice or to receive one or other of two styles of antismoking booklets. By the end of the pregnancy, 2 per cent of the control group had stopped smoking and 7 per cent had reduced smoking. One of the booklets was associated with cessation of smoking in 6 per cent of patients and reduction in 14 per cent, whilst the other style was associated with cessation of smoking in 14 per cent of patients and a further reduction in 17 per cent. The advice does not seem to carry over significantly into subsequent pregnancies. Thus MacArthur *et al.* (1987) reported the effect of intervention by advice and leaflet to 493 smokers when compared with a control group of 489 smokers who received no specific advice. During the pregnancy under study, 3.6 per cent of the control group stopped smoking, but only 2.1 per cent of them stopped smoking in a subsequent pregnancy. Some 7 per cent of the intervention group stopped smoking during the study pregnancy, but only 2.2 per cent of them stopped smoking in a later pregnancy.

Although an analysis of intervention demonstrates that most techniques of advice were associated with a reduction of smoking during pregnancy in a minority of women (10 per cent of advice group compared with 5 per cent), it has yet to be shown that the overall benefit from the resulting increase in infant birthweight is of any clinical benefit (Hjalmarson *et al*. 1991; Lumley 1991).

The mechanism by which smoking exerts its effect on the fetus is partially understood and has been likened to a chronic hypoxic state. Cole *et al*. (1972) reported that cigarette smoke contains up to 5 per cent of carbon monoxide by volume, and that fetal levels of carboxyhaemoglobin, estimated from cord samples at delivery, were, on average, 1.8 times greater than maternal levels in women who smoked during late pregnancy, suggesting an adverse effect on oxyhaemoglobin dissociation. Lehtovirta and Forss (1978) demonstrated that during smoking there is an acute decrease in intervillous (maternal) placental blood flow lasting approximately 15 minutes, from a presmoking mean of 105 ml per 100 ml/minute based on isotope studies, this being a possible vasoconstriction effect due to nicotine. Goodman *et al*. (1984) studied 10 patients who smoked but who had otherwise unremarkable pregnancies. Judged ultrasonographically during the last three weeks of pregnancy, smoking was associated with a significant reduction in fetal trunk movements but not in fetal breathing movements. There were significant reductions in the number of fetal heart accelerations for a period of approximately 15 minutes following each cigarette.

Christianson (1979) compared the placentae of 2890 smokers and 4761 non-smokers. Whilst there were no differences in placental weights, there were significantly greater amounts of subchorionic fibrin deposits in the placentae of smokers compared with non-smokers and a higher incidence of 'true infarcts'. Buchan (1983) demonstrated an increase in viscosity in fetal blood collected from the umbilical veins of 40 infants born to mothers who smoked 20 or more cigarettes per day throughout pregnancy compared with 40 matched non-smoking controls. This combination of decreased intervillous blood flow with increased intravillous blood viscosity and reduced oxyhaemoglobin dissociation could explain the potential for IUGR.

The effect of alcohol

In 1973, Jones *et al*. reported eight unrelated children born to mothers who were known to be chronic alcoholics and who had similar patterns of cranio-facial, limb, and cardiovascular defects associated with an antenatal onset of growth retardation and development delay. There were short palpebral fissures, maxillary hypoplasia, microcephaly, a systolic heart murmur associated with delayed closure of an atrial or ventricular septal defect, a single palmar skin crease, limited mobility sometimes associated with hypoplastic fingers and toes, birthweight and body length below the 10th centile for gestational age, linear growth during the first year of life that was 65 per cent of normal, weight gain during the first year of life of 38 per cent of normal, head circumference below the 3rd centile at one year, and a reduction in motor skills and eye–hand co-ordination. In 1974, Jones *et al.* reported a further 23 pregnancies associated with a perinatal mortality of 17 per cent and, in the survivors, 32 per cent had the facial appearance of fetal alcohol syndrome as described above, whilst 44 per cent had evidence of mental deficiency. The problems are not confined to chronic alcoholics, however, and alcohol-related problems during pregnancy may represent a dose-response, differing levels of problems associated with differing levels of alcohol intake (see p. 422 Table 15.15). Like smoking, the problem may also be complicated by a less than exact account from the patient as to her alcohol intake.

With this caveat, the drinking habits of pregnant women have been assessed by Harlap and Shiono (1980) who reported the results of a questionnaire to over 32 000 pregnant women. Some 51.7 per cent reported that they had not taken alcohol in early pregnancy, 44.7 per cent had less than one drink per day, 2.4 per cent had one or two drinks per day, 0.4 per cent had between three and five drinks per day, and 0.1 per cent had six or more. Lumley *et al.* (1985), in a review of almost 15 000 births in Tasmania, demonstrated that drinking, unlike smoking, was more likely to occur during pregnancy in the higher socio-economic groups, thus 64.5 per cent of all professional women drank during pregnancy as compared with 45.5 per cent of women of social class V. Social class I women also drank more when they did drink, thus 14.5 per cent of social class I women drank between three and six alcoholic drinks per week compared with 4.6 per cent of social class V women.

Kline *et al.* (1980) compared the drinking habits of 616 women with spontaneous abortions with 632 women who delivered beyond the 28th week of pregnancy (controls). Some 8.1 per cent of the controls admitted drinking twice a week or more during pregnancy compared with 17.0 per cent of the cases. Following a logistic regression analysis, the relative risk for drinkers for spontaneous abortion was 2.62. Harlap and Shiono, from the questionnaire described above, and following adjustment for other risks, including smoking, estimated that the relative risk for first trimester abortion was unchanged in women who drank alcohol, but there was an increase in the relative risk for second trimester abortions, this risk being 1.01, 1.98, and 3.53 for women drinking less than one drink per day, one or two drinks per day, or more than three drinks per day, respectively. This trend is comparable to that shown in Table 15.11.

Thus moderate alcohol consumption (or paternal alcohol consumption) does not increase the risk of miscarriage (Halmesmaki *et al.* 1989).

The effect of alcohol intake during pregnancy upon birthweight has also been widely studied. Wright *et al.* (1983), in a prospective study of 900 pregnant women adjusted for social class and smoking, demonstrated that drinking more than 100 g of alcohol per week (10 standard measures) was associated with a risk of IUGR twice that of those drinking less than 50 g per week. The effects of alcohol and smoking were synergistic, with 17 per cent of heavy drinking, non-smoking women having a baby with IUGR compared with 38 per cent of heavy smoking, heavy drinking women. Those women who drank heavily dur-

Table 15.14   Smoking, drinking, and Intrauterine growth retardation (IUGR)

Relative risks for intrauterine growth retardation

Drinking	Non-smoker	Smoker	All
Moderate vs. light	0.96	2.00	1.24
Heavy vs. light	1.71	3.43	2.27

From Wright *et al.* (1983)

ing early pregnancy but who reduced drinking to below 50 g per week during the second trimester had a 10 per cent risk of IUGR, that is, there was no increased risk. The data taken from Wright's study (Table 15.14) suggest that smoking is a greater risk factor for IUGR than is drinking.

In the Tasmanian study (Lumley *et al.* 1985), drinking less than 30 g of alcohol per week (three drinks) had no effect on birthweight, whilst 5.6 per cent of women drinking between three and six drinks per week delivered a baby weighing less than 2.5 kg, and 14 per cent of those having two or more drinks per day delivered a baby weighing less than 2.5 kg. There was no association between alcohol intake and the incidence of congenital abnormality even in women having up to three drinks per day. Similarly, Sulaiman (1988) obtained antenatal information on smoking and drinking from 901 primigravidae in Dundee. When corrections were made for age, parity, and social class, there was no detrimental effect from smoking upon birthweight, although there was some association between excessive alcohol intake and a shortened gestational age. At the current state of information, pregnant women should be reassured that the regular taking of one or two units of alcohol per day during pregnancy is unlikely to reduce potential fetal birthweight.

There is evidence to associate excessive alcohol intake with an increase in congenital abnormality. In one study, Lumley *et al.* (1985) could find no evidence of an increase in congenital abnormality in women having up to three drinks per day but did find an increase in congenital abnormality with a larger alcohol intake. In a larger prospective study on alcohol consumption in 32 873 pregnancies, there was no increase in the incidence of fetal abnormality unless six or more units of alcohol were taken daily (Mills and Graublrd 1987). These results are illustrated in Table 15.15.

It may be that the advice of the Surgeon General of the USA and the Royal College of Psychiatrists of the United Kingdom who warn that women should 'avoid all alcohol during pregnancy' is excessive (Edwards, 1983).

Conclusions

Although it might be difficult to prove, scientifically, to the cynic that antenatal care may significantly alter the outcome of pregnancy, there is much evidence to demonstrate that certain aspects of both prepregnancy care and antenatal

Table 15.15 Alcohol and risk of fetal anomaly

Alcohol units per day	Relative risk of fetal anomaly
None	1.0
<1	0.99
1-2	1.07
3-5	0.9
>6	1.39

From Mills and Grauberd (1987)

care will have a direct effect on pregnancy outcome, whilst some other traditional aspects of antenatal care are without scientific value. Perhaps the best example of the effect of intervention on fetal outcome relates to the management of rhesus isoimmunization discussed in a later chapter. The problems of prenatal diagnosis, the assessment of intrauterine growth retardation, and the management of labour will be discussed in their own chapters.

Perhaps one lesson which has been learned from an analysis of our antenatal care is the need to make a detailed assessment of the benefits and/or hazards of any given intervention before it is introduced into routine clinical practice.

References

Acheson, D. and Poole, A. A. B. (1991). Folic acid in the prevention of neural tube defects. *Department of Health Circular*, pL-CMO (91) 11.

Adelstein, P. and Fedrick, J. (1978). Antental identification of women at increased risk of being delivered of a low birthweight infant at term. *British Journal of Obstetrics and Gynaecology* **85**, 8-11.

Alberman, E. (1989). Perinatal mortality. In *Obstetrics* (ed. A. Turnbull and G. Chamberlain), pp. 1111-19. Churchill Livingstone, Edinburgh.

Anderson, M. (1993). Changing childbirth. *British Journal of Obstetrics and Gynaecology* **100**, 1071-2.

Andrews, J. and McGarry, J. M. (1972). A community study of smoking in pregnancy. *Journal of Obstetrics and Gynaecology of the British Commonwealth* **79**, 1057-73.

Backe, B. and Nakling, J. (1993). Effectiveness of antenatal care. *British Journal of Obstetrics and Gynaecology* **100**, 727-32.

Balarajan, R. and Botting, B. (1989). Perinatal mortality *in England and Wales*. Health Trends **21**, 79-84.

Banatvala, J. E. (1985). Rubella—continuing problems. *British Journal of Obstetrics and Gynaecology* **92**, 193-6.

Blondel, B., Pusch, D., and Schmidt, E. (1985). Some characteristics of antenatal care in 13 European Countries. *British Journal of Obstetrics and Gynaecology* **92**, 365-8.

Brooke, O. G., Brown, I. R. F., Bones, C. D. M., Carter, N. D., Cleeve, H. J. W., Maxwell, J. D., *et al.* (1980). Vitamin D supplements in pregnant Asian women. *British Medical Journal* **280**, 751-4.

Brooke, O. G., Butters, F., and Wood, C. (1981*a*). Intrauterine vitamin D nutrition and postnatal growth in Asian infants. *British Medical Journal* **283**, 1024.

Brooke, O. G., Brown, I. R. F., and Cleeve, H. J. W. (1981b). Observations on the Vitamin D state of pregnant Asian women in London. *British Journal of Obstetrics and Gynaecology* **88**, 18–26.

Bryce, R. (1990). Social and midwifery support. *Ballière's Obstetrics and Gynaecology* **4**, 77–88.

Buamah, P. K., Russell, M., Bates, G., Milford-Ward, A., and Skillen, A. W. (1984). Maternal zinc status. *British Journal of Obstetrics and Gynaecology* **91**, 788–90.

Buchan, P. C. (1983). Cigarette smoking in pregnancy and fetal hyperviscosity. *British Medical Journal* **236**, 1315.

Buckley, J. D., Hobbie, W. L., Ruccione, K., Sather, H. N., Woods, W. G., and Hammond, G. D. (1986). Maternal smoking during pregnancy and the risk of childhood cancer. *Lancet* **ii**, 519–20.

Bucknell, E. W. C. and Wood, B. S. B. (1985). Wessex perinatal mortality survey. *British Journal of Obstetrics and Gynaecology* **92**, 550–8.

Butler, N. R. and Bonham, D. (1963). *Perinatal mortality*, pp. 60–1. E. and S. Livingstone, Edinburgh.

Campbell-Brown, M., Ward, R. J., Haines, A. T., North, W. R. S., Abraham, R., and McFadyen, I. R. (1985). Zinc and copper in Asian pregnancies. *British Journal of Obstetrics and Gynaecology* **92**, 886–91.

Centres for Disease Control (1991). Use of folic acid for the prevention of spina bifida and other neural tube defects. *Morbidity and Mortality Weekly Report* **40**, 512–16.

Chamberlain, G. (1978). Background to perinatal health. *Lancet* **ii**, 1061–3.

Chng, P. K., Hall, M. K., and MacGillivray, I. (1980). An audit of antenatal care: the value of the first antenatal visit. *British Medical Journal* **281**, 1184–6.

Christianson, R. E. (1979). Growth differences observed in the placentas of smokers and non-smokers. *American Journal of Epidemiology* **110**, 178–87.

Clarke, M., Mason, E. S., MacVicar, J., and Clayton, D. G. (1993). Evaluating perinatal mortality rates—effects of referral case mix. *British Medical Journal* **306**, 824–7.

Cnattingius, S., Forman, M. R., Berendes, H. W., Graubard, B. I., and Isotalo, L. (1993). Effect of age, parity and smoking on pregnancy outcome. *American Journal of Obstetrics and Gynecology* **168**, 16–21.

Cole, P. V., Hawkins, L. H., and Roberts, D. (1972). Smoking during pregnancy and its effects on the fetus. *Journal of Obstetrics and Gynaecology of the British Commonwealth* **79**, 782–7.

Czeizel, A. E. (1993). Prevention of congenital abnormalities by periconceptual multivitamin supplementation. *British Medical Journal* **306**, 1645–8.

Donovan, J. W. (1977). Randomised controlled trial of antismoking advice in pregnancy. *British Journal of Preventative and Social Medicine* **31**, 6–12.

Drug and Therapeutics Bulletin (1993). Routine iron supplements in pregnancy are unnecessary. *Drug and Therapeutics Bulletin* **32**, 30–1.

Dunlop, W. (1993). Changing childbirth. *British Journal of Obstetrics and Gynaecology* **100**, 1072–4.

Edwards, G. (1983). Alcohol and advice to the pregnant woman. *British Medical Journal* **286**, 247–8.

Elbourne, D., Robertson, M., Chalmers, I., Waterhouse, I., and Holt, E. (1987). The Neubury Maternity Care Study. *British Journal of Obstetrics and Gynaecology* **94**, 612–19.

Epstein, S. and Vedder, J. S. (1960). Acrodermatitis enteropathica persisting into adulthood. *Archives of Dermatology* **82**, 189–90.

Evans, D. R., Newcombe, R. G., and Campbell, H. (1979). Maternal smoking habits and congenital malformations. *British Medical Journal* **2**, 171–3.

Fletcher, J., Gurr, F., Fellingham, F. R., Prankerd, T. H. A., Brant, H. A., and Menzies, D. M. (1971). The value of folic acid supplements in pregnancy. *Journal of Obstetrics and Gynaecology of the British Commonwealth* **78**, 781–5.

Ghosh, A., Fong, L. Y. Y., Wan, C. W., Liang, S. T., Woo, J. S. K., and Wong, V. (1985). Zinc deficiency is not a cause for abortion, congenital abnormality or small for gestational age infants in Chinese women. *British Journal of Obstetrics and Gynaecology* **92**, 886–94.

Goodman, J. D. S., Visser, F. G. A., and Dawes, G. S. (1984). Effect of maternal cigarette smoking on fetal trunk movements, fetal breathing movements and the fetal heart rate. *British Journal of Obstetrics and Gynaecology* **91**, 657–61.

Hall, M. H. (1990). Identification of high-risk and low-risk. *Ballières Obstetrics and Gynaecology* **44**, 65–76.

Hall, M. H., Chng, P. K., and MacGillivray, I. (1980). Is routine antenatal care worthwhile? *Lancet* ii, 78–80.

Halmesmaki, E., Valimaki, M., Roine, R., Ylikahri, R., and Ylikorkala, O. (1989). Maternal and paternal alcohol consumption and miscarriage. *British Journal of Obstetrics and Gynaecology* **96**, 188–91.

Harlap, S. and Shiono, P. H. (1980). Alcohol, smoking and the incidence of spontaneous abortions in the first trimester of pregnancy. *Lancet* ii, 173–6.

Hathcock, J. N., Hatlan, D. J., Jenkins, M. Y., McDonald, J. T., Sundaresan, P. R., and Wilkening, V. W. (1990). Evaluation of vitamin A toxicity. *American Journal of Clinical Nutrition* **52**, 183–202.

Hemminki, E. and Starfield, B. (1978). Routine administration of iron and vitamins during pregnancy: a review of controlled clinical trials. *British Journal of Obstetrics and Gynaecology* **85**, 404–10.

Hepburn, M. (1990). Social problems. *Ballières Obstetrics and Gynaecology* **4**, 149–64.

Heringa, M. P. and Huisjes, H. J. (1988). Antenatal care: current practices in debate. *British Journal of Obstetrics and Gynaecology* **95**, 836–40.

Himmelberger, D. U. (1978). Cigarette smoking during pregnancy and the occurrence of spontaneous abortion and congenital abnormality. *American Journal of Epidemiology* **108**, 470–9.

Hjalmarson, A. I. M., Hahn, L., and Svanberg, B. (1991). Stopping smoking in pregnancy: effects of a self-help manual in a controlled trial. *British Journal of Obstetrics and Gynaecology* **98**, 260–4.

Hobel, C. J. (1973). Pre-natal and intra-partum high-risk scoring. *American Journal of Obstetrics and Gynecology* **117**, 1–9.

Hytten, F. E. (1985). Do pregnant women need zinc supplements? *British Journal of Obstetrics and Gynaecology* **92**, 873–4.

Jones, K. L., Smith, D. W., Ulleland, C. N., and Streissguth, S. P. (1973). Patterns of malformation in offspring of chronic alcoholic mothers. *Lancet* ii, 1267–71.

Jones, K. L., Smith, D. W., Streissguth, S. P., and Myrianthopoulos, N. C. (1974). Outcome in offspring of chronic alcoholic women. *Lancet* i, 1076–8.

Kaunitz, A. M., Spence, C., Danielson, T. S., Rochat, R. W., and Grimes, D. A. (1984). Perinatal and maternal mortality in a religious group avoiding obstetric care. *American Journal of Obstetrics and Gynecology* **150**, 826–31.

Keirse, M. J. N. C. (1989). Interaction between primary and secondary care during pregnancy and childbirth. In *Effective care in pregnancy and childbirth* (ed. I. Chalmers, N. Enkin, and M. Keirse), pp. 197–201. Oxford University Press, Oxford.

Kline, J., Shrout, P., Stein, Z., Susser, M., and Warburton, D. (1980). Drinking during pregnancy and spontaneous abortion. *Lancet* ii, 176–80.

Knox, A. J., Sadler, L., Pattison, N. S., Mantell, C. D., and Mullins, P. (1993). An obstetric scoring system. *Obstetrics and Gynecology* **81**, 195-9.

Kudesia, G., Robinson, E. T., Wilson, W. D., Wilson, T. S., Stewart, I. M., Campbell, A. T., *et al.* (1985). Rubella: immunity and vaccination in school girls. *British Medical Journal* **290**, 1406-7.

Lancet (1985). Vitamin A and teratogenesis. *Lancet* **i**, 319-20.

Lancet (1991*a*). Perinatal mortality rates—time for a change? *Lancet* **337**, 331.

Lancet (1991*b*). Folic acid and neural tube defects. *Lancet* **338**, 153-4.

Laurence, K. M., James, N., Miller, N. H., Tennant, G. B., and Campbell, H. (1981). Double-blind randomised controlled trial of folate treatment before conception to prevent recurrence of neural tube defects. *British Medical Journal* **282**, 1509-11.

Lehtovirta, P. and Forss, M. (1978). The acute effect of smoking on the intervillous blood flow of the placenta. *British Journal of Obstetrics and Gynaecology* **85**, 729-31.

Lilford, R. J., and Chard, T. (1983). Problems and pitfalls of risk assessment in antenatal care. *British Journal of Obstetrics and Gynaecology* **90**, 507-10.

Lowe, C. R. (1959). Effects of mothers' smoking habits on birthweight of their children. *British Medical Journal* **2**, 673-6.

Lumley, J. (1988). The prevention of preterm birth. *Australian Paediatric Journal* **24**, 101-11.

Lumley, J. (1991). Stopping smoking—again. *British Journal of Obstetrics and Gynaecology* **98**, 847.

Lumley, J., Corrie, J. F., Newman, N. M., and Curran, J. T. (1985). Cigarette smoking, alcohol consumption and fetal outcome in Tasmania. *Australian and New Zealand Journal of Obstetrics and Gynaecology* **25**, 33-40.

MacArthur, C. and Knox, E. G. (1988). Smoking and pregnancy: effects of stopping at different stages. *British Journal of Obstetrics and Gynaecology* **95**, 551-9.

MacArthur, C., Newton, J. R., and Knox, E. G. (1987). Effect of anti-smoking health education on infant size at birth. *British Journal of Obstetrics and Gynaecology* **84**, 295-300.

MacFarlane, A., Cole, S., and Hey, E. (1986). Comparisons of data from regional perinatal mortality surveys. *British Journal of Obstetrics and Gynaecology* **93**, 1224-32.

McIlwaine, G. M., Howat, R. C. L., Dunn, F., and MacNaughton, M. C. (1979). The Scottish perinatal mortality survey. *British Medical Journal* **2**, 1103-6.

Mahomed, K., James, D. K., Golding, J., and McCabe, R. (1989). Zinc supplementation during pregnancy: a double-blind randomized control trial. *British Medical Journal* **299**, 826-30.

Malhotra, A. and Sawers, R. S. (1986). Dietary supplementation in pregnancy. *British Medical Journal* **293**, 465-6.

Marsh, G. A. (1985). New programme of antenatal care in general practice. *British Medical Journal* **291**, 646-8.

Meadows, N. J., Ruse, W., Smith, M. F., Day, J., Keeling, P. W. N., Scopes, J. W., *et al.* (1981). Zinc and small babies. *Lancet* **ii**, 1135-6.

Medical Research Council Vitamin Study Research Group (1991). Prevention of neural tube defects. *Lancet* **338**, 131-7.

Meyer, M. B., Jonas, B. S., and Tonaxia, J. A. (1976). Perinatal events associated with maternal smoking during pregnancy. *American Journal of Epidemiology* **103**, 464-76.

Mills, J. L. and Grauberd, B. I. (1987). Is moderate drinking during pregnancy associated with an increased risk for malformation? *Pediatrics* **80**, 309-14.

Mills, J. L., Rhodes, G. G., Simpson, J. L., Cunningham, T. C., Connley, M. R., Lassman, M. R., *et al.* (1989). The absence of a relation between the periconceptual use of vitamins and neural tube defects. *New England Journal of Medicine* **312**, 430–5.

Misra, R. and Anderson, D. C. (1990). Providing the fetus with calcium. *British Medical Journal* **300**, 1220–1.

Murphy, J. F., Drumm, J. E., Mulcahy, R., and Daly, L. (1980). Effect of maternal cigarette smoking on fetal birthweight and on growth of the fetal biparietal diameter. *British Journal of Obstetrics and Gynaecology* **87**, 462–6.

Neldner, K. H. and Hambidge, K. M. (1975). Zinc therapy of acrodermatitis enteropathica. *New England Journal of Medicine* **292**, 879–82.

O'Brien, M. and Smith, C. (1981). Women's views and experiences of antenatal care. *Practitioner* **225**, 123–5.

O'Shea, S., Best, J. M., Banatvala, J. E., Marshall, W. C., and Dudgeon, J. A. (1984). Persistence of rubella antibody 8–18 years after vaccination. *British Medical Journal* **288**, 1043.

Paintin, D. B., Thompson, W., and Hytten, F. E. (1966). Iron and the haemoglobin level in pregnancy. *Journal of Obstetrics and Gynaecology of the British Commonwealth* **73**, 181–90.

Peckham, C. S. (1978). Congenital rubella surveillance. *Journal of the Royal College of Physicians* **12**, 250–5.

Rabo, E. and Taranger, J. (1984). Scandinavian model for eliminating measles, mumps and rubella. *British Medical Journal* **289**, 1402–4.

Raman, L., Rajalakshmi, K., Krishnamachari, K. A. U. R., and Sastri, J. G. (1978). Effect of calcium supplementation to undernourished mothers during pregnancy on the bone density of the neonates. *American Journal of Clinical Nutrition* **31**, 466–9.

Report from an Expert Advisory Group (1992). *Folic acid and the prevention of neural tube defects*. Department of Health.

Rush, D., Stein, Z., and Susser, M. (1980). Randomized controlled trial of pre-natal nutritional supplementation in New York City. *Pediatrics* **65**, 683–97.

Sexton, M. and Hebel, J. R. (1984). A clinical trial of change in maternal smoking and its effect on birthweight. *Journal of the American Medical Association* **251**, 911–15.

Smithells, R. W., Sheppard, S., Schorah, C. J., Seller, M. J., Nevin, N. C., Harris, R., *et al.* (1980). Possible prevention of neural tube defects by periconceptual vitamin supplementation. *Lancet* **i**, 339–40.

Smithells, R. W., Nevin, N. C., Seller, M. J., Sheppard, S., Harris, R., Read, A. P., *et al.* (1983). Further experience of vitamin supplementation for prevention of neural tube defect recurrences. *Lancet* **i**, 1027–31.

Solton, M. H. and Jenkins, D. M. (1982). Maternal and fetal plasma zinc concentrations and fetal abnormality. *British Journal of Obstetrics and Gynaecology* **85**, 56–8.

Soothill, P. W., Ajay, I. R., Campbell, S., Gibb, S., Chandran, R., Gibb, D., *et al.* (1991). The effect of a fetal surveillance unit on admission for antenatal patients to hospital. *British Medical Journal* **303**, 269–71.

Steer, P. (1993). Rituals in ante-natal care — do we need them? *British Medical Journal* **307**, 697–8.

Stjernfeld, T. M., Berglund, K., Lindsten, J., and Ludwigsson, J. (1986). Maternal cigarette smoking during pregnancy and risk of childhood cancer. *Lancet* **i**, 1350–2.

Street, P., Gannon, M. J., and Holt, E. M. (1991). Community obstetric care in West Berkshire. *British Medical Journal* **302**, 698–700.

Sulaiman, N. D. (1988). Alcohol consumption in Dundee primigravidas. *British Medical Journal* **296**, 1500–3.

Taylor, D. J. and Lind, T. (1976). Haematological changes during normal pregnancy. *British Journal of Obstetrics and Gynaecology* **83**, 760–7.

Terry, P. B. (1990). Routine testing and prophylaxis. *Ballières Obstetrics and Gynaecology* **4**, 25–43.

Thomas, H., Draper, J., and Field, S. (1983). An evaluation of the practice of shared antenatal care. *Journal of Obstetrics and Gynaecology* **31**, 157–60.

Tracy, T. A. and Miller, G. L. (1969). Obstetric problems of the massively obese. *Obstetrics and Gynecology* **33**, 204–8.

Tuffnell, D. J., Lilford, R. J., Buchan, P. C., Prendiville, V. M., Tuffnell, A. J., Holgate, M. P., *et al.* (1992). Randomized control trial of day care for hypertension in pregnancy. *Lancet* **339**, 224–7.

Wald, N. J. and Bower, C. (1994). Folic acid, pernicious anaemia, and prevention of neural tube defects. *Lancet* **343**, 307.

Wen, S. W., Goldenberg, S. L., Cutter, G. R., Hoffman, H. J., Clivers, S. P., Davies, R. L., *et al.* (1990). Smoking, maternal age, fetal growth, and gestational age at delivery. *American Journal of Obstetrics and Gynecology* **162**, 53–8.

Windsor, R. A., Cutter, G., Morris, J., Reese, Y., Manzella, B., Bartlett, E. E., *et al.* (1985). The effectiveness of smoking cessation methods for smokers in public health maternity clinics. *American Journal of Public Health* **75**, 1389–92.

Working Party on the Very Low Birthweight Infant (1990). European Community Collaborative Study of Outcome of Pregnancy between 22 and 28 Weeks' Gestation. *Lancet* **336**, 782–4.

Wright, J. L., Waterson, E. J., Barrison, I. J., Toplis, P. J., Lewis, I. G., Gordon, M. G., *et al.* (1983). Alcohol consumption, pregnancy and low birthweight. *Lancet* **i**, 663–5.

16   Prenatal diagnosis

Fetal abnormalities, either genetic or structural, occur in 2.5 per cent of deliveries; the techniques currently used in screening for such abnormalities are the subject of this chapter. Structural abnormalities are diagnosed (almost exclusively) by ultrasound. They are usually polygenetic but sometimes they are the result of genetic chromosomal abnormalities. Genetic and chromosomal diseases themselves are diagnosed by invasive tests in which the benefit of diagnosis has to be balanced against the known (and sometimes unknown) risks.

Chromosome abnormalities

There are four major indications for karyotyping of the fetus during pregnancy:

(1) the result of a positive screening for chromosome abnormality;

(2) a previous child with a chromosomal abnormality;

(3) parental chromosomal abnormality;

(4) the determination of fetal sex,

The result of a positive screening for chromosome abnormality

The influence of maternal age upon chromosomal abnormality is thought to be the result of an increase in the incidence of maternal non-dysjunction, especially during the first meiotic division. Trisomy 21 (Down syndrome), Trisomy 13 (Patau syndrome), and Trisomy 18 (Edward syndrome) are all age-related (Clark *et al*. 1993; Wenstrom *et al*. 1993). The sex chromosome trisomies (47XXX and 47XXY) are also maternal age-related but not as strongly as are the autosomal trisomies (Hassold *et al*. 1980). Hook *et al*. (1983) devised maternal age-specific rates based on 1000 abnormal karyotypes obtained following amniocentesis in approximately 20 000 pregnancies (Table 16.1).

Down syndrome is the most important chromosomal abnormality among viable pregnancies, affecting 1 per 1000 total births in the UK and Europe. Up to 96 per cent of patients with Down syndrome have a Trisomy 21, the remainder having a translocation (Nevin 1991). The extra chromosome is maternally derived in over 90 per cent of cases. Traditionally, screening for Down syndrome is on the basis of maternal age yet 70 per cent of all fetuses affected by Down syndrome occur in women below the age of 35 years (Merkatz *et al*. 1984; Mutton *et al*. 1991). The majority of fetuses with Down syndrome have not been diagnosed before birth (62 per cent) (Mutton *et al*. 1993).

Table 16.1 Chromosomal abnormality and maternal age

Chromosomal abnormality per 1000 amniocenteses

Maternal age	Trisomy 21	Trisomy 18	Trisomy 13	47XXY	47XXY	Others	All
35	4.0	1.0	0.5	0.6	1.3	1.3	8.0
38	8.7	2.1	0.7	1.0	1.2	1.5	15.2
40	14.5	3.3	1.0	1.4	1.9	1.7	23.8
42	24.1	5.2	1.3	2.0	3.0	1.9	37.5
45	51.8	10.6	2.0	3.4	5.9	2.3	76.0
47	86.2	16.9	2.7	4.9	9.3	2.6	122.6
49	143.5	26.9	3.6	7.0	14.6	2.9	198.5

From Hook *et al.* (1983)

In an attempt to offer genetic screening of the fetus to a greater population of pregnant women at risk, there is a growing interest in the relationship between genetic abnormality and maternal serological screening during the second trimester of pregnancy. It is recognized that the distribution of maternal serum alphafetoprotein levels (AFP) is significantly lower in women with a fetus affected by Trisomy 21 when compared with those with a normal fetus (Merkatz *et al.* 1984; Murday and Slack 1985). In a review of 11 published series, Wald and Cuckle (1989) reported that the mean maternal serum AFP was 0.68 multiples of the mean (MoM) in the presence of a Down fetus compared with a normal fetus. Using such information, the age-related risk of Down syndrome may be modified by correcting the age-related risk for the results of maternal serological analysis, this may then increase the risk of a Down syndrome affected infant such that a woman below the age of 35 years might then wish to have a genetic test, for example an amniocentesis.

Other maternal serological markers are influenced by the presence of a fetus with Down syndrome. Thus, maternal serum unconjugated oestriol in a fetus with Down syndrome is 0.73 MoM of that of unaffected controls, whilst maternal serum hCG concentrations are 1.5 MoM that of unaffected controls (Wald *et al.* 1988*a*, 1988*b*).

By combining maternal age with the three maternal serum markers described above (AFP, hCG, and unconjugated oestriol) the so-called 'triple test' would enable 60 per cent of all fetuses with Down syndrome to be detected should a risk of greater than 1 in 250 be followed by an amniocentesis for genetic determination. This would result in amniocentesis being offered to 5 per cent of the pregnant population, the same proportion as would be offered invasive testing on the basis of maternal age 35 years or greater. By this means, approximately 550 additional fetuses affected by Down syndrome would be diagnosed every year in England and Wales in women below the age of 35 years and, assuming a miscarriage rate of 0.5 per cent following amniocentesis, some

Table 16.2 Chromosomal abnormality and paternal age

Paternal age (years)	Maternal age (years)			
	35–40		41–46	
	Trisomy 21 (%)	All trisomies (%)	Trisomy 21 (%)	All trisomies (%)
⩽34	0.4	1.3	0.8	1.7
35–40	0.6	1.6	1.2	2.8
41–46	1.3	2.1	2.8	5.6
⩾47	2.0	2.3	4.1	6.5

From Stene *et al.* (1981)

17 unaffected fetuses would be lost every year. Of those women who underwent amniocentesis, 1.3 per cent would have an affected baby, a much higher proportion than on maternal age alone (Sheldon and Simpson 1991; Wald *et al.* 1988*b*).

Although it has yet to be proved by larger clinical trials, it is possible that additionally measuring maternal serum urea resistant neutrophil alkaline phosphatase similarly allows 80 per cent of Down syndrome infants to be detected for the same 5 per cent incidence of amniocentesis — the 'triple plus test' (Cuckle *et al.* 1990).

Since maternal serum alphafetoprotein screening is weight-sensitive, the result of the triple test should also be adjusted for maternal weight (Macri *et al.* 1986).

Whilst it is clear that the use of the triple test will detect greater numbers of infants affected by Trisomies 21 and 18, the test may not detect, reliably, other chromosomal abnormalities which occur more frequently with increasing maternal age. Because of this, and because of the delay imposed by waiting for the results of the biochemical test, some patients will elect to go straight to invasive testing (Heyl *et al.* 1990; MacDonald *et al.* 1991).

There is also some evidence that a first trimester triple test in which hCG is replaced by a protein called PAP-A will be developed with the advantages of an earlier genetic diagnosis and termination (Brock *et al.* 1990; Cuckle *et al.* 1988).

The effect of paternal age in the calculation of risk for Down syndrome was studied by Stene *et al.* (1981). In an analysis of 5014 prenatal diagnoses in women aged 35 or more, there were 117 chromosomal abnormalities (2.3 per cent). When the effect of maternal age was eliminated, paternal age *over* the age of 39 years exerted some effect to increase the risk of Trisomy 21 in all the maternal ages studied (Table 16.2). In societies in which consanguinity is prevalent, chromosomal aberrations are also increased. Naguib (1989) compared 401 patients with trisomies with 403 normal infants born in Kuwait. Increases in both maternal age and paternal age increased the risk for chromosomal aberration, but once corrections were made for these two variables, consanguinity was also a significant factor.

Ultrasound may also be used in screening for Down syndrome, although this is a less valuable method than is biochemical screening. There are two possible ways in which ultrasound could be used as a guide to Down syndrome. The first would identify abnormalities known to be associated with Down syndrome, such as duodenal atresia and cardiac abnormalities. In one series, 33 per cent of 92 fetuses with Trisomy 21 had a structural abnormality identified by ultrasound, of which cardiac defects, duodenal atresia, and cystic hygroma were the most common (Nyberg et al. 1990). The second method is the subject of current interest and relates to ultrasonic quantitative measurements of the ratio between the biparietal diameter and the occipitofrontal diameter of the fetal head (cephalic index), the nuchal thickness, and the femur length.

The ultrasonic measurement of aspects of the anatomy of the fetal head has been widely studied but would appear to be of limited value in the detection of Down syndrome. The biparietal diameter of a Down syndrome infant during the mid-trimester is similar to that of the normal population and may, therefore, be used as a guide to gestational age (Cuckle and Wald 1987). The brachycephaly associated with Down syndrome is unusual in Caucasians and may be measured by a shortening of the occipitofrontal diameter. Buttery (1979) reported one fetus with Down syndrome in whom there was a shortening of the occipitofrontal diameter during the mid-trimester of pregnancy. Perry et al. (1984) compared the occipitofrontal index during the mid-trimester of eight fetuses known to be affected by Down syndrome with 308 fetuses who were normal. The occipitofrontal diameter was not shorter during the mid-trimester in the infants with Down syndrome when compared with the normal fetuses, suggesting that the brachycephaly may not become apparent until later in pregnancy. Other authors have also been unable to detect any difference in the occipitofrontal diameter between normal fetuses and those with Down syndrome (Lockwood et al. 1987; Shah et al. 1990). Diameters of the fetal head may, therefore, be used for gestational age determination in the presence of Down syndrome.

An increase in nuchal skin thickness may also be measured using ultrasound. Although some 43 per cent of 21 Down syndrome affected infants had thickened soft tissue, that is 6 mm or more, at the back of the neck under the occiput compared with 0.1 per cent of almost 4000 unaffected infants, nuchal thickening generally only occurred when Down syndrome coexisted with hydrops, and, hence, nuchal skin thickness alone is a poor predictive test when applied to the whole population (Benacerraf et al. 1987; Nicolaides et al. 1992; Nyberg et al. 1990; Toi et al. 1987; Watson et al. 1994).

The single most useful ultrasound measurement in the ultrasonic prediction of Down syndrome relates to femur length measurement (Cuckle et al. 1989; Lockwood et al. 1987). However, other authors have failed to confirm a reduction in femur length in fetuses affected with Down syndrome (Shah et al. 1990). There have now been several recent studies which have confirmed the shortening of long bones, both femur and humerus in fetuses affected with Down syndrome, suggesting not only that this is a useful screening test, but also that it should not be used to date pregnancies for triple test screening (Hill *et al.* 1989; Johnson *et al.* 1993; Nyberg *et al.* 1993; Wenstrom *et al.* 1993).

A previous child with a chromosomal abnormality

Women who have produced a child with non-dysjunction trisomy have an increased risk of recurrence of trisomy, generally double that of the overall risk for the age-matched general population. When a more detailed analysis of risk is made, the younger the mother, the greater the risk of recurrence relative to other mothers of the same age; thus at maternal age 40 the risk of recurrence of Down syndrome is 40 per cent greater than the age-related risk alone, whereas at the age of 30 the risk is increased by over 400 per cent, from 1 in 960 to 1 in 224 (Wald and Cuckle 1989). Such patients may not wish to wait for a mid-trimester biochemical test or amniocentesis but rather elect for an early amniocentesis or a chorion villus sampling (Thornton *et al.* 1991).

Parental chromosomal abnormalities

Parents who have a chromosomal abnormality, yet no phenotypic abnormality, require formal genetic counselling in order that any risks are assessed. They usually have chromosomal rearrangements in which no DNA has been lost but in which a gene or a control sequence has moved. A typical example is a balanced translocation.

If the parents have an unbalanced chromosomal abnormality, then the risk to the fetus is high. Thus, Bovicelli *et al.* (1982) reported that 30 pregnancies in 26 parents themselves affected by Trisomy 21 resulted in ten children with Down syndrome (33 per cent), eighteen normal children (60 per cent), and three spontaneous abortions.

The determination of fetal sex

The determination of fetal sex may be indicated in the selective abortion of a male fetus with an X-linked recessive disorder, such as Duchenne muscular dystrophy or, in other X-linked conditions, such as retinitis pigmentosa or fragile X syndrome. In the latter, a break in a consistent portion of the X chromosome of affected individuals may allow the diagnosis to be made: the syndrome is associated with mental deficiency, delayed speech, and a variety of phenotypic abnormalities (Giraud *et al.* 1976).

Recent advances in gene probe technology and genetic engineering may ultimately allow for treatment of such conditions at an early embryonic level (Super 1990).

Techniques for invasive diagnosis

In general, diagnosis is made by the karyotyping of cells obtained by amniocentesis or chorion villus sampling. Should a satisfactory genetic culture not be obtained by these techniques, then either ultrasound, or fetal blood sampling guided by fetoscopy or ultrasound, may be used to determine either dysmorphic features or fetal karyotype. Fetal blood sampling may also be used to accelerate the diagnostic process in association with late presentation by a patient with the need for a possible genetic termination of pregnancy (Daffos *et al*. 1985). In general, however, amniocentesis and chorion villus sampling will be the commonest methods for obtaining fetal genetic material.

Amniocentesis

The classical method of obtaining material for fetal genetic analysis is by amniocentesis after the 14th week of gestation. A sample of amniotic fluid will be obtained in 94 per cent of cases and cell growth will be sufficient for culture in 98 per cent of samples obtained. The risk of maternal cell contamination is in the region of 1 in 1000 samples. (Benn and Hsu 1983; Milunsky *et al*. 1972).

The hazards of amniocentesis are now well documented. In a series of large non-randomized studies, the incidence of spontaneous abortion following amniocentesis was 1.4 per cent in the Netherlands (Galjaard 1976), 4.7 per cent in Canada (Simpson *et al*. 1976), and 2.4 per cent in Scotland (Philip and Bang 1978).

The Medical Research Council Study in the UK (1978) compared the outcome of pregnancy following 2428 amniocenteses with the outcome for 2428 pregnancies in which amniocentesis was not performed. Although the controls were matched for age, parity, and obstetric history, the matching has been criticized for not being close enough. The incidence of spontaneous abortion following amniocentesis was 2 per cent and the incidence of spontaneous abortion without amniocentesis was 1 per cent, suggesting an excess risk in the region of 1 per cent. There was no excess risk of preterm delivery, but there was an excess risk of placental abruption. In the Danish Study (Tabor *et al*. 1986) 4606 women, between the ages of 25 and 34 years, were randomized to receive an amniocentesis or not. The spontaneous abortion rate following entry to the trial in the control group was 1.3 per cent and in the study group 2.1 per cent, suggesting an excess in the region of 0.8 per cent. It would, therefore, seem that the risk of miscarriage following an amniocentesis is not in excess of 1 per cent and may be as low as 0.2 per cent (Halliday *et al*. 1992).

Although it was not statistically significant, there was a trend towards orthopaedic postural deformities in the infants of women who underwent amniocentesis in the MRC study. However, in a case-controlled study involving 1342 infants, there were no differences in the incidences of talipes or hip malformations in normal babies, normal babies following amniocentesis, or abnormal babies (Wald *et al.* 1983). Other risks related to amniocentesis include fetomaternal microhaemorrhage which occurs in up to 1.3 per cent of amniocenteses performed under ultrasonic control, and, hence, women who are Rhesus group did require prophylactic anti-D (Curtis *et al.* 1973; Lachman 1977). There are also reports of dimple-like scars, believed to be puncture scars, in infants following amniocentesis together with more serious injuries such as corneal perforation and limb gangrene (Raimer and Raimer 1984).

Chorion villus sampling (CVS)

Chorion villus sampling carries the advantage that it may be performed during the late first trimester giving a karyotype result within 24 hours, and hence allowing a first trimester termination to be carried out should it be indicated, whereas after amniocentesis, a termination is likely to be carried out at the 18th week or even later. With experience, it is possible to obtain villi in 93 per cents of attempts with successful karyotyping in 95 per cent of cultured villi (Maxwell *et al.* 1985).

There has been debate whether transabdominal CVS is preferable to transcervical CVS, since the former would avoid the theoretical risk of bacterial contamination associated with passage through the potentially infected endocervical canal (Maxwell *et al.* 1986). In randomized trials which have compared these two routes of sampling, there have been no statistical differences in fetal wastage, although transcervical CVS appears to allow a larger size of sample to be obtained whilst transabdominal CVS is considered to be easier to learn (Bovicelli *et al.* 1986; Brambati *et al.* 1990). However, Lilford *et al.* (1987) obtained sufficient tissue to allow for a chromosomal diagnosis to be made in 99 out of 100 cases of transabdominal CVS, suggesting that both techniques are applicable to clinical practice and the choice perhaps depends upon the preference of the operator rather than any other factor.

However, there are three aspects of CVS which require discussion and which have influenced the place of the technique in clinical practice. These are the accuracy of cytogenetic diagnosis, the risk of miscarriage, and the risk of fetal abnormality.

The accuracy of the cytogenetic diagnosis is as important, if not more so, than the safety aspects. Both CVS and amniocentesis result in very few false-negative results for trisomy. Thus, the incidence of producing a child with a trisomy after a diploid karyotype has been reported is in the region of 1 in 1000 cases, and this may be due to the presence of either placental mosaicism or maternal contamination (Eichenbaum *et al.* 1986; Gosden 1991; Lilford 1991). A greater problem is that of a false-positive result, generally due to a chromosomal abnormality being present in the placenta but not in the fetus. In such a situation, a direct placental chromosomal preparation shows a mosaicism with both a normal and an abnormal karyotype being represented. Placental chromosomal mosaicism is reported in 1.1 per cent of chorionic villus samples, but when the mosaicism is present a chromosomal abnormality is only found in the fetus in 16 per cent of cases, the remaining 84 per cent representing a potential source of error (Johnson *et al.* 1990). The risk of misinterpretation due to mosaicism is reduced by laboratory experience in the karyotyping of direct preparation and short-term culture, the use of longterm cultured preparations, and the use of either amniocentesis or cordocentesis (*Lancet* 1991).

The risk of miscarriage following CVS has to be interpreted with care. CVS tends to be performed between the 9th and 12th weeks of pregnancy, a common time for spontaneous abortion also to occur. Moreover, spontaneous abortion occurs more often in patients of higher maternal age. Gustavii (1984) reported that one-third of 105 pregnant women aged 40 or more miscarried, whilst Cohen-Overbeek *et al.* (1990) reported that the spontaneous abortion rate between the 6th and 10th weeks of gestation rose from 1.9 per cent in women aged 36 years to 10.9 per cent for those aged 40 years or over, largely due to chromosomal abnormalities.

The excess fetal wastage due to CVS has been estimated from two large randomized trials of CVS versus amniocentesis. In the Canadian Multicentre Trial (1989) 2787 women were randomized to undergo either CVS at 9–12 weeks' gestation or amniocentesis at 15–17 weeks' gestation for the detection of fetal chromosomal abnormality. The total pregnancy loss was 15.1 per cent in the group randomized to amniocentesis and 16.8 per cent in that randomized for CVS, suggesting an excess loss due to CVS of 1.7 per cent. The larger Medical Research Council European Trial (1991) reported an excess loss of 4.6 per cent in the CVS group compared with the amniocentesis group in 3248 women randomized to undergo one or other procedure. There would, therefore, appear to be an excess fetal loss associated with CVS compared with amniocentesis.

There may also be a direct link between CVS and fetal limb reduction abnormalities, (generally absent or shortened fingers or toes), especially if CVS is performed before the 9th week of gestation. The size of this risk has been estimated at between 1 in 200 and 1 in 1500 chorion villus samples (Firth *et al.* 1991; Lilford 1991; Mastrioacovo and Cavalcanti 1991; Monni *et al.* 1993). The cause of the fetal limb reduction abnormalities is probably a haemodynamic insult (Burton *et al.* 1992; Quintero *et al.* 1992).

In clinical practice, therefore, chorion villus sampling has both advantages and disadvantages compared with amniocentesis and, when performed, should be done after the 9th week of gestation. Since the risks to the fetus are increased by this technique, it is perhaps more appropriate for women with a higher risk of genetic abnormality than that based on maternal age alone; for instance, in those women at a high risk of a single gene defect, an unbalanced translocation, or in those women who would accept the increased risks for an earlier result (Lilford 1991).

Early amniocentesis

Early amniocentesis (before 15 weeks) would seem to be a safe alternative to both CVS and mid-trimester amniocentesis. In a non-randomized trial, the incidence of miscarriage following early amniocentesis was 3.1 per cent while the risk following CVS was 5 per cent (Godmilow *et al.* 1988). The authors were able to obtain a sample in 98 per cent of attempted early amniocenteses. Hackett *et al.* (1991) reported a series of 106 early amniocenteses in which clear liquor was obtained in 96 per cent of attempts. In a recent series, the spontaneous abortion rate in 222 patients who underwent amniocentesis between the 9th and 14th week of pregnancy was 1.4 per cent (Nevin *et al.* 1990).

Before early amniocentesis is introduced into routine clinical practice, women should be offered entry into randomized clinical trials comparing this technique with CVS and/or conventional amniocentesis. It is possible that the risk of mosaicism is lower with early amniocentesis than with CVS but this has yet to be proven. It is also suggested, from animal experimentation, that earlier amniocentesis has a greater inhibitory effect on fetal lung maturation than does later amniocentesis, and this will also have to be assessed. It should also be noted that most reports of early amniocentesis refer to amniocentesis after the 12th week of pregnancy, and it may be that these should be assessed separately from very early amniocentesis performed before the 12th week of pregnancy.

Screening for single gene diseases

Haemoglobinopathies

Haemoglobinopathies may be subdivided into the thalassaemias and the haemoglobin variants.

Beta-thalassaemia, particularly common in Mediterranean populations, India, and SE Asia, is found in the carrier state (beta-thalassaemia minor) in up to 20 per cent of such populations. Beta-thalassaemia major, the homozygous condition, may be amenable to blood transfusion, iron chelation, splenectomy, or bone marrow transplantation. Alpha-thalassaemia is less common, but the homozygous state generally results in the intrauterine death of a hydropic fetus.

Sickle cell trait does not carry serious antenatal problems, the babies are of normal birthweight but are subject to an increased incidence of fetal distress, 17 per cent in patients and 12 per cent in controls based on a series of 344 patients (Tuck *et al.* 1983). Tuck *et al.* also analysed 74 pregnancies in 42 patients with sickle cell disease, they found a spontaneous abortion rate of 23 per cent in anaemic patients, an incidence of IUGR of 28 per cent, a stillbirth rate of 5 per cent, a neonatal death rate of 5 per cent, and an incidence of pre-eclampsia of 14 per cent. These events were generally related to anaemia with episodes of infection; however, the liberal use of blood transfusion may help to improve fetal survival.

Previously, fetal blood samples were obtained using fetoscopy and aspiration from a fetal vein on the placental surface and then later by ultrasound-guided sampling directly from the umbilical cord. The newer technique of chorion villus sampling coupled with a genetic analysis using recombinant DNA now allows a first-trimester diagnosis. Thus, Old *et al.* (1986) reported a first-trimester prenatal diagnosis by DNA analysis in 80 per cent of 281 families at risk of having a child with beta-thalassaemia major, with only one misdiagnosis. Moreover, the specific genetic mutation can now be investigated in the parents using the polymerase chain reaction (PCR) which then allows for a more accurate diagnosis on chorion villus sampling.

Tay–Sachs disease

Tay–Sachs disease is an autosomal recessive condition due to the deficiency of a lysosomal enzyme (hexosaminidase A) which results in an accumulation of the ganglioside GM2. It is found predominantly in Ashkenazim Jews at an incidence of 0.4 per 1000 births, but the carrier state may be as high as 1 in 30. The disease is associated with progressive neurological degeneration from the sixth month of life and there is no cure; the classical cherry-red macular spot may be visible on the retina before the first year of life and death generally occurs between the third and fourth years.

The antenatal diagnosis of Tay–Sachs disease may be made on either amniotic fluid or fetal blood. Hexosaminidase A activity in amniotic fluid has been shown to be a correct predictor of Tay–Sachs disease in eight samples with low activity, and, although the levels in the liquor were generally lower in carriers than in normal fetuses, there was too great a range to allow for this distinction to be made (Grebner and Jackson 1979). Perry *et al.* (1979) reported the diagnosis of Tay–Sachs disease made on a single fetus following fetal blood sampling, demonstrating a significantly reduced percentage of hexosaminidase A activity compared with total hexosaminidase activity.

Nowadays, this and most other lyssosomal enzyme deficiencies are diagnosed by direct biochemical analysis of chorion villus samples.

Cystic fibrosis

Cystic fibrosis is the most common autosomal recessive disorder found in the Caucasian population, with an incidence of 1 in 2000 births. Until recently, there were no satisfactory easily applied tests available to screen the population for carrier status, although the finding of decreased levels of amniotic fluid protease activity in liquor was available for the diagnosis of an affected fetus (Nadler and Walsh 1980).

The genetic defect in the majority of CF patients has recently been identified (McIntosh *et al.* 1989; Rommens 1989). This has allowed not only the prenatal diagnosis of CF by direct gene probing and polymerase chain reactions, but also the possibility of population screening for CF heterozygotes in the detection of carrier status within an asymptomatic population. The utility of this whole population screening has yet to be established (Brock *et al.* 1991; *Lancet* 1990) and may allow screening of both partners from saliva samples with a view to amniocentesis or chorionic villus sampling, should both partners screen positive (Asche *et al.* 1993; Mennie *et al.* 1992).

Screening for structural abnormalities in the fetus

Screening for neural tube defects

Neural tube defects represent a major cause of fetal abnormality and are associated with significant mortality and morbidity. There is a marked geographical variation in the prevalence rates for neural tube defects. In the absence of selective abortion, the prevalence for neural tube defects in the UK mainland is 1.2 per 1000 births compared with 3.5 per 1000 births in Ireland (Nevin 1991). There may also be a decline in the prevalence of neural tube defects even in the absence of antenatal screening. Thus, during 1974–85, the prevalence of anencephaly fell by 50 per cent, whilst the prevalence of spina bifida fell by 38 per cent (Stone *et al.* 1988). The significance of being born with a neural tube defect has been highlighted by many authors, including Hunt (1990). Clearly no infant with anencephaly survives. Over a 20-year study of 117 consecutive children born with open spina bifida, 93 per cent either died or survived with significant handicap. Only 7 per cent of these infants had little or no disability.

Anencephaly and spina bifida are detectable by routine ultrasound screening. Clearly, anencephaly should have a 100 per cent sensitivity and specificity on ultrasound screening, but the diagnosis of spina bifida cannot reach this accuracy. Campbell and Pearce (1983) identified 93 per cent of 15 fetuses with either spina bifida or an encephalocoele. Wald *et al.* (1991) reported the results from all published series on the detection of neural tube defects by ultrasound. From this meta-analysis, ultrasound detected 100 per cent of 207 cases of anencephaly but only 88 per cent of 261 cases of spina bifida, with a false-positive detection rate of 1.2 per cent in 5185 ultrasound examinations.

Fetuses with spina bifida also tend to have an abnormal cephalic appearance on ultrasound screening even in the absence of anencephaly, but these appearances are very gestation specific. Thus, of 107 fetuses with an open spina bifida diagnosed before the 24th week of gestation, 98 per cent had a 'lemon sign' (frontal bone scalloping), whilst 96 per cent had abnormal cerebellar findings including the 'banana sign' (abnormal anterior curvature of the cerebellar hemispheres) or an absent cerebellum. Beyond the 24th week, only 13 per cent of fetuses with spina bifida had a 'lemon sign' although 91 per cent had abnormal cerebellar signs (Van den Hof *et al.* 1990).

The association between raised amniotic and maternal serum alphafetoprotein and anencephaly (Brock *et al.* 1973) and open spina bifida (Leek *et al.* 1974) is now well recognized. Alphafetoprotein is a glycoprotein, with a molecular weight of 70 000, and is synthesized by the embryonic yoke sac, fetal gastrointestinal tract, and liver. Brock and Scrimgeour (1975) reported that maternal serum AFP only deviated significantly from normal levels in the presence of an open neural tube defect after the 13th week of pregnancy, suggesting the possibility of population screening for this abnormality.

The principles of population screening currently in practice have arisen from the findings of the UK Collaborative Study Group (1977).

The UK Collaborative Study Group (1977) assessed maternal serum AFP screening for neural tube defects between the 10th and 24th weeks' gestation based on data from 18 684 singleton pregnancies without neural tube defects, and pregnancies in the presence of 146 anecephalic fetuses, 142 with open spina bifida, and 13 with encephalocoele. Gestation-specific levels of maternal serum AFP were calculated, and the group reported that the 'best time' for detecting an open neural tube defect was between the 16th and 18th week of pregnancy, when a balance between a high detection of abnormal fetuses with a low detection of unaffected singletons would be possible. At this gestational age, maternal serum AFP would detect 88 per cent of anencephalic fetuses, 79 per cent of those with open spina bifida, and 3.3 per cent of unaffected singletons. The group also suggested that the most convenient unit was not the centile but the 'multiple of the median' (MoM), and the above figures could be expected using a cut-off level for maternal serum AFP of 2.5 MoM. If a cut-off level of 2.0 MoM was taken, 90 per cent of anencephalics would be detected, as would 91 per cent of fetuses with open spina bifida, but so would 7.2 per cent of normal singletons, whilst if a cut-off point was taken of 3.0 MoM, 84 per cent of anencephalics would be detected, as would 70 per cent of spina bifida babies, and 1.4 per cent of normal singletons. In a smaller series, it has been claimed that maternal serum AFP screening will detect up to 97 per cent of all open spina bifida lesions (Macri *et al.* 1986).

The second report of the UK Collaborative Study Group (1979) assessed amniotic fluid alphafetoprotein levels on samples taken between the 13th and 24th weeks of pregnancy based on 13 105 singleton pregnancies without a neural tube defect, 222 samples from fetuses with anencephaly, 123 with open spina bifida, 11 with encephalocoele, and 18 with closed spina bifida. Again, liquor serum alphafetoprotein increased with gestational age and, again, a measure of 2.5 MoM was the 'best buy' detecting 98 per cent of anencephalic fetuses and 98 per cent with spina bifida. If the liquor was bloodstained, this level would also detect 0.48 of normal singleton fetuses, but if the liquor was clear this figure fell to 0.27 per cent. Thus, the risk of the fetus having an open spina bifida in the presence of a raised liquor alphafetoprotein and clear liquor was 18: 1, or 35: 1 for all neural tube defects. If the cut-off level for multiples of the median was increased, there was a greater pick-up for open spina bifida, approaching 100 per cent, but no further increase in detection of anencephalic fetuses.

Wald *et al.* (1982) demonstrated the refinement which could be made in alphafetoprotein screening if routine ultrasound dating was used. In a study of 1268 pregnant women with a singleton fetus without a neural tube defect,

Table 16.3 AFP screening

Outcome	Raised liquor AFP		Raised liquor acetylcholinesterase	
	No. pregnancies	% group	No. pregnancies	% group
Anencephaly	478	43.5	476	52.6
Open neural tube defect	335	30.5	333	36.8
Anterior abdominal wall defect	63	5.7	47	5.2
Congenital nephrosis	11	1.0	0	0
Other serious FA	14	1.4	7	0.8
Spontaneous abortion	73	6.6	34	3.7
No abnormality or abortion	125	11.3	8	0.9
Total	1099	100	905	100

From United Kingdom Collaborative Acetylcholinesterase Study Group (1981)

2.3 per cent of patients had a raised maternal serum AFP (2.5 MoM) if gestational age was based on the date of the last period, but only 1.8 per cent if it was based on ultrasound cephalometry. Whilst the accuracy for the use of ultrasound cephalometry for dating gestational age in the normal fetus is known, Wald *et al.* (1980) demonstrated that the biparietal diameter in the mid-trimester in 20 fetuses with spina bifida was 0.83 cm less than that of 186 unaffected fetuses at the same gestational age. Thus, if biparietal diameters from the normal population are used to estimate gestational age for any given level of alphafetoprotein there will be an artificial elevation in the maternal serum alphafetoprotein level in the presence of a neural tube defect over and above the level associated with the defect. Because of this, Wald *et al.* estimated that had all patients in the UK Collaborative Study of 1977 had a gestational age estimation based on ultrasound cephalometry performed, the detection of spina bifida would have increased from 79 to 91 per cent, thus increasing the sensitivity of the screening procedure.

The presence of a neural tube defect in the presence of a raised liquor alphafetoprotein may be confirmed by either ultrasound or by the estimation of acetylcholinesterase assay on the liquor, cerebrospinal fluid being rich in acetylcholine. Wald and Cuckle (1989) combined the results of three large published series to show that only nine out of 5021 (0.2 per cent) of liquor samples from normal fetuses had a raised acetylcholinesterase activity. The United Kingdom Collaborative Acetylcholinesterase Study Group (1981) reported on amniotic fluid acetylcholinesterase levels between the 13th and 24th week of gestation in women with a raised liquor AFP level. There were 1099 pregnancies with a raised liquor alphafetoprotein level and 905 with a raised level of acetylcholinesterase. As can be seen from Table 16.3, when allowances were made for patients who miscarried spontaneously, there were no serious fetal abnormalities detected in 11 per cent of the raised liquor AFP group and the false-positive level in the raised liquor acetylcholinesterase group was only 0.9 per cent. Of the 194 women who had a raised liquor alphafetoprotein but a normal liquor acetylcholinesterase, 19.6 per cent had a serious fetal abnormality, 20.1 per cent miscarried, and 60.3 per cent had no abnormality. Acetylcholinesterase was raised in over 99 per cent of all the open neural tube defects, 75 per cent of the anterior abdominal wall defects, but in none of the cases of congenital nephrosis.

Since neither ultrasound screening nor maternal serum AFP screening can possibly be both 100 per cent specific and 100 per cent sensitive, there is debate as to how both these techniques should fit into clinical practice. Ultrasound is considered to be a safe method of investigation (see below), but the incidence of a false-positive diagnosis of spina bifida of 1.2 per cent has already been stated (Wald *et al.* 1991). The finding of a raised maternal serum alphafeto-protein requires further investigation by either ultrasound or by amniocentesis, the latter carrying a risk of miscarriage of up to 0.5 per cent. Since most units now offer routine ultrasound screening during the mid-trimester, the place of maternal serum AFP screening has been questioned. Tyrrell *et al.* (1988) calculated that, for open spina bifida, routine ultrasound screening in most units (as opposed to the best units) would diagnose 80 per cent of lesions, whereas a combination of ultrasound and maternal AFP would diagnose 90 per cent of lesions if amniocentesis were performed for a maternal serum AFP level of 2.5 MoM for gestational age. This means that for every 20 fetuses with open spina bifida, this combination would diagnose 18 rather than 16 cases. However, in order to achieve this, 142 amniocenteses would need to be performed, and one fetus would be lost from abortion following the amniocentesis causing some degree of maternal distress in those patients who had a raised serum AFP yet no fetal abnormality. Many units, therefore, have chosen to screen for open neural tube defects by ultrasound alone and only offer combined ultrasound and maternal serum AFP screening to patients with a past history of neural tube defect, or to those patients who specifically request combined screening, or as part of a Down syndrome screen. Perhaps, ultrasound and maternal serum AFP screening should be considered to be complimentary rather than options (Wald *et al.* 1991).

Other uses of AFP

Other than screening for Down syndrome and neural tube defect, maternal serum AFP screening during the mid-trimester may be used as a predictor of poor fetal outcome. In a series of 54 singleton pregnancies in whom the mid-trimester maternal serum AFP was greater than 3.0 MoM, the mean birthweight of the babies was 350 g less than controls and the perinatal mortality rate was increased by 350 per cent (Wald *et al.* 1977). In a prospective trial involving 103 fetuses in the presence of a maternal serum AFP of greater than 2.3 MoM and in the absence of fetal abnormality, 11 per cent of infants weighed

2.5 kg at birth (Brock *et al.* 1977). There have been three large prospective studies to show the effect of serum alphafetoprotein screening on an obstetric population overall. In a prospective study of over 1300 singleton pregnancies in Boston, 3.9 per cent had a raised alphafetoprotein during the mid-trimester and this was associated with a relative risk for a neural tube defect of 224, for other fetal abnormalities of 4.7, for stillbirth 8.1, for neonatal death 4.7, for IUGR 4.0, for placental abruption 3.0, and for pre-eclampsia 2.3 (Milunsky *et al.* 1989). In a study of 176 000 women screened by mid-trimester maternal serum AFP in California, 22 per cent of patients with a high maternal AFP delivered a preterm infant whilst 3 per cent delivered a stillborn infant (Cowan *et al.* 1989). In a case-controlled study of women with a raised maternal serum AFP during the mid-trimester, there was a 10-fold risk of subsequent fetal death *in utero* (Waller *et al.* 1991).

There is an association between low circulating levels of maternal AFP and an anembryonic pregnancy, which is not surprising since the major site of AFP production is the fetal liver. Jarvis and Johnson (1981), in a series of 96 pregnant women whose serum AFP levels at the 16th week of pregnancy were less than 10 µg/litre, described a subgroup of 3 per cent with an anembryonic pregnancy and a second subgroup of 3 per cent with undiagnosed fetal death *in utero*. Similarly, Bennett *et al.* (1978) reported an association between low maternal serum AFP levels and anembryonic pregnancy, including hydatidiform mole. However, since maternal serum AFP screening now generally involves coincidental ultrasonic examination, it is likely that these diagnoses will now be made by ultrasound rather than by a low AFP level.

It has already been stated that the prevalence of open neural tube defects appears to be falling in the population even in the absence of screening. The effect of screening in addition to the natural trend has been assessed by several authors. Stone *et al.* (1988) reported that screening resulted in the termination of 59 per cent of anencephalic fetuses and 23 per cent of those with spina bifida. These statistics would seem to be disappointingly low. The reasons for the continuing significant incidence of open neural tube defect at birth would seem to be either a failure to offer screening or the decision to continue the pregnancy because of a coexisting normal twin (Cuckle and Wald 1987).

Ultrasound screening for fetal anomaly

Ultrasound screening may be used during the mid-trimester to screen for fetal anomaly. Grisoni *et al.* (1986) reported that 25 per cent of abnormalities recognized in 122 abnormal fetuses by ultrasound were detected before the 20th week of pregnancy, thereby allowing the possibility of termination of pregnancy in the minority and maternal preparation, with or without paediatric surgical counselling, in the majority. Pearce and Campbell (1984) reported that, over a five-year period, the obstetric ultrasound department diagnosed, antenatally, 244 congenital anomalies correctly, with a further six false-positive

Table 16.4 Ultrasound screening

Congenital abnormalities diagnosed on ultrasound

Type	Number	Comments	
Craniospinal	166	includes	73 open spina bifida 41 anencephaly 16 isolated hydrocephaly
Gastrointestinal tract	30	includes	17 exomphalos 4 gastroschisis
Urinary tract	29	includes	11 obstructive uropathy 6 polycystic kidney
Fetal tumours	16	includes	8 cystic hygroma
Limb deformities	13	includes	4 achondroplasia
Cardiac abnormalities	8	includes	3 hypertrophic cardiomyopathy

From Pearce and Campbell (1984)

diagnoses, and 17 false-negative ones. The major anomalies diagnosed are shown in Table 16.4.

It would seem that an ultrasound scan for fetal anomaly performed at around the 18th week of pregnancy is a reasonable balance between the detection of abnormalities and the option to perform a termination of pregnancy should it be indicated. Thus, routine ultrasound screening at the 18th week of pregnancy detected 58 per cent of 93 malformed fetuses in a series of 3098 antenatal ultrasound screening examinations. The only false-positive cases in the study related to mild fetal hydronephrosis (Rosendahl and Kivinen 1989). In one recent survey, 1 in 340 pregnancies in which a mid-trimester ultrasound scan took place resulted in a termination being performed for major fetal anomaly (Luck 1992).

The role of ultrasound in the detection of neural tube defects and Down syndrome has already been discussed. Other anomalies will now be considered.

Microcephaly, in the absence of other fetal anomalies, must be distinguished from early IUGR, and, hence, more than one examination is needed in order that the rate of head growth may be compared with the rate of growth of either the abdominal circumference or the femur length (Campbell and Pearce 1983; Chervenak *et al.* 1987).

Ultrasound may now detect choroid plexus cysts in the lateral ventricles during mid-trimester screening. Cysts below 10 mm in size tend to disappear by the 24th week and are without clinical significance, occurring in 11 out of 3627 fetuses screened (0.3 per cent) (Ostlere *et al.* 1987). However, cysts which are larger than this tend to persist and are associated with fetal chromosomal abnormalities in up to 25 per cent of fetuses (Ostlere *et al.* 1990; Ricketts *et al.* 1987). Similarly, fetal nuchal translucency may also be used as a first trimester marker for fetal chromosomal abnormalities, such abnormalities being present in 6 per cent of fetuses with a nuchal translucency (Nicolaides *et al.* 1992).

Ultrasound screening, especially in the last trimester, in patients with poly-hydramnios will demonstrate fetal anomaly in 18 per cent of cases (Hobbins 1979).

Oesophageal atresia occurs in approximately 1 in 2000 births and may be suggested by the absence of a gastric echo, whilst duodenal atresia, occurring in between 1 in 2700 and 1 in 10 000 births may be recognized by the 'double bubble', representing dilated stomach and duodenum. However, diagnosis of both these conditions will be difficult before the 26th week, and may be associated with polyhydramnios and other fetal anomalies. Thus, 30 per cent of fetuses with duodenal atresia will also have Trisomy 21, whilst 20 per cent will have cardiovascular abnormalities. Conversely, 3 per cent of fetuses with Trisomy 21 will have duodenal atresia (Balcar *et al.* 1984). Miro and Bard (1988) reported that infants in whom duodenal atresia was recognized antenatally ($n = 13$) underwent earlier neonatal surgery with less metabolic complications than did infants in whom the condition was first diagnosed post-natally ($n = 33$).

Fetal abdominal wall defects occur with an incidence of approximately 1 in 4000 births, exomphalos being more common (1 in 10 000 births) than gastroschisis (1 in 29 000 births) (Baird and MacDonald 1981). Exomphalos is due to a failure of fusion of the cephalic, lateral, and caudal folds to form the umbilical ring, and in up to 80 per cent of fetuses may be associated with other anomalies, such as congenital heart defects, diaphragmatic hernia, imperforate anus, and extrophy of bladder (Vintzileos *et al.* 1987). There is also an associa-tion between exomphalos and chromosomal anomalies; Vintzileos *et al.* (1987) reported that 9 per cent of such fetuses have Trisomy 18, whereas Gilbert and Nicolaides (1987) reported that 54 per cent of 35 such fetuses had a chromo-somal abnormality, of which the commonest was Trisomy 18. Gastroschisis is due to a defect in the recti muscles and tends to involve only the bowel without other associated fetal anomalies.

Both these conditions are associated with a raised maternal serum AFP level and are diagnosable by ultrasound between the 16th and 18th weeks' gestation, the defect in gastroschisis generally being smaller than in exomphalos and of better prognosis with paediatric surgery. The overall neonatal mortality for newborns with exomphalos is 29 per cent and for newborns with gastro-schisis, 13.5 per cent (Kirk and Wah 1983). There would appear to be no advantage in Caesarean section over vaginal delivery for these infants purely on the basis of the abdominal wall defect (Carpenter *et al.* 1984; Sipes *et al.* 1990).

The overall incidence of congenital heart defects is 8 per 1000 pregnancies. Basic ultrasound fetal cardiac screening should consist of the four-chamber view together with the aortic and pulmonary trunks (Bronshtein *et al.* 1993). It is best performed between the 18th and 24th weeks of gestation, false-negative diagnoses occurring more frequently with earlier screening. Crawford *et al.* (1988) reported that ultrasound will detect a cardiac abnormality on antenatal screening in 82 per cent of affected fetuses. Davis *et al.* (1990) reviewed the outcome of 129 pregnancies in which the fetus was found to have a structural cardiac abnormality and in whom the prenatal diagnosis was fully or partially correct in 96 per cent of patients. During the same period, 11 major and 15 minor cardiac abnormalities were missed and four fetuses had an incorrect cardiac diagnosis, but all had a cardiac abnormality. The positive predictive value was thus 98.4 per cent and the negative predictive value 98.6 per cent. Of 82 pregnancies not terminated, only 16 per cent of infants survived one year, whilst only 17 per cent survived one year in the Crawford study (which came from the same unit). Other authors have quoted similar specificity with this examination (Achiron *et al.* 1992).

Limb reduction deformities may be recognized based on normograms of the long bones (Queenan *et al.* 1980) as may skeletal dysplasias and osteogenesis imperfecta (D'Ottavio *et al.* 1993; Sharony *et al.* 1993), whilst non-immune fetal hydrops, occurring in 1 in 3748 births, will generally be associated with predisposing problems such as fetal cardiac abnormalities in 40 per cent, chromosomal anomalies in 16 per cent, twin–twin transfusion in 10 per cent, skeletal abnormalities in 11 per cent, and congenital infections in 4 per cent (Allan *et al.* 1986; Hutchinson *et al.* 1982).

Fetal urological abnormalities may also be apparent on ultrasound, and they present one of the more difficult problems in clinical practice since a significant number of abnormalities seen antenatally do not appear to be associated with fetal or infant compromise. Greig *et al.* (1989) reported a series of 62 fetuses with renal abnormalities seen on ultrasound examination; only 71 per cent of these fetuses were liveborn, 24 per cent were subject to termination of pregnancy, and 5 per cent were stillborn. On assessment in infancy, 30 of the liveborn infants (48 per cent of the original series) had no evidence of renal disease. Arthur *et al.* (1989) reported an ultrasound diagnosis of fetal renal tract abnormality in 1 in 600 antenatal scans. The commonest abnormalities were posterior urethral valves which were associated with good renal function following corrective surgery in the neonatal period. Other abnormalities included primary vesicourethral reflux, renal dysplasia including polycystic disease, and pelviureteric obstruction. The presence of pelviureteric obstruction may be associated with a relatively poor outcome. In a series of 63 kidneys with antenatally detected pelviureteric junction obstruction, 51 per cent required surgery for deteriorating renal function, whilst 49 per cent did not require any intervention (Madden *et al.* 1991). When a renal tract abnormality is found antenatally, serial ultrasound scanning together with a paediatric urological opinion may help to assess the situation.

The possibility of intrauterine surgical intervention exists in this situation and perhaps should only be performed in the presence of deteriorating fetal renal function as assessed by the estimation of fetal urinary sodium and osmolality (Lipitz *et al.* 1993; Thomas 1990). It is possible that fetal surgery for deteriorating renal function is unnecessary, in that either the damage is so severe that the surgery is too late or the prognosis is so good that the surgery is not required (Adzick and Harrison 1994).

There has been concern expressed regarding the safety of ultrasound to the fetus. Early evidence that chromosomal aberrations could be induced by ultrasound were not reproduced by other investigators (Wells 1987). Although it is never possible to demonstrate that any technique has absolute clinical safety, there have been no confirmed biological affects on patients (or operators) caused by exposure to ultrasound at intensities typical of present diagnostic ultrasound instruments, moreover, the benefits from the prudent use of ultrasound must outweigh the risks, if any (Reece *et al.* 1990).

Conclusions

Prenatal diagnosis, based on chromosomal, biochemical, haematological, or structural investigations is a rapidly increasing field. The advantages of diagnosis have to be balanced against the risks of any invasive procedure and the sensitivity and specificity of the techniques. It is likely that, as time progresses, the diagnosis will extend to genetic defects in eggs and embryos, and perhaps into genetic manipulation. Advances in laboratory science will enable parents to receive results more rapidly. For instance, a recent report using a chromosome probe specific for chromosome 21 has suggested that a result could be available within three days after amniocentesis for the exclusion of Trisomy 21 (Bryndorf *et al.* 1992).

The technology needs to be combined with careful counselling at all levels. More difficult cases should perhaps be referred to a specialist regional unit which should embrace a multidisciplinary approach consisting of obstetrician, geneticist, ultrasonographer, and paediatrician.

The possible psychological effect arising from screening should also be borne in mind. Patients need to be adequately counselled before they enter a screening programme, whilst patients may need significant reassurance should investigations ultimately prove to be negative, whilst other patients may suffer adverse psychological effects related to late termination of pregnancy (Green 1990).

References

Achiron, R., Glaser, J., Gelernter, I., Hegesh, J., and Yagel, S. (1992). Extended fetal echocardiographic examination for detecting cardiac malformations in low risk pregnancies. *British Medical Journal* **304**, 671–4.
Adzick, N. S. and Harrison, M. R. (1994). Fetal surgical therapy, *Lancet* **343**, 897–902.
Allan, L. D., Crawford, D. C., Sheridan, R., and Chapman, M. G. (1986). Aetiology of non-immune hydrops. *British Journal of Obstetrics and Gynaecology* **93**, 223–5.
Arthur, R. J., Irving, H. C., Thomas, M. F. M., and Watters, J. K. (1989). Bilateral fetal uropathy. *British Medical Journal* **298**, 1419–20.
Asche, D. A., Patton, J. P., Hershey, J. C., and Mennuti, M. T. (1993). Reporting the results of cystic fibrosis carrier screening. *American Journal of Obstetrics and Gynecology* **168**, 1–6.
Baird, P. A. and MacDonald, E. C. (1981). An epidemiological study of congenital

malformations of the anterior abdominal wall. *American Journal of Human Genetics* **33**, 470–8.

Balcar, I., Grant, D. C., Miller, W. A., and Bieber, F. A. (1984). Antenatal detection of Down's syndrome by sonography. *American Journal of Roentology* **143**, 29–30.

Benacerraf, B. R., Frigoletto, F. D., and Cramers, D. W. (1987). Down's syndrome: sonographic sign for diagnosis in the second-trimester fetus. *Radiology* **163**, 811–13.

Benn, P. A. and Hsu, L. Y. F. (1983). Maternal cell contamination of amniotic fluid cell cultures. *American Journal of Medical Genetics* **15**, 297–305.

Bennett, M. J., Grudzinskas, J. G., Gordon, Y. B., and Turnbull, A. C. (1978). Circulating levels of AFP and pregnancy-specific beta 1-glycoprotein in pregnancies without an embryo. *British Journal of Obstetrics and Gynaecology* **85**, 348–50.

Bovicelli, L., Orsini, L. F., Rizzo, N., Montacuti, V., and Bacchetta, M. (1982). Reproduction in Down's syndrome. *Obstetrics and Gynecology* **59**, 13S–17S.

Bovicelli, L, Rizzo, N., Montacuti, V., and Morandi, R. (1986). Transabdominal versus transcervical routes for chorion villus sampling. *Lancet* **ii**, 290–1.

Brambati, B., Lanzani, A., and Tului, L. (1990). Transabdominal and transcervical chorion villus sampling. *American Journal of Medical Genetics* **35**, 160–4.

Brock, D. J. H. and Scrimgeour, J. B. (1975). Screening for neural tube defects. *Lancet* **i**, 745.

Brock, D. J. H., Bolton, A. E., and Monaghan, J. M. (1973). Prenatal diagnosis of anencephaly through maternal serum AFP measurement. *Lancet* **ii**, 923–4.

Brock, D. J. H., Barron, L., Jelen, P., Watt, M., and Scrimgeour, J. B. (1977). Maternal serum AFP measurements as an early indicator of low birthweight. *Lancet* **ii**, 267–8.

Brock, D. J. H., Barron, L., Holloway, S., Liston, W. A., Hillier, S. G., and Seppala, M. (1990). First-trimester maternal serium biochemical indicators in Down syndrome. *Prenatal Diagnosis* **10**, 245–51.

Brock, D. J. H., Mennie, M. E., McIntosh, I., Jones, C., and Shrimpton, A. E. (1991). Heterozygote screening for cystic fibrosis. In *Antenatal diagnosis of fetal abnormalities* (ed. J. O. Drife and D. Donnai), pp. 59–70. Springer–Verlag, London.

Bronshtein, M., Zimmer, E. Z., Gerlish, M., Lorber, A., and Drugan, A. (1993). Early ultrasound diagnosis of fetal congenital heart defects. *Obstetrics and Gynecology* **82**, 225–9.

Bryndorf, T., Christensen, B., Philip, G., Hansen, W., Yokobata, K., Bui N., *et al.* (1992). New rapid test for prenatal detection of trisomy 21. *British Medical Journal* **304**, 1536–9.

Burton, B. K., Schultz, C. J., and Burd, L. I. (1992). Limb anomalies associated with chorion villus sampling. *Obstetrics and Gynecology* **79**, 726–30.

Burton, B. K., Pring, G. S., and Verp, M. S. (1993). A prospective trial of pre-natal screening for Down syndrome. *American Journal of Obstetrics and Gynecology* **169**, 526–30.

Buttery, E. (1979). Occipitofrontal–biparietal diameter ratio. *Medical Journal of Australia* **2**, 662–4.

Campbell, S. and Pearce, J. M. (1983). Ultrasound visualisation of congenital malformations. *British Medical Bulletin* **39**, 322–31.

Canadian Collaborative Chorionic Villus Sampling–Amniocentesis Group (1989). Multicentre randomized trial of chorionic villus sampling and amniocentesis. *Lancet* **i**, 1–6.

Carpenter, M. W., Carci, M. R., Dibins, A. W., and Haddow, J. E. (1984). Perinatal management of ventral wall defects. *Obstetrics and Gynecology* **64**, 646–51.

Chervenak, F. A., Rosenberg, J., Brightman, R. C., Chitkara, U., and Geanty, P. (1987). A prospective trial of the accuracy of ultrasound in predicting fetal microcephaly. *Obstetrics and Gynecology* **69**, 908–15.

Clark, B. A., Kennedy, K., and Olson, S. (1993). The need to re-evaluate trisomy screening for advanced maternal age. *American Journal of Obstetrics and Gynecology* **168**, 812–16.

Cohen-Ooverbeek, T. E., Hop, W. C. T., Denouden, M., Pijpers, L., Jahoda, M. G. J., and Wladimiroff, J. W. (1990). Spontaneous abortion rate and advanced maternal age: consequences for prenatal diagnosis. *Lancet* **ii**, 27–9.

Cowan, L. S., Phelps-Sandall, B., Hanson, F. W., Peterson, A. G., and Tennant, F. R. (1989). A prenatal diagnostic centre's first year experience with the California AFP screening program. *American Journal of Obstetrics and Gynecology* **160**, 1496–1504.

Crawford, D. C., Chita, S. K., and Allan, L. D. (1988). Prenatal detection of congenital heart disease. *American Journal of Obstetrics and Gynecology* **159**, 352–6.

Cuckle, H. S. and Wald, N. J. (1987). The impact of screening for open neural tube defects in England and Wales. *Prenatal Diagnosis* **7**, 91–9.

Cuckle, H. S., Wald, N. J., and Thompson, S. G. (1987). Estimating a woman's risk of having a pregnancy associated with Down's syndrome using her age and serum AFP level. *British Journal of Obstetrics and Gynaecology* **94**, 387–402.

Cuckle, H. S., Wald, N. J., Barkai, G., Fuhrmann, W., Altland, K., Brambati, B., et al. (1988). First-trimester biochemical screening for Down syndrome. *Lancet* **ii**, 851–2.

Cuckle, H. S., Wald, N. J., Quinn, J., Royston, P., and Butler, L. (1989). Ultrasound fetal femoral length measurement in the screening for Down syndrome. *British Journal of Obstetrics and Gynaecology* **96**, 1373–8.

Cuckle, H. S., Wald, N. J., Goodburn, S. F., Sneddon, J., Amess, J. A. L., and Dunn, S. C. (1990). Measurement of activity of urea resistant neutrophil alkaline phosphatase as an antenatal screening test for Down syndrome. *British Medical Journal* **301**, 1024–6.

Curtis, J. D., Cohen, W. M., Richerson, H. B., and White, C. A. (1972). The importance of placental localization preceding amniocentesis. *Obstetrics and Gynecology* **44**, 1914–18.

Daffos, F., Capella-Pavlovasky, M., and Forestier, F. (1985). Fetal blood sampling during pregnancy with use of a needle guided by ultrasound. *American Journal of Obstetrics and Gynecology* **153**, 655–60.

Davis, G. K., Farquar, C. M., Allan, L. D., Crawford, D. C., and Chapman, M. (1990). Structural cardiac abnormalities in the fetus. *British Journal of Obstetrics and Gynaecology* **97**, 27–31.

D'Ottavio, G., Tamaro, L. F., and Mandruzzato, G. (1993). Early pre-natal ultrasound diagnosis of osteogenesis imperfecta. *American Journal of Obstetrics and Gynecology* **169**, 384–5.

Eichenbaum, S. Z., Krumins, E. J., Fortune, D. W., and Duke, J. (1986). False-negative finding on chorionic villus sampling. *Lancet* **ii**, 391.

Firth, H. V., Boyd, P. A., Chamberlain, P., MacKenzie, I. A., Lindenbaum, R. H., and Huson, S. M. (1991). Severe limb abnormalties after chorionic villus sampling at 56–66 days' gestation. *Lancet* **337**, 762–3.

Galjaard, H. (1976). European experience with prenatal diagnosis of congenital disease. *Cytogenics and Cellular Genetics* **16**, 453–67.

Gilbert, W. M. and Nicolaides, K. H. (1987). Fetal omphalocoele: associated malformations and chromosomal defects. *Obstetrics and Gynecology* **70**, 633–5.

Giraud, F., Ayme, S., Mattei, J. F., and Mattei, G. M. (1976). Constitutional chromosomal breakage. *Human Genetics* **34**, 125–36.

Godmilow, L., Weiner, S., and Dunn, L. K. (1988). Early genetic amniocentesis. *American Journal of Human Genetics* **43**, 9234.

Gosden, C. M. (1991). Fetal karyotyping using chorionic villus samples. In *Antenatal diagnosis of fetal abnormalities* (ed. J. O. Drife and D. Donnai), pp. 153–67. Springer–Verlag, London.

Grebner, E. E. and Jackson, L. G. (1979). Prenatal diagnosis of Tay–Sachs disease. *American Journal of Obstetrics and Gynecology* **134**, 547–50.

Green, J. M. (1990). Prenatal screening and diagnosis: some psychological and social problems. *British Journal of Obstetrics and Gynaecology* **97**, 1074–6.

Greig, J. D., Raine, P. A. M., Young, D. G., Azmy, A. F., MacKenzie, J. R., Danskin, F., *et al.* (1989). Value of antenatal diagnosis of abnormalities of the urinary tract. *British Medical Journal* **298**, 1417–19.

Grisoni, E. R., Gauderer, M. W. L., Wolfson, R. M., and Izant, R. J. (1986). Antenatal ultrasonography: the experience in a high-risk perinatal centre. *Journal of Pediatric Surgery* **21**, 358–61.

Gustavii, B. (1984). Chorionic biopsy and miscarriage in first trimester. *Lancet* **i**, 562.

Hackett, G. A., Smith, J. H., Rebello, M. T., Gray, C. T. H., Rooney, D. E., Beard, R. W., *et al.* (1991). Early amniocentesis at 11–14 weeks' gestation for the diagnosis of fetal chromosomal abnormality. *Prenatal Diagnosis* **11**, 311–15.

Halliday, J., Lumley, J., Sheffield, L. J., Robinson, H. P., Renou, P., and Carlin, J. P. (1992). Importance of complete follow-up of spontaneous fetal loss after amniocentesis and chorion villus sampling. *Lancet* **340**, 886–90.

Hassold, T., Jacobs, P., Kline, J., Stein, Z., and Warburton, D. (1980). The effect of maternal age on chromosomal trisomies. *Annals of Human Genetics* **44**, 29–36.

Heyl, P. S., Miller, W., and Canick, J. A. (1990). Maternal serum screening for aneuploid pregnancy by alphafetoprotein, hCG, and unconjugated oestriol. *Obstetrics and Gyneology* **76**, 1025–31.

Hill, L. M., Guzick, D., Belfar, H. L., Hixson, J., Rivello, D., and Rusnak, J. (1989). The current role of sonography in the detection of Down syndrome. *Obstetrics and Gynecology* **74**, 620–3.

Hobbins, J. C. (1979). Ultrasound in the diagnosis of congenital anomalies. *American Journal of Obstetrics and Gynecology* **134**, 331–45.

Hook, E. B., Cross, P. K., and Schreinemachers, D. M. (1983). Chromosomal abnormality rates at amniocentesis. *Journal of the American Medical Association* **249**, 2034–8.

Hunt, G. M. (1990). Open spina bifida: outcome for a complete cohort treated unselectively and followed into adulthood. *Developmental Medicine and Child Neurology* **32**, 108–18.

Hutchinson, A. A., Yu, V. Y., and Fortune, D. W. (1982). Non-immune hydrops. *Obstetrics and Gynecology* **59**, 347–52.

Jarvis, G. J. and Johnson, A. (1981). Low circulating levels of AFP and missed abortion. *Journal of Obstetrics and Gynaecology* **1**, 151–2.

Johnson, A., Wapner, R. J., Davis, G. H., and Jackson, L. G. (1990). Mosaicism in chorionic villus sampling. *Obstetrics and Gynecology* **75**, 573–7.

Johnson, M. P., Barr, M., Treadwell, M. C., Michaelson, J., Isada, N. B., Pryde, P. G., *et al.* (1993). Fetal leg and femur–foot length ratio. *American Journal of Obstetrics and Gynecology* **169**, 557–63.

Kirk, E. P. and Wah, R. M. (1983). Obstetric management of the fetus with omphalocoele or gastroschisis. *American Journal of Obstetrics and Gynecology* **146**, 512–18.

Lachman, E. (1977). Ultrasound screening during amniocentesis. *Lancet* ii, 832.

Lancet (1990). Cystic fibrosis: prospects for screening and therapy. *Lancet* 335, 79–80.

Lancet (1991). Chorionic villus sampling: valuable additional dangerous alternative? *Lancet* 337, 1513–15.

Leek, A. E., Leighton, P. C., Kitau, M. J., and Chard, T. (1974). Prospective diagnosis of spina bifida. *Lancet* ii, 1511.

Lilford, R. J. (1991). The rise and fall of chorionic villus sampling. *British Medical Journal* 303, 936–7.

Lilford, R. J., Irving, H. C., Linton, G., and Mason, M. Y. (1987). Transabdominal chorionic villus biopsy. *Lancet* i, 1415–16.

Lipitz, S., Ryan, G., Samuell, C., Haeusler, M. C. H., Robson, S. C., Dillon, H. K., *et al.* (1993). Fetal urine analysis for the assessment of renal tract in obstructive uropathy. *American Journal of Obstetrics and Gynecology* 168, 174–9.

Lockwood, C., Benacerraf, B., Krinsky, A., Blakemore, K., Belanger, K., Mahoney, M., *et al.* (1987). A sonographic screening method for Down's Syndrome. *American Journal of Obstetrics and Gynecology* 157, 803–8.

Luck, C. A. (1992). Value of routine ultrasound scanning at 19 weeks: a four year study of 8849 deliveries. *British Medical Journal* 304, 1474–8.

MacDonald, M. L., Wagner, R. M., and Slotnick, R. N. (1991). Sensitivity and specificity of screening for Down syndrome with alphafetoprotein, hCG, unconjugated oestriol, and maternal age. *Obstetrics and Gynecology* 77, 63–8.

McIntosh, I., Raeburn, J. A., Curtis, A., and Brock, D. J. H. (1989). First trimester prenatal diagnosis of cystic fibrosis by direct gene probing. *Lancet* ii, 972–3.

Macri, J. N., Kasturi, R. V., Krantz, D. A., and Koch, K. E. (1986). Maternal serum alphafetoprotein screening, maternal weight, and detection efficiency. *American Journal of Obstetrics and Gynecology* 155, 758–60.

Madden, N. P., Thomas, D. F. M., Gordon, A. C., Arthur, R. J., Irving, H. C., and Smith, S. E. W. (1991). Antenatally detected pelviureteric junction obstruction. *British Journal of Urology* 68, 305–10.

Mastroiacovo, P. and Cavalcanti, D. P. (1991). Limb reduction defects and chorionic villus sampling, *Lancet* 337, 1091.

Maxwell, D., Scepulkowski, B. H., Heaton, D. E., Coleman, D. V., and Lilford, R. (1985). A practical assessment of ultrasound guided transabdominal aspiration of chorionic villi and subsequent chromosomal analysis. *British Journal of Obstetrics and Gynaecology* 92, 660–5.

Maxwell, D., Lilford, R., Scepulkowski, B. H., Heaton, D. E., and Coleman, D. V. (1986). Transabdominal CVS. *Lancet* i, 123–6.

Medical Research Council (1978). An assessment of the hazards of amniocentesis. *British Journal of Obstetrics and Gynaecology* 85, supplement.

Medical Research Council Working Party (1991). Medical Research Council European Trial of chorionic villus sampling. *Lancet* 337, 1491–9.

Mennie, M. E., Gilfillan, A., Compton, M., Curtis, L., Liston, W. A., Pullen, W., *et al.* (1992). Pre-natal screening for cystic fibrosis. *Lancet* 340, 214–16.

Merkatz. I. R., Nitowsky, H. M., Marci, J. N., and Johnson, W. E. (1984). An association between low maternal serum alphafetoprotein and fetal chromosomal abnormalities. *American Journal of Obstetrics and Gynecology* 148, 886–94.

Milunsky, A., Atkins, L., and Littlefield, J. W. (1972). Amniocentesis for prenatal genetic studies. *Obstetrics and Gynecology* 40, 104–8.

Milunsky, A., Jick, S. S., Bruell, C. L., MacLaughlin, D. S., Tsung, Y. K., Jick, H., *et al.* (1989). Predictive values, relative risks, and overall benefits of high and low maternal serum AFP screening in singleton pregnancies. *American Journal of Obstetrics and Gynecology* 161, 291–7.

Miro, J. and Bard, H. (1988). Congenital atresia and stenosis of the duodenum. *American Journal of Obstetrics and Gynecology* **158**, 555–9.

Monni, G., Ibba, M. R., Lai, R., Cau, G., Mura, S., Olla, G., *et al.* (1993). Early transabdominal chorion villus sampling. *American Journal of Obstetrics and Gynecology* **168**, 170–3.

Murday, V. and Slack, J. (1985). Screening for Down's syndrome in the North East Thames Region. *British Medical Journal* **291**, 1315–18.

Mutton, D. E., Alberman, E., Ide, R., and Bobrow, M. (1991). Results of first year of a national register of Down's syndrome in England and Wales. *British Medical Journal* **303**, 1295–7.

Mutton, D. E., Ide, R., Alberman, E., and Bobrow, M. (1993). Analysis of national register of Down syndrome in England and Wales. *British Medical Journal* **306**, 431–2.

Nadler, H. L. and Walsh, M. M. J. (1980). Prenatal detection of cystic fibrosis on amniotic fluid. *Lancet* **ii**, 96–7.

Naguib, K. K. (1989). Effect of parental age, birth order, and consanguinity on nondysjunction in the population of Kuwait. *Journal of the Kuwait Medical Association* **23**, 37–47.

Nevin, J., Nevin, N. C., Dornan, J. C., Sim, B., and Armstrong, M. J. (1990). Early amniocentesis. *Prenatal Diagnosis* **10**, 79–83.

Nevin, N. C. (1991). Trends in prevalence of congenital abnormalities. In *Antenatal diagnosis of fetal abnormalities* (ed. J. O. Drife and D. Donnai), pp. 3–11. Springer-Verlag, London.

Nicolaides, K. H., Azar, G., Byrne, D., Mansur, C., and Marks, K. (1992). Fetal nuchal translucency: ultrasound screening for chromosomal defects in the first trimester of pregnancy. *British Medical Journal* **304**, 867–9.

Nicolaides, K. H., Snijders, R. J. M., Gosden, C. M., Berry, C., and Campbell, S. (1992). Ultrasonographically detectable markers of fetal chromosome abnormalities. *Lancet* **340**, 704–7.

Nyberg, D. A., Resta, R. G., Luthy, D. A., Hickok, D. E., Mahony, B. S., and Hirsch, J. H. (1990). Prenatal sonographic findings of Down syndrome. *Obstetrics and Gynecology* **76**, 370–7.

Nyberg, D. A., Resta, R. G., Luthy, D. A., Hickok, D. E., and Williams, M. A. (1993). Humerus and femur length shortening in the detection of Down syndrome. *American Journal of Obstetrics and Gynecology* **168**, 545–8.

Old, J. M., Ward, R. H. T., Petrou, M., Karagozou, F., Modell, B., and Weatherall, D. J. (1986). First-trimester fetal diagnosis for haemoglobinopathies. *Lancet* **ii**, 763–6.

Ostlere, S. J., Irving, H. C., and Lilford, R. J. (1987). Choroid plexus cysts in the fetus. *Lancet* **ii**, 1491.

Ostlere, S. J., Irving, H. C., and Lilford R. J. (1990). Fetal choroid plexus cysts, a report of 100 cases. *Journal of Radiology* **175**, 753–5.

Pearce, J. M. and Campbell, S. (1984). Ultrasound and fetal abnormalities. In *Progress in obstetrics and gynaecology* Vol. 4, (ed. J. Studd), pp. 52–81. Churchill Livingstone, Edinburgh.

Perry. T. B., Hechtman, P., and Chow, J. C. W. (1979). Diagnosis of Tay–Sachs disease of blood obtained at fetoscopy. *Lancet* **i**, 973–4.

Perry, T. B., Benzie, R. J., Cassar, N., Hamilton, E. F., Stocker, J., Toftager-Larsen, K., *et al.* (1984). Fetal cephalometry by ultrasound as a screening procedure for the prenatal detection of Down's syndrome. *British Journal of Obstetrics and Gynaecology* **91**, 138–43.

Philip, J. and Bang, J. (1978). Outcome of pregnancy after amniocentesis for chromosomal analysis. *British Medical Journal* **2**, 1183–4.

Queenan, J. T., O'Brien G. B., and Campbell, S. (1980). Ultrasound measurement of fetal limb bones. *American Journal of Obstetrics and Gynecology* **138**, 297–302.

Quintero, R. A., Romero, R., Mahoney, M. J., Vecchio, M., Holden, J., and Hobbins, J. C. (1992). Fetal haemorrhage after chorion villus sampling. *Lancet* **339**, 193.

Raimer, S. S. and Raimer, B. G. (1984). Needle puncture scars from mid-trimester amniocenteses. *Archives of Dermatology* **120**, 1360–2.

Reece, E. A., Assimakopoulos, E., Zheng, X. Z., Hagay, Z., and Hobbins, J. C. (1990). The safety of obstetric ultrasound. *Obstetrics and Gynecology* **76**, 139–46.

Ricketts, N. E. M., Lowe, E. M., and Patel, N. B. (1987). Prenatal diagnosis of choroid plexus cysts. *Lancet* **i**, 213–14.

Rommens, J. M., Ianuzzi, M. C., Kerem, B., Drumm, M. L., Melmer, G., Dean, M., *et al.* (1989). Identification of the cystic fibrosis gene: chromosome walking and jumping. *Science* **245**, 1059–65.

Rosendahl, H. and Kivinen, S. (1989). Antenatal diagnosis of malformations by routine ultrasonography. *Obstetrics and Gynecology* **73**, 947–51.

Shah, Y. G., Eckl, C. J., Stinson, S. K., and Woods, J. R. (1990). Biparietal diameter/ femur length ratio, cephalic index, and femur length measurements: not reliable screening techniques for Down syndrome. *Obstetrics and Gynecology* **75**, 186–8.

Sharony, R., Browne, C., Lachman, R. N., and Rimion, D. L. (1993). Pre-natal diagnosis of the skeletal dysplasias. *American Journal of Obstetrics and Gynecology* **169**, 668–75.

Sheldon, T. A. and Simpson, J. (1991). Appraisal of a new scheme for prenatal diagnosis for Down syndrome. *British Medical Journal* **302**, 1133–6.

Simpson, N. E., Dallaire, L., Miller, J. R., Siminovich, L., Hamerton, J. L., Miller, J., *et al.* (1976). Prenatal diagnosis of genetic disease in Canada. *Canadian Medical Association Journal* **115**, 739–45.

Sipes, S. L., Weiner, C. P., Sipes, D. R., Grant, S. S., and Williamson, R. A. (1990). Gastroschisis and omphalocoele. *Obstetrics and Gynecology* **76**, 195–9.

Spencer, K. and Carpenter, P. (1993). Prospective study of pre-natal screening for Down syndrome. *British Medical Journal* **307**, 764–9.

Spencer, K., Mallard, A. S., Coombes, E. J., and Macri, J. N. (1993). Pre-natal screening for trisomy 18. *British Medical Journal* **307**, 1455–8.

Stene, J., Stene, E., Stengel-Rutkowski, S., and Murken, J. D. (1981). Paternal age and Down syndrome. *Human Genetics* **59**, 119–24.

Stone, D. H., Smalls, M. J., Rosenberg, K., and Womersley, J. (1988). Screening for congenital neural tube defects in high-risk area. *Journal of Epidemiology and Community Health* **42**, 271–3.

Super, M. (1990). An introduction to modern genetics. In *Prenatal diagnosis and prognosis* (ed. R. Lilford), pp. 165–71. Butterworths, London.

Tabor, A., Philip, J., Madsen, M., Bang, J., Obel, M., and Norgaard-Pedersen, B. (1986). Randomized controlled trial of genetic amniocentesis in 4606 low-risk women. *Lancet* **i**, 1287–92.

Thomas, D. F. M. (1990). Fetal uropathy. *British Journal of Urology* **66**, 225–31.

Thornton, J. G., Cartmill, R. S. V., Williams, J., Holding, S., and Lilford, R. J. (1991). Clinical experience with the triple test for Down syndrome. *Journal of Perinatal Medicine* **19**, 151–4.

Toi, A., Simpson, G. F., and Filly, R. A. (1987). Ultrasonically evident fetal nuchal skin thickness. *American Journal of Obstetrics and Gynecology* **156**, 150–3.

Tuck, S., Studd, J. W. W., and White, J. M. (1983). Pregnancy in women with sickle traits. *British Journal of Obstetrics and Gynaecology* **90**, 108–11.

Tyrrell, S., Howel, D., Bark, M., Allibone, E., and Lilford, R. J. (1988). Should maternal AFP estimation be carried out in centres where ultrasound screening is routine? *American Journal of Obstetrics and Gynecology* **158**, 1092–9.

United Kingdom Collaborative Study on AFP (1977). Maternal AFP measurement in antenatal screening for anencephaly and spina bifida in early pregnancy. *Lancet* **i**, 1323–32.

United Kingdom Collaborative Study on AFP (1979). Amniotic fluid AFP measurement in antenatal diagnosis of anencephaly and open spina bifida in early pregnancy. *Lancet* **ii**, 651–61.

United Kingdom Collaborative Acetylocholinesterase Study Group (1981). Amniotic fluid acetylocholinesterase electrophoresis as a secondary test in the diagnosis of anenecephaly and open spina bifida in early pregnancy. *Lancet* **ii**, 321–4.

Van den Hof, M. C., Nicolaides, K. H., Campbell, J., and Campbell, S. (1990). Evaluation of the lemon and banana signs in 130 fetuses with open spina bifida. *American Journal of Obstetrics and Gynecology* **162**, 322–7.

Vintzileos, A. M., Campbell, W. A., Weinbaum, P. J., and Nochminson, D. J. (1987). Antenatal detection and management of ultrasonically detected fetal anomalies. *Obstetrics and Gynecology* **69**, 640–60.

Wald, N. J. and Cuckle, H. S. (1989). Biochemical detection of neural tube defects and Down's syndrome. In *Obstetrics* (ed. A. Turnbull and G. Chamberlain), pp. 269–90. Churchill Livingstone, Edinburgh.

Wald, N. J., Cuckle. H. S., Stirrat, G. M., Bennett, M. J., and Turnbull, A. C. (1977). Maternal serum alphafetoprotein and low birthweight. *Lancet* **ii**, 268–70.

Wald, N. J., Cuckle, H. S., Boreham, J., and Stirrat, G. (1980). Small biparietal diameter of fetuses with spina bifida. *British Journal of Obstetrics and Gynaecology* **87**, 219–21.

Wald, N. J., Cuckle, H., Boreham, J., and Turnbull, A. C. (1982). Effect of estimating gestational age by ultrasound cephalometry on the specificity of AFP screening. *British Journal of Obstetrics and Gynaecology* **89**, 1050–3.

Wald, N. J., Terzian, E., Vickers, P. A., and Weatherall, J. A. C. (1983). Congenital talipes and hip malformation in relation to amniocentesis. *Lancet* **ii**, 246–9.

Wald, N. J., Cuckle, H. S., Densem, J. W., Nanshahal, K., Canick, J. A., Haddow, J. E., *et al.* (1988*a*). Maternal serum and conjugated oestriol as an antenatal screening test for Down's syndrome. *British Journal of Obstetrics and Gynaecology* **95**, 334–41.

Wald, N. J., Cuckle, H. S., Densem, J. W., Nanshahal, K., Royston, P., Chard, T. *et al.* (1988*b*). Maternal serum screening for Down's syndrome in early pregnancy. *British Medical Journal* **297**, 883–7.

Wald, N. J., Cuckle, H. S., Haddow, J. E., Doherty, J. A., Knight, G. J., and Palomaki, G. E. (1991). Sensitivity of ultrasound in detecting spina bifida. *New England Journal of Medicine* **324**, 769–71.

Waller, D. K., Lustig, L. S., Cunningham, G. C., Globus, M. C., and Hook, E. B. (1991). Second-trimester maternal serum alphafetoprotein levels and the risk of subsequent fetal death. *New England Journal of Medicine* **325**, 6–10.

Watson, W. J., Miller, R. C., Menaro, M. K., Chescheir, N. C., Katz, V. L., Hansen, W. F., *et al.* (1994). Ultrasound measurement of fetal nuchal skin to screen for chromosome abnormalities. *American Journal of Obstetrics and Gynecology* **170**, 583–6.

Wells, P. N. T. (1987). The safety of diagnostic ultrasound. *British Journal of Radiology* **supp. 20**, 1.

Wenstrom, K. D., Williamson, R. A., Grant, S. S., Hudson, J. D., and Getshell, J. P. (1993). Evaluation of multiple marker screening for Down syndrome. *American Journal of Obstetrics and Gynecology* **169**, 793–7.

17 The diagnosis and assessment of intrauterine growth retardation

This chapter is concerned primarily with the screening for, and evaluation of, intrauterine growth retardation (IUGR). There are numerous terms which are often used synonymously, yet are not necessarily synonymous with the term IUGR, to describe the fetus who has failed to reach its growth potential due to some form of intrauterine constraint. This constraint may be physiological, such as sex, race, and birth order, as well as pathological. The phrase IUGR is to be preferred to 'small for dates', 'light for dates', or 'small for gestational age', which are descriptions of statistical distribution and do not imply either intrauterine constraint or 'starvation' (Whittle 1991). Studies on fetuses with IUGR should take into account these physiological constraints and try to distinguish them from pathological ones. Thus, Thompson *et al.* (1968) reported a survey based on over 52 000 singleton pregnancies and demonstrated that males were, on average, 150 g heavier than females at all gestational ages beyond the 38th week; that first babies were, on average, 100 g lighter than subsequent babies at all gestations but especially beyond the 38th week; and that for each sex and within each parity group, mean birthweights fall with decreasing social status with a mean difference between social class I and V of 150 g. Moreover, there is a distinction between fetal size and fetal growth such that growth retardation describes a dynamic event in which the fetus deviates progressively from a normal growth line, and, hence, true IUGR must require at least two measurements of size (Altman and Hytten 1989a).

The condition of IUGR is not homogeneous and similar presentations may have different aetiologies and different implications. Two large categories which have been described are symmetrically and asymmetrically small babies, but even here the overlap is very large (Campbell and Thoms 1977). In general, the asymmetrically small baby, which has a larger head–abdominal circumference ratio, may result from the reduced uterine perfusion often found in the hypertensive mother. Symmetrically small babies, however, may arise from factors likely to affect the overall fetal growth potential and may be found as a feature of chromosome anomalies or early infections such as rubella. However, they may also appear as the result of severe early intrauterine starvation. Perhaps a more useful modern concept depends upon the association between intrauterine growth retardation and the presence or absence of an abnormal umbilical artery Doppler study (Burke *et al.* 1990). This study reported 179 fetuses whose ultrasonically determined abdominal circumference was below

Table 17.1 Risk factors for IUGR

Condition	Relative risk for IUGP
Pre-eclampsia	14.6
Congenital abnormality	11.5
Sibling IUGR	5.7
Smoking	3.5
Hypertension	2.7
Low maternal weight (< 50 kg)	1.7
Low maternal height (< 51 cm)	1.3

the 5th centile. Of these, 124 fetuses had normal blood flow and resulted in four Caesarean sections for fetal distress with one baby having cerebral irritation. Among 55 women with abnormal umbilical artery studies, there were three perinatal deaths, one baby with cerebral irritation, and six Caesarean sections for fetal distress, suggesting that a normal Doppler study in the presence of growth retardation may result in some reassurance, whereas an abnormal study is more predictive of morbidity.

Since the use of the term IUGR is based upon the presumption of intrauterine constraint, then the morbidity and mortality associated with this condition will depend upon the definition below which IUGR is diagnosed. Traditionally a cut-off point of below the 10th centile is used, but a cut-off point of below the 5th centile (which approximates to two standard deviations below the mean) is tighter and, therefore, the definition should always be stated. A small number of studies still take 2.5 kg as the cut-off point, regardless of gestational age.

The aetiology of IUGR

The aetiology of IUGR has been studied by several authors, including Bakketeig *et al*. 1979, Dobson *et al*. 1982, Galbraith *et al*. 1979, Ounsted *et al*. 1985, and Wen *et al*. 1990. The strongest predictive factors would appear to be pre-eclampsia in the index pregnancy or a past history of IUGR. When severe pre-eclampsia occured, 31 per cent of fetuses were growth retarded, whereas 23 per cent of pregnancies in women in whom there was a past history of growth retardation resulted in a baby with IUGR.

Smoking, discussed more fully in Chapter 15 (Routine antenatal care), remains a significant risk factor in its own right when a multiple logistic regression is used to control for other known risk factors (Kleinman and Madans 1985). The association between fetal abnormality and IUGR was reported by Macafee *et al*. (1972) who reported IUGR occurring in 46 per cent of 115 pregnancies in the presence of a malformed infant. A list of known risk factors for IUGR is shown in Table 17.1.

The identification of such risk factors may allow for a increased clinical and technological vigilance in the identification of this condition. In a study of over 8000 births, IUGR occurred in 9.8 per cent of a group with known risk factors compared with 2.3 per cent in a group without known risk factors (Galbraith *et al.* 1979).

Intrauterine growth retardation, either idiopathic or secondary to a known aetiological agent, may be caused by a defect in placental development related to poor invasion of spiral arteries by trophoblast. Placental bed biopsies taken from patients with a growth-retarded infant have shown varying degrees of luminal occlusion by atheromatous-like lesions in the myometrial spiral arteries (Sheppard and Bonnar 1981). These lesions are said to represent a defect in the normal maternal vascular response to migratory trophoblast in the inner myometrium and resemble the changes found in pre-eclampsia (Khong *et al.* 1986).

The consequences of IUGR

Intrauterine growth retardation is a potentially lethal condition. McIlwaine *et al.* (1979) reported that 13.8 per cent of 1012 perinatal deaths in singleton births in Scotland were related to IUGR, of these 71 per cent died before labour, 7 per cent during labour, and 22 per cent after delivery. Dobson *et al.* (1981) compared fetal outcome in 500 pregnancies when the baby weighed less than the 10th centile for gestational age at birth with 500 pregnancies where birthweight was normal. The perinatal mortality rate in the growth-retarded group was 52 per 1000, whilst it was 12 per 1000 in the normal birthweight group. When severe growth retardation was considered (less than the 5th centile), the perinatal mortality rate became 187 per 1000, whilst the perinatal mortality rate was 22 per 1000 for babies between the 5th and 9th centile for birthweight. Some 17 per cent of the babies born below the 5th centile had a fetal malformation as compared with 4.2 per cent for the control group. Bucknell and Wood (1985) reported a survey of 335 perinatal deaths in the Wessex region of England in 1982; they found that 25 per cent of the deaths in singleton fetuses, without evidence of congenital abnormality, were related to IUGR.

The morbidity associated with growth-retarded infants has also been studied. Fancourt *et al.* (1976) reviewed 60 children whose birthweight was below the 10th centile for gestational age, corrected for fetal sex and maternal height and weight. At a mean age of four years (range 28–84 months) the majority of children had 'caught up', but those whose skull growth on antenatal cephalometry had begun to slow before the 26th week of pregnancy were more likely to have their height and weight below the 10th centile for their age than were those whose IUGR had not become apparent until after the 26th week of pregnancy. Overall, 16 of the 60 children (27 per cent) were below the 10th centile for height, 21 (35 per cent) were below the 10th centile for weight, and 20 (33 per cent) were below the 10th centile for head circumference. There was also a decrease in developmental quotient, based on the Griffiths extended scales, for infants whose IUGR was detected before the 26th week of gestation.

Chiswick (1985) reported that babies with symmetrical growth retardation and those with severe asymmetrical growth retardation were less likely to catch up in growth than those with lesser degrees of asymmetrical growth retardation. Between 10 and 35 per cent of such growth-retarded children had evidence of minimal cerebral dysfunction in the forms of speech and language problems, learning difficulties, and attention deficits. In a prospective study of 96 infants delivered at term and more than two standard deviations below the mean for gestational age (Fitzhardinge and Steven 1972) there was a 1 per cent incidence of cerebral palsy, a 6 per cent incidence of infantile convulsions, and a 25 per cent incidence of minimal cerebral dysfunction; speech defects reflecting immaturity of reception and expression were present in 33 per cent of severely growth-retarded boys and 26 per cent of severely growth-retarded girls, but there was no evidence of hearing or visual difficulties.

The prediction of IUGR

The clinical ability to detect IUGR is relatively poor and, indeed, the estimation of birthweight is notoriously inaccurate. Loeffler (1967) demonstrated that, in a total of 2868 predictions of fetal weight on 585 patients in labour by 106 members of the medical and nursing staff of Queen Charlotte's Maternity Hospital, only 80 per cent of observations were within 1 lb of infant birth-weight, the largest errors occurring in babies weighing less than 5 lb or greater than 9 lb. Moreover, only the minority of babies born with IUGR have been predicted antenatally. Most reported series have suggested that only between 26 and 44 per cent of growth-retarded infants have been so-predicted by abdominal palpation antenatally (Hall *et al.* 1980; Hepburn and Rosenberg 1986; Villar and Belizan 1986). For every infant with IUGR correctly predicted antenatally, there are 2.5 false-positive diagnoses (Hall *et al.* 1980).

There is some benefit in a risk scoring system (Galbraith *et al.* 1979). Although such a system increased the percentage of growth-retarded fetuses diagnosed to 69 per cent, clearly 31 per cent of growth-retarded infants were not suspected.

Tests for IUGR may be divided into those which may act as screening procedures and those which have diagnostic ability. Because routine clinical methods are so unreliable, the development of a sensitive screening test with which to identify a group of women at-risk of having an IUGR baby would be of great value. Clearly the previous delivery of a growth-retarded baby or the fact that the mother has hypertension would be a factor, but most often IUGR appears unexpectedly. Numerous techniques have, therefore, been tested to screen for IUGR and, in current clinical practice, consideration must be given to repeated maternal weighing, the measurement of fundal height, and the use of ultrasound.

Maternal weight

The prediction of IUGR based on the repeated assessment of maternal weight gain during pregnancy had a vogue in previous decades but is of little clinical value now. Several authors in the 1970s advised that maternal weight gain should be monitored regularly during pregnancy and kept 'near the average' by dietary advice, both for the prediction and prevention of IUGR (Niswander and Jackson 1974; Simpson *et al.* 1975). Although there is a correlation between maternal weight gain during pregnancy and infant birthweight, this relationship is weak. A retrospective survey of 1092 pregnant women showed that repeated maternal weight measurement during pregnancy was not a useful indicator of IUGR in that poor weekly maternal weight gain (less than 0.2 kg) had a positive predictive value of 13 per cent for IUGR, but maternal weight loss or failure to gain weight occurred at some stage in 46 per cent of all the pregnancies studied (Dawes and Grudzinskas 1991). The routine repeated weighing of women during pregnancy in order to detect IUGR cannot be recommended (Altman and Hytten 1989*b*; Dawes *et al.* 1992).

Fundal height measurement

Fundal height measurement ought to assess fetal growth more directly than maternal weight. Beazley and Underhill (1970) showed that the abdominal anatomy of pregnant women varies so greatly, especially in relationship to the position of the umbilicus, that whilst judging the height of the fundus related to anatomical landmarks was inaccurate, measurement was more likely to be a consistent predictor of fetal size than palpation alone. Calvert *et al.* (1982) demonstrated that the inter-observer error in measurement was 6.4 per cent but that the intra-observer error was 4.6 per cent, suggesting that only serial measurements by the same observer would be of real value. Belizan *et al.* (1978) reported 1508 measurements of symphyseal–fundal height in 298 pregnant women based on a normogram. Using this method, the authors predicted 38 out of 44 growth-retarded infants (86 per cent), whilst some 10 babies of normal birthweight had also been predicted as being growth retarded. Similarly, Quaranta *et al.* (1981), using a symphyseal–fundal height and gestational age chart, were able to predict 30 out of 41 infants (73.1 per cent) whose birthweight was below the 10th centile for gestational age.

Larger studies have failed to reach so favourable a conclusion on the predictive value of the symphyseal–fundal height measurement. Rosenberg *et al.* (1982) reported 761 pregnant women who delivered 50 babies weighing below the 10th centile for gestational age. Only 28 of the 50 (56 per cent) were predicted by measurement, whilst a further 108 normal babies had been designated growth retarded. Persson *et al.* (1986) reported approximately 50 000 measurements made by midwives of symphyseal–fundal height in 3197 pregnant women. Only seven of the 42 infants (17 per cent) whose birthweight was less than two standard deviations below the mean for gestational age were predicted,

Table 17.2 The place of symphyseal–fundal height measurement

	Measured group	Control group
Number	804	835
Birthweight < 10th centile (%)	7.6	5.7
Suspicion of IUGR (%)	10	10
Sensitivity (%)	27.9	47.9
Specificity (%)	96.6	96.7

From Lindhard *et al.* (1990)

whereas 382 fetuses were considered, falsely, to be growth retarded. Lindhard *et al.* (1990) randomized 1639 pregnant women, such that 804 women received symphyseal–fundal height measurements at each antenatal visit throughout the third trimester in addition to the usual care given, and 835 women received the usual care without the specific measurement. The measured group were no different from the control group as regards the prediction of IUGR, the number of interventions, or the conditions of the newborns (see Table 17.2). It may be that these studies demonstrate that serial symphyseal–fundal height measurements made by different observers on the same patients do not produce accurate predictions, whereas the smaller studies which involve less observers do. Mathai *et al.* (1987) showed that symphyseal–fundal height measurement was a more sensitive predictor of intrauterine growth retardation than was abdominal girth measurement. The positive predictive value for symphyseal–fundal height measurement was 77.5 per cent compared with 55 per cent for girth, whilst the false-positive predictive rate was 12 per cent for symphyseal–fundal height measurement compared with 25 per cent for abdominal girth.

The measurement of symphyseal–fundal height is, therefore, a simple clinical test which, whilst not absolute, will act as a reasonable screening procedure for the presence of intrauterine growth retardation.

Ultrasound

The use of ultrasound as a screening method for the detection of IUGR has a long history. Two main approaches have been used, namely sequential measurements or a two-stage procedure of an early dating scan and a later fetal measurement scan.

Under any circumstances the interpretation of measurements taken during the third trimester depends upon an accurate knowledge of gestational age. Bennett *et al.* (1982) reported that only 81 per cent of women who were 'sure' of the date of their last menstrual period had an appropriate biparietal diameter measurement during the second trimester. In a group of patients in whom a second trimester biparietal diameter measurement was determined but not revealed, there was a higher incidence of labour induction for either post-maturity or suspected IUGR than in a group where the information was

Table 17.3 The value of serial BPD measurement

Ultrasound growth rate	Fetal birthweight			
	Normal (> 10th centile)	Borderline (5–10th centile)	Retarded (< 5th centile)	Total (< 10th centile)
Normal (> 10th centile) (n = 266)	220 (83)	22 (8)	24 (9)	46 (17)
Borderline (5–10th centile) (n = 26)	18 (70)	4 (15)	4 (15)	8 (30)
Retarded (< 5th centile) (n = 114)	21 (18)	16 (14)	77 (68)	93 (82)
Total (n = 406)	259 (63.8)	42 (10.3)	105 (25.9)	147 (36.2)

Numbers in parentheses are percentages. From Campbell and Dewhurst (1971)

revealed. Similarly, Ewigman *et al.* (1990) altered the estimated date of confinement in 25 per cent of women who underwent a routine mid-trimester ultrasound examination in the absence of any specific clinical indication.

The classical ultrasonic determination of IUGR is by serial biparietal diameter measurements (Campbell and Dewhurst 1971). The correlation between serial biparietal diameter growth rate and fetal birthweight based on 406 pregnancies is shown in Table 17.3, from which it may be seen that 68 per cent of infants whose birthweight was below the 5th centile had an ultrasonic-determined growth rate below the 5th centile. Thus, serial biparietal diameter measurements alone will miss approximately 32 per cent of infants who are growth retarded because the fetal head continues to grow at a normal rate; hence, other measurements have been assessed. Neilson *et al.* (1980) reported the ability of a series of different measurements to predict growth retardation. As shown in Table 17.4, the least predictive of the third trimester measurements were the head measurements, whilst the most predictive was trunk circumference at the level of umbilical vein insertion. When a two-stage prospective study in order to assess fetal growth was performed (mid-trimester scan and third trimester scan), ultrasound correctly predicted 94 per cent of growth-retarded infants, but falsely suggested IUGR in 9 per cent of infants whose birthweight was above the 10th centile for gestational age (Neilson *et al.* 1984).

Table 17.4 The value of two ultrasound scans

Variable	% small fetuses detected	% false negatives	% false positives
Biparietal diameter	58	42	10
Head area	59	41	10
Head circumference	56	44	8
Trunk area	81	19	11
Trunk circumference	83	17	10
Transverse trunk diameter	61	39	12
Crown–rump length	69	31	12

From Neilson *et al.* (1980)

The assessment of the identified IUGR baby

In practical terms, the aim of investigation is to separate the small, healthy baby from the small but potentially sick one. Many techniques are available but none are definitive, although in combination they help to provide an overall view of the fetal condition. The following methods of assessment require consideration:

(1) fetal movement counting;

(2) hormonal tests;

(3) cardiotocography;

(4) ultrasound assessment;

(5) Doppler studies;

(6) fetal blood sampling.

Fetal movement counting

Fetal movement counting once had a vogue as a screening test for fetal well-being, including the prediction of intrauterine growth retardation.

Sadovsky and Yaffe (1973) reported that fetal movements are significantly reduced and then cease up to 12 hours before fetal death. Pearson and Weaver (1976) popularized the 12-hour daily fetal movement count, and reported that the lowest 2.5 per cent of 1654 daily fetal movement counts by 61 women who subsequently delivered healthy fetuses fell below ten movements per 12 hours. Of 14 subsequent patients whose daily fetal movement count fell below ten, five delivered fetuses below the 5th centile for birthweight (36 per cent), six were stillborn (43 per cent), two died during the neonatal period, and four of the surviving infants were acidotic at birth. This represented a mortality or severe morbidity of 86 per cent of this group. Jarvis and Macdonald (1979) reported that a daily fetal movement count of less than 21 movements identified 75 per cent of 12 low birthweight babies (less than two standard deviations below the mean for gestational age), although there was a coexisting false-positive rate of 83 per cent.

However, large randomized trials have failed to confirm any benefit from regular fetal movement counting. Grant *et al.* (1989) randomly allocated 68 654 women to a policy of routine counting or to standard care. The antepartum death rates for normally formed singletons were similar in both groups, and even in the 'counting' group most (82 per cent) of the fetuses were dead before the mother sought medical attention. By virtue of a high false-positive rate and a delay on behalf of patients in reporting reduced fetal movements despite advice to do so, the value of fetal movements counting is limited. Moreover, there is good evidence that mothers perceive only a minority (16 per cent) of ultrasonically detected fetal movements (Johnson *et al.*, 1990).

Hormonal tests

Various hormones, produced either by the placenta alone or by the fetoplacental unit, have been used as placental function tests. During the 1970s, when hormonal function tests were at their most popular, urinary oestriol assay was probably the most widely practised. However, in current practice, these tests are of little, if any, value.

Dickey *et al.* (1972) reported that when the urinary oestriol to creatinine ratio (OCR), measured in 563 women, fell below the 10th centile at any stage during pregnancy, 44 per cent of the patients delivered a baby whose birthweight was below the 10th centile for gestational age, whereas only 32 per cent of patients with a normal OCR delivered a growth-retarded baby. The perinatal mortality rate in the low oestriol group was 29.7 per 1000 compared with 2.2 per 1000 in the normal oestriol level group. Similarly, Dobson *et al.* (1981) reported a low oestriol excretion in 42 per cent of 500 fetuses of birthweight below the 10th centile compared with 15 per cent of controls. This investigation, therefore, gave some guide as to the fetus at risk but, as for all investigations of the fetoplacental unit, the limited specificity and sensitivity made it particularly important that the results were assessed in an overall clinical situation.

In the only controlled trial of oestriol estimation in the literature, Duenhoelter *et al.* (1976) studied a population of women with a fetus considered at 'high risk'. They randomly allocated them to either a group in whom oestriol reports would be revealed to the clinician ($n = 315$) or to a group in whom they would remain concealed ($n = 307$), a total of 4678 samples being measured. There were no statistically significant differences between perinatal mortality rates, induction of labour rates, or Caesarean section rates between the revealed and concealed groups. Moreover, Chamberlain (1984) reported that in 1981 and 1982 his unit performed 4953 oestriol estimations with a perinatal mortality rate of 23.2 per 1000, whilst, after abandoning oestriol assays, the perinatal mortality rate in 1983 was 17.3 per 1000, suggesting no detriment to care.

A similar situation relates to the estimation of human placental lactogen (HPL) which has also failed to stand the test of time.

Table 17.5 The value of CTGs

Condition	Reactive CTG (n = 261)	%	Non-reactive CTG (n = 39)	%
Perinatal death	1	0.4	6	15.4
Fetal distress	19	7.3	7	17.9
Meconium	23	8.8	6	15.4
IUGR	22	8.4	14	35.9
Apgar < 6 at 5 min	3	1.1	6	15.4
Admission to Special Care Baby Unit	33	12.6	15	38.5

From Flynn and Kelly (1977)

Other biochemical assays were also used to assess fetal well-being, but none reached the popularity of the two detailed above and none became accepted into universal practice. These tests included hCG, placental proteins, oxytocinase, heat-stable alkaline phosphatase, and pregnanediol.

Cardiotocography

Antenatal cardiotocography (CTG) has been used to assess fetal well-being, traces being defined as either reactive, that is accelerations of the fetal heart with movement and good variability, or non-reactive (Flynn and Kelly 1977). The differences in significance between reactive and non-reactive traces may be illustrated by the data in Table 17.5.

In an attempt to determine the value of antenatal CTGs in clinical practice, there have been four randomly allocated clinical trials, but it is doubtful whether any of the trials have proved or disproved the place for antenatal cardiotocography (Thacker and Berkelman 1986). These four trials (Brown *et al.* 1982; Flynn *et al.* 1982; Kidd *et al.* 1985; Lumley *et al.* 1983) involved a total of 1579 patients and one of these series (Lumley *et al.* 1983) estimated that there would need to be over 3000 patients in a trial if any statistically significant difference in fetal outcome, based on perinatal mortality, was to be shown. Hence, even taken together, these trials were much too small. Oates *et al.* (1987) reported, in 9849 women monitored by antenatal cardiotocography, that the perinatal mortality rate (excluding fetal abnormality), should delivery occur within seven days of a normal CTG, was 3 per 1000, whereas the perinatal mortality rate should delivery occur within seven days of a late deceleration was 195 per 1000.

There are several areas for caution when interpreting an antenatal CTG. There is an association between gestational age and the likelihood of reactive tests. Thus Druzin *et al.* (1985), in a longitudinal study, assessed 593 cardiotocographs on 41 obstetric patients and demonstrated that between 28 and 32 weeks only 82 per cent of tests were reactive, whereas between 32 and 36 weeks 95 per cent of tests were reactive, and between 36 and 40 weeks 99 per cent were reactive. Secondly, a test should not be accepted as being non-reactive unless

Table 17.6 A scoring system for CTGs

	Score		
	0	1	2
Baseline FHR	< 100 or > 180	100–120 160–180	120–160 —
Movements + FHR changes	no movement —	present and no change	present and acceleration
Contractions + FHR changes	no contraction deceleration	present and no change	present and acceleration

From Pearson and Weaver (1978)

it has been carried out for long enough. Brown and Patrick (1981) reported that a non-reactive trace may ultimately become reactive if the tracing is continued for long enough. In a study of 1102 CTGs on 343 fetuses, 25 per cent were non-reactive over a 20-minute period, whereas only 5 per cent were non-reactive over a 40-minute period, and 1 per cent over an 80-minute period. Thus, the length of time for a CTG to be assessed as truly non-reactive should probably exceed one hour, whilst any degree of time, however small, shows a good correlation between good fetal condition at delivery and a reactive trace. Thirdly, there is an association between an abnormal antenatal cardiotocograph and a fetal abnormality. Powell-Phillips and Towell (1980) reported a series of 3140 patients with antenatal and intrapartum cardiotocography. Of these patients, some 37 (1.2 per cent) had a major life-threatening fetal abnormality and 19 of these fetuses (51 per cent) had an abnormal CTG. The commonest fetal abnormality was cardiac, found in 59 per cent of the 37 fetuses.

Lastly, the interpretation of a CTG will show greater variability between observers if the assessment is subjective rather than using a formal scoring system (Trimbos and Keirse 1978). Many authors divide CTGs into reactive or non-reactive depending upon the presence or absence of accelerations or decelerations of the fetal heart associated with fetal movements or uterine activity, together with an assessment of baseline variability. Other authors have produced a formal scoring system. Pearson and Weaver (1978) reported a maximum six point score (Table 17.6), they demonstrated that patients who scored five or six on a CTG within 24 hours of delivery delivered a healthy fetus, whilst 46 per cent of patients with a score of four or less delivered an acidotic infant based on either scalp pH or cord blood estimation.

Patients no longer need to attend hospital in order that a CTG may be performed. Domiciliary antenatal CTGs may be transmitted to a central location using the national telephone system. Dawson *et al.* (1988) reported 1121 domiciliary recordings from 72 women, with unsuccessful transmission occurring in a further 147 readings, 12 per cent of the total attempts. A further 1 per cent of traces were uninterpretable. James *et al.* (1988) reported 825 recordings from 268 women with a 7 per cent incidence of unsuccessful transmission and a similar 1 per cent incidence of non-interpretable traces.

Table 17.7 The value of stress testing

Non-stress test (n = 300)		Stress test (n = 278)	
Result	% Fetal morbidity	Result	% Fetal morbidity
Reactive (n = 271)	28	Negative (n = 219)	27
Equivocal (n = 18)	44	Equivocal (n = 42)	31
Non-reactive (n = 11)	55	Positive (n = 17)	65

From Pratt *et al.* (1979)

There may be some additional benefit to be gleaned from oxytocin challenge test (stress test) as opposed to the non-stress tests discussed above. Pratt *et al.* (1979) compared 1000 non-stress tests with 919 oxytocin challenge tests performed on 362 high-risk obstetric patients. When the last test before delivery was compared with fetal outcome for 300 non-stress tests and 278 stress tests, there was good correlation between the two tests (as shown in Table 17.7) for fetal morbidity (as defined as either fetal distress during labour), an Apgar score of less than six at five minutes, or birthweight below the 10th centile. Of patients with both a non-reactive non-stress test and a positive stress test, 83 per cent showed some fetal morbidity. Both tests show poor sensitivity (with high false-negative rates) when fetal morbidity is considered. Weingold *et al.* (1975) reported 375 oxytocin challenge tests in 154 patients. For the 132 patients with a negative test, 3 per cent had late decelerations during labour and there was a perinatal mortality rate of 9.2 per 1000. Of eight patients with a suspicious test, 13 per cent had late decelerations during labour and the perinatal mortality rate was 125 per 1000. For the 14 patients with positive tests, 57 per cent had late decelerations during labour and a perinatal mortality rate of 214 per 100. However, there were five reports of uterine hypertonus (1.3 per cent), one of these patients requiring an emergency Caesarean section. The risk of death after a normal stressed or non-stressed cardiotocograph was 0.7 per cent for the next seven days (Odendaal 1980).

It may be that the place of a stress-test is in the assessment of a non-reactive, non-stress test. Keane *et al.* (1981) reported a prospective study of 1328 non-stress tests and sequential stress tests in which the uterine contractions were either spontaneous or oxytocin-induced in 566 patients. Overall, correlation was good in that no reactive non-stress test was followed by a positive stress test, and all positive stress tests were preceded by a non-reactive, non-stress test. However, 25 per cent of non-reactive, non-stress tests were followed by positive stress tests. As can be seen from Table 17.8., a positive stress test was more closely associated with overall morbidity than was a non-reactive, non-stress test. Stress testing may also be initiated using nipple stimulation rather than an oxytocin infusion. Lenke and Nemes (1984) reported 1312 non-stress tests of which 323 in 194 patients were non-reactive. In the 323, 25 per cent became reactive during nipple stimulation, but 4 per cent of patients developed uterine

Table 17.8 The value of stress testing

Condition	Non-stress test		Stress test	
	Non-reactive (n = 107) (%)	Reactive (n = 459) (%)	Positive (n = 52) (%)	Negative (n = 514) (%)
Fetal distress	44.8	8.5	80.8	8.9
Low Apgar score	40.2	7.8	69.2	8.4
Perinatal death	2.8	1.3	3.8	1.3

From Keane *et al.* (1981)

hypertonus, 16 per cent developed a suspicious stress test, and 3 per cent developed decelerations of the fetal heart. Should a stress test be planned, however, it seems more logical to rely upon an oxytocin infusion.

Ultrasound assessment

Ultrasonic techniques may be of value in two ways, the first by offering a measurement of fetal size and the second by providing a more detailed assessment, termed the biophysical profile. In addition, ultrasound may provide further evidence for the absence of a fetal anomaly.

The value of different measurements of fetal size have already been discussed. Ultrasound measurement may also be used in order to predict birthweight in a given fetus. Using fetal abdominal circumference and area, Campogrande *et al.* (1977) were able to predict fetal birthweight, but could not predict birthweights using biparietal diameter or transverse thoracic diameter. Brown *et al.* (1987) reported upon the predictive value of ultrasonically determined variables in fetal weight prediction (see Table 17.9). The best, predictor of intrauterine growth retardation was abdominal circumference, predicting 96 per cent of growth-retarded infants, but falsely predicting IUGR in 40 per cent of normal growth infants. More sophisticated formulae, based upon measurements of head size, abdominal circumference, and fetal length may give a better estimate of fetal weight than those based on head and abdominal measurements alone (Hadlock *et al.* 1985), whilst total intrauterine volume has also been used (Geirsson *et al.* 1985).

In 1980, Manning *et al.* devised a score based upon the five biophysical variables of fetal breathing movements, fetal movements, fetal tone, qualitative liquor volume estimation, and a non-stress test. These parameters were measured weekly in 216 patients with a high-risk pregnancy; the relationship between the biophysical profile within a week of delivery and fetal outcome in terms of fetal distress and perinatal mortality rate is shown in Table 17.10. For any single test, whilst the false-negative rate is low, the false-positive rate is high. However, the false-positive rate is lower when all five variables are considered, making this combination a better predictor than any single variable.

Table 17.9 The ultrasonic prediction of birthweight

Variable	% of IUGR fetuses detected	% false-positive	% false-negative
Biparietal diameter	67	33	30
Femur length	45	55	3
Abdominal circumference	96	4	40
FL: AC ratio	57	43	25
Ponderal index	54	46	29
Estimated weight	63	37	4

From Brown *et al.* (1987)

Table 17.10 The value of biophysical scoring

Variable (overall, n = 216)		% With fetal distress (12.5%)	PMR (50.9 per 1000)
Amniotic Fluid Volume	normal	6.1	6.9
	decreased	28.8	89.8
Fetal Breathing Movement	present	8.0	10.5
	absent	47.6	192.5
Fetal Tone	present	7.5	12.2
	absent	33.3	133.6
Cardiotocograph	reactive	8.8	12.8
	non-reactive	23.4	97.5
Fetal Movement	present	9.0	15.3
	absent	47.0	190.0
All five variables	good	2.9	0
	poor	85.5	400.0

From Manning *et al.* (1980)

In 1985, Manning *et al.* reported 26 257 tests on 12 620 high-risk patients with an overall perinatal mortality rate of 7.37 per 100 (93 deaths). Only eight fetuses without fetal abnormality died within one week of a normal test result (score eight or more), giving a perinatal mortality rate of 0.6 per 1000. With a biophysical score of four, the perinatal mortality rate was 22.0, with a score of two it was 24.6, and with a score of zero the perinatal mortality rate was 187. There is good correlation between a poor biophysical score, especially with absent fetal breathing, and a non-reactive, non-stress test, and fetal hypoxia and acidosis based upon umbilical cord blood samples (Manning *et al.* 1993; Vintzileos *et al.* 1987).

It can now be concluded that ultrasound screening improves the diagnosis of growth retardation but there is little evidence that it has improved the outcome once abnormal fetuses have been excluded (Bucher and Schmidt 1993; Larsen

Table 17.11 The value of Doppler studies

Fetal outcome	SD ratio			CTG		CTG	
	No.	low	high	reactive	non-reactive	>7	<7
Normal fetal outcome	117	99	18	113	4	104	13
Abnormal fetal outcome	53	21	32	44	9	34	19
Birthweight < 10th centile	47	16	31	38	9	32	15
Birthweight < 5th centile	24	7	17	19	5	17	7
Apgar < 7 at 5 minutes	10	6	4	8	2	3	7

From Trudinger *et al.* (1986)

et al. 1992). Furthermore, a recent study has suggested that frequent ultrasound examination may itself be an aetiological factor for growth retardation (Newnham *et al.* 1993). The Newnham trial itself has been severely criticized in its methodology and until a further trial confirms or refutes the results they will have to be treated with some degree of caution (James and Twining 1993; Whittle 1993; Zimmermann *et al.* 1993).

Doppler studies

Doppler ultrasound studies are being used increasingly to assess the velocity of blood flow in the uterine arteries, the placental circulation, the umbilical vessels, and the fetal vessels. Although the velocity may be studied quantitatively, there is an advantage in the assessment of wave-form analysis instead in that this is independent of the angle of insonation or the vessel diameter. Uteroplacental blood flow is reduced in IUGR when compared to average sized fetuses (Nylund *et al.* 1983) regardless of whether a fetal abnormality coexists or not. Jouppila and Kirkinen (1984) demonstrated that umbilical vein blood flow velocity was below the 10th centile for the normal range in all of 11 patients with an ultrasonic diagnosis of IUGR during pregnancy, mainly due to constriction of the umbilical vein in the compromised fetus.

Doppler studies may be used to assess both the fetoplacental and the uteroplacental wave forms. Whilst either may be abnormal in the presence of a growth-retarded fetus, the umbilical artery wave form is more likely to be abnormal than is the uterine (Trudinger *et al.* 1985). In a study of 53 growth-retarded infants, 64 per cent had an abnormal umbilical artery wave form, whereas 36 per cent had an abnormal uterine artery wave form. The umbilical artery velocity wave form is characteristic and has been quantified by various ratios including the SD ratio, that is, the peak systolic to end-diastolic value. Trudinger *et al.* (1986) compared the sensitivities of the SD ratio from the umbilical artery wave form, cardiotocograph (divided into reactive and non-reactive), and 'scored' cardiotocographs in 170 patients of whom 47 showed IUGR. The results, shown in Table 17.11, demonstrated that an abnormal

Table 17.12 The value of Doppler studies

	End-diastolic wave frequency	
Characteristic	Absent	Present
Number	26	20
Birthweight (g)	1045	1465
Below 5th centile (%)	88	35
Apgar < 6 at 5 min (%)	27	5
NND (%)	27	5
NEC (%)	27	0
RDS (%)	42	25
IVH (%)	23	0

From Hackett et al. (1987)

umbilical artery wave form occurred in 32 out of 53 (60 per cent) of compromised fetuses compared with only 9 out of 53 (17 per cent) and 19 out of 53 (36 per cent) for the two classifications of cardiotocograph.

The knowledge of the Doppler study may also influence clinical decision making. Trudinger et al. (1987) also performed a randomized controlled trial of Doppler umbilical artery wave-form studies in 300 high-risk patients, 127 being allocated to a revealed group and 162 to a concealed group, with 11 patients lost. The elective delivery date was similar in both groups (66 per cent), although the emergency Caesarean section rate was higher in the control group than the revealed group, the authors suggested that this was because the knowledge of the wave form 'allows improved obstetric decision making'. Whilst this may or may not be true, it is unlikely to be demonstrated by a series of less than 300 patients, a sample size of 20 000 would be needed in order to detect any difference in, say, perinatal mortality.

Particular emphasis should be given to a Doppler umbilical artery study which demonstrates poor, absent, or even reversed end-diastolic flow, since there is a correlation between such a result and fetal hypoxia and acidosis (Nicolaides et al. 1988). The clinical significance of absent as opposed to present end-diastolic wave frequency was demonstrated by Hackett et al. (1987), the result being shown in Table 17.12. In the presence of absent end-diastolic flow, 88 per cent of fetuses were below the fifth centile for birthweight, whilst 27 per cent died during the perinatal period. Other authors quote a survival rate of only 50 per cent when end-diastolic flow is absent (Brar and Platt, 1988). The absence of end-diastolic velocity would appear to be an accurate test for hypoxia, with a sensitivity of 78 per cent and a specificity of 98 per cent (Tyrrell et al. 1989).

A Doppler examination of the umbilical arteries may be used as a screening test for both IUGR and fetal distress during labour (Pattinson et al. 1991). However, used in this situation, a single Doppler scan is not a good predictor of low birthweight (Sijmons *et al.* 1989) and is a less good predictor for IUGR than is a single fetal abdominal circumference measurement during the third trimester (Chambers *et al.* 1989).

It has also been suggested that a uterine (arcuate) artery Doppler wave-form study performed during the mid-trimester may be predictive of pre-eclampsia, IUGR, or fetal asphyxia (Campbell *et al.* 1986). In this study, 42 per cent of pregnancies with an abnormal mid-trimester study became associated with one of the above problems, whereas only 13 per cent of pregnancies in which the study was normal became affected. Steel *et al.* (1990) reported a larger study of 1014 nulliparous pregnant women in whom the uteroplacental circulation was screened by Doppler ultrasound at a mean of 18 weeks' gestation. Some 12 per cent had an abnormal wave form, of whom 25 per cent became hypertensive later in pregnancy, compared with 5 per cent of patients with a normal wave form. It is possible, therefore, that such screening may identify a high-risk group of pregnancy-related hypertension and may, therefore, allow prophylactic therapy to be commenced. However, not all authors quote similar results. Hanretty *et al.* (1989) came to an opposite conclusion in a study of 543 unselected women attending an antenatal clinic. There were no differences in the outcome of pregnancy between normal and abnormal uteroplacental wave forms in terms of hypertension, fetal distress, or the need for paediatric care after delivery. The mean birthweight, however, was lower in the group, with an abnormal artery wave form (3.03 kg) compared with those with a normal wave form (3.39 kg). Future studies will be needed in order to assess the value of mid-trimester screening by Doppler as a predictive test of later obstetric problems. The routine use of Doppler ultrasound in the screening of low risk pregnancies is unlikely to be of value (Davies *et al.* 1992; Mason *et al.* 1993).

The main use of Doppler ultrasound in current practice, therefore, is the assessment of a fetus believed to be at risk of compromise following an ultrasound study which suggests reduced fetal body measurements. The finding of an abnormal umbilical artery study in this situation is predictive of morbidity, whereas a normal Doppler study may result in some reassurance (Burke *et al.* 1990). The association between an abnormal fetal umbilical artery velocity and subsequent neonatal pathology has been confirmed by Trudinger *et al.* (1991). As shown in Table 17.13 a high SD ratio was associated with a 5 per cent perinatal loss and a 46 per cent incidence of birthweight below the fifth centile.

The velocity of blood flow through other fetal vessels, especially the common carotid artery, has been used to assess fetal compromise. In one recent series, 89 per cent of fetuses with an abnormal carotid artery pulsality index had evidence of asphyxia based upon umbilical venous blood samples obtained by cordocentesis (Bilardo *et al.* 1990).

It is likely that Doppler studies will, in the future, allow for a more detailed assessment of fetal well-being by the use of colour flow Doppler (*Lancet* 1992).

Table 17.13 Umbilical artery studies and neonatal outcome

	Normal (< 95th centile)	SD ratio in umbilical artery		
		Elevated (95–99th centile)	High (> 99th centile)	Absent
Number	1650	194	23	96
Stillbirth or neonatal death (%)	1.4	4	5	16
Birthweight < 5th centile (%)	10	23	46	72
Major fetal abnormality (%)	1.6	4.7	6.7	9.4

From Trudinger *et al.* (1991)

Fetal blood sampling

The technique of fetal blood sampling allows a direct but invasive method of assessing fetal well-being. In the context of IUGR, the indication for fetal blood sampling (other than to exclude a fetal genetic abnormality) is to assess the degree of fetal hypoxia in selected cases where the need for delivery is either in doubt or has to be balanced against prematurity (Nicolaides *et al.* 1986). The technique has been used to distinguish between acidotic and non-acidotic fetuses with evidence of asymmetrical growth retardation and an abnormal cardiotocograph, allowing delivery to be expedited when the fetus was acidotic but delayed when it was not (Pearce and Chamberlain 1987).

The association between fetal acidosis and other invasive tests for fetal well-being has been the subject of some assessment. Nicolini *et al.* (1990) reported the results of fetal blood sampling by cordocentesis in 58 growth-retarded fetuses. The mean pH and P_{O_2} were both lower in fetuses with absent umbilical artery end-diastolic flow and Doppler studies compared with those fetuses in whom end-diastolic flow was present. It is likely that as time progresses, other biochemical parameters will be described which will allow a more accurate assessment of the *in utero* risk of a growth-retarded preterm fetus. Should the fetus be of such a gestational age that delivery need not be too great a cause for concern, (beyond the 32nd week), then delivery is probably preferable to fetal blood sampling.

The management of the IUGR baby

The use of the above investigation should confirm that a fetus is small and allow for some assessment of its current condition. The course of action will then depend upon the evidence of compromise and the gestational age. The small fetus which is active, is surrounded by plenty of amniotic fluid, and as normal Doppler studies can usually be monitored satisfactorily by twice-weekly cardiotocography, weekly biophysical profiles and Doppler studies, and two-weekly ultrasonic fetal measurement studies, the obstetrician may elect for delivery at the 38th week, but there is no consensus as to the best time for delivery. The small fetus associated with a reduction in amniotic fluid and/or an abnormal Doppler study should be considered for delivery certainly if it has reached a gestational age of 32 weeks and probably beyond 30 weeks. The real management problem concerns the growth-retarded fetus before the 30th week of gestation. Outcome here is often unsatisfactory and attempts at prolonging the pregnancy may be worthwhile.

Numerous attempts have been made to improve fetal growth *in utero*, including physical methods, for example compression suits, and pharmacological methods, for example heparin. Recent interest relates to the possible benefits of low-dose aspirin, which has been tested both as a treatment in the presence of growth retardation and as a prophylaxis in patients in whom there is a high risk of growth retardation. A discussion discussing the safety of aspirin during pregnancy may be found in the chapter on pre-eclampsia (Chapter 24).

There has been a small randomized trial of aspirin in patients who have an elevated SD ratio on umbilical artery Doppler studies during the third trimester of pregnancy (Trudinger *et al.* 1988). In this trial the mean birthweight of babies born to the 14 women receiving 150 mg of aspirin per day was 2551 g compared with a mean birthweight of 2035 g for the 20 women receiving a placebo. Whether or not aspirin will really help re-establish growth seems relatively unlikely and a larger clinical trial will be needed in order to confirm or refute the above results.

There is a greater volume of evidence concerning the place of aspirin as a prophylactic agent in women who are considered to be high risk for the delivery of a growth-retarded infant. Earlier non-randomized studies suggested that women with a past history of delivering a growth-retarded infant were less likely to deliver a growth-retarded infant in a pregnancy during which they had taken low-dose aspirin compared with a similar group who took a placebo (Wallenberg and Rutmans 1987). However, the results from more recent and larger randomized trials are conflicting. McParland *et al.* (1990) reported a controlled trial of 100 nulliparous women with abnormal Doppler wave forms diagnosed at the 18th week of pregnancy. These patients were randomly allocated to receive either low-dose aspirin (75 mg per day $n = 48$ patients) or placebo ($n = 52$) for the remainder of the pregnancy. There were no statistical significant differences between the treated and the placebo group for the incidence of growth retardation, whether defined as birthweight below 2.5 kg or birthweight below the 5th centile for gestational age. However, Uzan *et al.* (1991) suggested that there was benefit from the use of prophylactic aspirin. In a randomized, double-blind, placebo-controlled trial, 229 women with a past history of delivering a growth-retarded infant received either placebo, or aspirin 150 mg per day, or aspirin 150 mg per day plus dipyridamole. As can be seen from Table 17.14, the mean birthweight of infants in the active treatment group was higher than that in the placebo group and the incidence of both stillbirth and abruptio placentae were reduced; there was no benefit from adding

Table 17.14 The prevention of IUGR

	No	Mean birthweight (g)	IUGR (%)	Stillborn (%)	Abruptio (%)
Placebo	73	2526	26	5	8
Active treatment	156	2751	13	1	5

From Uzan *et al.* (1991)

dipyridamole to the aspirin. There have now been two large recent studies which have assessed the value of low dose aspirin either as prevention against intrauterine growth retardation or in the treatment of growth retardation, compared with placebo. In neither of these larger studies was there any evidence of benefit compared with placebo (CLASP 1994; Italian Study of Aspirin in Pregnancy 1993).

The treatment of growth retardation *in utero* has yet to be described.

Conclusions

Intrauterine growth retardation is a major cause of morbidity, mortality, and intervention in obstetrics. Whilst there have been major advances in the diagnosis of growth retardation and in the assessment of the well-being of the growth-retarded fetus, delivery remains the only real treatment option.

If prevention is to take place, it will need to be commenced in early pregnancy since growth retardation is probably the result of a defect in maternotrophoblastic interaction at the time of placentation (Khong 1991).

References

Altman, D. G. and Hytten, F. E. (1989*a*). Intra-uterine growth retardation; let's be clear about it. *British Journal of Obstetrics and Gynaecology* **96**, 1127–32.

Altman, D. G. and Hytten, F. E. (1989*b*). Assessment of fetal size and fetal growth. In *Effective care in pregnancy and childbirth* (ed. I. Chalmers, M. Enkin, and M. J. N. C. Keirse), pp. 411–18. Oxford University Press, Oxford.

Bakketeig, L. S., Hoffman, H. J., and Harley, E. E. (1979). The tendency to repeat gestational age and birthweight in successive pregnancies. *American Journal of Obstetrics and Gynecology* **135**, 1086–103.

Beazley, J. M. and Underhill, R. A. (1970). Fallacy of the fundal height. *British Medical Journal* **4**, 404–6.

Belizan, J. M., Villar, J., Nardin, J. C., Malmud, J., and Vicuna, L. S. (1978). Diagnosis of intra-uterine growth retardation by a simple clinical method. *American Journal of Obstetrics and Gynecology* **131**, 643–6.

Bennett, M. J., Little, G., Dewhurst, C. J., and Chamberlain, G. (1982). Predictive value of ultrasound measurement in early pregnancy. *British Journal of Obstetrics and Gynaecology* **89**, 338–41.

Bilardo, C. M., Nicolaides, K. H., and Campbell, S. (1990). Doppler measurements of fetal and uteroplacental circulations. *American Journal of Obstetrics and Gynecology* **162**, 115–20.

Brar, H. S. and Platt, L. D. (1988). Reversed end-diastolic flow velocity on umbilical artery velocimetry in high-risk pregnancies. *American Journal of Obstetrics and Gynecology* **159**, 559–61.

Brown, H. L., Miller, I. M., Gabert, H. A., and Kissing, G. (1987). Ultrasound recognition of the small for gestational age fetus. *Obstetrics and Gynecology* **69**, 631–5.

Brown, R. and Patrick, J. (1981). The non-stress test: how long is long enough? *American Journal of Obstetrics and Gynecology* **141**, 646–51.

Brown, V. A., Sawers, R. S., Parsons, R. J., Duncan, S. L. B., and Cooke, I. D. (1982). The value of antenatal cardiotocography in the management of high-risk pregnancy. *British Journal of Obstetrics and Gynaecology* **89**, 716–22.

Bucher, H. C. and Schmidt, J. G. (1993). Does routine ultrasound scanning improve outcome in pregnancy? *British Medical Journal* **307**, 13–17.

Bucknell, E. W. C. and Wood, B. S. B. (1985). Wessex perinatal mortality study, 1982. *British Journal of Obstetrics and Gynaecology* **92**, 550–8.

Burke, G., Stuart, B., Crowley, S., Scanaill, S. N., and Drumm, J. (1990). Is intrauterine growth retardation with normal umbilical artery blood flow a benign condition? *British Medical Journal* **300**, 1044–5.

Calvert, J. P., Crean, E. E., Newcombe, R., and Pearson, J. F. (1982). Antenatal screening by measurement of symphyseal–fundal height. *British Medical Journal* **285**, 846–9.

Campbell, S. and Dewhurst, C. J. (1971). Diagnosis of the small for dates fetus by serial ultrasound cephalometry. *Lancet* **ii**, 1002–6.

Campbell, S. and Thoms, A. (1977). Ultrasound measurement of the fetal head to abdominal circumference ratio in the assessment of growth retardation. *British Journal of Obstetrics and Gynaecology* **84**, 165–74.

Campbell, S., Pearce, J. M. F., Hackett, G., Cohen-Overbeek, T., and Hernandez, C. (1986). Qualitative assessment of uteroplacental blood flow. *Obstetrics and Gynecology* **68**, 649–53.

Campogra* nde, M., Todros, T., and Brizolara, M. (1977). Prediction of birthweight by ultrasound measurement of the fetus. *British Journal of Obstetrics and Gynaecology* **84**, 175–8.

Chamberlain, G. V. P. (1984). An end of antenatal oestrogen monitoring? *Lancet* **ii**, 1171–2.

Chambers, S. E., Hoskins, P. R., Haddad, N. G., Johnstone, F. D., McDicken, W. N., and Muir, B. B. (1989). A comparison of fetal abdominal circumference measurement and Doppler ultrasound in the prediciton of small for dates babies and fetal compromise. *British Journal of Obstetrics and Gynaecology* **96**, 803–8.

Chiswick, M. L. (1985). Intra-uterine growth retardation. *British Medical Journal* **291**, 845–8.

CLASP (1994). A randomized trial of low dose aspirin for the prevention and treatment of pre-eclampsia. *Lancet* **343**, 619–29.

Davies, J. A., Gallivan, S., and Spencer, J. A. D. (1992). Randomized controlled trial of Doppler ultrasound screening of placental perfusion during pregnancy. *Lancet* **340**, 1299–303.

Dawes, M. G. and Grudzinskas, J. G. (1991). Repeated measurement of maternal weight during pregnancy. Is this a useful practice? *British Journal of Obstetrics and Gynaecology* **98**, 189–94.

Dawes, M. G., Green, J., and Ashurst, H. (1992). Routine weighing in pregnancy. *British Medical Journal* **304**, 487-9.

Dawson, A. J., Middlemiss, C., Jones, E. J., and Gough, N. A. J. (1988). Fetal heart monitoring by telephone. *British Journal of Obstetrics and Gynaecology* **95**, 1018-23.

Dickey, R. P., Grannis, G. F., Hanson, F. W., Schumacher, A., and Ma, S. (1972). Use of oestrogen–creatinine ratio and oestrogen index for screening of normal and high-risk pregnancy. *American Journal of Obstetrics and Gynecology* **113**, 880-6.

Dobson, P. C., Abell, D. A., and Beischer, N. A. (1981). Mortality and morbidity of fetal growth retardation. *Australian and New Zealand Journal of Obstetrics and Gynaecology* **21**, 69-76.

Dobson, P. C., Abell, D. A., and Beischer, N. A. (1982). Antenatal pregnancy complications and fetal growth retardation. *Australian and New Zealand Journal of Obstetrics and Gynaecology* **22**, 203-5.

Druzin, M. L., Fox, A., Cogut, E., and Carlson, C. (1985). The relationship of the non-stress test to gestational age. *American Journal of Obstetrics and Gynecology* **153**, 386-9.

Duenhoelter, J. H., Whalley, P. J., and MacDonald, P. C. (1976). An analysis of the utility of plasma immunoreactive oestrogen measurements in determining delivery time of gravidas with a fetus considered at high risk. *American Journal of Obstetrics and Gynecology* **125**, 889-98.

Ewigman, D., Le Fevre, M., and Hesser, J. (1990). A randomized trial of routine prenatal ultrasound. *Obstetrics and Gynecology* **76**, 189-94.

Fancourt, R., Campbell, S., Harvey, D., and Norman, A. P. (1976). Follow-up study of small for dates babies. *British Medical Journal* **1**, 1435-7.

Fitzhardinge, P. M. and Steven, E. M. (1972). The small for dates infant. *Pediatrics* **50**, 50-7.

Flynn, A. M. and Kelly, J. (1977). Evaluation of fetal well-being by antepartum cardiotocography. *British Medical Journal* **1**, 936-9.

Flynn, A. M., Kelly, J., Mansfield, H., Needham, P., O'Connor, M., and Viegas, O. (1982). A randomized controlled trial of non-stress antepartum cardiotocography. *British Journal of Obstetrics and Gynaecology* **89**, 427-33.

Galbraith, R. S., Karchmar, E. J., Piercy, W. N., and Low, J. A. (1979). The clinical prediction of intra-uterine growth retardation. *American Journal of Obstetrics and Gynecology* **133**, 281-6.

Geirsson, R. T., Patel, M. B., and Christie, A. D. (1985). Efficacy of intra-uterine volume, fetal abdominal area, and biparietal diameter measurements with ultrasound in screening for small-for-dates babies. *British Journal of Obstetrics and Gynaecology* **92**, 929-35.

Grant, A., Elbourne, D., Valentine, L., and Alexander, S. (1989). Routine formal fetal movement counting and risk of antepartum late death in normally formed singletons. *Lancet* **ii**, 345-9.

Hackett, G. A., Campbell, S., Gamsu, H., Cohen-Overbeek, T., and Pearce, J. M. F. (1987). Doppler studies in the growth retarded fetus and prediction of neonatal morbidity. *British Medical Journal* **294**, 13-16.

Hadlock, F. P., Harris, T. R. B., Sharmar, R. S., Deter, R. L., and Park, S. K. (1985). Estimation of fetal weight with the use of head, body, and femur measurements. *American Journal of Obstetrics and Gynecology* **151**, 33-7.

Hall, M., Chng, P. K., and MacGillivray, I. (1980). Is routine antenatal care worthwhile? *Lancet* **ii**, 78-80.

Hanretty, K. P., Primrose, M. H., Neilson, J. P., and Whittle, J. (1989). Pregnancy screening by Doppler uteroplacental and umbilical artery wave forms. *British Journal of Obstetrics and Gynaecology* **96**, 1163–7.

Hepburn, M. and Rosenberg, K. (1986). An audit of the detection and management of small for gestational age babies. *British Journal of Obstetrics and Gynaecology* **93**, 212–16.

Italian Study of Aspirin in Pregnancy (1993). Low dose aspirin in the prevention and treatment of intra-uterine growth retardation and pregnancy-induced hypertension. *Lancet* **341**, 396–400.

James, D. and Twining, P. (1993). Effects of frequent ultrasound during pregnancy. *Lancet* **342**, 1359.

James, D., Peralta, B., Porter, S., Darvill, D., Walker, J., McCall, M., *et al.* (1988). Fetal heart rate monitoring by telephone. *British Journal of Obstetrics and Gynaecology* **95**, 1024–9.

Jarvis, G. J. and MacDonald, H. N. (1979). Fetal movements in small for dates babies. *British Journal of Obstetrics and Gynaecology* **86**, 724–7.

Johnson, T. R. B., Jordan, E., and Laine, L. L. (1990). Doppler recording of fetal movement. *Obstetrics and Gynaecology* **76**, 42–3.

Jouppila, P. and Kirkinen, P. (1984). Umbilical vein blood flow as an indicator of fetal hypoxia. *British Journal of Obstetrics and Gynaecology* **91**, 107–10.

Keane, M. W. D., Horger, E. O., and Vice, L. (1981). Comparative study of stressed and non-stressed antepartum fetal heart rate tracing. *Obstetrics and Gynecology* **57**, 320–4.

Khong, T. Y. (1991). The Robertson–Brosens–Dixon hypothesis. *British Journal of Obstetrics and Gynaecology* **98**, 1195–9.

Khong, T. Y., De Wolf, F., Robertson, W. B., and Brosens, I. (1986). Inadequate maternal vascular response to placentation in pregnancies complicated by pre-eclampsia and by small-for-gestational-age infants. *British Journal of Obstetrics and Gynaecology* **93**, 1049–59.

Kidd, L. C., Patel, N. B., and Smith, R. (1985). Non-stress antenatal cardiotocography. *British Journal of Obstetrics and Gynaecology* **92**, 1156–9.

Kleinman, J. C. and Madans, J. H. (1985). The effects of maternal smoking, physical stature, and educational attainment on the incidence of low birthweight. *American Journal of Epidemiology* **121**, 843–5.

Lancet (1992). Doppler ultrasound in obstetrics. *Lancet* **339**, 1083–4.

Larsen, T., Larsen, J. F., Petersen, S., and Greisen, G. (1992). Detection of small for gestational age fetuses by ultrasound screening in a high risk population. *British Journal of Obstetrics and Gynaecology* **99**, 469–74.

Lenke, R. R. and Nemes, J. M. (1984). Use of nipple stimulation to obtain contraction stress test. *Obstetrics and Gynecology* **63**, 345–8.

Lindhard, A., Neilsen, P. V., Mouritsen, L. A., Zackariassen, A., Sorensen, H. U., and Roseno, H. (1990). The implications of introducing the symphyseal–fundal height measurement. *British Journal of Obstetrics and Gynaecology* **97**, 675–80.

Loeffler, F. F. (1967). Clinical fetal weight prediction. *Journal of Obstetrics and Gynaecology of the British Commonwealth* **74**, 675–7.

Lumley, J., Lester, A., Anderson, I., Renou, P., and Wood, C. (1983). A randomized trial of weekly cardiotocography in high-risk obstetric patients. *British Journal of Obstetrics and Gynaecology* **90**, 1018–26.

Macafee, C. A. J., Beischer, N. A., Brown, J. B., and Fortune, D. W. (1972). Fetoplacental function and antenatal complications when the fetus is malformed. *Australian and New Zealand Journal of Obstetrics and Gynaecology* **12**, 71–85.

McIlwaine, G. M., Howat, R. C. L., Dunn, F., MacNaughton, M. C. (1979). The Scottish perinatal mortality survey. *British Medical Journal* **2**, 1103–6.

McParland, P., Pearce, J. M., and Chamberlain, G. V. P. (1990). Doppler ultrasound and aspirin in recognition and prevention of pregnancy-induced hypertension. *Lancet* **i**, 1552-5.

Manning, F. A., Platt, T. D., and Sipos, L. (1980). Antepartum fetal evaluation: development of a fetal biophysical profile. *American Journal of Obstetrics and Gynecology* **136**, 787-95.

Manning, F. A., Morrison, I., Lange, I. R., Harman, C. R., and Chamberlain, P. F. (1985). Fetal assessment based on fetal biophysical profile scoring. *American Journal of Obstetrics and Gynecology* **151**, 343-50.

Mason, G. C., Lilford, R. J., Porter, J., Nelson, E., and Tyrell, S. (1993). Randomized comparison of routine versus highly selective use of Doppler ultrasound in low risk pregnancies. *British Journal of Obstetrics and Gynaecology* **100**, 130-3.

Mathai, M., Jairaj, P., and Muthurathnam, S. (1987). Screening for light for gestational age infant. *British Journal of Obstetrics and Gynaecology* **94**, 217-21.

Neilson, J. P., Whitfield, C. R., and Aitchison, T. C. (1980). Screening for the small for dates fetus. *British Medical Journal* **280**, 1203-6.

Neilson, J. P., Munjanja, S. P., and Whitfield, C. R. (1984). Screening for small for dates fetuses. *British Medical Journal* **289**, 1179-82.

Newnham, J. P., Evans, S. F., Michael, C. A., Stanley, F. J., and Landau, L. I. (1993). Effects of frequent ultrasound during pregnancy. *Lancet* **342**, 887-91.

Nicolaides, K. H., Soothill, P. W., Rodeck, C. H., and Campbell, S. (1986). Ultrasound-guided sampling of umbilical cord and placental blood to assess fetal well-being. *Lancet* **i**, 1065-7.

Nicolaides, K. H., Billardo, C. M., Soothill, P. W., and Campbell, S. (1988). Absence of end-diastolic frequencies in umbilical artery: a sign of fetal hypoxia and acidosis. *British Medical Journal* **297**, 1026-7.

Nicolini, U., Nicolaides, K. H., Fisk, N. M., Vaughan, J. I., Fusi, L., Gleeson, R., *et al.* (1990). Limited role of fetal blood sampling in prediction of the outcome of intra-uterine growth retardation. *Lancet* **336**, 768-72.

Niswander, K. and Jackson, E. C. (1974). Physical characteristics of the gravida and their association with birthweight and perinatal death. *American Journal of Obstetrics and Gynecology* **119**, 306-13.

Nylund, L., Lunell, N. O., Lewander, R., and Sarby, B. (1983). Uteroplacental blood flow index in intra-uterine growth retardation of fetal or maternal origin. *British Journal of Obstetrics and Gynaecology* **90**, 16-20.

Oates, J. N., Shew, F. T. K., and Latten, V. J. (1987). Antepartum cardiotocography — an audit. *Australian and New Zealand Journal of Obstetrics and Gynaecology* **27**, 82-6.

Odendaal, H. J. (1980). Intra-uterine death after suspicious, uncertain, and normal antenatal fetal heart rate monitoring. *South African Medical Journal* **57**, 904-8.

Ounsted, M., Moar, V. A., and Scott, A. (1985). Risk factors associated with small for dates and large for dates infants. *British Journal of Obstetrics and Gynaecology* **92**, 226-32.

Pattinson, R., Dawes, G., Jennings, J., and Redman, C. (1991). Umbilical artery resistance index as a screening test for fetal wellbeing. *Obstetrics and Gynaecology* **78**, 353-8.

Pearce, J. M. and Chamberlain, G. V. P. (1987). Ultrasonically guided percutaneous umbilical blood sampling in the management of intra-uterine growth retardation. *British Journal of Obstetrics and Gynaecology* **94**, 318-21.

Pearson, J. F. and Weaver, J. B. (1976). Fetal activity and fetal well-being. *British Medical Journal* **1**, 1305-7.

Pearson, J. F. and Weaver, J. B. (1978). A six-point scoring system for antenatal cardiotocographs. *British Journal of Obstetrics and Gynaecology* **85**, 321–7.

Persson, B., Stangerberg, M., Lunell, N. O., Brodin, U., Holmberg, N. G., and Vaclavinkov, A. V. (1986). Prediction of size of infants at birth by measurement of symphyseal–fundal height. *British Journal of Obstetrics and Gynaecology* **93**, 206–11.

Powell-Phillips, W. D. and Towell, M. E. (1980). Abnormal fetal heart associated with congenital abnormalities. *British Journal of Obstetrics and Gynaecology* **87**, 270–4.

Pratt, D., Diamond, F., Yen, H., Bieniarz, J., and Burd, L. (1979). Fetal stress and non-stress tests. *Obstetrics and Gynecology* **54**, 419–23.

Quaranta, P., Currell, R., and Robinson, J. S. (1981). Prediction for small for dates infants by measurement of symphyseal–fundus height. *British Journal of Obstetrics and Gynaecology* **88**, 115–19.

Rosenberg, K., Grant, J. M., Tweedle, I., Aitchinson, T., and Gallagher, F. (1982). Measurement of fundal height as a screening test for fetal growth retardation. *British Journal of Obstetrics and Gynaecology* **89**, 447–50.

Sadovsky, E. and Yaffe, H. (1973). Daily fetal movement recording and fetal prognosis. *Obstetrics and Gynecology* **41**, 845–50.

Sheppard, B. L. and Bonnar, J. (1981). An ultrastructural study of uteroplacental spiral arteries in hypertensive and normotensive pregnancies and fetal growth retardation. *British Journal of Obstetrics and Gynaecology* **88**, 695–705.

Sijmons, E. A., Reviver, P. J. H. M., Beck, E. V., and Bruinse, H. W. (1989). The validity of screening for small for gestational age and low-weight-for-birth infants by Doppler ultrasound. *British Journal of Obstetrics and Gynaecology* **96**, 557–61.

Simpson, J. W., Lawless, R. W., and Mitchell, A. C. (1975). Responsibilities of the obstetrician to the fetus. *Obstetrics and Gynecology* **45**, 481–7.

Steel, S., Pearce, J. M., McParland, P., and Chamberlain, G. V. P. (1990). Early Doppler ultrasound screening in prediction of hypertensive disorders of pregnancy. *Lancet* **335**, 1548–51.

Thacker, S. B. and Berkelman, R. L. (1986). Assessing the diagnostic accuracy and efficacy of selected antepartum fetal surveillance techniques. *Obstetrics and Gynecological Survey* **41**, 121–41.

Thompson, A. M., Billewicz, W. Z., and Hytten, F. E. (1968). The assessment of fetal growth. *Journal of Obstetrics and Gynaecology of the British Commonwealth* **75**, 903–16.

Trimbos, J. B. and Keirse, M. J. N. C. (1978). Observer variability in assessment of antepartum cardiotocographs. *British Journal of Obstetrics and Gynaecology* **85**, 900–6.

Trudinger, B. J., Giles, W. B., and Cook, C. M. (1985). Flow velocity wave forms in the maternal uteroplacental and fetal umbilical placental circulations. *American Journal of Obstetrics and Gynecology* **152**, 155–63.

Trudinger, B. J., Cook, C. M., Jones, L., and Giles, W. B. (1986). A comparison of fetal heart rate monitoring and umbilical artery wave forms in the recognition of fetal compromise. *British Journal of Obstetrics and Gynaecology* **93**, 171–5.

Trudinger, B., Cook, C. M., Giles, W. B., Connelly, A., and Thompson, R. S. (1987). Umbilical artery flow velocity wave forms in high-risk pregnancy. *Lancet* **i**, 188–90.

Trudinger, B. J., Cook, C. M., Thompson, R. S., Giles, W. B., Connelly, A. (1988). Low–high dose aspirin therapy improves fetal weight in umbilical placental insufficiency. *American Journal of Obstetrics and Gynecology* **159**, 681–5.

Trudinger, B. J., Cook, C. M., Giles, W. B., Ng, S., Fong, E., Connelly, A., *et al.* (1991). Fetal umbilical artery velocity wave-form and subsequent neonatal outcome. *British Journal of Obstetrics and Gynaecology* **98**, 378–84.

Tyrrell, S., Obain, A. L., and Lilford, R. J. (1989). Umbilical artery Doppler velocimetry as a predictor of fetal hypoxia and acidosis at birth. *Obstetrics and Gynecology* **74**, 332–6.

Uzan, S., Beaufils, M., Breart, G., Bazin, B., Capitan, T. C., and Paris, J. (1991). Prevention of fetal growth retardation with low dose aspirin. *Lancet* **337**, 1427–31.

Villar, J. and Belizan, J. M. (1986). The evaluation of methods used in the diagnosis of intra-uterine growth retardation. *Obstetric and Gynecological Survey* **41**, 187–99.

Vintzileos, A. M., Gaffney, S. E., Selinger, L. M., Kontopoulous, V. G., Campbell, W. A., and Nochimson, D. J. (1987). The relationships among the fetal biophysical profile, umbilical cord pH, and Apgar scores. *American Journal of Obstetrics and Gynecology* **157**, 627–31.

Wallenburg, H. C. S. and Rutmans, N. (1987). Prevention of recurrent idiopathic fetal growth retardation by low-dose aspirin and dypyridamole. *American Journal of Obstetrics and Gynecology* **157**, 1203–5.

Weingold, A. D., De Jesus, T. P. S., and O'Keiffe, J. (1975). Oxytocin challenge test. *American Journal of Obstetrics and Gynecology* **123**, 466–72.

Wen, S. W., Goldenberg, R. L., Cutter, G. R., Hoffman, H. J., and Cliver, S. P. (1990). Intra-uterine growth retardation and preterm delivery: prenatal risk factors in an indigent population. *American Journal of Obstetrics and Gynecology* **162**, 213–18.

Whittle, M. (1991). Antenatal assessment of intra-uterine growth retardation. *British Journal of Hospital Medicine* **46**, 42–5.

Whittle, M. J. (1993). Effects of frequent ultrasound during pregnancy. *Lancet* **342**, 1359.

Zimmermann, R., Hebisch, G., Huch, R., and Huch, A. (1993). Effects of frequent ultrasound during pregnancy. *Lancet* **342**, 1359.

18   The management of labour

This chapter deals with two major areas of debate concerning the first stage of labour. The first relates to the assessment of fetal well-being during labour; the second relates to the practice of acceleration of labour. A third area of debate, which relates to a critical assessment of common procedures performed during labour will be discussed in Chapter 26 (Natural childbirth).

Fetal monitoring during labour

The traditional method for assessment of fetal well-being during labour is a combination of intermittent auscultation of the fetal heart and observation for the presence of meconium in the liquor. Walker (1959) reported that fetal distress, as judged by fetal heart abnormalities on auscultation and/or the passage of thick meconium in the liquor, occurred in 5.5 per cent of 12 000 labours but, when nature was allowed to take its course, only 4.5 per cent of these babies died during or after delivery.

The ability to assess fetal well-being during labour, with accuracy, has become increasingly important in recent years. The specialty of obstetrics, both in the UK and in the USA, has been associated with some of the largest claims for professional malpractice, and many of these claims have concerned fetal monitoring during labour.

Meconium staining of the liquor

Meconium staining of the liquor is not uncommon, occurring in 6–10 per cent of labours (Barrett *et al*. 1992; Fujikura and Klionsky 1975; Matthews and Martin 1974).

The aetiology and consequences of the passage of meconium during labour warrant discussion.

The correlation between the presence of meconium and delivery of a baby asphyxiated at birth is poor. Whilst intrapartum death due to asphyxia may occur more commonly in the presence of meconium staining of the liquor than in its absence, asphyxia and death may still occur in the presence of clear liquor (Fujikura and Klionsky 1975: Matthews and Martin 1974). However, there is a correlation between the degree of meconium staining of the liquor and condition at birth. Thus, Meis *et al*. (1978) reported a low 5-minute Apgar score in 2 per cent of labours associated with 'light meconium' but in 6 per cent of labours associated with 'heavy meconium'. This observation was confirmed in another study in which it was found that thick meconium was more likely to

Table 18.1 The passage of meconium

Umbilical artery pH	% Of labours with clear liquor	% Of labours with meconium
< 7.2	18	31
< 7.15	5	11

From Yeomans *et al.* (1989)

be associated with an abnormal cardiotocograph than was thin meconium or clear liquor (Starks 1980). Thick meconium is usually a sign of oligohydramnios which, in itself, is related to an increased risk for the development of fetal distress (Boylan 1991).

The evidence for a correlation between meconium and fetal acidosis in scalp or umbilical artery blood is poor (Starks 1980; Yeomans *et al.* 1989). Although, as can be seen in Table 18.1, fetal acidosis is more likely to be associated with the presence of meconium, however, the absence of meconium cannot be taken to indicate an uncompromised fetus (Yeomans *et al.* 1989).

The presence of meconium during labour may enable the obstetrician to anticipate the complication of meconium aspiration syndrome (Nathan *et al.* 1994). In a survey of over 38 000 births, the incidence of this syndrome was 0.2 per cent and, when it occurred, was associated with a mortality rate of 8 per cent (Coltart *et al.* 1989). The syndrome is particularly associated with pregnancies continuing beyond the 42nd week of gestation (Meis *et al.* 1978).

The presence of meconium staining of the liquor should, therefore, constitute an indication for fetal monitoring by continuous cardiotocography (Starks 1980: Yeomans *et al.* 1989).

The case for and against continuous fetal heart monitoring

Intermittent fetal heart monitoring is a relatively poor predictor of fetal well-being. Wood and Pinkerton (1961) reported that fetal heart abnormalities on auscultation were noted in only 60 per cent of 30 intrapartum anoxic stillbirths. Moreover, a low fetal scalp pH in the presence of an abnormal cardiotocograph during labour occurred in 7 per cent of complicated pregnancies and 5 per cent of uncomplicated ones, which was taken to indicate that selective monitoring was inappropriate and that all labours should be monitored (Edington *et al.* 1975). The introduction of continuous fetal heart rate monitoring during labour was accompanied by a fall in the perinatal mortality rate. Thus, Edington *et al.* (1975) reported that, in the two-year period before the introduction of widespread continuous fetal heart rate monitoring in their unit, the perinatal mortality rate was 29.3 per 1000, whereas the following year, when 85 per cent of patients were monitored, the perinatal mortality rate was 15.8 per 1000, and in the year after that, when 92 per cent of patients were monitored, the perinatal mortality rate dropped to 11.7 per 1000. Other authors have found a similar effect. Thus, Paul and Hon (1974) reported, in a non-random retrospective

Table 18.2 The significance of CTG changes

CTG	No.	Mean fetal scalp pH	Mean 1 min Apgar score	% with pH ⩽ 7.25
Normal	68	7.34	7.8	1.5
Accelerations	20	7.34	8.0	0
Early decelerations	25	7.33	8.2	8
Baseline bradycardia (uncomplicated)	34	7.33	8.4	3
Baseline tachycardia (uncomplicated)	43	7.31	8.1	14
Variable deceleration—normal baseline	30	7.31	8.5	10
Variable deceleration—abnormal baseline	23	7.22	6.2	61
Loss of beat-to-beat variation (uncomplicated)	15	7.30	8.0	20
Loss of beat-to-beat variation (complicated)	19	7.24	6.2	42
Late decelerations—normal baseline	2	7.28	4.0	0

From Beard *et al.* (1971)

series, that the intrapartum death rate was 4.4 per 1000 in 21 525 unmonitored 'low risk' labours compared with 1.3 per 1000 in 6750 'high risk' monitored labours, and concluded that 'fetal monitoring is of benefit in decreasing intrapartum fetal deaths'.

However, not all authors have reported such a result, and the association between widespread monitoring and a decrease in perinatal mortality rate has been questioned. Chalmers *et al.* (1976) reviewed the pregnancy outcome in almost 40 000 pregnancies in Wales and were unable to show any alteration in perinatal mortality related to the introduction of fetal monitoring, the induction of labour, or antenatal monitoring.

The significance of intrapartum fetal heart rate patterns obtained with electronic cardiotocography was originally reported in high-risk pregnancies. Beard *et al.* (1971) related data on continuous electronic fetal heart rate changes to fetal blood pH in 279 labours and found that not all deviations from the normal carried the same significance. A pattern of variable decelerations from an abnormalbaseline had the highest incidence of fetal acidosis, namely 61 per cent (Table 18.2). In addition to their descriptions should be added 'end-stage deceleration' and 'sinusoidal' fetal heart rate patterns. End-stage decelerations are deep and sustained episodes of fetal bradycardia occurring during the second stage of labour. Some 11 per cent of fetuses delivered after an end-stage deceleration of ten or more minutes were acidotic (Katz *et al.* 1982). Sinusoidal fetal heart rate patterns occur in up to 2 per cent of labours (Murphy *et al.*

1991). Such sinusoidal patterns, defined as undulating wave forms associated with loss of beat-to-beat variability, may be classified as minor (an amplitude of acceleration of less than 25 beats per minute) and major (amplitude of acceleration greater than 25 beats per minute). Minor sinusoidal fetal heart rate patterns are not considered to be of particular significance, but major patterns may relate to fetal anaemia (either associated with rhesus isoimmunization or placental abruption), and, in one series, 67 per cent of fetuses with a major sinusoidal fetal heart rate pattern died before, during, or after delivery (Katz *et al.* 1983). Pseudosinusoidal patterns, defined as undulating wave forms with episodes of normal baseline variability or reactivity, may be found in up to 15 per cent of labours and are associated with analgesia (both opiate and epidural) and tend to be associated with a normal fetal outcome (Murphy *et al.* 1991).

The variation in interpretation of cardiotocographs, both inter-and intra-observer, is a matter for concern. Nielson *et al.* (1987) asked experienced obstetricians to evaluate 55 cardiotocographs on two occasions, the assessment being a comparison between each cardiotocograph and a clinical outcome. Agreement between observers varied from 50 to 60 per cent, but only 11 of the cardiotocographs (20 per cent) were assessed the same way twice by all four obstetricians.

Trials of cardiotocograph in labour

There have now been several trials of continuous electronic fetal heart rate monitoring during labour. The early, small, randomized trials were contradictory, some failing to show any benefit (Haverkamp *et al.* 1976; Kelso *et al.* 1978; Wood *et al.* 1981), whilst others showed a benefit (Renou *et al.* 1976). Haverkamp *et al.* (1976), in Denver, performed a prospective randomized study of 483 high-risk patients in which the continuous electronic heart rate monitoring record was revealed in 242 and concealed in 241. There were no differences in outcome as judged by intrapartum deaths (none in either group), neonatal deaths, Apgar scores, cord blood gases, or neonatal morbidity. Kelso *et al.* (1978), in Sheffield, admitted 504 low-risk patients to a prospective randomized trial in which 253 had continuous electronic fetal heart rate monitoring and 251 had intermittent auscultation. Again, there were no differences in the cord blood gases, Apgar scores, admission rates to the neonatal unit, neonatal deaths, or in the abnormal neurological behaviour of the neonates. Wood *et al.* (1981) also failed to demonstrate any difference between Apgar scores and abnormal neurological signs after labours where either continuous electronic fetal heart rate monitoring or intermittent auscultation had been employed. Renou *et al.* (1976), in Melbourne, allocated 350 high-risk patients to a randomized trial of continuous electronic fetal heart rate monitoring and auscultation. There were no intrapartum deaths in either group and no differences in neonatal death rate, but there was a significantly higher rate of abnormal neurological behaviour (convulsions) in neonates in the auscultation group (0.5 per cent) compared with the electronically monitored group (0 per cent).

Although three of these four trials failed to show any obvious benefit from continuous cardiotocography, it is possible that none of them were of sufficient size. The *British Medical Journal* (1976) stated that 'possibly 5000 patients' would be needed in any trial of intrapartum cardiotocography, whilst MacDonald *et al.* (1985) estimated that, in order to show differences in an intrapartum death rate of 1 per 1000, a neonatal death rate of 2 per 1000, and a neonatal seizure rate in the survivors of 3 per 1000, a trial of 10 000 women would be required to have an 80 per cent chance of observing a statistically significant difference at the 5 per cent level.

There have now been three large trials of continuous electronic fetal heart rate monitoring (Leveno *et al.* 1986; Luthy *et al.* 1987; MacDonald *et al.* 1985). Leveno *et al.* (1986) reported a prospective trial of over 20 000 monitored labours comparing selective with universal monitoring. There were no statistically significant differences in the intrapartum stillbirth rates, neonatal death rates, or the incidence of neonatal seizures between the two groups. Luthy *et al.* (1987) reported a randomized, multicentre trial of continuous electronic fetal heart rate monitoring in 246 *preterm* singleton labours. Again, there were no significant differences in outcome between the two groups. MacDonald *et al.* (1985) reported the Dublin trial of fetal monitoring in which 12 964 patients were randomly allocated to either continuous electronic fetal heart rate monitoring or intermittent auscultation. The perinatal mortality rates, the incidence of low Apgar scores, the need for resuscitation, and incidence of admission to the neonatal unit were similar in the two groups (Table 18.3). Meta-analysis of all trials has not shown any benefit from continuous monitoring of the fetus (Grant 1989).

However, the Dublin trial (MacDonald *et al.* 1985) showed that electronic fetal heart rate monitoring reduced the incidence of abnormal neonatal neurological behaviour. They reported that the incidence of neonatal seizures in the intermittent auscultation group was more than double that in the continuous electronic fetal heart rate monitoring group, 27 babies in the intermittent auscultation group having neonatal seizures compared with 12 from the electronic monitoring group. However, this difference was not found to be of clinical significance. Grant *et al.* (1989) identified the children with cerebral palsy who had, or had not, participated in the Dublin trial of fetal monitoring (MacDonald *et al.* 1985). At the age of 4 years, the incidence of cerebral palsy was the same in each group (3.4 per 1000 children) suggesting that continuous monitoring, as opposed to intermittent auscultation, during labour had no protective effect against subsequent cerebral palsy. Similarly, Shy *et al.* (1990) reassessed, at the age of 18 months, the preterm infants from the study of Luthy *et al.* (1987). There were no differences in neurological development between those children who had undergone continuous as opposed to periodic monitoring. In fact, there was a higher incidence of cerebral palsy in the continuously monitored group (20 per cent of 93 children) as compared with the intermittently

Table 18.3 The value of continuous monitoring

Mate	Electronic monitoring	Intermittent auscultation
Perinatal deaths	14	14
Intrapartum stillbirth	3	2
Neonatal deaths	11	12
Caesarean sections	2.4%	2.2%
Intubated	1.2%	1.1%
Apgar < 3 at 5 minutes	0.2%	0.1%
Admission to special care nursery	8.4%	8.3%
Umbilical vein pH— < 7.05	0.4%	0.4%
— < 7.20	8.6%	9.6%
Neonatal seizures	12	27
Relative risk	0.45	1.0
Survivors	9	21.0
Severe neurological disability at one year	3	3
Other cerebral palsy of children	8	7

From MacDonald *et al.* (1985) (The Dublin Trial)

auscultated group (8 per cent of 96 children). It seems unlikely, therefore, that continuous electronic fetal heart rate monitoring results in an improvement in the neonatal or post-neonatal condition. In a review of 10 studies, there was no consistent association between any given CTG finding during labour and subsequent brain damage in the infant (Rosen and Dickinson 1993).

Some trials have demonstrated an increased Caesarean section rate in the groups which had continuous electronic fetal heart rate monitoring (Haverkamp *et al.* 1976; Renou *et al.* 1976), whilst other trials have failed to show any difference (MacDonald *et al.* 1985; Wood *et al.* 1981). Edington *et al.* (1975) reported that when abnormal cardiotocography was followed by fetal scalp pH sampling, the Caesarean section rate in fact fell, from 9.7 to 5.8 per cent. Meta-analysis suggests that there is a small increase in the incidence of Caesarean section for 'fetal distress' in patients who have continuous electronic fetal heart rate monitoring (Grant 1989).

There is, therefore, very little evidence that continuous fetal heart rate monitoring is associated with a better outcome than intermittent auscultation, and it is possible that the major reason why continuous fetal heart rate monitoring should now be performed is a medico-legal one rather than a clinical one (Spencer 1991*a*). Whilst there is undoubtedly a risk of umbilical artery metabolic acidosis associated with cardiotocographic abnormalities, the relationship is not consistent. In one series of 33 asphyxiated infants, 87 per cent had an abnormal cardiotocograph but 13 per cent had a normal one (Murphy *et al.* 1990). These authors also found that 29 per cent of 120 healthy controls had an abnormal cardiotocograph. The presence of abnormalities on the intrapartum cardiotocograph is relatively sensitive but is not specific for fetal and neonatal acidaemia. In order for the specificity to be increased, fetal scalp blood sampling is recommended for further evaluation (Fisk and Bower 1993; Spencer 1993; Westgate and Greene 1994).

Other tests of fetal well-being in labour

In view of the lack of evidence for any benefit from continuous fetal heart rate monitoring, with or without confirmatory fetal blood sampling, alternative methods for the assessment of fetal well-being during labour have been reported. The simplest of these is the short cardiotocograph, or 'admission test', lasting approximately 20 minutes. Ingemarsson *et al.* (1986) advocated an admission test for screening women when admitted in labour. In 94 per cent of 1041 patients, the test was reactive and fetal distress (as defined by an operative delivery for that indication or an Apgar score of less than seven at five minutes) was 1.3 per cent. In 1 per cent of patients the test was ominous and there was one intrapartum death (10 per cent) and one case of fetal distress (10 per cent). In 5 per cent of the patients the test was equivocal and the incidence of fetal distress, as defined above, was 8 per cent. Other authors have confirmed that an admission screening test has value for the prediction of a subgroup of patients at increased risk of Caesarean section for 'fetal distress' (Pello *et al.* 1988).

The fetal ECG wave form has also been evaluated, but preliminary results suggest that it has poorer predictive value for fetal acidaemia than the cardiotocograph (MacLachlan *et al.* 1992; Newbold *et al.* 1991).

The continuous measurement of fetal scalp pH and P_{O_2} has been studied, although the delicacy of the equipment as well as possible errors resulting from stasis in an area of caput, limit applicability. Huch *et al.* (1977) have shown a relationship between the severity of fetal heart deceleration and cardiotocography during labour and the fall in fetal P_{O_2}, but no association with baseline bradycardia or tachycardia provided that these lay between 100 and 180 beats per minute, suggesting that these should be the normal range rather than 120–160 beats per minute. The fetal P_{O_2} also fell when the mother moved from the lateral to the supine position. Aarnoudse *et al.* (1985) measured intrapartum fetal heart rates and subcutaneous scalp P_{O_2} continuously during labour in 34 patients. When the scalp P_{O_2} was equal or greater than 25 mmHg, only 0.8 per cent of cardiotocographs were abnormal, but during periods of time when the scalp P_{O_2} was less than 10 mmHg, 53 per cent of the cardiotocographs showed some abnormality. It may prove more valuable to assess fetal scalp oxygen saturation continuously during labour using a pulse oximeter, although scalp fixation remains a problem (Johnson *et al.* 1991). A fall in oxygen saturation during labour was associated with cardiotocographic decelerations, suggesting that the technique, with further assessment and development, may allow for the prediction of fetal distress during labour.

Fetal acoustic stimulation has also been used to assess fetal condition. In one series, a reactive fetal heart response to fetal acoustic stimulation occurred in 93 per cent of fetuses during labour. This group had a lower incidence of cardiotocographic abnormalities and Caesarean section for fetal distress than did the smaller group with a non-reactive cardiotocographic tracing following stimulation (Sarno *et al.* 1990). This technique requires further assessment. It has been known for some time that fetal heart rate accelerations in labour, either spontaneous or provoked, are an indication that the fetus is unlikely to be acidaemic (Spencer 1991*b*).

There is, as yet, no good evidence to show clinical value for the measurement of fetal electroencephalograms during labour.

Continued monitoring and the treatment of suspected fetal distress

If 'fetal distress' occurs, the cause should be sought by re-assessing the clinical situation in the light of the progress of labour. Management, in the absence of immediate delivery, is aimed at increasing uteroplacental perfusion by the correction of aortocaval compression and reduction of uterine activity (by reducing oxytocin infusion or commencing an infusion of a tocolytic). Administration of oxygen to the mother is commonly practised, although its value is uncertain. Accidents, such as uterine rupture or abruption, or cord prolapse, need to be excluded.

In terms of general measures, the evidence is often incomplete. There is very little evidence to suggest that maternal administration of oxygen is anything more than of marginal value, whilst the benefits of ceasing oxytocin infusion are clear. Eckstein and Marx (1974) demonstrated 'significant' femoral artery hypotension in 60 per cent of supine women during late pregnancy when compared with their femoral artery blood pressure in the left lateral position. Arbitol (1985) noted that 19 per cent of 126 women with fetal heart decelerations only demonstrated these decelerations in the supine position and turning to the left lateral position would abolish these decelerations. Should cardiotocographic changes persist, fetal scalp sampling is recommended in order to assess the degree of fetal hypoxia and acidosis. If acidosis is confirmed then either immediate delivery or tocolysis and reassessment should take place.

Recently, replacement of fluid within the uterine cavity by amnioinfusion has been shown to reduce those fetal heart rate changes suggestive of umbilical cord compression.

Amnioinfusion is an easy technique to perform, normal saline at 37 °C being infused into the uterine cavity via an intrauterine catheter at a rate of approximately 10 ml per minute for up to one hour. In a randomized trial of saline amnioinfusion ($n = 49$) compared with non-infusion ($n = 47$), 51 per cent of cardiotocographs returned to normal in the infusion group compared with 4 per cent in the non-infusion group (Miyazaki and Nevarez 1985). However, the incidence of Caesarean section and the incidence of low Apgar scores were statistically similar in both the infusion and the non-infusion group, suggesting that amnioinfusion may dispel fetal heart decelerations yet not improve fetal condition. Similarly, in a randomized trial of amnioinfusion against non-infusion, Owen *et al.* (1990) reported a reduction in the incidence of Caesarean section for fetal distress in the infusion group, although the reduction was not statistically significant. This technique requires greater evaluation before its place in clinical practice can be assessed.

The use of beta-sympathomimetic agents has been advocated for the treatment of fetal distress. There is evidence from randomized trials that beta-sympathomimetic administration will improve the acid–base status of the fetus (Patriarco *et al.* 1987). In this trial, terbutaline reduced uterine activity, abolished fetal heart decelerations, and resulted in a higher mean umbilical artery pH. In another series, 36 patients with an abnormal cardiotocograph and a mean fetal scalp pH of 7.16 were given a bolus intravenous injection (0.25 mg) of terbutaline and the scalp pH estimation repeated (at an average of 13 minutes later). Some 56 per cent of fetuses had an improved pH and labour was allowed to continue, but as 94 per cent of the fetuses were ultimately delivered by Caesarean section, the technique may allow for a delay in the performance of the Caesarean section but not its avoidance (Sherkarloo *et al.* 1989). Provided that a maternal tachycardia is not present before treatment, sympathomimetic agents may prove to be a useful treatment for fetal distress, but further information is required.

Monitoring the fetus and neurological handicap

Neurological handicap may occur as a consequence of obstetric complications, the severity of early onset neonatal encephalopathy being the best predictor of neurological damage. It has been estimated that 27 per cent of neonates with seizures will not survive, whilst a further 25 per cent will survive but with a 'severe or moderate handicap' (Dennis and Chalmers 1982). Of these handicaps, cerebral palsy is the one which is most likely to be associated with adverse perinatal events (Paneth and Stark 1983).

There is a poor correlation between obstetric events, birth asphyxia, and subsequent cerebral palsy (Hull and Dodd 1991; Painter *et al.* 1988; Spencer 1991c). Although cerebral palsy, with or without mental retardation, may result from neurological damage antenatally or during labour, the majority of cases are idiopathic or caused by cerebral vascular abnormalities, cerebral infarction, metabolic disorders, dysmorphic syndromes, or chromosomal defects (Hall 1989). Various estimates in the literature relate the percentage of cases of cerebral palsy which may result from intrapartum hypoxia. Paneth and Stark (1983) suggest that no more than 15 per cent of cases of cerebral palsy are due to adverse perinatal events, whilst other authors quote lower figures, such as 11 per cent (Nelson and Ellenburg 1986), 8 per cent (Nelson 1988), and 6 per cent (Naeye *et al.* 1989). Moreover, the occurrence of abnormal cardiotocographic changes cannot be taken to mean that asphyxia was the cause of cerebral palsy should this subsequently develop (Grant 1990). *The Lancet* (1989) described the promotion of the poor relationship between the standard of obstetric care and the occurrence of cerebral palsy as 'shooting the specialty of obstetrics in the foot'. Although there is an association between low Apgar scores, fetal acidosis, and neonatal outcome, the relationship is loose and no single clinical or biochemical measurement is as good a predictor of neonatal morbidity as is a combination of these indicators (Portman *et al.* 1990). In one series of 125 babies who were severely acidotic at birth (defined as an umbilical artery blood pH of less than 7.1 and a base deficit above 12 mmol/l), only 14 per cent had a 5-minute Apgar score of less than seven (Sykes *et al.* 1982). Two studies have suggested that the failure of the fetus to mount an appropriate response to hypoxia (an inability to become acidaemic) is more predictive of subsequent neurodevelopmental handicap in the presence of a low Apgar score at birth (Dennis *et al.* 1989; Dijxhoorn *et al.* 1986). A diagnosis of birth-related neonatal encephalopathy (the term birth asphyxia should be avoided since it does not imply damage but does imply aetiology) requires clinical circumstances compatible with the production of severe hypoxia substantiated by objective confirmation of asphyxia followed by early onset neonatal encephalopathy.

The progress of labour

Since there is no objective marker from which to time the onset of labour, it is traditional to time the commencement of labour from the admission to the labour ward.

Progressive cervical dilatation and progressive descent of the presenting part are the methods by which the progress of labour is judged. Cervical dilatation is now almost always assessed by vaginal rather than rectal examination. The reluctance to perform vaginal examination for fear of infection was said to have originated with Oliver Wendell Holmes in 1843 and to have been reinforced by Semmelweis in 1847. Bertelsen and Johnson (1963) analysed 1057 consecutive labours, of which 543 were managed with vaginal and 514 with rectal examinations. Puerperal pyrexia, excluding urinary tract infection, occurred in 2 per cent of patients in the vaginal examination group and 2 per cent in the rectal examination group. Patients also prefer vaginal to rectal examination (Murphy *et al.* 1986).

The rate of cervical dilatation was described by Friedman (1954 and 1955) in a study of 500 primigravidae at term. He divided the first stage of labour into four parts. An initial latent phase was followed by an accelerated phase, a phase of maximal slope, and a decelerated phase. These last three phases were combined as the active phase of labour. The duration of these phases, the mean rate of cervical dilatation, and the range of cervical dilatation for each phase is shown in Table 18.4. The mean duration of labour for primigravidae was 7.3 hours in the latent phase and 4.4 hours in the active phase, with a mean rate of cervical dilatation of 3.7 cm/hour during the active phase of labour. The same author reported that the rates of cervical dilatation during the three parts of the active phase were inter-related, the phase of maximum slope being

Table 18.4 The rate of cervical dilatation

Phase	Mean duration (h)	Mean rate of cervical dilatation (cm/h)	Range of cervical dilatation (cm)
Late phase	7.3	0.35	0–2.5
Accelerated phase	1.9 ⎫		2.5–3.5
Phase of maximum slope	1.6 ⎬ 3.7		3.5–8.5
Decelerated phase	0.9 ⎭		8.7–10

From Friedman (1954, 1955)

especially governed by the rate of cervical dilatation during the accelerated phase of labour.

Subsequently, there have been numerous assessments of the mean lengths of the first and second stages of labour and one such assessment has demonstrated that, for nulliparous patients, the mean length of the first stage of labour was 8.1 hours whilst the mean length of the first stage of labour in multiparous patients was 5.7 hours (Kilpatrick and Laros 1989). Since 95 per cent of nulliparous patients have a first stage of labour of less than 16.6 hours and 95 per cent of multiparous patients have a first stage of labour of less than 12.5 hours, it is reasonable to accept these times as a working definition of prolonged labour (Kilpatrick and Laros 1989).

The mean length of the second stage of labour have been estimated as being 58 minutes and 19 minutes, respectively, for nulliparous and multiparous patients in the absence of an epidural, but 97 minutes and 54 minutes, respectively, in the presence of an epidural (Kilpatrick and Laros 1989; Patterson *et al.* 1992). This is discussed further in Chapter 26. However, it is inappropriate to extrapolate the concept of prolonged labour to the second stage, since the second stage of labour should be allowed to continue as long as there is progress in the absence of complications (Kilpatrick and Laros 1989).

The use of a partogram

A graphic recording of labour, described by Philpott and Castle in 1972, forms the basis of the partogram currently in use throughout much of the obstetric world. Taking zero time as the time of admission to hospital, it records the cervical dilatation and descent of the fetal head in the concept of 'fifths' (and not fixed or engaged) as well as the fetal heart rate, liquor (I for intact membranes, C for clear, and M for meconium), moulding by a series of pluses (+), the quality and quantity of contractions denoted by shading, the administration of drugs, maternal pulse, blood pressure and temperature, and urine volume with urinalysis. Philpott (1974) then added an 'alert line' for cervical dilatation, allowing patients with poor cervical dilatation to be recognized more easily so that, when indicated, alterations in management are instigated early.

Table 18.5 The importance of the rate of cervical dilatation

	% Patients faster than average progress (n = 164)	% Patients slower than average progress (n = 128)
Spontaneous delivery	82.9	53.1
Non-rotational forceps	11.7	27.3
Rotational forceps	3.0	9.4
Ventouse	2.4	7.8
Caesarean section	0	2.4

From Studd (1973)

Studd (1973) used a modified graphic record, based upon Philpott's partogram, in 15 000 labours in order to construct normograms for normal progressive cervical dilatation in primigravidae admitted at different cervical dilatations. Such a stencil, used retrospectively, was able to separate normal labour from labour destined to result in an abnormal outcome (Table 18.5). Studd *et al.* (1975) then assessed the predictive value of the normogram stencil in a prospective study of 741 consecutive spontaneous labours with cephalic presentation in both primigravidae and multigravidae. Using the stencil, 159 patients (21.5 per cent) required augmentation with oxytocics because cervical progress fell two hours to the right of the normogram. Some 82 per cent of the 741 patients had normal vaginal deliveries, and this included 69 per cent of all primigravidae and 93 per cent of all multigravidae. Of patients whose cervimetric progress kept to the left or within two hours of the right of the partogram, normal vaginal delivery occurred in 81 per cent of primigravidae and 96 per cent of multigravidae.

The use of such graphic records may allow for abnormal labour to be predicted with the possibility of correction by either amniotomy or the use of oxytocin. Thus, Cardozo *et al.* (1982) reported on 684 primigravidae and 847 multigravidae in spontaneous labour. A normal cervimetric pattern, found in 64 per cent of patients, was associated with vaginal delivery in 98 per cent of cases; the classification of abnormalities together with their incidences and the resulting Caesarean section rates is shown in Table 18.6.

The place of early amniotomy

It is generally believed that early amniotomy is an effective method of reducing the duration of labour. However, randomized controlled trials have produced conflicting results. In one randomized trial involving 68 patients, four underwent Caesarean section for cephalopelvic disproportion. The outcome for the remaining 64 patients suggested that early amniotomy reduced the mean length of the first stage, reduced the number of patients requiring augmentation, and increased the percentage of patients who underwent a spontaneous vaginal

Table 18.6 The importance of the rate of cervical dilatation

	No.	%	Caesarean section rate (%)
Total primigravidae	684	100	8.7
Normal labour	437	63.9	1.6
Prolonged latent phase	24	3.5	16.7
Primary dysfunction labour —improved by oxytocin	145	21.2	6.2
—not improved by oxytocin	35	5.1	77.3
Secondary arrest —improved by oxytocin	26	3.8	11.6
—not improved by oxytocin	17	2.5	54.0

From Cardozo *et al.* 1982

Table 18.7 The effect of amniotomy

	Early amniotomy	Late amniotomy
No.	34	30
Mean length 1st stage (hours)	4.9	7.0
% Requiring Syntocinon	23.5	49.7
Normal vaginal delivery	73.5	56.7
Forceps delivery	26.5	43.3

From Stewart *et al.* (1982)

delivery (Table 18.7) (Stewart *et al.* 1982). In a second randomized controlled trial involving 97 nulliparous women in spontaneous labour at term with a cephalic presentation, there were no differences between the lengths of the first and second stages, the occurrence of cardiotocographic abnormalities, abnormal Apgar scores, or low umbilical arterial pH measurements between an early amniotomy group and a group in whom the membranes were left intact (Fraser *et al.* 1991). In a larger study involving 362 patients, early amniotomy again resulted in a significant reduction in the mean length of the first stage in nulliparous patients, but made no difference to the length of the first stage in multiparous patients or the length of the second stage in either nulliparous or multiparous patients (Table 18.8) (Barrett *et al.* 1992).

Whilst it would seem that early amniotomy may reduce the length of the first stage in nulliparous patients, the need for a larger randomized controlled trial is apparent.

The active management of labour

O'Driscoll *et al.* (1973) enumerated three principles for active management of labour, namely that every woman admitted in her first pregnancy will deliver

Table 18.8 The effect of amniotomy

Duration of labour (hours)	Amniotomy (n = 183)	Spontaneous rupture (n = 179)
1st stage		
All women (n = 362)	7.4	7.7
Nulliparae (n = 156)	8.3	9.7
2nd stage		
All women (n = 362)	0.5	0.5
Nulliparae (n = 156)	0.8	0.8

From Barrett *et al.* (1992)

within 12 hours, every woman will have a personal nurse, and every labour will be controlled. In a prospective study of 1000 consecutive primigravid labours, intervention occurred if progress, as judged by cervical dilatation, failed to exceed 1 cm/hour. Stimulation was by amniotomy followed by intravenous oxytocin one hour later, unless progress was appropriate. Oxytocin was given in a dosage of 10 units/litre increasing until appropriate progress was made, synthetic oxytocin being required by 55 per cent of patients. Some 955 patients (95.5 per cent) delivered within 12 hours and, when 38 patients not in labour were excluded, only 0.7 per cent of patients were undelivered within 12 hours. The Caesarean section rate was 5 per cent, the forceps rate 19.5 per cent, the Ventouse was not used, and the perinatal mortality 25 per 1000. Some 42 per cent of women did not require any analgesia, and this series compares with the previous series by O'Driscoll *et al.* (1969). The authors stated that the primigravid uterus is almost immune to rupture, except by manipulation.

In a third study of 1000 consecutive primigavidae, O'Driscoll *et al.* (1977) reported a Caesarean section rate of 3.8 per cent with no intrapartum deaths and a perinatal mortality rate of 16 per 1000. All surviving infants were assessed for neurological dysfunction which was considered to be present in two; in one infant it was related to diazepam given to the mother for eclampsia and in the other to meconium aspiration syndrome. No case of cerebral dysfunction related to labour (hypoxia or trauma) was found. The forceps rate was 20 per cent and rotational forceps or Ventouse were not used in this group. Of the 16 perinatal deaths, none were intrapartum and two were neonatal, one related to prematurity, and one to meconium aspiration. The other deaths all occurred before labour. O'Driscoll *et al.* (1984) suggested that the active management not only treats but actually prevents 'dystocia' such that the incidence of Caesarean section for dystocia in Dublin was 0.7 per cent whereas it was 4.7 per cent in the United States.

Not all authors have found the augmentation of labour to be as effective as the above studies from Dublin, probably because of the delay before intervention. Bidgood and Steer (1987*a*, *b*) randomly allocated 60 women in labour, progressing slowly with a vertex presentation, to receive either no specific management, low-dose oxytocin, or high-dose oxytocin. Although the 'delay-to-delivery' intervals were shorter in the high-dose group than the control group (mean 7.8 hours compared with 11.1 hours), the rates of Caesarean section were not statistically significantly different between the three groups (45 per cent, 35 per cent, and 26 per cent, respectively). However, there was a clear trend towards a lower Caesarean section rate in the high-dose oxytocin group, and this observation needs to be taken in the context that the above trial consisted of 60 patients compared with the results from several thousand women in Dublin (Stronge and Connolly 1988; Turner and Gordon 1988).

The active management of labour has been successfully introduced into other centres with associated reductions in Caesarean section rates (Akoury *et al.* 1988; Lopez-Zemo *et al.* 1992; Turner *et al.* 1988). In one such controlled randomized trial, the Caesarean section rate for 351 patients managed actively was 10.5 per cent, whereas the Caesarean section rate for 354 patients managed traditionally was 14.1 per cent (Lopez-Zemo *et al.* 1992).

Should augmentation of labour be practised, the important complication of uterine hyperstimulation remains a major anxiety. It was recorded in between 33–37 per cent of patients in series from outside of Dublin (Bidgood and Steer 1987*b*; Hemminki *et al.* 1985; Seitchik and Castillo 1982) yet in none out of 3181 patients in Dublin (Stronge and Connolly 1988). The explanation of this apparent discrepancy may depend, in part, upon the criteria for the diagnosis of uterine hypertonus, but Stronge and Connolly (1988) stated that 'there was no case of uterine hyperstimulation because no woman in labour had more than seven palpable uterine contractions in any 15-minute period'.

Conclusions

A major debate regarding management of labour revolves around the question of continuous fetal heart rate monitoring in a low-risk population (Spencer 1991*a*, *b*, and *c*). Probably all the trials have been too small to detect any benefit, should a benefit be present. This could mean that either the benefit is small or that the overall assessment of the patient allows for the same assessment of fetal well-being to be made. Active management of labour is not practised in many units, probably because its actual title leads to the belief that such a policy is too aggressive and more interfering than is desirable. The benefits, especially in terms of lower Caesarean section rates, have not been successfully conveyed to women or accepted by obstetricians.

References

Aarnoudse, J. G., Huisjes, H. J., Gordon, H., Oeseburg, B., and Zijlstra, W. G. (1985). Fetal subcutaneous scalp P_{O_2} and abnormal heart rate during labour. *American Journal of Obstetrics and Gynecology* **153**, 565–6.
Akoury, H. A., Brodie, G., Caddick, R., McLaughlin, V. D., and Pugh, P. A. (1988).

Active management of labour and operative delivery in nulliparous women. *American Journal of Obstetrics and Gynecology* **158**, 255–8.

Arbitol, M. M. (1985). Supine position in labour and associated fetal heart rate changes. *Obstetrics and Gynecology* **65**, 481–6.

Barrett, J. F., Savage, J., Phillips, K., and Lilford, R. J. (1992). Randomized trial of amniotomy in labour versus the intension to leave membranes intact until the second stage. *British Journal of Obstetrics and Gynaecology* **99**, 5–9.

Beard, R. W., Filshie, G. M., Knight, C. A., and Roberts, G. M. (1971). The significance of changes in the continuous fetal heart rate in the first stages of labour. *Journal of Obstetrics and Gynaecology of the British Commonwealth* **78**, 865–81.

Bertelsen, H. H. and Johnson, D. B. (1963). Routine vaginal examinations during labour. *American Journal of Obstetrics and Gynecology* **85**, 527–31.

Bidgood, K. A. and Steer, P. J. (1987*a*). A randomized controlled study of oxytocin augmentation of labour: obstetric outcome. *British Journal of Obstetrics and Gynaecology* **94**, 512–17.

Bidgood, K. A. and Steer, P. J. (1987*b*). A randomized controlled study of oxytocin augmentation of labour: uterine outcome. *British Journal of Obstetrics and Gynaecology* **94**, 518–22.

Boylan, P. C. (1991). Liquor measurements; meconium and oligohydramnios. In *Fetal monitoring* (ed. J. A. D. Spencer), pp. 133–7, Oxford University Press, Oxford.

British Medical Journal (1976). Intra-partum fetal monitoring for all? *British Medical Journal* **2**, 1466.

Cardozo, L. D., Gibb, D. M. F., Studd, J. W. W., Vasant, R. Z., and Cooper, D. J. (1982). Predictive value of cervimetric labour patterns in primigravidae. *British Journal of Obstetrics and Gynaecology* **89**, 33–8.

Chalmers, I., Zlosnik, J. E., Johns, K. A., and Campbell, H. (1976). Obstetric practice and outcome of pregnany in Cardiff residents. *British Medical Journal* **1**, 735–8.

Coltart, T. M., Byrne, D. I., and Bates, S. A. (1989). Meconium aspiration syndrome. *British Journal of Obstetrics and Gynaecology* **96**, 411–14.

Dennis, J. and Chalmers, I. (1982). Very early neonatal seizure rate. *British Journal of Obstetrics and Gynaecology* **89**, 418–26.

Dennis, J., Johnson, A., Muteh, L., Yudkin, P., and Johnson, P. (1989). Acid–base status at birth and neurodevelopmental outcome at four and one-half years. *American Journal of Obstetrics and Gynecology* **161**, 213–20.

Dijxhoorn, M. J., Visser, G. H. A., Fidler, V. J., Touwen, B. C. L., and Huisjes, H. J. (1986). Apgar score, meconium and acidaemia at birth in relation to neonatal neurological morbidity in term infants. *British Journal of Obstetrics and Gynaecology* **93**, 217–22.

Eckstein, K. L. and Marx, G. (1974). Aortocaval compression and uterine displacement. *Anaesthesiology* **40**, 92–6.

Edington, P. T., Sibanda, J., and Beard, R. W. (1975). Influence on clinical practice of routine intra-partum fetal monitoring. *British Medical Journal* **3**, 341–3.

Fisk, N. M. and Bower, S. (1993). Fetal blood sampling in retreat. *British Medical Journal* **307**, 143–4.

Fraser, W. D., Sauve, R., Parboosingh, I. J., Fung, T., Sokol, R., and Persaud, D. (1991). A randomized controlled trial of early amniotomy. *British Journal of Obstetrics and Gynaecology* **98**, 84–91.

Friedman, E. A. (1954). The graphic analysis of labour. *American Journal of Obstetrics and Gynecology* **68**, 1568–75.

Friedman, E. A. (1955). Primigravid labour. *Obstetrics and Gynecology* **6**, 567–89.

Fujikura, T. and Klionsky, B. (1975). The significance of meconium staining. *American Journal of Obstetrics and Gynecology* **121**, 45–50.

Grant, A. (1989). Monitoring the fetus during labour. In *Effective care in pregnancy and childbirth* (ed. I. Chalmers, N. Enkin, and M. J. N. C. Keirse), pp. 846–82, Oxford University Press, Oxford.

Grant, A. (1990). Cerebral palsy in infants born during trial of intrapartum monitoring. *Lancet* **335** 660.

Grant, A., O'Brien, N., Joy, M. T., Hennessey, E., and MacDonald, D. (1989). Cerebral palsy among children born during the Dublin randomized trial of intrapartum monitoring. *Lancet* **ii**, 1233–5.

Hall, D. M. B. (1989). Birth asphyxia and handicap. *British Medical Journal* **299**, 279–82.

Haverkamp, A. D., Thompson, H. E., McFee, J. G., and Cetrulo, C. (1976). The evaluation of continuous fetal heart monitoring in high-risk labour. *American Journal of Obstetrics and Gynecology* **125**, 310–20.

Hemminki, E., Lenck, M., Saarikoski, S., and Henriksson, L. (1985). Ambulation versus oxytocin in protracted labour. *European Journal of Obstetrics, Gynaecology, and Reproductive Biology* **20**, 199–208.

Huch, A., Huch, R., Schneider, H., and Rooth, G. (1977). Continuous transcutaneous monitoring of fetal oxygen tension during labour. *British Journal of Obstetrics and Gynaecology* **84**, (supp.), 1–39.

Hull, J. and Dodd, K. (1991). What is birth asphyxia? *British Journal of Obstetrics and Gynaecology* **98**, 953–5.

Ingemarsson, I., Arulkumaran, S., Ingemarsson, E., Tambyraja, R. L., and Ratnan, S. S. (1986). Admission test. *Obstetrics and Gynecology* **68**, 800–6.

Johnson, N., Johnson, V. A., Fisher, J., Jobbings, B., Bannister, J., and Lilford, R. J. (1991). Fetal monitoring with pulse oximetry. *British Journal of Obstetrics and Gynaecology* **98**, 36–41.

Katz, M., Shani, N., Meizner, I., and Insler, V. (1982). Is end-stage deceleration of the fetal heart ominous? *British Journal of Obstetrics and Gynaecology* **89**, 186–9.

Katz, M., Meizner, I., Shani, N., and Insler, V. (1983). Clinical significance of sinusoidal fetal heart rate pattern. *British Journal of Obstetrics and Gynaecology* **90**, 832–6.

Kelso, I. M., Parsons, R. J., Lawrence, G. F., Arora, S. S., Edmonds, D. K., and Cooke, I. D. (1978). An assessment of continuous fetal heart rate monitoring in labour. *American Journal of Obstetrics and Gynecology* **131**, 526–32.

Kilpatrick, S. J. and Laros, R. K. (1989). Characteristics of normal labour. *Obstetrics and Gynecology* **74**, 85–7.

Lancet (1989). Cerebral palsy, intra-partum care, and a shot in the foot. *Lancet* **ii**, 1251–2.

Leveno, K. J., Cunningham, F. G., Nelson, S, Roark, M., Williams, M. L., Guzick, D., *et al.* (1986). A prospective comparison of selective and universal electronic fetal heart monitoring in 34 995 pregnancies. *New England Journal of Medicine* **315**, 615–19.

Lopez-Zemo, J. A., Peaceman, A. M., Adashek, J. A., and Socol, M. L. (1992). A controlled trial of a programme for the active management of labour. *New England Journal of Medicine* **326**, 450–4.

Luthy, D. A., Shy, K. K., Van Belle, G., Larson, E. B., Hughes, J. P., Benedetti, T. J., *et al.* (1987). A randomized trial of electronic fetal heart monitoring in preterm labour. *Obstetrics and Gynecology* **69**, 687–95.

MacDonald, D., Grant, A., Sheridan-Pereira, M., Boyland, P., and Chalmers, I.

(1985). The Dublin randomized controlled trial of intra-partum fetal heart rate monitoring. *American Journal of Obstetrics and Gynecology* **152**, 524–39.

MacLachlan, N. A., Spencer, J. A. D., Harding, K., and Arulkumaran, S. (1992). Fetal acidaemia, the cardiotocograph, and the T/QRS ratio of the fetal ECG in labour. *British Journal of Obstetrics and Gynaecology* **99**, 26–33.

Matthews, E. D. and Martin, M. R. (1974). Early detection of meconium-stained liquor during labour. *American Journal of Obstetrics and Gynecology* **120**, 808–11.

Meis, P. J., Hall, M., Marshall, J. R., and Hobel, C. J. (1978). Meconium passage. *American Journal of Obstetrics and Gynecology* **131**, 509–13.

Miyazaki, F. S. and Nevarez, F. (1985). Saline amnio-infusion for relief of repetitive variable decelerations. *American Journal of Obstetrics and Gynecology* **153**, 301–6.

Murphy, K., Grieg, V., Garcia, J., and Grant, A. (1986). Maternal considerations in the use of pelvic examinations in labour. *Midwifery* **2**, 93–7.

Murphy, K. M., Johnson, P., Moorcroft, J., Pattinson, R., Russell, V., and Turnbull, L. A. (1990). Birth asphyxia and the intrapartum cardiotocograph. *British Journal of Obstetrics and Gynaecology* **97**, 470–9.

Murphy, K. M., Russell, V., Collins, A., and Johnson, P. (1991). The prevalence, aetiology, and clinical significance of pseudo-sinusoidal fetal heart rate patterns in labour. *British Journal of Obstetrics and Gynaecology* **98**, 1093–101.

Naeye, R. L., Peters, E. C., Bartholomew, M., and Landis, J. R. (1989). Origins of cerebral palsy. *American Journal of Diseases of Children* **143**, 1154–61.

Nathan, L., Leveno, K. J., Carmody, T. J., Kelly, M. A., and Sherman, M. L. (1994). Meconium—a 1990s perspective on an old hazard. *Obstetrics and Gynecology* **83**, 329–32.

Nelson, K. B. (1988). What proportion of cerebral palsy is related to birth asphyxia? *Journal of Pediatrics* **112**, 572–4.

Nelson, K. B. and Ellenburg, J. H. (1986). Antecedent of cerebral palsy. *New England Journal of Medicine* **315**, 81–6.

Newbold, S., Wheeler, T., and Clewlow, F. (1991). Comparison of the T/QRS ratio of the fetal electrocardiogram and the fetal heart rate during labour and the relation of these variables to condition at delivery. *British Journal of Obstetrics and Gynaecology* **98**, 173–8.

Nielson, P. V., Stigsby, B., Nichelsen, C., and Nim, J. (1987). Intra-and inter-observer variability in the assessment of intra-partum cardiotocographs. *Acta Obstetrica et Gynaecologica Scandinavica* **66**, 421–4.

O'Driscoll, K., Jackson, R. J. A., and Gallagher, J. T. (1969). Prevention of prolonged labour. *British Medical Journal* **2**, 477–80.

O'Driscoll, K., Stronge, J. M., and Minogue, M. (1973). Active management of labour. *British Medical Journal* **3**, 135–7.

O'Driscoll, K., Coughlan, M., Fenton, V., and Skelly, M. (1977). Active management of labour. *British Medical Journal* **2**, 1451–3.

O'Driscoll, K., Foley, M., and MacDonald, D. (1984). Active management of labour as an alternative to Caesarean section for dystocia. *Obstetrics and Gynecology* **63**, 485–90.

Owen, J., Henson, B. V., and Hauth, J. C. (1990). A prospective randomized study of saline solution amnioinfusion. *American Journal of Obstetrics and Gynecology* **162**, 1146–9.

Painter, M. J., Scott, M., Hirsch, R. P., O'Donoghue, P. D., and Deep, R. (1988). Fetal heart rate patterns during labour. *American Journal of Obstetrics and Gynecology* **159**, 854–8.

Paneth, N. and Stark, R. I. (1983). Cerebral palsy and mental retardation in relation to indicators of perinatal asphyxia. *American Journal of Obstetrics and Gynecology* **147**, 960–6.

Paterson, C. M., Saunders, N. S. G., and Wadsworth, J. (1992). The characteristics of the second stage of labour in 25 069 singleton deliveries in the North West Thames Health Region, 1988. *British Journal of Obstetrics and Gynaecology* **99**, 377–80.

Patriarco, M. S., Viechnicki, B. M., Hutchinson, T. A., Klasko, S. K., and Yeh, S. Y. (1987). A study of intrauterine fetal resuscitation with terbutaline. *American Journal of Obstetrics and Gynecology* **118**, 529–33.

Paul, R. H. and Hon, E. H. (1974). Clinical fetal monitoring. *American Journal of Obstetrics and Gynecology* **118**, 529–33.

Pello, L. C., Dawes, G. S., Smith, J., and Redman, C. W. G. (1988). Screening of the fetal heart in early labour. *British Journal of Obstetrics and Gynaecology* **95**, 1128–36.

Philpott, R. H. (1974). Graphic records in labour. *British Medical Journal* **4**, 163–5.

Philpott, R. H. and Castle, W. A. (1972). Cervicographs in the management of labour in primigravidae. *Journal of Obstetrics and Gynaecology of the British Commonwealth* **79**, 592–8.

Portman, R. J., Carter, B. S., Gaylord, M. S., Murphy, M. G., Thieme, R. E., and Merenstein, G. B. (1990). Predicting neonatal morbidity after perinatal asphyxia. *American Journal of Obstetrics and Gynecology* **162**, 174–82.

Renou, P., Chany, A., Anderson, I., and Wood, C. (1976). Controlled trial of fetal intensive care. *American Journal of Obstetrics and Gynecology* **126**, 470–6.

Rosen, M. G. and Dickinson, J. C. (1993). The paradox of fetal heart monitoring. *American Journal of Obstetrics and Gynecology* **168**, 745–51.

Sarno, A. P., Anh, M. O., Phelan, J. P., and Paul, R. H. (1990). Fetal acoustic stimulation in the early intrapartum period as a predictor of acceptable fetal condition. *American Journal of Obstetrics and Gynecology* **162**, 762–7.

Seitchik, J. and Castillo, M. (1982). Oxytocin augmentation of dysfunctional labour. *American Journal of Obstetrics and Gynecology* **144**, 899–905.

Shekarloo, A., Mendez-Bauer, C., Cook, V., and Freese, U. K. (1989). Terbutaline for the treatment of acute intrapartum fetal distress. *American Journal of Obstetrics and Gynecology* **160**, 615–18.

Shy, K. K., Luthy, D. A., Bennett, F. C., Whitfield, M., Larson, E. B., von Belle, G., *et al.* (1990). Effects of electronic fetal heart rate monitoring, as compared with periodic auscultation, and the neurological development of preterm infants. *New England Journal of Medicine* **322**, 588–93.

Spencer, J. A. D. (1991a). Monitoring in labour. *Journal of Obstetrics and Gynaecology* **11**, supp. 1, S16–19.

Spencer, J. A. D. (1991b). Predictive value of the fetal heart rate acceleration at the time of fetal blood sampling in labour. *Journal of Perinatal Medicine* **19**, 207–15.

Spencer, J. A. D. (1991c). Intrapartum hypoxia, birth asphyxia, and handicap. In *Fetal monitoring* (ed. J. A. D. Spencer), pp. 223–32. Oxford University Press, Oxford.

Spencer, J. A. D. (1993). Clinical over view of cardiotocography. *British Journal of Obstetrics and Gynaecology* **100**, supp. 9, 4–7.

Starks, G. C. (1980). Correlation of meconium-stained amniotic fluid, intrapartum pH, and Apgar scores. *Obstetrics and Gynecology* **56**, 604–9.

Stewart, P., Kennedy, J. H., and Calder, A. A. (1982). When should the membranes be ruptured? *British Journal of Obstetrics and Gynaecology* **89**, 39–43.

Stronge, J. and Connolly, R. (1988). Oxytocin augmentation of labour. *British Journal of Obstetrics and Gynaecology* **95**, 105–6.

Studd, J. (1973). Partograms and normograms of cervical dilatation in management of normal labour. *British Medical Journal* **4**, 451–5.

Studd, J., Clegg, D. R., Sanders, H. H., and Hughes, A. O. (1975). Identification of high-risk labours by labour normogram. *British Medical Journal* **2**, 545–7.

Sykes, G. S., Molloy, P. M., Johnson, P., Gu, W., Ashworth, P., Stirratt, G. M., *et al.* (1982). Do Apgar score indicate asphyxia? *Lancet* **i**, 494–6.

Turner, M. J. and Gordon, H. (1988). Oxytocin augmentation of labour. *British Journal of Obstetrics and Gynaecology* **95**, 104–5.

Turner, M. J., Brassil, M., and Gordon, H. (1988). Active management of labour associated with a decrease in the Caesarean section rate in nulliparas. *Obstetrics and Gynecology* **71**, 150–4.

Walker, N. (1959). The case for conservatism in management of fetal distress. *British Medical Journal* **2**, 1221–6.

Westgate, J. and Greene, K. (1994). How well is fetal blood sample used in clinical practice? *British Journal of Obstetrics and Gynaecology* **101**, 250–1.

Wood, C. and Pinkerton, J. H. M. (1961). Clinical aspects of hypoxia stillbirth. *Journal of Obstetrics and Gynaecology of the British Commonwealth* **68**, 552–6.

Wood, C., Renou, P., Oats, J., Farrell, E., Beischer, N., and Anderson, I. (1981). A controlled trial of fetal heart rate monitoring in a low-risk obstetric population. *American Journal of Obstetrics and Gynecology* **141**, 527-34.

Yeomans, E. R., Gilstrap, L. C., Leveno, K. J., and Burris, J. S. (1989). Meconium in the amniotic fluid and fetal acid–base status. *Obstetrics and Gynecology* **73**, 175–8.

19　The induction of labour

The induction of labour has been subject to certain trends, partly due to the use of newer methods of fetal monitoring during the late antenatal period, partly due to the accumulation of scientific data, and partly due to the pressure of media opinion. The frequency with which labours were induced increased from 13.4 per cent in 1964 to 39.4 per cent in 1977 and then fell, from 37 per cent in 1978 to 18.8 per cent in 1982 (Tew 1986). In our own unit, approximately 15 per cent of all labours are induced and this incidence is continuing to fall. The indications for the induction of labour fall into three broad categories (Calder 1991). These may be summarized as follows:

1. It is perceived that either the fetus or mother is at risk from a complication, such as placental insufficiency, red cell alloimmunization, hypertension, etc. In this category should also be included intrauterine death where the major indication for induction is an attempt to minimize parental grief.
2. The fetus is perceived to be at risk based upon epidemiological evidence rather than demonstrable compromise. These situations would include prolonged pregnancy.
3. There is a social indication for induction in order that the baby may be delivered for the convenience of the patient, her partner, or her obstetrician.

This chapter will examine the scientific basis behind obstetric intervention for the commonest indication regarding the induction of labour, namely prolonged pregnancy, and will examine the techniques for the induction of labour, and for the ripening of a cervix prior to that induction. The chapter will also examine induction of labour in the presence of an intrauterine death since the induction of labour in this situation differs from that in the presence of a live fetus.

Prolonged pregnancy

Prolonged pregnancy may be defined as pregnancy lasting 42 completed weeks or 294 days from the first day of the last period. It occurs in approximately 5 per cent of all pregnancies (Cotta and Cibils 1993). Post-maturity is a less well-defined term, and perhaps is based upon the concept of a 'post-maturity syndrome' described by Clifford (1954), this consists of loss of vernix, parchment-like skin (with meconium staining), respiratory difficulty at birth, and atelectasis. Some 7 per cent of all pregnancies are prolonged (Vorherr 1975; Zwerdling 1967). Eden et al. (1987) compared the infants born after 42 weeks in 3457 pregnancies with 8135 infants born at 40 weeks. The overall perinatal mortality rate was comparable, but there were statistically significant increases

Table 19.1 The effects of prolonged pregnancy

	Delivery at 40 weeks	Prolonged pregnancy
No. of infants	8135	3457
Perinatal mortality rate	2.8	4.9
Corrected PMR	2.7	4.2
Mean birthweight (g)	3452	3636
% > 4000 g Birthweight	0.8	2.8
% Meconium present	19.4	26.5
% Meconium aspiration	0.6	1.6
% Caesarean section	8.3	17.6
% Apgar ≤ 3 at 5 min	0.3	0.6
% Shoulder dystocia	0.7	1.3

From Eden *et al.* (1987)

in birthweight, operative delivery, shoulder dystocia, meconium aspiration, and reduced Apgar scores in the prolonged pregnancy group (see Table 19.1). More recent studies show similar findings (Grant 1992).

Possible influences in prolonged pregnancy

Prolonged pregnancy is not necessarily a pathological state. Minor variations may, in fact, be physiological. The following possible influences have been implicated:

(1) racial factors;

(2) fetal causes;

(3) individual variation.

Racial factors

Tuck *et al.* (1983) analysed 2632 consecutive pregnancies in white (*n* = 1885), black (*n* = 572), and Asian women (*n* = 175). Pregnancy was prolonged in 2 per cent of the black women, 2.3 per cent of the Asian women, and 5 per cent of the white women.

Fetal causes

There is no longer considered to be an association between fetal abnormality and prolonged pregnancy. Zwerdling (1967) reported that lethal congenital abnormalities, including anencephaly, occurred in 5.7 per 1000 prolonged pregnancies but in only 1.4 per 1000 pregnancies which terminated between the 37th and 42nd weeks, but more recent evidence has shown that no such association exists, even for neural tube defects (Bakketeig and Bergsjo, 1989).

Table 19.2 The risks of prolonged pregnancy

Gestation (completed weeks)	No. of patients	Stillbirths		First week deaths	Perinatal mortality rate (per 1000)
		Antepartum	Intrapartum		
40	32 856	188 (0.6)	298 (0.9)	214 (0.7)	14
41	24 208	133 (0.6)	241 (1.0)	171 (0.7)	16
42	10 752	89 (0.8)	147 (1.4)	111 (1.0)	23
43	3080	45 (1.5)	65 (2.1)	33 (1.1)	32
44	1008	32 (3.2)	25 (2.5)	26 (2.6)	56

Numbers in parentheses are percentages
From Butler and Alberman (1969)

Individual variation

There is a tendency towards repeated prolonged pregnancy in women with a previous prolonged pregnancy. Bakketeig *et al.* (1979) analysed 453 358 singleton births. In the analysis of 11 540 prolonged pregnancies, the relative risk for a prolonged pregnancy in the presence of a previous prolonged one was 2.2 compared with no previous prolonged pregnancy. The length of pregnancy tends to be greater in women below the age of 20 years than above (Mittendorf *et al.* 1993).

Possible risks of prolonged pregnancy

The possible risks associated with prolonged pregnancy should be examined from the point of view of the fetus, the labour, the placenta, and the infant.

Traditional teaching has suggested that prolonged pregnancy is associated with an increased perinatal mortality rate. Butler and Alberman (1969), in a study of over 200 000 births, reported that the perinatal death was increased in prolonged pregnancy (Table 19.2). Thus, the perinatal mortality rate after 42 weeks of pregnancy is 1.6 times that after 40 completed weeks. Vorherr (1975) reported that the perinatal mortality rate of term pregnancy was 14 per 1000, but rose to 15 at 42 weeks, 25 at 43 weeks, and 35 in those pregnancies which extended beyond 44 weeks. Chamberlain *et al.* (1978) reported, in a survey of 16 815 singleton pregnancies, that the perinatal mortality rate was 7.6 per 1000 for 4603 singleton pregnancies which lasted between 41 and 42 weeks and 17.6 per 1000 for 739 singleton pregnancies which lasted beyond this. It has, therefore, been extrapolated that such deaths might be prevented by the induction of labour.

There is evidence that the fetus continues to grow beyond term. Boyd *et al.* (1983) reported that macrosomia (defined as birthweight of greater than 4000 g) occurred in 16 per cent of 1271 infants delivered between the 41st and 42nd weeks of pregnancy compared with 21 per cent of 447 infants delivered after the 42nd week. Associated with this was the complication of shoulder dystocia which occurred in 4 per cent of 1897 infants whose birthweight was in excess of 4000 g.

There is also evidence that the placenta continues to grow beyond the 40th week of gestation. The average weight of the term placenta is 578 g, whilst the average weight of a placenta associated with prolonged pregnancy is 600 g (Vorherr 1975). There is also evidence that total placenta DNA levels rise in a linear fashion beyond the 40th week of gestation, demonstrating that placental growth continues, albeit at a reduced rate (Fox 1983).

The presence of meconium is associated with prolonged pregnancy. Freeman *et al.* (1981) reported the presence of meconium in 25 per cent of 167 prolonged pregnancies and in 13 per cent of 63 controls, but the incidence of meconium aspiration was not increased. There is no good evidence that fetal distress is more common in prolonged pregnancies. Those controlled trials which compared the elective induction of labour at or beyond term with spontaneous labour in prolonged pregnancy were unable to find any difference in fetal heart abnormality during labour between the two groups (Crowley 1989).

There is no good evidence that the rate of operative delivery is increased in prolonged pregnancy. It used to be argued that the incidence of Caesarean section was, in fact, double that in prolonged pregnancy compared with pregnancy in general (Freeman *et al.* 1981; Schneider *et al.*1978). However, in a meta-analysis of 12 controlled trials which compared elective induction at or beyond term with spontaneous labour in prolonged pregnancy, the incidence of Caesarean section was the same in both groups (Crowley 1989; Grant 1994).

The classical description of an infant following a prolonged pregnancy has already been given (Clifford 1954). Controlled trials of elective induction have demonstrated that the incidences of low Apgar scores and neonatal jaundice are similar whether or not labour in a prolonged pregnancy is induced or is spontaneous (Crowley 1989). Shime *et al.* (1986) reported a prospective study of 89 infants of prolonged pregnancy and 130 term controls at the age of one year, and 76 infants of prolonged pregnancy and 111 term controls at two years. There were no differences between the infants of prolonged pregnancy and the term controls in general intelligence assessment, the attainment of physical milestones, and the incidence of intercurrent illness.

The place of routine induction for prolonged pregnancy

There have now been several comparisons, both retrospective and in the form of controlled trials, of routine induction in prolonged pregnancy. However, no convincing benefits in terms of either a reduction in morbidity or mortality have been demonstrated. Cardozo *et al.* (1986) reported a randomly allocated, prospective trial of routine induction at the 42nd week of pregnancy compared with conservative management in otherwise uncomplicated pregnancies. As can be seen in Table 19.3, there was no statistically significant differences in perinatal mortality, Apgar scores, the need for admission to a special care baby unit, or in the incidence of meconium aspiration. However, there was a statistically

Table 19.3 The value of routine induction

	Induced group	Conservative group
No. of patients	195	207
Perinatal mortality rate	2.5	2.5
% Caesarean section	13	11
% Intubated neonates	15	8
Mean cord pH	7.29	7.32
% Admission to special care unit	3	1.5
% Meconium aspiration	0.5	0.5
% Apgar score < 5 at 5 min	1.0	1.9

From Cardozo *et al.* (1986)

significant increase in the occurrence of acidosis and the need for intubation in the induced group. Miller and Read (1981) found no significant difference in the mean umbilical artery pH estimation in 250 control patients and 88 prolonged pregnancies.

There is no convincing evidence that the induction of labour in prolonged pregnancy will reduce perinatal death. Crowley (1989) reported the results of 13 such controlled trials of elective versus spontaneous labour in prolonged pregnancies. Even a meta-analysis of the results could not demonstrate any mortality consequences from one or other action. There were eight perinatal deaths in 3422 randomized pregnancies. If the mortality risk from prolonged pregnancy was as high as 0.5 per cent, a trial of 70 000 such pregnancies would be needed in order to give an 80 per cent chance of showing a 25 per cent reduction in perinatal mortality. On the basis of the evidence which is available so far, there would seem to be no real advantage from routine induction. However, such a policy may just reduce the Caesarean section rate (Grant 1994).

Surveillance and prolonged pregnancy

In the trials outlined above, the conservative management, in which spontaneous labour was awaited, was generally accompanied by some degree of additional antenatal surveillance over and above a routine antenatal clinic visit. Such surveillance, by these and other authors, have included fetal movement counting (Gibb *et al.* 1982), cardiotocography (Cario 1984; Gibb *et al.* 1982; Keegan and Paul 1980), oxytocic challenge tests (Schneider *et al.* 1978), twice-weekly biophysical profile studies (Johnson *et al.* 1986), and a cocktail of several investigations (Bergsjo *et al.* 1989; Homburg *et al.* 1979).

Should any of the above investigations be abnormal, labour is generally induced. Although there may be an increased incidence in 'fetal distress' in this situation, there would appear to be no detrimental effect on outcome. The benefit of mass induction of pregnancies in week 42 remains to be proven and weighed against possible hazards (Bakketeig and Bergsjo 1989).

Table 19.4 The place of amniotomy

	No. of patients	% Not in labour within 24 hours
Unripe	131	51.9
Intermediate	482	28.8
Ripe	384	9.4
All	997	24.4

From Turnbull and Anderson (1967)

Table 19.5 The induction of labour

	No. of patients	% Caesarean section
Amniotomy + oxytocin	31	32
Amniotomy + extra-amniotic PGE_2	56	9
Prostaglandin in tylose gel	52	12

From Calder and Embrey (1975)

Induction and the unripe cervix

All obstetricians are aware that the induction of labour by amniotomy in the presence of an unripe cervix is associated with an increased incidence of failure and of Caesarean section. These difficulties would appear to be particularly pronounced should the patient be nulliparous. In one series, 65 per cent of nulliparous women with a Bishop's score of three or less underwent a Caesarean section following induction of labour. The commonest indication for this Caesarean section (46 per cent) was 'failed induction' (Arulkumaran *et al.* 1985). Turnbull and Anderson (1967) reported 997 patients who underwent amniotomy alone in order to induce labour. As can be seen from Table 19.4, the more unripe was the cervix, the greater was the percentage of patients not in labour within 24 hours. Similarly, Calder and Embrey (1975) reported a Caesarean section rate of 32 per cent for 31 women when amniotomy and oxytocin were used to induce labour in the presence of an unfavourable cervix, as compared with 9 per cent for 56 women with an unfavourable cervix in whom labour was induced using extra-amniotic prostaglandin followed by amniotomy (see Table 19.5).

The commonest method used to mature or ripen the uterine cervix involved the use of prostaglandin (Calder 1991). Various vehicles exist in which prostaglandin might be applied to the cervix and the use of a prostaglandin E_2 has been the most widely used. A study of 3313 pregnancies from 59 prospective trials in which intravaginal PGE_2 gel was used to ripen the cervix prior to induction of labour indicated that local prostaglandin gel was superior to placebo or no treatment in enhancing cervical effacement, reducing induction

Table 19.6 The induction of labour

	Extra-amniotic PGE$_2$	Intravenous oxytocin	Intravaginal PGE$_2$	Oral PGE$_2$
No. of patients	15	15	14	15
Mean initial Bishop's score	3.5	3.4	3.4	3.3
Mean post-treatment score	8.0	4.5	5.9	4.9
Vaginal delivery	93.3	66.7	80.0	73.3

From Wilson (1978)

failure, shortening the induction–delivery interval, and lowering the incidence of Caesarean section. Uterine hyperstimulation or pathological fetal heart rate patterns following administration occurred in less than 1 per cent of cases (and were generally self-correcting or corrective by tocolytic therapy) (Rayburn 1989).

From an overview of 27 placebo-controlled trials of the use of prostaglandin for cervical ripening, it was apparent that a patient treated with prostaglandin was seven times more likely to ripen her cervix than one treated with placebo, three times less likely to have a 'failed induction of labour', was almost twice as likely to have delivered within 12 hours of induction of labour (66 per cent compared with 39 per cent), was less likely to be delivered by Caesarean section (18 per cent compared with 22 per cent), and was less likely to require operative vaginal delivery (14 per cent compared with 25 per cent) (Keirse and van Oppen 1989*a*).

Prostaglandin E$_2$ would appear to be more effective than PGF$_{2\alpha}$ (MacKenzie and Embrey 1979), whilst intravaginal or extra-amniotic PGE$_2$ is superior to either oral prostaglandin or oxytocin for ripening the cervix (Table 19.6; Wilson 1978). The effect upon the cervix is also dose-related (Graves *et al.* 1985). Should the cervix remain unfavourable, the prostaglandin is generally repeated within six hours of the initial administration (Calder 1991).

Current practice favours the administration of prostaglandin in the form of a vaginal gel rather than a vaginal pessary. Prostaglandin E$_2$ is equally effective for cervical ripening whether administered in the form of a pessary or in a gel (Perryman *et al.* 1992; Smith *et al.* 1990). However, hyperstimulation of the uterus will occur in 0–3 per cent of patients receiving prostaglandin E$_2$ in a gel but in 20–24 per cent of patients who receive prostaglandin E$_2$ in the form of a vaginal pessary (Perryman *et al.*; Smith *et al.* 1990). More recently, the prostaglandin E$_1$ (misoprostol) has been advocated for vaginal use (Fletcher *et al.* 1993).

Mechanical methods of cervical ripening are again being reported and include the use of laminaria tents and lamicel. These methods are said to stimulate local release of prostaglandins (Wei and Lan 1988). However, although laminaria tents are effective in reducing the duration of labour following their use for cervical ripening, they are associated with infection and, hence, are of limited value. Thus, 60 per cent of 25 women who used laminaria tents for cervical

Table 19.7 The induction of labour

	Nulliparous patients		Multiparous patients	
	Amniotomy alone	Amniotomy + oxytocin	Amniotomy alone	Amniotomy + oxytocin
No. of patients	80	82	120	118
% In labour within 6 hours	10	96.3	40	98.3
In labour within 12 hours	55	100	59.2	100

From Patterson (1971)

ripening had evidence of endometritis after delivery compared with 11 per cent in a control group, the incidence of Caesarean section being similar in both groups (Kazzi *et al.* 1982). Lamicel, a synthetic polyvinyl sponge containing magnesium sulfate, has been used for cervical ripening. In a randomized trial, lamicel was shown to be as effective as PGE_2 gel in nulliparous women and, since it caused less uterine activity, may be less associated with the risk of uterine hypertonus (Johnson *et al.* 1985). However, it remains more convenient to both patients and doctors to insert a pessary or gel into the vagina rather than a lamicel tent into an unfavourable cervix.

Techniques for the induction of labour

Several options are now available for the induction of labour and these will now be discussed, together with their associated complications.

Stretch and sweep

This technique is now of historical interest. Swann (1958) reported that 69 per cent of 147 women who underwent this procedure daily for three days went into labour during the 72 hours of the study (29 per cent within 24 hours) compared with 26 per cent of 74 controls. The effect of the technique is considered to be due to the release of local prostaglandins (Mitchell *et al.* 1977). More recent studies, including randomized trials, have shown that sweeping the membranes significantly reduces the subsequent duration of pregnancy in post-mature women with a favourable cervix from a mean of five days to a mean of two days following the procedure, yet without harmful side-effects (Allott and Palmer 1993; Grant 1993).

Amniotomy

Amniotomy is the traditional technique for the induction of labour. The efficacy of amniotomy was described by Turnbull and Anderson (1967). This study has already been referred to and the results are illustrated in Table 19.4. Patterson (1971) reported that amniotomy alone resulted in labour in 10 per cent of nulliparous women within six hours and in 55 per cent within 12 hours, whereas the technique resulted in labour in 40 per cent of 120 multiparous women within six hours and in 60 per cent within 12 hours. These results are shown in Table 19.7.

The mechanism by which amniotomy induces labour is not clear. There have been conflicting studies which claim to demonstrate either an increase in plasma oxytocin levels (Chard and Gibbens 1983) or no increase in these levels (Thornton *et al.* 1989). It is likely that the effect is mediated by the local release of prostaglandin, especially, PGF (Husslein *et al.* 1983).

There are several complications of amniotomy. These are:

(1) cord prolapse;

(2) rupture of a vasa praevia;

(3) infection;

(4) increased intervention.

Cord prolapse

The incidence of cord prolapse has been assessed by various authors and would appear to be in the range of 0.1 to 0.2 per cent of all amniotomies. Niswander and Patterson (1963) reported cord prolapse in 0.1 per cent of 2862 amniotomies, whilst Fields (1960) reported this complication in 0.2 per cent of 3324 amniotomies, and Setna *et al.* (1967) reported this complication in 0.2 per cent of 3130 amniotomies. This figure is not dissimilar from that reported in spontaneous labours with a cephalic presentation.

Rupture of vasa praevia

This complication is potentially fatal for the fetus and occurs in less than 1 in 3000 amniotomies (Setna *et al.* 1967).

Infection

Infection, as judged by maternal pyrexia during labour, was present in 9 per cent of 297 primigravid labours and in 2 per cent of 703 multiparous labours (MacDonald 1970). Several authors have demonstrated a relationship between the incidence of infection during labour and the induction–delivery interval. Muldoon (1968) reported that maternal pyrexia occurred in 1 per cent of 286 women who delivered within 24 hours, in 10 per cent of 122 women who delivered within 24–48 hours, and in 13 per cent of 75 women who delivered with 48–72 hours. Patterson (1971) correlated the incidence of infection with the induction–delivery interval. As shown in Table 19.8, the incidence of infection became particularly significant once the induction–delivery interval exceeded 24 hours.

Table 19.8 Induction and infection

Induction–delivery interval (h)	No. of patients delivered	% With infection
0–6	75	0
6–12	150	0
12–18	70	2.8
18–24	36	5.5
24–30	27	34.0
30–36	36	29.0
36 +	17	30.0

From Patterson (1971)

Table 19.9 Induction and delivery

	Induced	Spontaneous	Total
No. of pregnancies	350 030	1 375 790	1 725 820
% Forceps	16.9	9.6	11.1
% Caesarean section during labour	7.8	4.0	4.8

From Tew (1986)

Increased intervention

The association between induction of labour and the need for increased intervention of delivery is not necessarily a cause and effect. Tew (1986) used national statistics to compare the incidences of different forms of operative delivery in 350 030 induced labours and 1 375 790 spontaneous labours. There was an increased incidence of operative delivery, both vaginal and abdominal, in the induced group (see Table 19.9). It was not apparent, however, whether it was the induction, or the indication for the induction, which resulted in the increased need for intervention.

Other authors have attempted to separate the indications for induction from the process of induction. Yudkin *et al.* (1979) reported a retrospective survey of 200 induced labours and 200 spontaneous labours in patients well-matched for age, parity, social class, and obstetric complications prior to labour. The results, shown in Table 19.10, suggested that the outcome was less likely to be complicated following spontaneous rather than induced labour.

Amniotomy and oxytocin

As can be seen from Table 19.7, Patterson (1971) demonstrated that amniotomy and oxytocin together were a more efficient method of inducing labour than was amniotomy alone, both in nulliparous and multiparous patients. Similarly, Saleh (1975) reported that all 25 patients induced by amniotomy and oxytocin

Table 19.10 Induction and outcome

	Induced	Spontaneous
% Intrapartum Caesarean section	5	0
% Forceps	30	1
% Epidural	49	13.5
Mean length first stage of labour (h)	5.4	6.2
Mean length second stage of labour (h)	0.48	0.4
% Forceps in non-epidural group	6	0.5
% Babies intubated	7.5	2

From Yudkin *et al.* (1979)

infusion delivered within 24 hours compared with 68 per cent of 25 patients induced by amniotomy alone.

A randomized trial of induction by amniotomy alone and amniotomy and oxytocin combined was reported by Bakos and Backstrom (1987). In a trial involving 223 patients, 49 per cent induced with oxytocin alone delivered within 24 hours, compared with 98 per cent induced by amniotomy alone and 100 per cent induced by amniotomy with an oxytocin infusion. Oxytocin alone, without amniotomy, is not an efficient method of inducing labour. Lilienthal and Ward (1971) reported that with an oxytocin infusion alone, the mean induction-delivery interval was 70 hours in 154 patients, with 48 per cent of patients being delivered within 24 hours.

Numerous regimes by which oxytocin is administered in order to induce (and maintain) labour have been described, but there is little evidence that any one regime is superior to any other. Some units use an automatic feedback oxytocin infusion system in which the dose of oxytocin infused intravenously is controlled by the strength and frequency of uterine contractions (Cardiff pump). Thomas and Blackwell (1974) reported a randomized prospective trial of the Cardiff infusion system in 17 patients compared with a control infusion system in 19 patients. There were no significant differences in the incidence of fetal distress or in the length of labour between the two groups. Steer *et al.* (1985) reported a prospective randomized control trial of the Cardiff infusion system and conventional intravenous infusion in 84 patients. There were no differences as regards the modes of delivery, Apgar scores, or the need for analgesia between either system in either nulliparous or multiparous patients. However, the automatic infusion system used less oxytocin, and, hence, this infusion system may be specifically indicated in patients in whom there is particular clinical anxiety concerning fluid balance.

There is also debate as to the optimum starting dose of oxytocin. Wein (1989) reported that each of three regimes (commencing with 2, 5, or 10 units/litre of oxytocin) were equally effective in inducing labour and with similar delivery outcomes in a non-randomized study of 1020 patients. On general principles, it seems more appropriate to use a lower total dosage of drug. The American College of Obstetricians and Gynecologists recommend an initial dosage of 0.5 mU per minute, increased by between 1 and 2 mU per minute every 30–60 minutes (American College of Obstetricians and Gynecologists 1987). There is no advantage in increasing the dose of oxytocin every 15 minutes rather than every 60 minutes (Blakemore *et al.* 1990).

The complications of oxytocin infusion may include the following:

(1) uterine hypertonus;

(2) uterine rupture;

(3) fetal hypoxia;

(4) water retention;

(5) neonatal hyperbilirubinaemia.

Uterine hypertonus

Uterine hypertonus due to overstimulation with oxytocin is well recognized and may lead to either uterine rupture or fetal hypoxia. Oxytocin should not be administered within six hours of vaginal prostaglandin (Calder 1991).

Uterine rupture

Uterine rupture with oxytocin infusion, even in the primigravida, has been reported (Daw 1973).

Fetal hypoxia

Uterine stimulation or overstimulation may lead to profound bradycardia; this is relieved by stopping the infusion (Thomas and Blackwell 1974).

Water retention

Water retention is an uncommon complication of oxytocin infusion, but the antidiuretic action of oxytocin may lead to water retention, water intoxication, maternal hyponatraemia, and oligouria. This complication may result in neonatal hyponatraemia and convulsions (Mwambingo 1985; Schwartz and Jones 1978).

Neonatal hyperbilirubinaemia

Reports of neonatal hyperbilirubinaemia in infants whose mothers had received oxytocin during labour were commonplace in the 1970s. Numerous case reports appeared to link the two events and numerous mechanisms were proposed to explain this relationship, including some interference by oxytocin in the hepatic conjugation of bilirubin (Ghosh and Hudson 1972; O'Driscoll 1972). The most unusual feature stressed by these authors was the observation of increased neonatal hyperbilirubinaemia in mature infants.

However, the association is probably apparent rather than real. Calder *et al.*

Table 19.11 The technique of induction

	No amniotomy		Amniotomy	
	PGE$_2$	Syntocinon	PGE$_2$	Syntocinon
No. of patients	54	50	53	50
% In labour within 4 hour	39	66	92	98
% Delivered within 12 hours	81	90	77	84

From Ratnam *et al.* (1974)

(1974) reported a prospective trial of 120 primigravidae. Some 30 patients were allocated to each of four groups. The first group went into spontaneous labour, whilst the other three groups were induced by amniotomy and intravenous oxytocin, amniotomy and intravenous prostaglandin, or extra-amniotic prostaglandin, respectively. The mean neonatal bilirubin levels on the fifth days were higher following the induced labours than the spontaneous ones, but there were no significant differences in neonatal bilirubin levels following induction by oxytocin or prostaglandin. There were no differences between gestational age and birthweight in any group, and no specific explanation of the findings could be given. Similarly, Sivasuriya *et al.* (1978) compared 114 patients allocated to amniotomy, amniotomy with intravenous oxytocin, amniotomy with oral prostaglandin, or spontaneous labour. No significant differences in neonatal bilirubin levels on the fifth day could be found between any of these four groups. Campbell *et al.* (1975) reported that the incidence of neonatal hyperbilirubinaemia had increased from 8 per cent of 3499 live births in 1971 to 15 per cent of 3575 live births in 1973, but could not implicate induction, the use of oxytocin, epidural analgesia, or artificial feeds as the causative agent. The implication that oxytocin in general, or induction in particular, is a cause of neonatal hyperbilirubinaemia in term infants has to remain unproven.

Prostaglandins

Although the use of prostaglandins is established for cervical ripening, and clearly some of these patients progress into labour, these agents have found only a limited place in the induction of labour despite their efficacy.

The intravenous administration of prostaglandin is rarely used because of the complications of maternal pyrexia (in 20 per cent of patients) or erythema at the infusion site (Naismith *et al.* 1973). The oral administration of PGE$_2$ augmented by amniotomy, would appear to be as effective as intravenous oxytocin augmented by amniotomy. Ratnam *et al.* (1974) randomized 207 patients to have labour induced by oral PGE$_2$ or intravenous oxytocin, half in each group also having an amniotomy. The results, shown in Table 19.11, demonstrated the efficacy of both techniques. Some 9 per cent of patients who received oral prostaglandins developed gastrointestinal side-effects, especially diarrhoea, whilst no side-effects were observed following intravenous oxytocin.

Similarly, prostaglandins are as effective as intravenous oxytocin in inducing labour following spontaneous rupture of the membranes. Chapman *et al.* (1984) reported 63 such consecutive patients given intravenous oxytocin and 62 consecutive patients given a vaginal 3 mg PGE_2 tablet. There were no differences in the mean induction–delivery intervals for either group. Westergaard *et al.* (1983) gave oral PGE_2 tablets to 109 women with spontaneous rupture of the membranes at term and who were not in labour. Induction was successful in 84 per cent of patients, the rest receiving intravenous Syntocinon (synthetic oxytocin). All patients delivered within 24 hours. Gastrointestinal side-effects occurred in 21 per cent of patients.

An overview of 11 trials which compared oral prostaglandins with intravenous oxytocin in order to induce labour when the state of the membranes was similar in both arms of the study was reported by Keirse and van Oppen (1989*b*). There were no significant differences between these regimes for the length of labour or the need for an operative delivery, either vaginal or abdominal. Oral prostaglandin, however, did allow for greater maternal mobility during labour and this is preferred by some patients.

In current clinical practice, therefore, vaginal prostaglandins will be used in order to ripen an unripe cervix prior to the induction of labour. The induction of labour is then likely to be by amniotomy, generally augmented by either intravenous oxytocin or oral prostaglandins either from the time of amniotomy or after four hours should labour not be well established (Calder 1991). Which of these options is chosen would appear to relate to personal preference rather than to any specific benefit.

Induction of labour after fetal death

Since 81 per cent of all stillbirths occur before labour (Macfarlane *et al.* 1986), the induction of labour after fetal death *in utero* is of clinical importance. It presents certain additional problems in that 'failed induction' is not an acceptable option. Before the diagnosis is accepted and labour induced, there should be at least one 'long and careful' ultrasound examination (Keirse and Kanhai 1989).

There are two broad possible approaches to delivery in this situation, either expectant, awaiting spontaneous labour or active, inducing labour. The decision as to which of these is pursued will depend largely upon the wishes of the woman concerned. The main advantage of an active approach is the emotional benefit from terminating 'a pregnancy which has lost its purpose'. The risk that a conservative approach may leave the woman at risk of a disseminated intravascular coagulopathy is not a real one in clinical practice so long as the fetal death was not caused by a placental abruption (Keirse and Kanhai 1989).

The option for active management really arose with the advent of prostaglandin therapy. Previous methods which included high-dose oxytocin infusion with or without prior oestrogen were unpredictable, slow, and associated with iatrogenic risks including water intoxication (Mwambingo 1985). The administration of intravenous prostaglandin, extra-amniotic prostaglandin, or vaginal prostaglandin resulted in delivery of 97 per cent of 1584 dead fetuses within a range of 6 to 20 hours (Keirse and Kanhai 1989).

The use of a vaginal or oral agent to induce labour in the presence of an intrauterine death has specific advantages to the mother in terms of mobility, and probably psyche, when compared with intravenous or extra-amniotic use. Scher *et al.* (1980) described their experience of the use of 20 mg PGE_2 vaginal pessary which induced delivery in a mean of 9.2 hours in 91 per cent of 23 women with an intrauterine death. However, this series demonstrated the principle that potentially large doses of PGE_2 were required (a mean of 45.2 mg) which resulted in a 44 per cent incidence of pyrexia and a 57 per cent incidence of gastrointestinal tract side-effects.

More modern management tends to utilize prostaglandin analogues, such as sulprostone and gemeprost. These have the advantage over the parent compounds of greater uterine stimulation related to a longer half-life, an effect which precludes their use in the presence of a live fetus.

Sulprostone, based on PGE_2, has the disadvantage of the inconvenience of intravenous infusion, but Kanhai and Keirse (1989) found that it resulted in the delivery of all 85 women with an intrauterine death within 72 hours of the commencement of an infusion, some 98 per cent of patients delivering within 36 hours. Side-effects were mild but included pyrexia, diarrhoea and/or vomiting in 32 per cent of patients.

The prostaglandin analogue gemeprost, based on PGE_1, has the advantage of being efficiently absorbed via the vagina. Using between one and three pessaries, 10 patients with an intrauterine death all delivered at a mean induction–delivery interval of 11.7 hours (6–19 hours) and with a mean active phase of the first stage of labour of 1.7 hours (Shaft *et al.* 1989). Side-effects, which were not significant, included pyrexia, nausea, and vomiting. The use of a vaginal pessary to induce labour in the presence of an intrauterine death would seem to be a significant advantage over other methods, but caution concerning its safety has to prevail until the results of larger series are available (Bamber 1980; Moran 1989).

There have also been some reports on the use of the antiprogesterone agent mifepristone. A double-blind controlled trial of 94 patients with an intrauterine death resulted in the delivery of 63 per cent of patients within 72 hours of commencing the agent (at a dosage of 600 mg per day for two days) compared with 17 per cent following a placebo (Cabrol *et al.* 1990). Again, however, large studies will be needed in order that the efficacy and safety may be assessed but, on theoretical grounds, prostaglandin analogues should be more successful than an antiprogesterone agent alone.

Conclusions

The induction of labour has been the cause of many debates between obstetricians and their patients. The rising trend of induction noted in the 1970s is now falling, and the perceived need to interfere in an otherwise uncomplicated prolonged pregnancy has also decreased. Both these events would appear to be without detriment; however, this is not an indication for decreased vigilance. There would appear to be a specific need to monitor those pregnancies which would previously have been induced.

The advent of vaginal and oral prostaglandin therapy has had a significant impact upon obstetric practice, and there is a need to include, somewhere in the statistics for the induction of labour, all those labours which followed cervical ripening with prostaglandins. This will become particularly important as more potent prostaglandins are synthesized.

References

Allott, H. A. and Palmer, C. R. (1993). Sweeping the membranes – a valuable procedure in stimulating the onset of labour? *British Journal of Obstetrics and Gynaecology* **100**, 898–903.

American College of Obstetricians and Gynecologists (1987). Induction and augmentation of labour. *Technical Bulletin, no. 110*. American College of Obstetricians and Gynecologists, Washington DC.

Arulkumaran, S., Gibb, D. M. F., Tamby Raja, R. L., Heng, S. H., and Ratnan, S. S. (1985). Failed induction of labour. *Australian and New Zealand Journal of Obstetrics and Gynaecology* **25**, 190–3.

Bakketeig, L. S. and Bergsjo, L. (1989). Post-term pregnancy: magnitude of the problem. In *Effective care in pregnancy and childbirth* (ed. I. Chalmers, M. Enkin, and M. J. N. C. Keirse), pp. 765–75. Oxford University Press, Oxford.

Bakketeig, L. S., Hoffman, H. J., and Harley, E. E. (1979). The tendency to repeat gestational age and birthweight in successive pregnancies. *American Journal of Obstetrics and Gynecology* **135**, 1086–103.

Bakos, O. and Backstrom, T. (1987). Induction of labour. *Acta Obstetrica et Gynaecologica Scandinavica* **66**, 537–41.

Bamber, M. (1990). Gemeprost vaginal pressaries for inducing third-trimester intrauterine death. *British Journal of Obstetrics and Gynaecology* **97**, 366.

Bergsjo, P., Gui-dan, H., Su-qin, Y., Zhi-zeng, G., and Bakketeig, L. S. (1989). Comparison of induced versus non-induced labour in post-term pregnancy. *Acta Obstetrica et Gynaecologica Scandinavica* **68**, 683–7.

Blakemore, K. J., Qin, N. G., Petrie, R. H., and Paine, L. L. (1990). A prospective comparison of hourly and quarter-hourly oxytocin dose increase intervals for the induction of labour at term. *Obstetrics and Gynecology* **75**, 757–61.

Boyd, M. E., Usher, R. H., and McLean, F. H. (1983). Fetal macrosomia. *Obstetrics and Gynecology* **61**, 715–22.

Butler, N. R. and Alberman, E. D. (1969). *Perinatal problems*, pp. 163–83. E. and S. Livingstone, Edinburgh.

Cabrol, D., Dubois, C., Cronje, H., Gonnet, J. M., Guillot, M., Maria, B., *et al.* (1990).

Induction of labour with mifepristone in fetal death. *American Journal of Obstetrics and Gynecology* **163**, 540–2.

Calder, A. A. (1991). Reasons for, and methods of, induction. *Journal of Obstetrics and Gynaecology* **supp. 1**, S2–5.

Calder, A. A. and Embrey, M. P. (1975). Induction of labour. In *The management of labour* (ed. R. Beard, M. Brudenell, P. Dunn, and D. Fairweather, pp. 62–9. Royal College of Obstetricians and Gynaecologists, London.

Calder, A. A., Moar, A. A., Ounsted, M. K., and Turnbull, A. C. (1974). Increased bilirubin level in neonates after induction of labour by intravenous prostaglandin E_2 or oxytocin. *Lancet* **ii**, 139–42.

Campbell, N., Harvey, D., and Norman, A. P. (1975). Increased frequency of neonatal jaundice in a maternity hospital. *British Medical Journal* **2**, 548–52.

Cardozo, L. D., Fysh, J., and Pearce, J. M. (1986). Prolonged pregnancy: the management debate. *British Medical Journal* **293**, 1059–63.

Cario, G. M. (1984). Conservative management of prolonged pregnancy using fetal heart rate monitoring only. *British Journal of Obstetrics and Gynaecology* **91**, 23–30.

Chamberlain, G., Philips, E., Howlett, B., and Masters, K. (1978). *British births, 1970*, Vol. 2, p. 180. Heinemann Medical, London.

Chapman, M., Lawrence, D., Sims, C., and Bennett, M. (1984). Induction of labour by prostaglandin pessary or oxytocin infusion after spontaneous rupture of the membranes. *Journal of Obstetrics and Gynaecology* **4**, 185–7.

Chard, T. and Gibbens, G. L. D. (1983). Spurt release of oxytocin during surgical induction of labour in women. *American Journal of Obstetrics and Gynecology* **147**, 678–80.

Clifford, S. H. (1954). Postmaturity—with placental dysfunction. Clinical syndrome and pathological findings. *Journal of Paediatrics* **44**, 1–13.

Crowley, P. (1989). Post-term pregnancy: induction or surveillance? In *Effective care in pregnancy and childbirth* (ed. I. Chalmers, M. Enkin, and M. J. N. C. Keirse), pp. 776–91. Oxford University Press, Oxford.

Daw, E. (1973). Oxytocin-induced rupture of the primigravid uterus. *Journal of Obstetrics and Gynaecology of the British Commonwealth* **80**, 374–5.

Eden, R. D., Seifert, L. S., Winegar, A., and Spellacy, W. N. (1987). Perinatal characteristics of uncomplicated postdate pregnancies. *Obstetrics and Gynecology* **69**, 296–9.

Fields, H. (1960). Complications of elective induction. *Obstetrics and Gynecology* **15**, 476–80.

Fletcher, H. M., Mitchell, S., Simeon, D., Frederick, J., and Brown, D. (1993). Intravaginal misoprostol as a cervical ripening agent. *British Journal of Obstetrics and Gynaecology* **100**, 641–4.

Fox, H. (1983). Placental pathology. In *Progress in obstetrics and gynaecology* (ed. J. Studd), Vol. 3, pp. 47–56. Churchill Livingstone, Edinburgh.

Freeman, R. K., Garite, T. J., Modanlou, H., Dorchester, W., Rommal, C., and Devaney, M. (1981). Postdate pregnancy. *American Journal of Obstetrics and Gynecology* **140**, 128–35.

Ghosh, I. and Hudson, F. P. (1972). Oxytocic agents and neonatal hyperbilirubinaemia. *Lancet* **ii**, 823.

Gibb, D. M. F., Cardozo, L. D., Studd, J. W., and Cooper, J. W. W. (1982). Prolonged pregnancy: is induction of labour indicated? *British Journal of Obstetrics and Gynaecology* **89**, 292–5.

Grant, J. M. (1993). Sweeping the membranes in prolonged pregnancy. *British Journal of Obstetrics and Gynaecology* **100**, 889–90.

Grant, J. M. (1994). Induction of labour confers benefits in prolonged pregnancy. *British Journal of Obstetrics and Gynaecology* **101**, 99–102.

Graves, G. R., Baskett, T. F., Gray, J. H., and Luther, E. R. (1985). The efficacy of vaginal administration of various doses of prostaglandin E$_2$ gel on cervical ripening and induction of labour. *American Journal of Obstetrics and Gynecology* **151**, 178–81.

Homburg, R., Ludomirski, A., and Insler, B. (1979). Detection of fetal risk in postmaturity. *British Journal of Obstetrics and Gynaecology* **86**, 759–64.

Husslein, P., Kofler, E., Rasmussen, A., Sumulong, L., Fuchs, A. R., and Fuchs, F. (1983). Oxytocin and initiation of human parturition. *American Journal of Obstetrics and Gynecology* **147**, 503–7.

Johnson, I. R., Macpherson, M. B. A., Welch, C. C., and Filshie, T. M. (1985). A comparison of lamicel and prostaglandin E$_2$ vaginal gel for cervical ripening prior to induction of labour. *American Journal of Obstetrics and Gynecology* **151**, 604–7.

Johnson, J. M., Harman, C. R., Lange, I. R., and Manning, F. A. (1986). Biophysical profile scoring in the management of the post-term pregnancy. *American Journal of Obstetrics and Gynecology* **154**, 269–73.

Kanhai, H. H. H. and Keirse, M. J. N. C. (1989). Induction of labour after fetal death. *British Journal of Obstetrics and Gynaecology* **96**, 1400–4.

Kazzi, G. M., Bottoms, S. F., and Rosen, M. G. (1982). Efficacy and safety of Laminaria Digitata for pre-induction ripening of the cervix. *Obstetrics and Gynecology* **60**, 440–3.

Keegan, K. A. and Paul, R. H. (1980). Antepartum fetal heart rate testing. *American Journal of Obstetrics and Gynecology* **136**, 75–80.

Keirse, M. J. N. C. and Kanhai, H. H. H. (1989). Induction of labour after fetal death. In *Effective care in pregnancy and childbirth* (ed. I. Chalmers, M. Enkin, and M. J. N. C. Keirse), pp. 1118–26. Oxford University Press, Oxford.

Keirse, M. J. N. C. and van Oppen, A. C. C. (1989a). Preparing the cervix for induction of labour. In *Effective care in pregnancy and childbirth* (ed. I. Chalmers, M. Enkin, and M. J. N. C. Keirse), pp. 988–1056. Oxford University Press, Oxford.

Keirse, M. J. N. C. and van Oppen, A. C. C. (1989b). Comparison of prostaglandin and oxytocin for induction of labour. In *Effective care in pregnancy and childbirth* (ed. I. Chalmers, M. Enkin, and M. H. N. C. Keirse), pp. 1080–111. Oxford University Press, Oxford.

Lilienthal, C. M. and Ward, J. P. (1971). Medical induction of labour. *Journal of Obstetrics and Gynaecology of the British Commonwealth* **78**, 317–21.

MacDonald, D. (1970). Surgical induction of labour. *American Journal of Obstetrics and Gynecology* **107**, 908–11.

Macfarlane, A., Cole, S., and Hey, E. (1986). Comparison of data from Regional Perinatal Mortality Surveys. *British Journal of Obstetrics and Gynaecology* **93**, 1224–32.

MacKenzie, I. Z. and Embrey, N. P. (1979). A comparison of PGE$_2$ and PGF$_{s\alpha}$ vaginal gel for ripening the cervix before induction of labour. *British Journal of Obstetrics and Gynaecology* **86**, 167–70.

Miller, F. C. and Read, J. A. (1981). Intrapartum assessment of the postdate fetus. *American Journal of Obstetrics and Gynecology* **141**, 516–20.

Mitchell, M. D., Flint, A. P. F., Bibby, J., Brunt, J., Anderson, A. B. M., and Turnbull, A. C. (1977). Rapid increases in plasma prostaglandin concentration after vaginal examination and amniotomy. *British Medical Journal* **2**, 1183–5.

Mittendorf, R., Williams, M. A., Berkey, C. S., Lieberman, E., and Monson, R. (1993). Prediction of human gestation length. *American Journal of Obstetrics and Gynecology* **168**, 480–4.

Moran, D. J. (1989). Gemeprost vaginal pessaries for inducing third-trimester intrauterine deaths. *British Journal of Obstetrics and Gynaecology* **96**, 1245–6.

Muldoon, M. J. (1968). A prospective study of intrauterine infection following surgical induction of labour. *Journal of Obstetrics and Gynaecology of the British Commonwealth* **75**, 1140–5.

Mwambingo, F. T. (1985). Water intoxication and oxytocin. *British Medical Journal* **290**, 113.

Naismith, W. C. M. K., Barr, W., and MacVicar, J. (1973). Comparison of intravaginal $PGF_{2\alpha}$ and E_2 with intravenous oxytocin in the induction of labour. *Journal of Obstetrics and Gynaecology of the British Commonwealth* **80**, 531–5.

Niswander, K. R. and Patterson, R. J. (1963). Induction hazards. *Obstetrics and Gynecology* **22**, 228–33.

O'Driscoll, D. (1972). Oxytocic agents and neonatal hyperbilirubinaemia. *Lancet* **ii**, 1150.

Patterson, W. M. (1971). Amniotomy, with or without simultaneous oxytocin infusion. *Journal of Obstetrics and Gynaecology of the British Commonwealth* **78**, 310–16.

Perryman, D., Yeast, J. D., and Holst, V. (1992). Cervical ripening: a randomized study comparing prostaglandin E_2 gel to prostaglandin E_2 suppository. *Obstetrics and Gynecology* **79**, 670–2.

Ratnam, S. S., Khew, K. S., Chen, C., and Lim, T. C. (1974). Oral prostaglandin E_2 induction of labour. *Australian and New Zealand Journal of Obstetrics and Gynaecology* **14**, 26–30.

Rayburn, W. F. (1989). Prostaglandin E_2 gel for cervical ripening and induction of labour. *American Journal of Obstetrics and Gynecology* **160**, 529–34.

Saleh, Y. Z. (1975). Surgical induction of labour with and without oxytocin infusion. *Australian and New Zealand Journal of Obstetrics and Gynaecology* **15**, 80–3.

Scher, J., Jeng, D. Y., Moshirpur, J., and Kerenyi, T. D. (1980). A comparison between vaginal prostaglandin E_2 suppositories and extra-amniotic prostaglandins for the management of fetal death *in utero*. *American Journal of Obstetrics and Gynecology* **137**, 769–72.

Schneider, J. M., Olsen, R. W., and Curet, L. B. (1978). Screening for fetal and neonatal risk in the postdate pregnancy. *American Journal of Obstetrics and Gynecology* **131**, 473–8.

Schwartz, R. H. and Jones, R. W. A. (1978). Transplacental hyponatraemia due to oxytocin. *British Medical Journal* **1**, 152–3.

Setna, F., Chatterjee, T. K., and Black, M. D. (1967). An assessment of the safety of surgical induction of labour. *Journal of Obstetrics and Gynaecology of the British Commonwealth* **74**, 262–5.

Shafi, M. I., Byrne, P., Luesley, D. M., and Pogmore, J. R. (1989). Gemeprost vaginal pessaries for inducing third-trimester intrauterine death. *British Journal of Obstetrics and Gynaecology* **96**, 745–6.

Shime, J., Librach, C. L., Gare, D. J., and Cook, C. J. (1986). The influence of prolonged pregnancy on infant development at one and two years of age. *American Journal of Obstetrics and Gynecology* **154**, 341–5.

Sivasuriya, M., Tan, K. L., Salmon, Y. M., and Karim, S. M. M. (1978). Neonatal serum bilirubin levels in spontaneous and induced labour. *British Journal of Obstetrics and Gynaecology* **85**, 619–23.

Smith, C. V., Rayburn, W. F., Cunnar, R. E., Fredston, G. R., and Phillips, C. B. (1990). Double-blind comparison of intravaginal prostaglandin E_2 gel and 'chip' for preinduction cervical ripening. *American Journal of Obstetrics and Gynecology* **163**, 845–7.

Steer, P. J., Carter, N. C., Choong, K., Hanson, M., Gordon, A. J., and Pradhen, P.

(1985). A multicentre prospective randomized controlled trial of induction of labour with an automatic closed-loop feedback controlled oxytocin infusion system. *British Journal of Obstetrics and Gynaecology* **92**, 1127–33.

Swann, R. O. (1958). Induction of labour by stripping membranes. *Obstetrics and Gynecology* **11**, 74–8.

Tew, M. (1986). Do obstetric interventions make birth safer? *British Journal of Obstetrics and Gynaecology* **93**, 659–74.

Thomas, G. and Blackwell, R. J. (1974). A controlled trial of the Cardiff automated infusion system in the management of induced labour. *British Journal of Clinical Practice* **28**, 203–6.

Thornton, S., Davison, J. M., and Baylis, P. H. (1989). Amniotomy-induced labour is not mediated by endogenous oxytocin. *British Journal of Obstetrics and Gynaecology* **96**, 945–8.

Tuck, S. M., Cardozo, L. D., Studd, J. W. W., and Gibb, D. M. F. (1983). Obstetric characteristics in different racial groups. *British Journal of Obstetrics and Gynaecology* **90**, 892–7.

Turnbull, A. C. and Anderson, A. B. M. (1967). Induction of labour. *Journal of Obstetrics and Gynaecology of the British Commonwealth* **74**, 849–54.

Vorherr, H. (1975). Placental insufficiency in relation to post-term pregnancy and fetal postmaturity. *American Journal of Obstetrics and Gynecology* **123**, 67–107.

Votta, R. A. and Cibils, L. A. (1993). Active management of prolonged pregnancy. *American Journal of Obstetrics and Gynecology* **168**, 557–63.

Wei, J. S. and Lan, S. L. (1988). Cervical ripening. *Australian and New Zealand Journal of Obstetrics and Gynaecology* **28**, 52–61.

Wein, P. (1989). Efficacy of different starting doses of oxytocin for induction of labour. *Obstetrics and Gynecology* **74**, 863–8.

Westergaard, J. G., Lang, A. P., Pederson, G. T., and Sesher, N. J. (1983). Use of oral oxytocics for stimulation of labour in cases of premature rupture of the membranes at term. *Acta Obstetrica et Gynaecologica Scandinavica* **62**, 111–16.

Wilson, P. D. (1978). A comparison of four methods of ripening the unfavourable cervix. *British Journal of Obstetrics and Gynaecology* **85**, 941–4.

Yudkin, P., Frumar, A. N., Anderson, A. B. M., and Turnbull, A. C. (1979). A prospective study of induction of labour. *British Journal of Obstetrics and Gynaecology* **86**, 257–65.

Zwerdling, M. A. (1967). Factors pertaining to prolonged pregnancy and its outcome. *Paediatrics* **40**, 202–12.

20 The management of breech presentation

Breech presentation is the commonest malpresentation and is associated with increased fetal morbidity and mortality, partly due to the association with congenital malformations, partly due to the association with prematurity, and partly due to trauma associated with the delivery. There is also an association with an increased maternal operative delivery rate. This chapter examines these issues in detail.

The incidence of breech presentation

The incidence of breech presentation at delivery lies between 1 and 4 per cent. A range of estimates quoted in the literature includes 1.1 per cent (De Crespigny and Pepperell 1979) 2.5 per cent, (Bingham *et al*. 1987) 2.7 per cent (Christian *et al*. 1990) 3.5 per cent (Kaupilla 1975) and 4.1 per cent (Rovinsky *et al*. 1973).

These statistics require modification for there are numerous factors associated with an increased risk of breech presentation. It is more appropriate that these factors are considered to be associations with an increased incidence of breech presentations rather than to consider such factors as aetiological.

They include:

(1) fetal abnormality;

(2) previous breech presentation;

(3) prematurity;

(4) extended fetal legs;

(5) placenta praevia;

(6) cornual placenta;

(7) short cord;

(8) small pelvis.

The association between breech presentation and congenital malformation will be discussed in the next subsection (p. 521).

A woman who has previously delivered a baby presenting by the breech has an increased risk of breech presentation at delivery in a subsequent pregnancy, possibly related to the association between breech presentation and uterine abnormality. Thus, Hall *et al*. (1965) reported that whilst the incidence of breech delivery was 3.2 per cent of an overall singleton population of almost

Table 20.1 The influence of gestational age

Weeks of pregnancy	Presentation		
	Cephalic (%)	Breech (%)	Other (%)
25	56	22	22
28	66	24	10
32	81	13	6
36	91	6	3
40	92	5	3

From Scheer and Nubar (1976)

200 000 births, 14 per cent of women with breech presentation at delivery had previously delivered a baby by the breech.

The association between breech presentation and preterm delivery is well recognized; Scheer and Nubar (1976), classifying presentation by gestational age, demonstrated the decreasing incidence of breech presentation noted antenatally as pregnancy progresses. This is illustrated in Table 20.1. Thus, the earlier preterm delivery occurs, the more likely it is that the fetus will present by the breech. Brenner *et al.* (1974) reported that 35 per cent of 1016 consecutive singleton breech deliveries had occurred by the 36th week of pregnancy compared with only 7 per cent of 29 343 singleton non-breech deliveries, whilst Hall *et al.* (1965) reported that 24 per cent of their 6044 singleton breech deliveries resulted in babies weighing less than 2500 g.

The presence of extended fetal legs will make it more difficult for a fetus to rotate spontaneously to a cephalic presentation, whilst a small pelvis will keep the head in the abdomen. However, such 'classical explanations' may only be present in 15 per cent of breech presentations (Tompkins 1946).

The placental site is considered to be an important factor in the aetiology of breech presentation. Thus, breech presentation co-exists with placenta praevia in 1.2 per cent of all breech presentations, whilst the presence of a cornual placenta, as demonstrated by ultrasound, may be found in 73 per cent of breech presentations near term compared with 5 per cent of cephalic presentations near term (Fianu and Vaclavinkova 1978; Tompkins 1946). There is also evidence that the mean umbilical cord length is shorter in breech presentations, by a mean of 4.6 cm, than in cephalic presentations (Soernes and Bakke 1986).

Congenital malformations

There is an increased incidence of congenital malformation in babies who present by the breech rather than by the head. Thus, Rovinsky *et al.* (1973) reported that 2.1 per cent of 2145 term breech deliveries were associated with major lethal congenital malformations compared with 0.8 per cent of almost 85 000 cephalic presentations, whilst Brenner *et al.* (1974) reported that 6.3 per cent of 1016 consecutive single breech deliveries were associated with a fetal malformation compared with 2.4 per cent of 29 343 consecutive single non-breech deliveries. The major abnormalities appear to include central nervous system lesions (hydrocephaly and anencephaly, especially), cardiovascular abnormalities, gastrointestinal tract abnormalities, and multiple congenital malformations.

Bingham and Lilford (1987) reviewed 19 studies from the literature and reported that the mortality due to congenital malformations in 7219 term breech presentations was 8.59 per 1000, whereas the mortality due to congenital malformations in a total population of 586 278 live births over the same period of time was only 1.34 per 1000. They suggested that the vast majority of these abnormalities could be detected before birth using ultrasound, and that the incidence of lethal fetal abnormality in term breeches not detectable by ultrasound was only 0.55 per 1000, trisomy and pulmonary hypoplasia being the major two undetected problems.

There is also an increased incidence of congenital dislocation of the hip associated with breech presentation. Thus, Kaupilla (1975) reported that 5 per cent of breech deliveries resulted in babies with congenital dislocation of the hip, whereas the incidence of this condition for the overall population was less than 1 per cent. However, this abnormality was as common in those babies delivered vaginally by the breech as in those delivered abdominally, suggesting that it is the breech presentation rather than the mode of delivery which is the associated factor. This association has been confirmed by other authors (Clausen and Nielsen 1988).

Mortality, morbidity, and breech presentation

The association between lethal fetal malformations and breech presentation has already been described, as has the association between breech delivery and prematurity. Both of these factors are major contributors to perinatal mortality. Thus, Kaupilla (1975) found that the complications of prematurity accounted for 25 per cent of the perinatal mortality associated with preterm delivery, whereas fetal abnormality accounted for 10 per cent of the perinatal mortality associated with preterm delivery and 32 per cent of the mortality associated with term breech delivery.

De Crispigny and Pepperell (1979) reported that whilst breech delivery accounted for only 1 per cent of 62 998 births, it was associated with 24 per cent of perinatal deaths. The perinatal mortality rate for their 664 breech deliveries was 104 per 1000, some five times that for the population in general. Of their 69 perinatal deaths, two-thirds were stillborn and one-third died in the neonatal period. The major causes of perinatal abnormality in this series were fatal abnormality (29 per cent), death *in utero* before labour (27.5 per cent), death during labour (14.5 per cent), and neonatal death (29 per cent). Kaupilla (1975) reported that trauma and asphyxia accounted for a greater proportion of deaths in term breeches than in preterm breeches. Thus, 5 per cent of preterm

Table 20.2 Breech presentation and mortality

Type of breech	No.	Perinatal mortality per 1000
All	6044	123
Frank	3630	102
Complete	285	144
Footling	1567	148
Not stated	562	171

From Hall *et al.* (1965)

breech mortality was due to intraventricular cerebral haemorrhage, whilst 20 per cent of deaths in term breeches were due to asphyxia, and a further 14 per cent were due to trauma.

The perinatal mortality rate in breech presentation is greater for multiparous patients than for primiparous ones. Thus, the perinatal mortality rate in 3707 multiparous breech deliveries was 145 per 1000 compared with 87 in 2337 primiparous deliveries. These authors also classified mortality by the type of breech presentation, the overall mortality being 123 per 1000 for 6044 breech deliveries, and lower for frank breeches than for complete (or full) breeches, or footling breeches, as shown in Table 20.2 (Hall *et al.* 1965). These figures are, in part, explained by the prolapse of either the umbilical cord or fetal body associated with breech presentation in general and non-frank breeches in particular. Hall *et al.* (1965) reported that prolapse of the cord occurred in 0.3 per cent of non-breech presentations but in 5.2 per cent of breech presentations. Hay (1959) reported that a prolapse of the cord occurred in 3.6 per cent of 165 singleton breech presentations and Kaupilla (1975) stated that cord accidents accounted for 10 per cent of the perinatal mortality of the term breech. Rovinsky *et al.* (1973) noted that cord prolapse occurred in 1.7 per cent of 1632 frank breeches, with a mortality of 11 per cent, and 10.9 per cent of 513 complete breeches, with a mortality of 5 per cent.

The perinatal mortality associated with vaginal breech delivery will be due to either hypoxia or trauma, or both. In a review of the literature, Duignan (1982) concluded that intraventricular cerebral haemorrhage, generally due to hypoxia, was more common than intracranial haemorrhage due to trauma and accounted for 7 per cent of perinatal deaths.

There is also an increased perinatal morbidity associated with vaginal breech delivery. Alexopoulos (1973) reported an eight-year follow-up study of 443 infants surviving vaginal breech delivery and weighing over 1500 g at birth. Some degree of morbidity, including hypoxia, asphyxia, and neurological damage, was reported in 15.8 per cent of the infants during the neonatal period. Some eight children (all asphyxiated at birth) had developmental delay and/or spasticity, whilst 2.7 per cent, of infants had evidence of brachial nerve damage at birth, this was still present at eight years of age in 1.1 per cent of the children.

Soft tissue trauma relating to breech delivery is anecdotally described, including fracture of the skull, long bones, and clavicle, trauma to the spinal cord, and injury to the liver, spleen, kidney, adrenal glands, and back muscles (Coltart 1989).

The conclusion that such perinatal mortality and morbidity may, therefore, be avoided by the use of universal Caesarean section for the mature breech cannot be substantiated since longterm neurological problems would appear to be equally common after abdominal delivery as after vaginal delivery, suggesting that it is the breech presentation rather than the delivery which is the predisposing factor. Faber-Nijholt *et al.* (1983) studied 256 surviving children after breech delivery matched with controls delivered vaginally with a cephalic presentation. These children were assessed neurologically at various stages during their first ten years of life. There were no significant differences in neurological findings between those delivered abdominally by the breech (20 per cent) or vaginally by the breech (80 per cent). In a larger series of 1240 singleton breech infants without congenital abnormality, there was no increased risk for vaginal delivery compared with Caesarean section (Croughan-Minihane *et al.* 1990). From a literature review, Westgren and Ingermarsson (1988) concluded that, when selected breech delivery occurred, 'the rate of neurodevelopmental handicap will not be higher than in abdominally delivered breech infants or in cephalic presentations'.

External cephalic version

The practice of external cephalic version, initially popular in obstetric practice, lost popularity partly because of an apparent lack of influence upon the incidence of breech presentation at term and partly because of the dangers inherent in the technique. In recent years, the possible place of external cephalic version has become clearer. In summary, the practice of external cephalic version between 32 and 36 weeks' gestation is no longer indicated, but external cephalic version beyond the 37th week of gestation would appear to be indicated.

One major criticism of the practice of external cephalic version before the 37th week of pregnancy is that spontaneous cephalic version undoudtedly occurs in the majority of breech presentations and this has made the results of non-controlled trials of external cephalic version difficult to interpret (please see Table 20.1). Westgren *et al.* (1985) reported a prospective study of 310 singleton breech presentations identified at the 32nd week of pregnancy in whom spontaneous version occurred in 57 per cent overall, but in 76 per cent of multiparous patients and 24 per cent of primiparous ones. Moreover, spontaneous version from a cephalic version to a breech presentation also occurred in 5 per cent of an antenatal population during the third trimester. Spontaneous version may be encouraged by changes in maternal posture, including the adoption of the knee–chest position for a short period of time (Hofmeyr 1983).

Table 20.3 The value of external cephalic version

	External cephalic version	No external cephalic version
No.	278	282
% Cephalic at delivery	70.1	21.3
% Breech at delivery	29.9	78.7
% Caesarean section for breech	14.7	31.9

From Hofmeyr (1991)

The place of external cephalic version before term in non-randomized trials was assessed by Hofmeyr (1989) who performed a meta-analysis of nine trials involving 4177 patients in whom external cephalic version was attempted. There was a cephalic presentation at birth in 90 per cent and a fetal death rate of 0.4 per cent related to the version. The conclusion from this meta-analysis of non-randomized trials together with three randomized trials was that external cephalic version before the 37th week of pregnancy failed to demonstrate any beneficial effect upon either the incidence of breech presentation at delivery or the incidence of Caesarean section for delivery.

External cephalic version is not without its complications and these have to be balanced against the risks of either vaginal delivery or Caesarean section. Fetal death *in utero* is said to occur in between 0.4 per cent and 0.9 per cent of all fetuses who undergo external cephalic version. Other complications include antepartum haemorrhage (3 per cent), preterm labour (1.2 per cent), and premature rupture of the membranes (0.6 per cent) (Bradley-Watson 1975; Hofmeyr 1989).

There is no longer a case for performing external cephalic version before the 37th week of pregnancy.

External cephalic version would appear to be more useful when performed after the 37th week of pregnancy (Hofmeyr 1989, 1991; Mahomed *et al.* 1991; Marchick 1988). Hofmeyr (1991) assessed the results from five randomized controlled trials of external cephalic version beyond the 37th week of pregnancy. From a meta-analysis of these studies, external cephalic version was associated with an incidence of breech presentation in 30 per cent of patients at delivery compared with 79 per cent of controls, a reduction in the incidence of breech presentation of 60 per cent. Similarly, the need for Caesarean section in those patients who had undergone external cephalic version was 15 per cent compared with 32 per cent in controls, a reduction of 54 per cent. The data from which the statistics are derived are shown in Table 20.3.

External cephalic version has even been used during labour, Ferguson and Dyson (1985) turning 11 out of 15 breech presentations at term in labour with intact membranes without complication (73.3 per cent). None of the above randomized trials at term involved tocolysis using betasympathomimetics, but Morrison *et al.* (1986) advocated tocolysis, enabling them to turn 68 per cent

Table 20.4 The outcome of delivery

Type of breech delivery	%	Mortality due to trauma (%)
Caesarean section	23.4	0
Assisted breech delivery	68.4	0.9
Breech extraction	8.2	6.0

From Todd and Steer (1963)

of breech presentations without serious complication at term. Whilst the utility of external cephalic version during labour has yet to be proven in larger studies, there can be no doubt that external cephalic version beyond the 37th week of pregnancy in patients not in labour and in whom there is a breech presentation should be selectively performed.

The mode of delivery—the mature breech

The dilemmas faced in breech delivery relate to whether or not selected vaginal breech delivery is more hazardous to the baby than would be universal Caesarean section and, if this were so, would there be a price to pay in terms of increased maternal morbidity and mortality from Caesarean section for this indication. The Caesarean section rate in breech presentation is currently increasing without any apparent fall in the perinatal mortality rate in mature babies (Olan *et al.* 1988).

It has already been stated that the universal use of Caesarean section in breech presentation will not have a dramatic effect upon perinatal mortality or morbidity. However, some mature babies presenting by the breech will be better delivered abdominally, and the case for selected vaginal breech delivery will be discussed below. It should also be considered whether elective abdominal delivery increases the maternal risks or whether, in fact, the potential benefits are maternal as well as fetal.

Older series from the literature support the premise that the trauma from vaginal breech delivery will be avoided by Caesarean section. Thus, Todd and Steer (1963) reported a series of 1006 breech deliveries and, as can be seen from Table 20.4, there were a greater number of deaths related to trauma from spontaneous or assisted breech delivery compared with abdominal delivery. Such studies also demonstrate that there is a highly significant increase in mortality associated with breech extraction, suggesting that this procedure should not be performed except in a dire emergency in the presence of a singleton breech. Even in carefully selected contemporary series, vaginal breech delivery is associated with a significant incidence of intra-partum and neonatal death in the absence of congenital anomalies, perhaps up to the 1 per cent level (Cheng and Hannah 1993; Thorpe-Beeston *et al.* 1992).

The question to be answered is whether or not there is a safe place in current practice for selective vaginal breech delivery. From the literature, the typical criteria used to select patients for abdominal delivery, in the absence of other obstetric pathology, would include:

(1) elderly primigravida:

(2) fetal weight estimate greater than 3.6 kg;

(3) unsatisfactory maternal pelvimetry;

(4) extension of fetal head;

(5) full or footling breech.

These criteria require further discussion. Although it has already been stated that the perinatal mortality rate for multiparous breech delivery exceeds that for primiparous, the 'elderly primigravida' may be at specific risk. Thus, Racker (1943) reported two retrospective series of breech presentations in primigravidae aged 30 years or more. In the first, the perinatal mortality in 128 vaginal deliveries was 33.5 per cent and the perinatal mortality for 62 such patients delivered by Caesarean section was zero. However, Hall and Kohl (1956), also in a retrospective series, reported 30 primigravidae aged 35 years or over with a breech presentation and, although 13 per cent of the fetuses died, they all died before labour and no death could be attributed to the mode of delivery (vaginal, $n = 18$; abdominal, $n = 12$). Perhaps the most important criteria which will determine whether or not selective vaginal breech delivery is safe is fetal weight. The effect of fetal weight was examined by Neilson (1970), who reported 203 singleton term breech presentations all of whom were of birthweight 3.8 kg or more. Vaginal delivery was associated with trauma sufficient to cause death in two babies and fracture in three. Neonatal neurological damage (twitching or severe irritability) occurred in 16, giving an overall incidence of trauma of 10.3 per cent. Rovinsky *et al.* (1973) reported that the least birth trauma occurred in fetuses of birthweight less than 3399 g (1.5 per cent mortality due to trauma) delivered vaginally by the breech ($n = 1050$), whereas for 71 babies weighing 4000 g or over, the mortality from trauma was 5.6 per cent. In a more recent study, a trial of vaginal delivery was successful in 36 per cent of breech fetuses weighing greater than 3500 g compared with 66 per cent of breech fetuses weighing less than 3500 g (Bingham *et al.* 1987).

Many authors suggest that the use of pelvimetry will define a patient with a potentially hazardous pelvis. Tatum *et al.* (1985) reported a retrospective study of 174 patients who delivered vaginally and who were selected from a total group of 580 term breech presentations (30 per cent). The only mortality was due to fetal abnormality, none being due to the mode of delivery. Those selection criteria used to define a 'satisfactory pelvis' were:

(1) anteroposterior diameter of the inlet, 11.0 cm or greater;

(2) transverse diameter of the inlet, 12.0 cm or greater;

(3) midspinous diameter, 10.0 cm or greater;

(4) hollow sacrum;

(5) normal subpublic arch.

Table 20.5 The value of pelvimetry

| Pelvimetry result | No. | Outcome | No. | Mortality due to birth trauma | |
				No.	%
AP inlet less than 11.0 cm	131	Caesarean section	79	0	0
		vaginal delivery	52	3	6
AP inlet 11.0 cm or more	233	Caesarean section	34	0	0
		vaginal delivery	199	1	0.5

From Todd and Steer (1963)

Table 20.6 The value of pelvimetry

| Model of delivery | No. | Antenatal pelvimetry | No. with evidence of birth trauma | |
			Pelvimetry	No pelvimetry
Caesarean section (elective)	31	12	0	1
Caesarean section (in labour)	81	37	0	3
Vaginal delivery	116	37	3	10

From Ridley *et al.* (1982)

However, from a study of the literature, the belief is that selection based upon pelvimetry measurements is not forthcoming, save perhaps to identify a pelvis which is unexpectedly small. Some series do suggest that antenatal pelvimetry will be helpful. Thus, Todd and Steer (1963) reviewed 1006 term breech deliveries, of whom 76.6 per cent were delivered vaginally. Some 364 patients had a pelvimetry estimate performed antenatally, the results of which are summarized in Table 20.5. This would suggest that the avoidance of vaginal delivery in the presence of a pelvis below average size should reduce birth trauma. Ridley *et al.* (1982) reported a series of 228 patients with singleton term breech presentations of whom 86 underwent antenatal pelvimetry. There were no statistically significant differences in the neonatal condition of those babies delivered by Caesarean section compared with those delivered vaginally in the presence of a 'favourable pelvimetry', but trauma was significantly increased in those patients delivered vaginally without antenatal pelvimetry (see Table 20.6).

However, other series have suggested that a knowledge of the pelvic diameters will not be helpful. Thus, Rovinsky *et al.* (1973) were unable to demonstrate that erect lateral pelvimetry was associated with a lower mortality or morbidity in a non-randomized retrospective series of 1720 cases of vaginal breech delivery. These results are shown in Table 20.7, but it is possible that those patients who were known to have a large pelvis, based on clinical examination or past obstetric history, may not have had a pelvimetry performed. Bingham

Table 20.7 The value of pelvimetry

Group	No. of cases	Perinatal mortality rate (per 1000)	% With neonatal morbidity
Pelvimetry			
Primigravidae	387	5.2	1.8
Multigravidae	233	17.2	2.2
Total	620	9.7	1.9
No pelvimetry			
Primigravidae	438	4.6	0.7
Multigravidae	662	0.0	1.1
Total	1100	1.8	0.9

From Rovinsky *et al.* (1973)

et al. (1987) could find no relationship between the mean conjugate of those delivered vaginally (12.7 cm) or abdominally (12.8 cm).

It would seem that the use of pelvimetry may be to exclude selected vaginal delivery in the presence of a small pelvis, whilst the presence of a larger pelvis does not allow for the accurate prediction of vaginal delivery but may allow for a trial of descent of the breech.

The size of the maternal pelvis may be assessed by more modern techniques, and it is yet to be proven whether or not these will have a beneficial effect on the selection of patients for vaginal breech delivery. Gimovsky *et al.* (1985) recommend X-ray pelvimetry by computerized tomography scanning which is associated with a lower exposure to irradiation than conventional X-ray pelvimetry, and may be more accurate. In a prospective series, 81 per cent of 85 women who had a satisfactory pelvis based upon computerized tomography scanning delivered vaginally without complication (Christian *et al.* 1990). The use of magnetic resonance imaging, which gives reliable pelvimetry results without any ionizing radiation, is also described (van Loon *et al.* 1990).

There is good evidence to suggest that a deflexion attitude of the fetal head is a relative contraindication to vaginal delivery. Ballas *et al.* (1978) radiologically assessed the deflexion attitude of the fetal head in 233 consecutive breech presentations during labour, and recommended Caesarean section for those which were hyperextended, that is, the angle of cervical spine compared with thoracic spine of greater than 90 ° (0.8 per cent of breeches). They allowed those fetuses with an extended head, but an angle of less than 90 °, to deliver vaginally (15.6 per cent), without trauma. Westgren *et al.* (1981) reported hyperextension in 7.4 per cent of 445 breech presentations, and in view of the neurological sequelae, including paraplegia, detected between 2–4 years of age in 22 per cent of such patients delivered vaginally, Caesarean section was recommended.

The principles upon which selection is based having been discussed, one should now examine the effect of that selection in clinical practice. It has already been stated that the perinatal mortality rate for a frank breech is less than that for either a complete or a footling breech (Hall *et al*. 1965). A randomized trial of selected vaginal delivery in the presence of a frank breech has demonstrated the relative safety of this policy. Collea *et al*. (1980) randomly allocated 208 women with a singleton frank breech presentation to deliver vaginally ($n = 115$) or abdominally ($n = 93$). Of the 115 patients scheduled for vaginal delivery, 45 per cent underwent elective Caesarean section based on unsatisfactory pelvimetry results. Of the 63 remaining, 82.5 per cent delivered vaginally without perinatal death (but with two brachial plexus injuries), whilst 17.5 per cent underwent Caesarean section for either poor progress or fetal distress during labour. The maternal morbidity for Caesarean section was 49 per cent compared with 7 per cent for vaginal delivery.

The situation for non-frank breech presentations is less satisfactory. Gimovský *et al*. (1983) randomized 70 patients with a non-frank breech to a trial of labour and 35 to elective Caesarean section. Of those in the labour arm, 44 per cent delivered vaginally, the rest by Caesarean section for which poor progress was the commonest indication. There were three fetal deaths, two due to fetal abnormality and one due to 'inadequate resuscitation' after vaginal delivery. Prolapse of the cord occurred in 4 per cent of labouring patients and prolapse of the body in a further 3 per cent. Febrile morbidity occurred in 2.9 per cent of mothers who delivered vaginally and 46 per cent of those who delivered abdominally. Although the authors of the above study concluded that selected trial of labour in non-frank breech presentation was acceptable, clearly the risks are greater than for a frank breech and the increased risk of fetal compromise and emergency Caesarean section may make this policy unacceptable to patients.

If selected vaginal breech delivery is a safe alternative in selected patients with a frank breech at term, those women who then need an intrapartum Caesarean section will then need an 'emergency' rather than an 'elective' procedure, and this difference may influence the risk of maternal mortality, especially related to the anaesthetic. In a cohort study of 313 singleton breech deliveries, 52.5 per cent underwent an elective Caesarean section and 18.8 per cent underwent an emergency Caesarean section, the commonest indication being 'poor progress' (Bingham and Lilford 1987) (please see Table 20.8). Bingham and Lilford (1987) have estimated that, whilst the overall risk of maternal mortality for abdominal delivery was 0.4 per 100, the risk following emergency Caesarean section was three times that after elective Caesarean section. Once correction is made for the indication for that Caesarean section, the excess risk for emergency Caesarean section increased to six-fold. Moldin *et al*. (1984) also allowed for the indication for Caesarean section, and quoted a 'Caesarean-attributed' maternal mortality of 0.13 per 1000 overall, and although the distinction between emergency and elective procedures is not always clear, their best estimate was a risk of 0.04 per 1000 for elective procedures and 0.18 per 1000 for emergency procedures. This excess risk with emergency procedures may be reduced by the elective siting of an epidural catheter in labour allowing

Table 20.8 The mode of delivery

Group	Number
No.	313
% Elective Caesarean section	52.5
% Emergency Caesarean section	18.8
% Vaginal delivery	28.7
Reason for emergency Caesarean section	
—% fetal distress	3
—% poor progress	14.1
—% prolapsed cord	1.7

From Bingham and Lilford (1987)

extension of the block to an appropriate level for surgery should it be necessary (Morgan *et al*. 1990).

However, this advantage from epidural analgesia has to be balanced against the possible increase in Caesarean section rate during the second stage of labour associated with this technique (24 versus 4 per cent) presumably due to inadequate maternal expulsive effort (Chadha *et al*. 1992).

Using decision analysis, Bingham and Lilford (1987) demonstrated that there was no excess risk to the mother from elective Caesarean section for all breech presentations, and a reduced morbidity to the baby. It is possible that, as greater patient involvement in the decision process takes place, the incidence of elective Caesarean section for breech delivery at term will increase, even though the bulk of the evidence supports the safety of *selected* vaginal breech delivery at term.

The mode of delivery—the preterm breech

There is debate concerning the route of delivery of a preterm infant presenting by the breech. It is generally accepted that the mortality following vaginal delivery of a preterm breech infant is greater than that following the vaginal delivery of a preterm infant presenting by the vertex or for the abdominal delivery of a preterm infant regardless of presentation (Smith *et al*. 1980). The data produced by these authors is reproduced in Table 20.9.

Such a statement, however, requires further amplification. Such statistics only suggest a survival benefit in preterm breech babies weighing less than 1500 g at birth, whilst preterm babies weighing more than 1500 g at birth have similar survival rates regardless of whether the presentation was breech or vertex (Effer *et al*. 1983; Kiely 1991; Lamont *et al*. 1983; Rosen and Chik *et al*. 1984; Yu *et al*. 1984). One of these series, for example, demonstrated that the neonatal mortality rate following vaginal delivery in a preterm baby with a breech presen-

Table 20.9 Mortality of babies 751–2000 g at birth

Route of delivery and presentation	No. of infants	% survival
Vaginal—vertex	401	86
Vaginal—breech	102	65
Abdominal—any	225	90

From Smith *et al*. (1980)

tation was 70 per cent higher than that associated with abdominal delivery when the birthweight was less than 1750 g (Kiely 1991).

From such studies, the obstetrician might conclude that potentially viable fetuses in premature labour, presenting by the breech, and of estimated weight less than 1500 g should be delivered by Caesarean section (Gravenhorst *et al*. 1993). However, no series has been controlled for other obstetric factors. These studies undoubtedly contain an in-built bias towards the benefit from Caesarean section since infants considered, for whatever reason, to be unsalvagable will be delivered vaginally. The proponents of Caesarean section, however, would argue that the policy avoids the danger of head entrappment through a partially dilated cervix, a cause of death in smaller fetuses presenting by the brech (Bodmer *et al*. 1986). In order to resolve the question of route of delivery for the preterm breech fetus weighing less than 1500 g, a randomized trial is needed, but such a trial would be difficult to perform and may never take place (Penn and Steer 1991).

Conclusions

Recent practice has seen two major modifications in the management of breech presentation in a mature fetus. The first change relates to the increasing evidence for the benefit of external cephalic version beyond the 37th week of pregnancy, whereas it is of limited, if any, value before this gestation. Secondly, whilst it is appropriate that there is an increasing use of elective Caesarean sections for the non-frank mature breech, the evidence from the literature allows for safe selected vaginal breech delivery preferably in the presence of an epidural catheter, for the frank breech. The most important dilemma to be solved is the route of delivery for the potentially viable preterm fetus presenting by the breech during labour. It is still disappointing to note that approximately 25 per cent of all singleton breech presentations are not diagnosed prior to admission in labour (Nwosu *et al*. 1993).

References

Alexopoulos, K. A. (1973). The importance of breech delivery in the pathogenesis of brain damage. *Clinical Paediatrics* 12, 248-9.

Ballas, S., Toaff, R., and Jaffa, A. J. (1978). Deflexion of the fetal head in breech presentation. *Obstetrics and Gynecology* 52, 653-5.

Bingham, P. and Lilford, R. J. (1987). Management of the selected term breech presentation. *Obstetrics and Gynecology* 69, 965-78.

Bingham, P., Hird, V., and Lilford, R. J. (1987). Management of the mature selected breech presentation. *British Journal of Obstetrics and Gynaecology* 94, 746-52.

Bodmer, B., Benjamin, A., McLean, F. H., and Usher, R. H. (1986). Has the use of Caesarean section reduced the risk of delivery in the preterm breech presentation? *American Journal of Obstetrics and Gynecology* 154, 244-50.

Bradley-Watson, P. J. (1975). The decreasing value of external cephalic version in modern obstetric practice. *American Journal of Obstetrics and Gynecology* 123, 237-40.

Brenner, W. E., Bruce, R. D., and Hendricks, C. H. (1974). The characteristics and perils of breech presentation. *American Journal of Obstetrics and Gynecology* 118, 700-12.

Chadha, Y. C., Mahmood, T. A., Dick, M. J., Smith, N. C., Campbell, D. M., and Templeton, A. (1992). Breech delivery and epidural analgesia. *British Journal of Obstetrics and Gynaecology* 99, 96-100.

Cheng, M. and Hannah, M. (1993). Breech delivery at term. *Obstetrics and Gynecology* 82, 605-18.

Christian, S. C., Brady, K., Read, J. A., and Copelman, J. N. (1990). Vaginal breech delivery: a five-year prospective evaluation of a protocol using computerized tomography pelvimetry. *American Journal of Obstetrics and Gynecology* 163, 848-55.

Clausen, I. and Nielsen, K. T. (1988). Breech presentation delivery rate and congenital dislocation of the hip. *Acta Obstetrica et Gynaecologica Scandinavica* 67, 595-7.

Collea, J. V., Chein, C., and Quilligan, E. J. (1980). A randomized management of term frank breech presentation. *American Journal of Obstetrics and Gynecology* 137, 235.

Coltart, T. M. (1989). Management of breech presentation. In *Contemporary obstetrics* (ed. G. Chamberlain), pp. 126-34. Churchill Livingstone, Edinburgh.

Croughan-Minihane, J., Petitti, D. B., Gordis, L., and Golditch, I. (1990). Morbidity among breech infants according to method of delivery. *Obstetrics and Gynecology* 75, 821-5.

De Crespigny, L. J. C. and Pepperell, R. J. (1979). Perinatal mortality and morbidity in breech presentation. *Obstetrics and Gynecology* 53, 141-5.

Duignan, N. (1982). The management of breech presentation. In *Progress in obstetrics and gynaecology* Vol. 2, (ed. J. Studd), pp. 73-84. Churchill Livingstone, Edinburgh.

Effer, S. B., Saigal, S., Rand, C., Hunter, D. J. S., Stoskops, B., Harper, A. C., et al. (1983). Effect of delivery method on outcome in very low birthweight breech infants. *American Journal of Obstetrics and Gynecology* 145, 123-8.

Faber-Nijholt, R., Huisjes, H. J., Touwen, B. C. L., and Fidler, V. J. (1983). Neurological follow-up of 281 children born in breech presentation. *British Medical Journal* 286, 9-12.

Ferguson, J. E. and Dyson, D. C. (1985). Intrapartum external cephalic version. *American Journal of Obstetrics and Gynecology* 152, 297-8.

Fianu, S. and Vaclavinkova, V. (1978). The site of placental attachment as a factor in the aetiology of breech presentation. *Acta Obstetrica et Gynaecologica Scandinavica* **57**, 371–2.

Gimovsky, M. L., Wallace, R. L., Schifrin, B. S., and Paul, R. H. (1983). Randomized management of the non-frank breech presentation at term. *American Journal of Obstetrics and Gynecology* **153**, 887–8.

Gimovsky, M. L., Willard, K., Neglio, M., Howard, T., and Zerne, S. (1985). X-ray pelvimetry in a breech protocol: a comparison of digital radiology and conventional methods. *American Journal of Obstetrics and Gynecology* **153**, 887–8.

Gravenhorst, J. B., Schreuder, A. M., Veen, S., Brand, S., Verloove-Vanhorick, S. P., Verweij, R. A., *et al.* (1993). Breech delivery in very pre-term and very low birthweight infants in the Netherlands. *British Journal of Obstetrics and Gynaecology* **100**, 411–15.

Hall, J. E. and Kohl, S. G. (1956). Breech presentation. *American Journal of Obstetrics and Gynecology* **72**, 977–90.

Hall, J. E., Kohl, S. G., O'Brien, F., and Ginsberg, M. (1965). Breech presentation and perinatal mortality. *American Journal of Obstetrics and Gynecology* **91**, 665–83.

Hay, D. (1959). Observations on breech presentation and delivery. *Journal of Obstetrics and Gynaecology of the British Empire* **66**, 529–47.

Hofmeyr, G. J. (1983). Effect of external cephalic version in late pregnancy on breech presentation and Caesarean section rate. *British Journal of Obstetrics and Gynaecology* **90**, 392–9.

Hofmeyr, G. J. (1989). Breech presentation and abnormal lie in late pregnancy. In *Effective care in pregnancy and childbirth* (ed. I. Chalmers, M. Enkin, and M. J. N. C. Keirse), pp. 653–63.Oxford University Press.

Hofmeyr, G. J. (1991). External cephalic version at term: how high are the stakes? *British Journal of Obstetrics and Gynaecology* **98**, 1–3.

Kaupilla, O. (1975). The perinatal mortality in breech deliveries and observations on affecting factors. *Acta Obstetrica et Gynaecologica Scandinavica* **Supp. 39**, 1–79.

Kiely, J. L. (1991). Mode of delivery and neonatal death in 17587 infants presenting by the breech. *British Journal of Obstetrics and Gynaecology* **98**, 898–904.

Lamont, R. F., Dunlop, P. D. M., Crowley, P., and Elder, M. G. (1983). Spontaneous preterm labour and delivery under 34 weeks' gestation. *British Medical Journal* **286**, 454–7.

Mahomed, K., Seeres, R., and Coulson, R. (1991). External cephalic version at term. *British Journal of Obstetrics and Gynaecology* **98**, 8–13.

Marchick, R. (1988). Antepartum external cephalic version with tocolysis. *American Journal of Obstetrics and Gynecology* **158**, 1339–46.

Moldin, P., Hokegard, K., and Nielsen, T. F. (1984). Caesarean section and maternal mortality in Sweden. *Acta Obstetrica et Gynaecologica Scandinavica* **63**, 7–11.

Morgan, B. M., Magni, V., and Goroszenvik, T. (1990). Anaesthesia for emergency Caesarean section. *British Journal of Obstetrics and Gynaecology* **97**, 420–4.

Morrison, J. C., Myatt, R. E., Martin, J. N., Meeks, G. R., Martin, R. W., Bucovaz, E. T., *et al.* (1986). External cephalic version of the breech presentation under tocolysis. *American Journal of Obstetrics and Gynecology* **154**, 900–3.

Neilson, D. R. (1970). Management of the large breech infant. *American Journal of Obstetrics and Gynecology* **107**, 345–8.

Nwosu, E. C., Walkinshaw, S., Chia, P., Manasse, P. R., and Atlay, R. D. (1993). Undiagnosed breech. *British Journal of Obstetrics and Gynaecology* **100**, 531–5.

Olan, P., Skramm, I., Hannisdal, E., and Bjoro, K. (1988). Breech delivery. *Acta Obstetrica et Gynaecologica Scandinavica* **67**, 75–9.

Penn, Z. J. and Steer, P. J. (1991). How obstetricians manage the problem of preterm delivery with special reference to the preterm breech. *British Journal of Obstetrics and Gynaecology* **98**, 531–4.

Racker, D. C. (1943). Breech presentation in the elderly primipara. *Journal of Obstetrics and Gynaecology of the British Empire* **50**, 352–8.

Ridley, W. J., Jackson, P., Stewart, J. H., and Boyle, P. (1982). Role of antenatal radiography in the management of breech deliveries. *British Journal of Obstetrics and Gynaecology* **89**, 342–7.

Rosen, M. G. and Chik, L. (1984). Delivery route in breech presentation. *American Journal of Obstetrics and Gynecology* **148**, 909–14.

Rovinsky, J. J., Miller, J. A., and Kaplan, S. (1973). Management of breech presentation at term. *American Journal of Obstetrics and Gynecology* **115**, 497–513.

Scheer, K. and Nubar, J. (1976). Variation of fetal presentation with gestational age. *American Journal of Obstetrics and Gynecology* **125**, 269–70.

Smith, M. L., Spencer, S. A., and Hull, D. (1980). Mode of delivery and survival in babies weighing less than 2000 g at birth. *British Medical Journal* **281**, 118–19.

Soernes, T. and Bakke, T. (1986). The length of the human umbilical cord in vertex and breech presentation. *American Journal of Obstetrics and Gynecology* **154**, 1086–7.

Tatum, R. K., Orr, J. W., Soony, S., and Huddleston, J .F. (1985). Vaginal breech delivery of selected infants weighing more than 2000 grams. *American Journal of Obstetrics and Gynecology* **152**, 145–55.

Thorpe-Beeston, J. G., Banfield, P. J., and Saunders, N. J. S. (1992). Outcome of breech delivery at term. *British Medical Journal* **305**, 746–7.

Todd, W. D. and Steer, C. M. (1963). Term breech. *Obstetrics and Gynecology* **22**, 583–95.

Tompkins, P. (1946). An enquiry into the causes of breech presentation. *American Journal of Obstetrics and Gynecology* **51**, 595–606.

van Loon, A. J., Manteingh, A., Thijn, C. H. P., and Mooyaart, E. L. (1990). Pelvimetry by magnetic resonance imaging in breech presentation. *American Journal of Obstetrics and Gynecology* **163**, 1256–60.

Westgren, L. M. and Ingermarsson, I. (1988). Breech delivery and mental handicap. *Ballière's Obstetrics and Gynaecology* **2**, 187–94.

Westgren, M., Grundsell, H., Ingermarsson, I., Muhlow, A., and Svenningsen N. W. (1981). Hyperextension of the fetal head in breech presentation a study with long-term follow-up. *British Journal of Obstetrics and Gynaecology* **88**, 101–4.

Westgren, M., Edvall, H., Nordstrom, L., Svalenivs, E., and Ranstam, J. (1985). Spontaneous cephalic version of breech presentation in the last trimester. *British Journal of Obstetrics and Gynaecology* **92**, 19–22.

Yu, V. Y. H., Bajuk, B., Cutting, D., Orgill, A. A., and Astbury, I. (1984). Effect of mode of delivery on outcome of very low birthweight infants. *British Journal of Obstetrics and Gynaecology* **91**, 633–9.

21   Specific infections during pregnancy

This chapter is concerned with the interrelationships between specific infections and pregnancy. Some of the infections, especially candidosis, trichomoniasis, and the sexually transmitted diseases were discussed in Chapter 6, but specific aspects of these infections in pregnancy are in this chapter. The chapter also discusses viral infections during pregnancy.

Viral infections

Viral infection is a common event, and, although it is usually only a minor illness or may pass unnoticed, the risk of severe congenital malformation with certain viral infections makes this an important event. Sever and White (1968) reported that 5.2 per cent of 30 059 pregnancies were complicated by a viral infection (Table 21.1). The prevalence of transplacental infections was reported by Alford (1971) who took cord blood samples at 5951 deliveries and found significantly raised levels of IgM in 3.2 per cent, the commonest infection being cytomegalovirus (1 in 400 deliveries). The results are shown in Table 21.2.

Cytomegalovirus (CMV)

CMV is now the most common congenital infection. It is probably also the commonest cause of severe brain disease in neonates. Stern and Tucker (1973) calculated that, based on the worst estimates, if 0.5 per cent of the pregnant women of England and Wales developed CMV infection, then approximately 4000 CMV-infected babies would be delivered each year. If 10 per cent of these babies were mentally retarded, then CMV infection would be the cause of severe brain damage in 400 infants annually.

CMV is a DNA-containing member of the herpes virus family, characterized by intranuclear and intracytoplasmic inclusion bodies. It is clearly able to cross the placenta.

The incidence of CMV infection during pregnancy has to be assessed serologically since many of the maternal infections are subclinical. In a recent study, serological evidence of CMV infection was found in 1 in 8000 neonates (Griffiths *et al*. 1991). There are, however, racial differences in this incidence. Stern and Tucker (1973) reported serological testing at the booking antenatal visit and again after delivery. Some 42 per cent of native white English women were seropositive at the start of pregnancy and 3 per cent of the susceptible

Table 21.1 Viral infections during pregnancy

	Rate per 10 000 pregnancies
Influenza	310
Herpes simplex	120
Viral gastroenteritis	45
Mumps	10
Rubella	8
Varicella	5

From Sever and White (1964)

Table 21.2 Viral infections and IgM in cord blood samples at delivery

	Incidence of raised IgM
Cytomegalovirus	1 in 400
Toxoplasmosis	1 in 682
Rubella	1 in 938
Syphillis	1 in 1250
Any	1 in 178

From Sever and White (1964)

women seroconverted during pregnancy. Some 90 per cent of immigrant Asian women were seropositive at the start of pregnancy and 16 per cent of the susceptible women seroconverted.

Past infection does not confer immunity. Reactivation of latent infection occurred in 0.7 per cent of white women in 2.9 per cent of the Asian women (Stern and Tucker 1973), and may result in a handicapped child (Peckham *et al*. 1983).

The diagnosis of CMV infection is generally made upon the *in vitro* culture of urine inoculated on to human fibroblasts or myometrial cells (Weller 1971*a*). Positive serological tests for CMV-IgG may be found in neonates in the absence of maternal CMV-specific IgM, presumably due to reactivation of infection, whilst maternal seroconversion is not necessarily associated with congenital infection (Griffiths *et al*. 1991). Screening for CMV by serological testing during pregnancy is, therefore, of limited value. When an accurate assessment concerning fetal infection is required, fetal blood sampling under ultrasound control may be performed (Forestier *et al*. 1988; Doner *et al*. 1993), to look for CMV-specific IgM. At present, however, we cannot correlate infection with handicap, although the risk may be as high as 50 per cent.

The major route of infection of the infant is transplacental. However, infection may also be transmitted directly from the mother to her infant, or to

Table 21.3 Handicap and CMV

Clinical manifestation	Weller and Hanshaw (1962) (n = 17) (%)	Tobin (1970) (n = 36) (%)
Hepatomegaly	100	36.1
Splenomegaly	100	41.7
Microcephaly	82.4	16.7
Mental retardation	82.4	19.4
Motor disability	76.5	11.1
Jaundice	64.7	30.6
Thrombocytopenic purpura	52.9	30.6
Chorioretinitis	29.4	2.8
Cerebral calgification	23.5	11.1
Possible deafness	not stated	8.3

others, post-natally, by excretion of the virus in urine. In a prospective study of 81 CMV-negative infants, based on cord blood estimations, delivered to mothers with cytomegaloviruria, 26 per cent seroconverted during the first year of life, all without apparent detriment in the short-term (Kumar *et al.* 1984*a*). Although the virus may be found in human breast milk, this is not considered to be an important source of post-natal transmission (Weller 1971*b*).

Handicap and CMV

The consequences to the infant from congenital CMV infection were described Weller and Hanshaw (1962) and by Tobin (1970). As can be seen from Table 21.3, the incidence of serious handicap varies greatly between the series, with a minimum incidence of mental retardation of 19 per cent and a maximum risk of handicap of 82 per cent. Although handicap may follow maternal re-infection, almost all cases of serious handicap follow a primary maternal infection (Embril *et al.* 1970; Stagno *et al.* 1982).

There is good evidence to suggest that congenital CMV infection is more serious a problem than post-natally acquired CMV infection. Kumar *et al.* (1984*b*) assessed children with CMV infection based upon excretion of the virus in urine. They assessed 17 children with congenital CMV, 10 with post-natal CMV, and 21 seronegative controls, all at a mean age of 7–11 years. The only abnormalities were in four children in the congenitally acquired infection group, all having sensorineural hearing difficulties, one being profoundly deaf.

More recent studies, generally prospective, have demonstrated lesser than expected risks from congenital CMV infection. Saigal *et al.* (1982) followed 50 children with evidence of congenital CMV infection. Three died from causes unrelated to CMV infection and only one of the 47 surviving infants developed cerebral palsy, none developed microcephaly, but 17 per cent had evidence of sensorineural deafness. Peckham *et al.* (1983) reported 43 infants who were congenitally infected with CMV. Some 7 per cent had serious handicaps, 33 per cent had minor ones, and the others were free of problems. Pearl *et al.* (1986) assessed the neurodevelopmental state of 41 children with congenital CMV at the age of two years and found that 90 per cent of these children were neurologically and developmentally normal. Other authors have found similar results (Griffiths and Baboonian 1984). These studies have suggested that serious handicap will occur in some 2–20 per cent of infants whose mothers have seroconverted and, as a generalization, termination of pregnancy for maternal CMV infection would need to be discussed.

There is no effective treatment for CMV infection, but vaccination of susceptible adolescent girls may be the best way to reduce CMV infection during pregnancy (Griffiths *et al.* 1991).

Rubella

The association between antenatal rubella infection and congenital malformation is well-known, the classical triad of cataracts, deafness, and cardiac defects being termed 'rubella syndrome'. Although the incidence of congenital rubella syndrome has been falling, largely due to successful vaccination programmes, there is recent evidence that an increase in congenital rubella syndrome is occurring (Centers for Disease Control 1991). This is due, in part, to the observation that between 6 and 11 per cent of adolescent girls are still seronegative and hence at risk of infection (Stehr-Green *et al.* 1990).

The diagnosis of a rubella infection during pregnancy may be difficult, despite the characteristic appearance of the maculopapular rash on the first day of illness. An IgG titre may demonstrate immunity at the time of contact, but only the absence of IgM can exclude infection with any degree of certainty. Cord blood IgM may confirm the diagnosis of congenital rubella. Miller *et al.* (1985) reported that 0.8 per cent of 899 women who had been in contact with rubella, and who had no symptoms, showed IgM evidence of active rubella infection. The most useful technique for identification of rubella anti bodies is the haemagglutination inhibition antibody test which can detect rubella-specific IgM as well as IgG. IgM appears in the serum immediately after the rash, reaching a peak in some 7–14 days.

Rubella — the risks

The risk of infection is dependent upon the stage of pregnancy at which infection occurs. In a series of 578 pregnancies complicated by rubella, 6 per cent of children had a major congenital abnormality as compared with 2 per cent of children in a control group. Of those pregnancies complicated by rubella, 5 per cent were considered to be congenital rubella syndrome and, in 96 per cent of these pregnancies, the infection was acquired during the first 16 weeks'

Table 21.4 Risks of congenital rubella defects

Gestation defects (weeks)	% Fetuses infected	Overall risk (% of those infected)	Main defect
< 11	100	90	Multiple defects
11–12	67	33	deafness
13–14	67	11	deafness
15–16	47	24	deafness
17–36	37	0	none
> 36	100	0	none

From Miller *et al.* (1982)

gestation. The other congenital abnormalities, which were not considered to be congenital rubella syndrome, included spina bifida, oesophageal atresia, pyloric stenosis, imperforate anus, and cardiac murmurs, there being no specific association with any gestational age (Manson *et al.* 1960).

The comparative risk from congenital rubella infection at different stages of pregnancy have been confirmed by other authors (Lundstrom 1962; Miller *et al.* 1982). As can be seen from Table 21.4, the most significant risk from rubella occurred when infection arose during the first trimester, in contrast no specific risk arose when infection occurred beyond the 16th week of pregnancy.

Diagnosis of fetal infection

This may be performed by cordocentesis at 18–20 weeks' gestation when the infected fetus will demonstrate rubella-specific IgM. There is a high correlation between fetal infection and the rubella syndrome if the timing of the primary infection is known. Alternatively, there have been isolated case reports of the virus being demonstrated by electron microscopy or the polymerase chain reaction (PCR) following chorion villus sampling at the end of the first trimester.

Rubella vaccination and pregnancy

The effect of the rubella vaccination policy has been to reduce the number of women susceptible to rubella prior to pregnancy, whilst women who are susceptible during pregnancy may be offered vaccination during the puerperium (Miller *et al.* 1985).

It occasionally occurs that rubella vaccination takes place inadvertently during early pregnancy. Since the vaccine is a live attenuated one, a theoretical risk of congenital rubella syndrome could be present. However, the *Morbidity and Mortality Weekly Report* (1986) reported 1142 pregnant women who received rubella vaccine either in the three months prior to conception or within the first three months following the presumed date of conception. Although there was evidence of seroconversion in the infant in 8.5 per cent of such pregnancies, this report failed to identify a single infant with congenital rubella syndrome amongst 794 such infants delivered alive. It would seem that, although some theoretical risk may be present, it must be small and should not be considered as an indication for termination of pregnancy.

Varicella–zoster infections in pregnancy

Unlike most other viruses varicella–zoster (VZ) not only has the potential to cause profound effects on the fetus but may also result in serious or fatal maternal effects. Management, therefore, needs to include both patients.

Chickenpox in the mother

Primary VZ results in chickenpox and is highly contagious such that most adults have acquired the infection prior to reaching reproductive age. The attack rate in pregnancy is estimated at 1–5 cases per 10 000 pregnancies, but pregnant women are not excessively prone to attack (Brunell 1967; Hermann 1982; Pearson 1964) as was previously claimed. VZ is acquired by droplet infection, and some 10–21 days later results in a crop of intensely pruritic vesicles with constitutional upset. The skin lesions start on the face and spread to the trunk with relative sparing of the extremities. They are initially macules, but rapidly become vesicles and pustules, healing by crusting and then scabbing.

Although uncommon in children, varicella pneumonia affects up to a third of adults with chickenpox (Paryani and Arvin 1986). There are few large series of VZ pneumonia in pregnant women but mortality rates of up to 45 per cent have been reported (Harris and Rhoades 1965); death only occurred in those women who developed pneumonia. A non-productive cough occurs within a few days of the rash and in severe cases leads to high fever, pleuritic chest pain, haemoptysis, dyspnoea, and cyanosis. Headaches, of sufficient severity to warrant a lumbar puncture, may occur. Recovery is usually rapid in mild cases but death occurs from respiratory failure in the severe cases. Survivors of severe cases show diffuse pulmonary fibrosis. The respiratory failure is the result of interstitial pneumonitis with subsequent alveolar haemorrhage that leads to a perfusion–ventilation mismatch. The chest X-ray shows diffuse nodular densities that range from 2 to 20 mm scattered throughout the lung fields. The appearances are far more severe than suggested by early symptoms or physical examination.

Any pregnant woman with chickenpox should be specifically questioned for respiratory symptoms and if present she should have a chest X-ray. If the above changes are present the woman should be admitted to intensive care and her respiratory status should be carefully monitored and supported, by positive pressure ventilation if necessary. Acyclovir, in a dose of 10 mg/kg, should be given intravenously eight-hourly (Eder 1988; Hankins *et al.* 1987; Landsberger *et al.* 1986). Although experiences are limited the outlook appears to be improved with the use of acyclovir (Gilbert 1993). It has also been used in non-pregnant women for the treatment of VZ encephalitis, myocarditis, and pericarditis.

If a pregnant woman reports contact with chickenpox or shingles then

Table 21.5 Varicella embryopathy syndrome

Symmetrical intrauterine growth retardation
Limb aplasia
Chorioretinitis
Micropthalmia
Cataracts
Severe CNS defects
Skin manifestations

VZ-IgG should be estimated. As more than 95 per cent of women will have had chickenpox (even if they deny infection in childhood) and because a result can be obtained within 24 hours using modern techniques it is unnecessary to immunize every pregnant women who reports a contact. The administration of VZ immune gamma-globulin (VZIG) has been shown to substantially reduce the symptoms of susceptible women exposed to chickenpox if administered within 72 hours of contact (Brunnell *et al.* 1969). The dose is 1.25 ml given intramuscularly.

Chickenpox in the fetus

VZ causes a collection of congenital abnormalities known as varicella embryopathy (VE), but it also causes a severe infection in the newborn infant if it is acquired in the last few weeks of pregnancy.

Varicella embryopathy (VE)

VZ may result in the anomalies listed in Table 21.5 if it is acquired early in pregnancy. The virus appears to have a predisposition for the fetal central nervous system and causes cerebellar and cortical atrophy as well as focal calcification (Srabstein *et al.* 1974).

The skin manifestations are most commonly linear scars that involve the aplastic limb but extend on to the trunk. Discrete lesions that are typical of VZ are also seen.

Higa *et al.* (1987) reported on 52 cases of VZ in pregnancy. In those women who had contracted the disease before 20 weeks all 27 infants had congenital abnormalities, whereas the remaining 25 all developed herpes zoster after birth. The incidence of VZ in the first 20 weeks of pregnancy is unknown but small studies suggest that the risk of transplacental infection is 10–35 per cent (Paryani and Arvin 1986).

Transplacental passage of VZ has been demonstrated by electron microscopy on chorionic villus samples and by finding VZ specific IgM in the fetus after 18 weeks' gestation. It should also be possible to demonstrate the virus in chorionic villi by means of the polymerase chain reaction (PCR). There is no data on the relationship of transplacental passage to the occurrence of the embryopathy, but it is likely that most if not all fetuses will be affected in the first half of pregnancy. There is no data available for the use of VZIG (given to the mother or the fetus) or acyclovir in the prevention of the embryopathy.

VZ infections in the newborn

These may be serious with up to a third of the infants dying (Meyers 1974). The risk, however, is related to the timing of the maternal infection and the acquisition of maternal antibodies by the fetus and is summarized below.

The risk to the neonate is highest if it is born after the maternal viraemia has occurred but before antibody formation. Viraemia occurs 12–48 hours prior to the onset of the rash which is 10–17 days after exposure; antibodies are formed 4–5 days after the rash. Babies born two days before the onset of the rash to five days afterwards are most likely to die, with deaths being unknown outside the period of five days before to ten days after the development of the rash (Meyers 1974).

Maternal administration of VZIG does not affect the rate of transmission, in that half of the babies born to 95 mothers who receive prophylaxis will get a neonatal infection (Hanngren *et al.* 1985), but it may influence the severity of the neonatal disease for those at highest risk (Readett 1961). No infant died or had longterm sequelae following maternal VZIG, although half of 82 infants born in the high-risk period had a neonatal infection. Regardless of maternal treatment, all infants born within two weeks of infection or where the timing of the infection is not known should receive 1.25 ml of VZIG at birth. Data on specific treatment of such infants with acyclovir or vidarabine is limited.

Infants born prior to the maternal viraemia and rash need to be isolated from their mothers until five days after the onset of the rash and should not be breastfed. They should also be isolated from other infants until one week after development of the rash or 20 days after exposure (Music *et al.* 1971).

Herpes genitalis

Maternal herpes genitalis infection is said to occur in 1 in 1600 pregnancies (Brown *et al.* 1991).

The major hazard lies with neonatal herpes. Neonatal herpes infection in the UK occurs in 0.003 per cent of births or 1 in 33 000 live births, but, in the USA, it occurs in 0.2 per cent or 1 in 5000 live births (Lissauer and Jeffries 1989). Infant mortality is the major complication of this disease. Kelly (1988) reported 111 laboratory indentifications of the virus in neonates and this was associated with a mortality of 16.2 per cent.

There are two major dilemmas concerning maternal herpes genitalis and neonatal infection. The first relates to the observation that neonatal infection may occur from an asymptomatic mother, and the second, and interrelated, dilemma relates to the screening of high-risk mothers as a guide to their mode of delivery.

The risks to the neonate were assessed by Nahmias *et al.* (1971*a*) in a series of 283 pregnant women with herpes genitalis. Some 43 per cent of patients who were shedding virus were asymptomatic. Spontaneous abortion occurred in 34 per cent of pregnancies and preterm delivery in 21 per cent. For 42 patients delivered vaginally, the overall risk of neonatal herpes was 9.5 per cent. However, this figure warrants further explanation depending upon whether the infection was primary or recurrent. Of nine patients with primary herpes and who delivered vaginally, 33 per cent of the neonates became infected, whilst for 23 patients with recurrent genital herpes, only 3 per cent of the neonates developed infection. Abdominal delivery with either intact membranes or within four hours of membrane rupture was not associated with any neonatal herpes infection. Prober *et al.* (1987) reported 34 neonates born vaginally to mothers with a history of recurrent genital herpes simplex virus infection. Even though 56 per cent of the women had evidence of clinical herpes at the time of vaginal delivery, no infant developed neonatal herpes. The authors concluded that the risks for neonatal herpes in the presence of recurrent maternal herpes must be low and, based upon confidence limits, could not exceed 8 per cent. Similarly, Vontner *et al.* (1982) reported 80 pregnant patients with recurrent genital herpes and, although 16.3 per cent of the patients had asymptomatic shedding of the virus at some stage during the pregnancy, none of the infants showed any evidence of herpetic infection. Recurrent maternal genital herpes is, therefore, less of a risk to the neonate than is primary maternal genital herpes.

Since abdominal delivery would seem to be protective against neonatal herpes infection, there has been a trend towards abdominal delivery for such women. Binkin *et al.* (1984) assessed the theoretical risks and benefits of such a policy. Assuming that Caesarean section was performed for all patients with asymptomatic viral shedding in a cohort of 3.6 million women (the number of women delivering annually in the USA), screening would probably avert 11.3 neonatal deaths, 3.7 cases of severe retardation, but 3.3 women would die as a result of operative delivery. Furthermore, intact membranes prior to Caesarean section do not totally preclude the risk of neonatal herpes. Kelly (1988) reported that 19 cases of neonatal herpes infection have been reported in patients delivered by Caesarean section before membrane rupture.

Screening of the high-risk population antenatally does not seem to identify all the fetuses at risk since asymptomatic shedding of the virus occurs (Arvin *et al.* 1986). This study also demonstrated that patients who shed the virus asymptomatically during labour did not necessarily shed the virus asymptomatically during the antenatal period, suggesting that antenatal screening of asymptomatic women is a relatively inefficient way of predicting viral shedding during labour. Consequently, the majority of neonates with herpes are born to mothers without a history of herpes genitalis infection (Whitley *et al.* 1980; Yeager and Arvin 1984). Moreover, neonatal infection of an infant may occur despite negative maternal cervical cultures during labour (Brown *et al.* 1991).

The advice given in the literature concerning screening has, therefore, changed over the last decade. Amstey *et al.* (1979) and Grossman *et al.* (1981) recommended weekly viral culture screening of high-risk pregnant women from the 32nd week of gestation onwards, high risk being defined as a past history of genital herpes or a male contact with genital herpes. These authors recommended Caesarean section for those with virus demonstrated during the week prior to delivery. However, Gibbs *et al.* (1988) assessed the available evidence on behalf of the US Infection Disease Society for Obstetrics and Gynaecology and advised that, in women with a history of genital herpes but without lesions:

1. Weekly prenatal cultures should be abandoned.
2. In the absence of clinical lesions, vaginal delivery should be expected (unless, of course, other indications for Caesarean section are present).
3. A culture should be taken from both mother and neonate on the day of delivery.

In women with herpetic lesions when labour begins or membrane rupture occurs:

1. Caesarean section should be considered as it will reduce the risk of neonatal herpes infection.
2. Caesarean section should ideally be performed within 4–6 hours of membrane rupture, but may be of benefit regardless of the length of time since membrane rupture.

The consequences to the neonate from herpes infection are potentially serious. In one series of 56 such neonates, 46 per cent were born prematurely. Of these 56 infants, 71 per cent had evidence of herpetic skin lesions, 39 per cent had systemic disease, and 29 per cent had central nervous system disease (Whitley *et al.* 1980). The mortality from untreated disseminated or central nervous system disease was 74 per cent and for treated disease (adenine arabinoside) 38 per cent.

There is a school of thought which advocates treatment of pregnant women with acyclovir, especially when herpes genitalis occurs near to term, in the hope that both Caesarean section or neonatal infection may be reduced (Brown and Baker 1989; Stray-Pedersen 1990). Andrews *et al.* (1992) reported 312 pregnancies in which acyclovir had been prescribed, in 239 pregnancies during the first trimester. There was no evidence for an increased incidence of either spontaneous abortion or fetal abnormality. Although there is no reason to suspect that acyclovir carries specific problems for the fetus when administered to a mother during pregnancy, the safety and efficacy of such a policy has yet to be established. As herpes is acquired during delivery it may be logical to treat the at-risk infant immediately after delivery, thereby removing the need for Caesarean section. This policy has not yet been subjected to appropriate trials since the administration of acyclovir to mothers does not seem to prevent transmission of the virus to the fetus (Haddad *et al.* 1993).

Genital warts

Genital warts are not themselves a particular problem during pregnancy, although wart virus infection of the neonate may occur following delivery, or even rarely *in utero* (Tang *et al.* 1978). There is also an association between childhood laryngeal warts and maternal condylomata (Quick *et al.* 1980). Genital warts in a child should not be considered to be evidence of sexual abuse since close non-sexual contact between parent and child may transmit the virus (Oriel 1992).

In order to treat the maternal symptoms due to warts, and perhaps to prevent neonatal infection, physical rather than chemical methods of treatment should be used. Both podophyllin and 5-fluorouracil are relatively contraindicated because of their possible absorption (Ferenczy 1984; Slater *et al.* 1978). These chemicals have been associated with toxicity, including liver damage, neurological sequelae, and coma. Cryosurgery or carbon dioxide laser treatment are probably the most appropriate method of treatment during pregnancy, should treatment be indicated (Ferenczy 1984; D. B. Schwartz *et al* 1988). Most warts, however, resolve after pregnancy.

Parvovirus

Human parvovirus causes a mildly erythematous disease, occasionally associated with arthralgia. Animal parvovirus has been implicated in fetal infection, death, and abortion, hence there is reason to examine these possibilities in humans. This infection does not seem to be a common cause of congenital abnormality, no specific IgM being found in the sera of 253 abnormal infants (Mortimer *et al.* 1985), but there is some association with the spontaneous abortion of a hydropic fetus (Anand *et al.* 1987) and late intrauterine death (Knott *et al.* 1984), although maternal infection, confirmed serologically, may occur without pregnancy complication (Wright *et al.* 1985).

Mumps

There is little evidence to link mumps with congenital abnormality. St Geme *et al.* (1966) drew attention to an association between mumps during pregnancy and cutaneous delayed hypersensitivity to mumps virus in children born with primary endocardial fibroelastosis. However, other authors (for example Dudgeon 1976) do not accept a causal relationship.

Echovirus

Echovirus is a known cause of upper respiratory tract infection, especially in children, and is known to cause severe diarrhoea and meningitis. Nagington *et al.* (1978) described an outbreak of echovirus infection in a special care baby unit in which 12.5 per cent of 24 infected neonates died. There is no evidence that echovirus causes an increased incidence of abortion or congenital abnormalities (Kovar and Harvey 1981).

Coxsackie group B

This virus may cause mild infections in mothers and, rarely fatal myocarditis and meningoencephalitis in neonates, but it is not a proven agent in abortion or congenital abnormality although some implication in congenital heart disease has been suggested (Kovar and Harvey 1981).

Influenza

Flu-like illnesses occur in 3.1 per cent of pregnancies (Sever and White 1968) and, although there have been suggestions that the influenza virus is a cause of congenital malformation, evidence is contradictory and has only been accumulated from the major influenza epidemics.

It has been suggested that maternal influenza is associated with fetal abnormality, but the evidence is that this is only a feature of virulent influenza epidemics. There were two prospective studies of the Asian influenza outbreak of 1957 which reported a congenital abnormality rate of between 3.6 and 3.9 per cent of pregnant women with influenza compared with 1.3 per cent of controls (Coffey and Jessop 1959). Influenza epidemics which occurred since have not been associated with an increased incidence of congenital abnormality (Manson *et al.* 1960). Leck (1963) reported 22 698 pregnancies following three influenza epidemics in which the incidence of major congenital abnormalities was 0.9 per cent compared with 1.1 per cent in 79 344 controls.

The TORCH syndrome

Because several transplacental viral (and protozoan) infections may cause similar clinical features of infection and handicap in the infant, the concept arose of TORCH, **T**oxoplasma, **R**ubella, **C**ytomegalovirus, and **H**erpes simplex (Nahmias *et al.* 1971*b*). These authors cited serological evidence to involve these four infections as the causative organism in 37 per cent of 192 cases of transplacental or post-natal infection, often difficult to distinguish clinically, as can be seen from Table 21.6.

However, this concept should be considered of limited value for three reasons.

1. These infections may cause other problems which do not become apparent until later development.
2. The effects of these infections are not necessarily indistinguishable clinically. For instance, cerebral calcification is rare in rubella, whilst cardiac lesions are rarely associated with toxoplasmosis.
3. Other viral agents, as have been discussed above, may tend to be forgotten if one merely relies upon 'a TORCH screen'. (*Lancet* 1990).

Table 21.6 The TORCH syndrome

	Infective agent			
	To	R	C	H
No. of patients	11	16	22	12
Involvement of:				
central nervous system	4	9	10	7
ocular	5	4	5	3
growth retardation	1	5	2	1
viscera	2	2	10	2
other features	2	1	1	2

From Nahmias *et al.* (1971*b*)

Human immunodeficiency virus infection

Women represent a minority of AIDS patients in the Western world. Of 4098 recorded cases of AIDS in the UK, 5 per cent were in women only 6.4 per cent of whom were considered 'low risk', the other 93.6 per cent belonging to a recognized high-risk group (Chartan 1991).

The overall incidence of HIV infection in the pregnant population is not yet known, but there is evidence that the incidence of infection is increasing in high-risk areas. In the United States, some 0.15 per cent of women of child-bearing age are HIV positive, although in the highest risk areas this figure reaches 8 per cent (Pizzo and Butler 1991). In 1988, only 1 in 1900 pregnant women at an antenatal clinic in Central London were HIV positive and none of 95 pregnant women who requested testing were HIV positive. At the same clinic in 1990, 1 in 228 pregnant women were HIV positive, almost a nine-fold increase, as was 1 in 52 requests for HIV testing (Banatvala *et al.* 1990, 1991). Similarly, another recent series demonstrated an increase in the incidence of HIV infection in neonates in Central London, from 1 in 2000 in 1988 to 1 in 500 in 1991. There was *no* comparable increase in the incidence of HIV infection in neonates outside Central London, where the incidence remained static at 1 in 1400 pregnancies (Ades *et al.* 1991). The high incidence of HIV infection in maternity units in Edinburgh has also been reported (Davison *et al.* 1989).

It would seem logical to offer serological screening for HIV infection to antenatal patients in high-risk areas. However, if this is to be done then it is only logical to offer HIV screening to all women and not just to those perceived as being high risk. Krasinski *et al.* (1988) reported that counselling and voluntary testing of 'high-risk' mothers failed to identify 86 per cent of 28 HIV infected mothers based upon the anonymous testing of cord blood samples. Landesman *et al.* (1987) reported that only 58.3 per cent of 12 women found to be HIV positive during pregnancy on a routine screening programme had any high-risk identification factors. In London, the obstetrician was aware of maternal HIV infection in only 20 per cent of infected neonates (Ades *et al.* 1991), whilst acknowledged risk factors were detected in only 57 per cent of another prospective study of women who were HIV positive (Barbacci *et al.* 1991).

The effect of HIV upon pregnancy

There is no evidence to suggest that, in asymptomatic HIV women, infection has a deleterious effect upon the pregnancy (Alger *et al.* 1993; European Collaborative Study 1991; Italian Multicentre Study 1988; Johnson and Webster, 1989). Selwyn *et al.* (1989) reported a prospective study of pregnancy in HIV-positive and HIV-negative intravenous drug abusers, studying 125 pregnancies in 97 women, 39 seropositive and 58 seronegative. No differences were observed between the groups in the frequencies of spontaneous or elective abortion, ectopic pregnancy, preterm delivery, stillbirth, or intrauterine growth retardation. It is more likely that the person who acquires HIV is the risk factor and not the HIV itself. Thus, Johnstone *et al.* (1988) in a study of 50 HIV-positive pregnant women and 64 high-risk but HIV-negative, pregnant women (45 intravenous drug abusers and 19 women with seropositive partners), found no differences between the two groups in pregnancy outcome, but both groups had a rate of prematurity and intrauterine growth retardation of between two and three times that of the Edinburgh population.

The effect of pregnancy on HIV infection

There is some evidence that pregnancy has an adverse effect upon the course of HIV infection based upon case reports of HIV-positive women developing AIDS during pregnancy (Scott *et al.* 1985), whereas several other studies have concluded that the rate of progression from the HIV-positive asymptomatic state to AIDS is, or is not, accelerated by pregnancy (Alger *et al.* 1993; Johnstone *et al.* 1992). Webster and Johnson (1990) reported the results of two case-control studies, presented at an international meeting on AIDS, which suggested that pregnancy may adversely affect the course of HIV disease. A prospective study of large numbers of HIV-positive women will be needed in order to determine the true effects of pregnancy on HIV infection.

Transmission to the fetus

That transplacental infection with HIV is possible is beyond doubt. Both p24 antigen and the HIV genome may be found in cord blood and the fetal spleen, respectively (Webster and Johnson 1990).

It is debated whether the fetus of an HIV-positive woman may develop a characteristic dysmorphic syndrome, or whether this is related to other maternal behavioural factors, or even to author selection bias. Marion *et al.* (1986) described 20 HIV-positive infants affected by growth failure microcephaly, craniofacial abnormalities — including a prominent 'box-like' forehead, flat nasal bridge, and patulous lips.

There have now been several large studies which have addressed the prevalence of both HIV infection and AIDS due to vertical transmission from mother to fetus. Not all children with evidence of perinatal HIV infection develop AIDS or an AIDS-related condition. Thus the European collaborative studies (1991, 1992) reported 721 children born to HIV-infected mothers in ten countries. Some 14 per cent of the children were HIV positive by the age of 18 months. The Italian Multicentre Study (1988) reported that 33 per cent of children born to HIV-positive women were themselves HIV positive and 20 per cent had evidence of AIDS or an AIDS-related condition. Other authors have also estimated that between 20 and 30 per cent of the infants born to HIV-positive mothers developed AIDS (Ades *et al.* 1993; Blanche *et al.* 1989; MacDonald *et al.* 1991; Newell and Peckham 1994; Pizzo and Butler 1991).

These figures may be an underestimate since AIDS has been diagnosed in children up to ten years of age following seroconversion diagnosed at birth (Aiuti *et al.* 1987; Auger *et al.* 1988).

Not all childhood HIV infection will be transplacental. Post-natal transmission may also occur, with breast milk being cited as an efficient route for the transmission of HIV from recently infected mothers to their infants. Van de Perre *et al.* (1991) reported a prospective study of 212 high-risk mother–infant pairs who were HIV negative at the time of delivery. Of nine infants who seroconverted, the authors estimated that 55 per cent acquired their infection during pregnancy or delivery and 45 per cent via breast milk. This should not constitute a contraindication to breast feeding, but patients should be given the appropriate information upon which to make a decision. It is now accepted that approximately one-third of the babies born to HIV infected women will become infected themselves (European Collaborative Study 1992; Senturia *et al.* 1987; Ziegler 1993). There may also be some HIV transmission by close contact, for example at the time of delivery (Ehrnst *et al.* 1991).

The management of HIV-positive women during pregnancy

Due consideration should be given to the following specific points of management.

1. Counselling and support should be given concerning the risk to the fetus.
2. The infant may show signs of opiate withdrawal after delivery if the mother is a drug addict.
3. Specific advice should be given to staff concerning protective clothing, the use of double gloves and eye protection, the disposal of blood-stained garments, and the autoclaving of instruments.
4. Abdominal electronic fetal heart monitoring should be used; the scalp clip (and fetal blood sampling) being contraindicated.
5. The use of a double-chamber neonatal oropharyngeal suction equipment should be employed.
6. Breast feeding should not be considered a contraindication.
7. Follow-up of the mother and child should take place.
8. Contraceptive advice, especially in the use of condoms, should be given.

Termination of pregnancy, purely on the grounds of the mother being HIV positive, should be considered but not necessarily encouraged.

These points have been discussed in detail by MacDonald *et al.* (1991) and the Revised Report of the RCOG Subcommittee (1990).

There is accumulating evidence that a woman who has AIDS or AIDS-related conditions should be treated during pregnancy, even though there is limited information on the effect of zidovudine upon the fetus or neonate (O'Sullivan *et al.* 1993; Sperling *et al.* 1992; Stratton *et al.* 1992). These authors recommend the use of zidovudine (100 mg five times daily) in this situation. There is no real evidence for fetal toxicity, but there is a theoretical risk of fetal bone marrow depression related to the transplacental transfer of the drug. Such patients should be managed in a specialist unit (Stratton *et al.* 1992). Trials are also underway for the use of zidovudine from birth in an attempt to prevent the development of AIDS in infants who remain HIV positive at six months.

Non-viral infections

Chlamydia

The importance of chlamydial infection during pregnancy relates to the risk of conjunctivitis and pneumonia in the neonates of infected mothers, but there may also be an increased incidence of premature rupture of the membranes (5 per cent) and low birthweight (20 per cent) in neonates born to mothers with untreated infection (Ryan *et al.* 1990). Conjunctivitis is said to occur in up to 73 per cent of infants born to culture-positive women, whilst pneumonia occurs in 18 per cent of their offspring (Frommell *et al.* 1979).

It would seem likely that chlamydial infection is an unusual cause of miscarriage. Whilst it cannot be considered as a common cause of miscarriage (Munday *et al.* 1984) there has been a report of abortion due to infection with *Chlamydia psittaci* in the wife of a sheep farmer. An ovine strain of *C. psittaci* was isolated from the placenta and the fetus following miscarriage in a woman who had been helping with lambing. It is, therefore, recommended that pregnant women in the farming community do not assist with lambing (Johnson *et al.* 1985).

The prevalence of chlamydial infection in pregnant women will depend in part upon the population being screened and in part upon the quality of cultures taken. However, some 4 per cent of the overall pregnant population have evidence of cervical chlamydial infection (Schachter *et al.* 1979).

The identification of chlamydial infection during pregnancy will generally follow the identification of the organism in a cervical culture taken from a woman with cervicitis or with a past history of chlamydial infection. Treatment may then be offered to the mother during pregnancy and prophylactic treatment given to the neonate, both in an attempt to reduce neonatal infection (McGregor and French 1991).

Maternal infection is generally treated with erythromycin, 400 mg four times daily for seven days (Magat *et al*. 1993). In one study of 59 pregnant women treated with this regime, 92 per cent became culture negative and 7 per cent of infants were culture positive. A further 24 pregnant women refused treatment. None of these women became culture negative and 50 per cent of the infants were culture positive, suggesting that such treatment might reduce neonatal morbidity (Schachter *et al*. 1986). Should side-effects occur with erythromycin, clindamycin may also be used during pregnancy (McGregor and French 1991).

Neonatal prophylaxis with topical tetracycline is generally aimed at the prevention of conjunctivitis, although there is no evidence that this is superior to silver nitrate (Hammerschlag *et al*. 1989). Infant pneumonia due to chlamydia tends to run a long and intermittent course but with spontaneous resolution and few sequelae (Hobson *et al*. 1983).

Toxoplasmosis

Toxoplasmosis is caused by the intracellular protozoan parasite *Toxoplasma gondii*, which causes congenital abnormalities in the fetus (often clinically indistinguishable from CMV infection) with chorioretinitis, cerebral calcification, hydrocephaly, and neurological damage, often with an asymptomatic mother. The domestic cat appears to be the definitive host, the oocysts passing on to the soil with the faeces. The risk of congenital abnormality seems to relate only to the infants of those mothers who acquire a primary infection during pregnancy, albeit asymptomatic (Desmonts and Couvreur 1974*a*).

The incidence of toxoplasmosis infection during pregnancy in the UK is low. Rouss and Bourne (1972) took serum from 3187 women at the booking-in antenatal clinic, and demonstrated a previous infection in 22.1 per cent based on dye test antibody titres. Based upon umbilical cord blood samples, 0.2 per cent of neonates had been exposed to maternal toxoplasmosis infection, however, none of the seven such infants in this series displayed any of the clinical signs of congenital toxoplasmosis. In France, however, 84 per cent of pregnant women have antibodies as do 32 per cent in New York (Desmonts and Couvreur 1974*a*). These authors demonstrated, on positive dye tests in cord blood samples, that a further 6 per cent of 2238 French pregnant women seroconverted during pregnancy. Only 11 per cent of these infants had clinical evidence of congenital toxoplasma infection. These same authors (1974*b*) reported that seroconversion occurred in 6.3 per cent of 183 susceptible pregnant women, 47.5 per cent of the infants of women who seroconverted having serological evidence of congenital toxoplasmosis. Of these 59 infants with congenital toxoplasmosis 3 per cent died, 12 per cent had severe disease (with cerebral and ocular involvement), 19 per cent had mild disease, and 66 per cent were disease-free. None of the infants of 195 mothers with toxoplasma antibodies prior to pregnancy had any evidence of congenital toxoplasma infection. The severe infections occurred during the first and second trimesters of pregnancy.

It is possible that short-term follow-up of affected infants may give an underestimate of the significance of the disease. Wilson *et al.* (1980) reported that, whilst the majority of infants with congenital toxoplasmosis were asymptomatic in the newborn period, 23 per cent of 13 such infants had unilateral blindness by the age of 8.5 years, 8 per cent had major neural sequelae, including fits and severe psychomotor retardation, whilst 23 per cent had some degree of sensorineural deafness. The mean IQ of the group was 88.6.

Joynson and Payne (1988) estimated that 2 per 1000 women seroconverted in the UK during pregnancy. Based on approximately 700 000 deliveries per year in England and Wales, there would be some 1400 maternal infections, 600 congenital infections, and 60 clinically apparent infections in neonates.

Screening for toxoplasmosis

The basic test for toxoplasma IgG is the antibody dye titre test. The diagnosis may be confirmed using the ELISA (enzyme-linked immunosorbent assay) to detect specific IgM against *T. gondii* (Payne *et al.* 1987; Roos *et al.* 1993), this test being 99 per cent sensitive and 99 per cent specific. Once the diagnosis is suspected immunologically in a pregnant woman, there is an approximately 11 per cent risk of the fetus being affected. Options are termination of pregnancy or the prevention of further transplacental passage by attempting treatment with spiramycin.

Confirmation of fetal infection can be made by cordocentesis to examine fetal blood for toxoplasma specific IgM, although a risk of death *in utero* of 1.1 per cent, spontaneous abortion of 0.8 per cent, and preterm labour of 5 per cent are known complications of this procedure (Daffos *et al.* 1985, 1988; Ghidini *et al.* 1993; Holliman *et al.* 1991). *T. gondii* may also be detected in liquor obtained by amniocentesis and then inoculated into a laboratory animal (Daffos *et al.* 1988; Foulon *et al.* 1990). It has also been detected by electron microscopy and polymerase chain reaction from chorion villus samples.

Antenatal screening has been used in France since 1976, and includes mandatory systematic serological tests on all pregnant women with monthly follow-up serological tests on all seronegative women (Jeannel *et al.* 1990). Those women who seroconvert are then offered treatment with spiramycin.

There are no randomized placebo-controlled trials of spiramycin treatment during pregnancy. Desmonts and Couvreur (1974*b*) estimated that congenital infection, based on antibody dye tests, occurred in 26 per cent of 98 treated women compared with 63 per cent of 85 untreated women, although the incidence of clinically congenital toxoplasmosis was 11 per cent in both groups. Jeannel *et al.* (1988) reported seroconversion during pregnancy in 1.6 per cent of 2216 non-immune women. Of 33 such mothers given spiramycin (1.5 g three times daily) 33 per cent of neonates had congenital toxoplasmosis; however, no longterm results are yet available. The longterm benefits of this screening programme are, therefore, yet to be proven. The main aim of spiramycin therapy (which is available on a named patient basis only) is to reduce parasitaemia and prevent further transplacental passage. Fetal infection may be treated by means

Table 21.7 Screening and pregnancy

Author	Cassie and Stevenson (1973)	Alder	Sparks et al. (1975)	Hurley et al. (1973)	Rees and Hamlett (1972)	Thin and Michael (1970)
No. of patients	1000	903	625	1031	319	56
% With yeasts	22.3	12.6	27.4	17.7	32.6	71.4
% With *T. vaginalis*	8.9	3.7	4.7	6.0	4.0	8.9
% With *N. gonorrhoeae*	0.2	0.3	0.16	—	0.6	0

of pyrimethamine and a sulfonamide, but this should probably only be used after there is definitive evidence for transplacental passage.

It is possible that congenital toxoplasmosis could be prevented by avoiding contamination during pregnancy. Infection may be acquired by eating under-cooked meat (containing cysts), raw vegetables, unwashed fruit, and contact with cats and cat litter. All the above have been identified as factors in a prospective study on seroconversion in Parisian women during pregnancy (Jeannel *et al.* 1990). Foulon *et al.* (1988) reported that a primary prevention campaign involving food hygiene reduced the seroconversion rate during pregnancy from 1.43 per cent of 2986 non-immune patients to 0.95 per cent of 3563 non-immune patients.

Candida

Pregnant women are more prone to candida infection than are the general population. Approximately 15 per cent of non-pregnant women have evidence of candida as compared to up to 35 per cent of pregnant women (please see Table 21.7; Milsom and Forssman 1985).

Although the treatment is essentially similar to that for the non-pregnant woman, Hurley and De Louvois (1979) drew attention to the relapse of 45 per cent during pregnancy once treatment had ceased. Samaranayake and MacFarlane (1982) demonstrated that the adhesion of *Candida albicans* in culture to a monolayer of epithelial cells was enhanced by the addition of reducing sugars. They proposed that the increased vaginal glycogen content during pregnancy explained the predeliction of thrush for the vagina of the pregnant woman.

Candida infection is also of importance in the neonate. Kozinn *et al.* (1957) reported the occurrence, based on mycological studies, of oral candida in 5 per cent of babies, an incidence some 10 times higher than that expected in older infants. However, colonization with candida would seem to increase in ill neonates. Thus, Lay and Russell (1977) reported that candida was isolated from 6 per cent of 99 neonates on arrival into a special care baby unit, but that by day 14, 70 per cent of these neonates had mycological evidence of oral candida.

Such colonization may be important. Systemic candidosis has been reported in association with low birthweight. Johnson *et al.* (1984) reported 31 cases of systemic candidosis in neonates weighing less than 1500 g, this complication occurring in 3 per cent of such infants. The mortality of this condition was 39 per cent and serious morbidity 13 per cent (including hydrocephaly and severe mental retardation).

Trichomonas

Trichomonas vaginalis was isolated from the vaginae of 6 per cent of 1031 pregnant women (Hurley *et al.* 1973), whilst 0.8 per cent of these patients had *T. vaginalis* coexisting with *C. albicans*. Vaginal candidiasis during pregnancy is, therefore, three times more common than trichomoniasis. Rees and Hamlett (1972) isolated *T. vaginalis* from the lower genital tract of 4 per cent of 319 pregnant women; some 77 per cent of the 13 women with *T. vaginalis* were symptomatic. Similarly, Adler *et al.* (1981) reported *T. vaginalis* in 3.7 per cent of 903 antenatal patients. There is no good evidence that metronidazole causes birth defects or neonatal side-effects (Piper *et al.* 1993).

Gonorrhoea

Gonorrhoea is not especially prevalent in the antenatal population. As can be seen from Table 21.7, it occurred in no more than 0.6 per cent of patients in six reports. Screening *per se* is clearly not indicated. Pregnant women with gonorrhoea may be treated with either a third generation cephalosporin or with erythromycin (Cavenee *et al.* 1993; Centers for Disease Control 1989).

However, when gonorrhoea does exist, the associated problem of ophthalmia neonatorum with its potential complication of blindness becomes important. At the beginning of the 20th century, gonococcal ophthalmia neonatorum affected 8 per 1000 live births, but the current figure is probably less than 1 per 1000 (Gray *et al.* 1984). Prophylaxis against gonococcal conjunctivitis is equally effective with either topical silver nitrate drops or with erythromycin ointment (Hammerschlag *et al.* 1989).

Syphilis

Syphilis is an unusual complication of pregnancy. Although there are still some 2203 new cases of syphilis annually in the UK (Public Health Laboratory Service Communicable Disease Surveillance Centre 1989), most cases appeared in men and were considered to be homosexually acquired. Recently, up to 19 cases of congenital syphilis were reported annually in children below the age of two years. In 1984 there were four cases of congenital syphilis and in 1986 there were nine reported cases. However, as recently as 1965, there were 300 reported cases of congenital syphilis, and this dramatic reduction is due to a decrease in the incidence of the disease in women and to antenatal screening. However, the incidence of congenital syphilis may again be rising, especially, in the USA,

Table 21.8 Screening for syphilis

	No.	%
Total	219	100
Syphilis	27	12.3
Yaws	14	6.4
Non-specific treponemal disease	127	58.0
Unclassified	2	0.9
Biological false-positive	49	22.4

From Hare (1973)

partly due to a failure to test antenatal women and partly due to the acquisition of the disease later in pregnancy, after a negative test (Berkawitz *et al.* 1990; Dorfman and Glaser 1990; Ricci *et al.* 1989).

Pregnancy in a woman with syphilis will terminate in abortion or stillbirth in approximately 33 per cent of cases, with a 33 per cent incidence of congenital abnormality, and a 33 per cent incidence of normal children (Guinness *et al.* 1988; Schofield 1979). There is also an association between maternal syphilis and an increased incidence of IUGR and premature delivery (Ricci *et al.* 1989). The problems to the child may include thrombocytopenia, hepatosplenomegaly, meningitis, the signs of congenital syphilis (Hutchinson's incisors, saddle nose, etc.), and all the problems of tertiary syphilis, including the cardiovascular, neurological, and joint problems. *Treponema pallidum* crosses the placenta as early as the first trimester. Harter and Benisschke (1976) found the organism in two (out of five) first trimester conceptuses following spontaneous abortion in women with a recent syphilitic infection, hence antenatal screening, if it is to be effective, should be performed as early as possible during pregnancy.

The effects of antenatal screening

Recent antenatal clinic surveys concerning the prevalence of syphilis are few. Cassie and Stevenson (1973) found two weakly positive VDRL tests in 100 unselected antenatal patients, the cause being yaws rather than syphilis in one patient and the second patient was known to have a past history of syphilis. Hare (1973) reported the serological results of 42 904 antenatal patients screened for syphilis at the booking clinic. Some 0.5 per cent of patients had a positive serological test and the cause of that positive test in this cohort is shown in Table 21.8. It will be seen that syphilis accounted for only 12.3 per cent of the positive test, whilst biological false-positive results accounted for 22.4 per cent. Bryce and Pritchard (1981) reported two cases of maternal syphilis diagnosed in 12 222 antenatal screens (0.02 per cent). There were also four cases of treated syphilis, 10 biological false-positive results, and nine inappropriately reported as being positive.

If the diagnosis of syphilis is to be made, at the very least, a second test must

Table 21.9 The results of treatment

When treated	No. of patients	% Stillborn infants	% Congenital syphilis live-borns
During pregnancy	463	11	1.5
Prior to pregnancy	379	13	1.3
Not treated	302	18.2	30.5

From Ingraham (1951)

also be positive if the incidence of biological false-positive diagnosis is to be avoided. Wright and Gerken (1981) reviewed the sera of 7140 antenatal patients. They concluded that, although a positive VDRL was probably the most appropriate screening test with a low incidence of biological false-positives (0.15 per cent of sera), they advocated the use of the TPHA (*Treponema pallidum* haemagglutination test) followed by the FTA-ABS (Fluorescent treponemal antibody absorption test) in order to confirm the diagnosis. The TPHA gave a positive result in 0.74 per cent of all sera and this was confirmed by the FTA-ABS in 0.59 per cent.

Since the disease is now unusual and since the vast majority of positive screening tests do not represent syphilis, the value of continuing to screen antenatal patients for syphilis has been questioned. Furthermore, Gilbert (1988) reported that 43 per cent of mothers whose infants have congenital syphilis did not present for antenatal care.

The main argument in favour of continued screening would appear to be a cost–benefit one.

Gilbert (1988) argued that, if the current incidence of the disease was 0.4 per cent, 40 maternal infections would be detected and treated and 16 cases of congenital syphilis be prevented for every 100 000 women screened. The author estimated that the cost of 100 000 screens was 200 000 Australian dollars (approximately £100 000 sterling), whilst it would have cost 4 000 000 Australian dollars to look after the handicapped children. Several other authors have performed a similar cost–benefit exercise and come to similar conclusions. Williams (1985) reported a benefit: cost ratio of between 9.2 and 82.8:1, with a 'best estimate' of 32.9:1 assuming that all women were screened before the 26th week of pregnancy, that 150 cases of maternal syphilis were diagnosed annually out of 600 000 deliveries, and that 29 children per year no longer needed lifelong institutional care.

The treatment of syphilis during pregnancy

The key to successful treatment would appear to be early diagnosis. Jackson *et al.* (1962) reported the treatment of 77 women with syphilis diagnosed during pregnancy using a single injection of 2.4 megaunits of benzylpenicillin. All 77 infants, tested within the first year of life, were seronegative. Ingraham (1951) reported 1144 women with syphilis. As can be seen from Table 21.9 treating syphilis either prior to pregnancy or during pregnancy would appear to have a significantly beneficial effect upon the incidence of stillbirth and of congenital syphilis. Guinness *et al.* (1988) reported that when 27 women with syphilis, detected by antenatal screening, were treated with penicillin, there were no perinatal losses. Penicillin is still considered to be the treatment of choice (Bout *et al.* 1992).

Treatment failure may occur. Mascola *et al.* (1984) analysed the causes of treatment failure in pregnant women with syphilis and found that true treatment failure occurred in 0.2 per cent of 1982 patients given 2.4 megaunits of benzylpenicillin. In patients with a penicillin allergy, erythromycin is used as the second choice antibiotic during pregnancy (Montgomery *et al.* 1961). However, erythromycin is less well able to cross the placenta than is penicillin, relatively lower fetal levels being obtained leading to failures of treatment (South *et al.* 1964). In view of this, it is recommended that patients with a penicillin allergy be admitted to hospital for desensitization followed by treatment with penicillin (Centers for Disease Control 1988). It is generally advised that the infant of any pregnant woman treated for syphilis during pregnancy is tested serologically as soon as possible after the birth.

Streptococcal infection

Whilst streptococcal septicaemia is no longer a major cause of puerperal sepsis, infection with β-haemolytic streptococcus still emerges as a potentially fatal cause of neonatal meningitis and septicaemia. Horn *et al.* (1974) reported a 50 per cent combined mortality and morbidity in 44 infants with neonatal group B streptococcal infection, with 18 deaths and 4 infants surviving with neurological sequelae, including poor speech and deafness. Greenspoon *et al.* (1991) assessed 7198 such infants with a mortality of 27 per cent and neurological sequelae from meningitis in 15 per cent of the survivors. The infection is found in 1 in 500 live births (Franciosi *et al.* 1973).

The organism may be commonly found in the vaginae of women in an incidence of 5–25 per cent (Easmon *et al.* 1985; Franciosi *et al.* 1973). Colonization of the fetus is said to occur during passage through the birth canal, but instances of infection in babies delivered by Caesarean section with intact membranes have been reported (Parker 1977).

One of the major problems with screening antenatal patients for this organism is that the colonization of the vagina by β-haemolytic streptococcus is not consistent. Ferrieri *et al.* (1977) reported that only 42 per cent of 63 women with a positive swab during labour had a positive swab during the mid-trimester period, whilst 16 per cent of 45 women with a positive swab during the third trimester had a negative culture during labour. Anthony *et al.* (1978) took 4–11 vaginal swabs from 1293 pregnant women during pregnancy and labour. Overall, 16 per cent of pregnant women had a positive culture on one of the first swabs, but 28 per cent had a positive culture on one of any swabs. Of the 108 carriers, the authors considered that 36 per cent were chronic, 20 per cent transient, and 44 per cent intermittent. Similarly, other series have demonstrated that 50 per cent of pregnant women who had positive vaginal cultures converted to negative cultures without any treatment (Lewin and Amstey 1981). It would, therefore, seem only logical to take swabs during the third trimester and not at other times, unless there is a vaginal discharge.

Antenatal screening for group B streptococcus will identify most, but not all, colonized women, and, hence, will not predict all those neonates at risk from infection (Greenspoon *et al.* 1991). In a prospective study of 1304 pregnant women, 7 per cent were colonized with the organism and three infants were infected in the neonatal period, all delivered by culture positive women (Iams and O'shaughnessey 1982). There would seem to be value in screening for the organism in women at particular risk (such as a previously affected infant) but not in total population screening (Greenspoon *et al.* 1991; Iams and O'Shaughnessey 1982).

Antibiotics and group B streptococci

Ideally, one should eradicate the organism from the vagina before labour occurs. However, this would seem not to be possible, partly because a single negative screen does not protect against streptococcal colonization of the vagina during labour and partly because of a recurrence of the organism in treated women. Gardner *et al.* (1979) treated women with oral penicillin following the isolation of group B streptococcus on vaginal swab. When these women were recultured three weeks later, 70 per cent were still colonized and 67 per cent were colonized at the time of delivery.

The value of intrapartum chemoprophylaxis with ampicillin or erythromycin is well recognized and is the treatment of choice for women with a positive culture. Yow *et al.* (1979) gave intravenous ampicillin (500 mg every six hours) to 34 women colonized with the organism during labour. None of the infants were colonized within 48 hours of birth, whereas 58 per cent of the infants of 24 women with the organism, but not given antibiotics, were colonized. Boyer *et al.* (1982) reported a randomized prospective trial of intravenous ampicillin (1 g every four hours) during labour. A positive culture was obtained from the neonate in 2.8 per cent of 71 women given ampicillin but in 37.5 per cent of 128 women who received no prophylaxis. Easmon *et al.* (1983) reported a group of pregnant women who were found to have group B streptococci in their vagina during the third trimester. They were randomly allocated to receive either 100 mg of intramuscular benzylpenicillin every eight hours during labour (erythromycin 500 mg if allergic to penicillin) or to receive no prophylaxis. Of the 38 women in the antibiotic group, no babies were colonized within 24 hours of birth, but 3 per cent of babies became colonized during the hospital stay. Of the 49 patients in the control group, 35 per cent of babies were colonized within 24 hours and 45 per cent by the time they were discharged home. Morales *et al.* (1986) randomized 263 women with a positive vaginal culture to receive antibiotics or no treatment. Of 135 women treated with 1 g ampicillin every six hours until delivery, no infant was colonized, whereas of 129 women not treated, 46 per cent of the infants were colonized.

Whilst it seems that antimicrobial prophylaxis in specific cases is of value, no one chemoprophylactic regime would seem to be superior to any other (Greenspoon *et al.* 1991). In patients who are allergic to penicillin, erythromycin would appear to be effective (Easmon *et al.* 1983).

Listeriosis

Listeria monocytogenes is a short, predominantly Gram positive, non-acid-fast bacillus that does not produce spores. The organism may be found in soil, plants, food, and human stools. It has the unusual ability to grow over a wide temperature range (2–42 °C), hence it will grow in food inside a refrigerator (*Lancet* 1989). There would appear to be a predeliction for pregnancy, causing either no ill-effects or a flu-like illness in the pregnant women yet crossing the placenta to kill the fetus or give rise to perinatal septicaemia or meningitis. B. Schwartz *et al.* (1988) reported 154 women with listeriosis, one-third of whom were pregnant and two-thirds either immunosuppressed or elderly. Some 28 per cent of the cases were fatal. In the presence of transplacental infection, the organism was cultured from the maternal surface of the placenta in 97 per cent of 30 cases (Relier 1975).

The annual incidence of infection with *Listeria* spp. in the UK is 1 per 230 000 head of population, but the annual incidence of perinatal or neonatal infection is 1 per 9700 births (McLauchlin *et al.* 1988). In France, the annual incidence of listeriosis is 1 per 91 000 head of population with a proportionate increase in the perinatal and neonatal infection rates (Buckdahl *et al.* 1990).

Congenital listeriosis may present with pneumonia, septicaemia, and meningitis as a later complication. Halliday and Hirata (1979) reported a mortality of 25 per cent of 12 patients with neonatal listeriosis, and occasional morbidity in the survivors, including chronic respiratory problems. Jacobs *et al.* (1978) reported a mortality of 44 per cent of nine neonates. This high mortality may reflect not just the disease but its association with prematurity, since infected fetuses have a tendency to deliver before term (Spencer 1987; Buckdahl *et al.* 1990).

There is evidence that listeriosis is increasing in incidence during pregnancy. Buckdahl *et al.* (1990) reported that between 30 and 40 per cent of all reported listeria infections occur in pregnant women and, in England and Wales, there were 291 reported cases of listeriosis in 1988, 259 in 1987, 137 in 1986, and 50 in 1967. Of those cases which occurred during pregnancy, some 34 per cent will be associated with abortion, stillbirth, or neonatal death.

The association between listeriosis and abortion is conflicting and out of date. Rappaport *et al.* (1960) isolated *Listeria* spp. from the genital tracts of 73.5 per cent of 34 women with a history of repeated abortion, but in none of 89 controls. These authors also found *Listeria* in some products of conception. Other workers have not been able to substantiate this view. Macnaughton (1962) was unable to isolate *Listeria* from an cervical swabs taken from 87 women with a threatened or incomplete abortion, whilst Ansbacher *et al.* (1966) were unable to isolate *Listeria* from swabs taken from the cervix and products of conception of 36 women with spontaneous abortions.

The treatment of listeriosis

Listeriosis is generally treated by a combination of ampicillin or penicillin with gentamicin or kanamycin (Gordon *et al*. 1972; Jacobs *et al*. 1978; Kalstone 1991; Spencer 1987). Gordon *et al*. 1972 stressed the possibility of *in vitro* synergism of antibiotic combinations based on studies of *Listeria* growth kinetics Hume (1976) advocated that ampicillin alone should be used for an infection during pregnancy, with evidence of fetal sparing from maternal infection following this treatment.

Listeria and food

Most outbreaks of listeriosis occur in clusters and many have been traced to particular foods. The following have been implicated:

(1) coleslaw made from contaminated cabbage (Schlech *et al*. 1983);

(2) supermarket prepacked salad (Sizmmur and Walker 1988);

(3) undercooked hot dogs (B. Schwartz *et al*. 1988);

(4) undercooked chicken, both fresh and frozen (B. Schwartz *et al*. 1988; *Lancet* 1989).

(5) cook–chill food (Kerr *et al*. 1988);

(6) milk, both pasteurized and unpasteurized, both cow and goat (Fleming *et al*. 1985);

(7) soft cheese; soft cheeses are 'fresh' and have not aged, whereas hard cheeses have been able to acquire a sufficiently low pH to discourage bacterial growth (Linnan *et al*. 1988; *Lancet* 1989).

It would seem sensible for pregnant patients to be given balance advice involving some precautions with the above food products (McLauchlin 1992).

Conclusions

Clearly, pregnant women can develop infection as can anyone, but certain infections, especially listeriosis, would appear to be more common in the pregnant woman. Other infections assume greater importance during pregnancy than they might otherwise in view of the possible associations with fetal abnormality. In order to give well-balanced and scientific advice to these patients, an appropriate knowledge of the statistics concerning their dangers and an appropriate knowledge of confirmatory tests, whether on maternal, fetal, or neonatal tissue, is mandatory. Lastly, although HIV infection occurs predominantly in the male population, the small, but significant, number of infected women who achieve pregnancy require some additional expertise and advice, and it may be that HIV infection during pregnancy will assume a greater importance over the next few years.

References

Ades, A. E., Parker, S., Berry, T., Holland, F. J., Davidson, C. F., Cubitt, D., *et al.* (1991). Prevalence of maternal HIV-1 infection in Thames regions. *Lancet* **337**, 1562–5.

Ades, A. E., Davison, C. F., Holland, F. J., Gibb, D. M., Hudson, C. N., Nicholl, A., *et al.* (1993). Vertically transmitted HIV infection in the British Isles. *British Medical Journal* **306**, 1296–9.

Adler, M. W., Belsey, E. M., and Rogers, J. S. (1981). Sexually transmitted diseases in a defined population of women. *British Medical Journal* **283**, 29–32.

Aiuti, F., Luzi, G., Messaroma, I., Scano, G., and Papetti, C. (1987). Delayed appearance of HIV infection in children. *Lancet* **ii**, 858.

Alford, C. A. (1971). Immunoglobulin determination in the diagnosis of fetal infection. *Pediatric Clinics of North America* **18**, 99–113.

Alger, L. S., Farley, J., Robinson, B. A., Hines, S. E., Birchin, J. M., and Johnson, J. P. (1993). Interaction of human immunodeficiency infection and pregnancy. *Obstetrics and Gynecology* **82**, 787–96.

Amstey, M. S., Monif, G. R. G., Nahmias, A. J., and Josey, W. E. (1979). Caesarean section and gestational herpes virus infection. *Obstetrics and Gynecology* **53**, 641–2.

Anand, A., Gray, E. S., Brown, T., Clewley, J. P., and Cohen, B. J. (1987). Human parvovirus infection in pregnancy and hydrops fetalis. *New England Journal of Medicine* **316**, 183–6.

Andrews, E. B., Yankaskas, B. L., Cordero, J. F., Schoeffler, K., Humpp, S., and the Acyclovir in Pregnancy Registry (1992). Acyclovir in Pregnancy. *Obstetrics and Gynecology* **79**, 7–13.

Ansbacher, R., Borchardt, K. A., Hannegan, M. W., and Boyson, W. A. (1966). Clinical investigations of listeria mycocytogenes as a possible cause of fetal wastage. *American Journal of Obstetrics and Gynecology* **94**, 386–90.

Anthony, B. F., Okada, D. M., and Hobel, C. J. (1978). Epidemiology of group B streptococcus. *Journal of Infectious Diseases* **137**, 524–30.

Arvin, A. M., Hensleigh, R. A., Prober, C. G., Au, D. S., Yasukawa, L. L., Wittek, A. E., *et al.* (1986). Failure of ante-partum maternal cultures to predict the infant's risk of exposure to herpes simplex at delivery. *New England Journal of Medicine* **315**, 796–800.

Auger, I., Thomas, P., DeGruttola, V., Morse, D., Moore, D., Willams, R., *et al.* (1988). Incubation period for paediatric AIDS patients. *Nature* **336**, 575–7.

Banatvala, J. E. Christie, I. L. Palmer, S. J., and Kenney, A. (1990). Retrospective study of HIV, hepatitis B and HTLV-1 infection at a London maternity clinic. *Lancet* **335**, 859–60.

Banatvala, J. E., Christie, I. L. Palmer, S. J. Sumner, D., Kennedy, J., and Kenney, A. (1991). HIV screening in pregnancy. *Lancet* **37**, 121–8.

Barbacci, M., Repke, J. T., and Chaisson, R. E. (1991). Routine prenatal screening for HIV infection. *Lancet* **337**, 709–11.

Berkowitz, K. M., Stamp, F. K., Baxi, L., and Fox, H. E. (1990). False negative screening tests for syphilis in pregnant women. *New England Journal of Medicine* **323**, 270–1.

Binkin, M. J., Koplan, J. P., and Kates, W. (1984). Preventing neonatal herpes. *Journal of the American Medical Association* **251**, 2816–21.

Blanche, S., Rouzioux, C., Moscato, M. L. G., Veber, F., Mayaux, M. J., Lacomet, C., *et al.* (1989). A prospective study of infants born to women seropositive for HIV, *New England Journal of Medicine* **320**, 1643–8.

Bout, J. M., Oranje, A. P., de Grout, R., Tan, G., and Stolz, E. (1992). Congenital syphilis. *International Journal of STD and AIDS* **3**, 161–7.

Boyer, K. M., Gadzala, C. A., Kelly, P. C., and Gotoff, S. P. (1982). Ampicillin prophylaxis of group B streptococcus transmission in high-risk parturient women. *Pediatric Research* **16**, 280A.

Brown, Z. A. and Baker, D. A. (1989). Acyclovir therapy during pregnancy. *Obstetrics and Gynecology* **73**, 526–31.

Brown, Z. A., Benedetti, J., Ashley, R., Burchett, S., Selk, E. S., Berry, S., *et al.* (1991). Neonatal herpes simplex infection *New England Journal of Medicine* **324**, 1247–52.

Brunnell, P. A. (1967). Varicella–zoster infections in pregnancy. *Journal of the American Medical Association* **199**, 315–17.

Brunnell, P. A., Roxx, A., Miller, L., Kuo, B. (1969). Prevention of varicella by zoster immune globulin. *New England Journal of Medicine* **280**, 1191.

Bryce, R. L. and Pritchard, R. C. (1991). The outcome of routine antenatal screening for syphilis. *Australian and New Zealand Journal of Obstetrics and Gynaecology* **21**, 211–13.

Buckdahl, R., Hird, M., Gamsu, H., Tapp, A., Gibb, D., and Tzannatos C. (1990). Listeriosis revisited. *British Journal of Obstetrics and Gynaecology* **97**, 186–9.

Cassie, R. and Stevenson, A. (1973). Screening for gonorrhoea, trichomonas, moniliosis, and syphilis in pregnancy. *Journal of Obstetrics and Gynaecology of the British Commonwealth* **80**, 48–51.

Cavenee, M. R., Farris, J. R., Spalding, T. R., Barnes, D. L., Castaneda, Y., and Wendel, G. D. (1993). Treatment of gonorrhoea in pregnancy. *Obstetrics and Gynecology* **81**, 33–8.

Centers for Disease Control (1988). Guide lines for the prevention and control of congenital syphilis. *Morbidity and Mortality Weekly Report* **37**, supp 1, 1–12.

Centers for Disease Control (1989). Sexually transmitted diseases treatment guidelines. *Morbidity and Mortality Weekly Report* **38**, supp 8, 4–36.

Centers for Disease Control (1991). Increase in rubella and congenital rubella syndrome in the United States. *Morbidity and Mortality Weekly Report* **40**, 93–9.

Charton, F. (1991). New AIDS figures. *British Medical Journal* **302**, 197–8.

Coffey, V. P. and Jessop, W. J. E. (1959). Maternal infection and congenital deformities. *Lancet* **ii**, 935–8.

Daffos, F., Capella-Pavlovsky, M., and Forestier, F. (1985). Fetal blood sampling during pregnancy with use of a needle guided by ultrasound. *American Journal of Obstetrics and Gynecology* **153**, 655–60.

Daffos, F., Forestier, F., Capella-Pavlovsky, M., Thulliex, P., Aufrant, C., Valenti, D., *et al.* (1988). Prenatal management of 746 pregnancies at risk for congenital toxoplasmosis. *New England Journal of Medicine* **318**, 271–5.

Davison, C. A., Ades, A. E., Hudson, C. N., and Peckham, C. S. (1989). Antenatal testing for HIV. *Lancet* **ii**, 1440–4.

Desmonts, G. and Couvreur, J. (1974a). Toxoplasma in pregnancy—its transmission to the fetus. *Bulletin of the New York Academy of Medicine* **50**, 146–59.

Desmonts, G. and Couvreur, J. (1974b). Congenital toxoplasmosis. *New England Journal of Medicine* **290**, 1110–16.

Doner, C., Leisnard, C., Content, J., Busine, A., Aderca, J., and Rodesch, F. (1993).

Pre-natal diagnosis of pregnancy at risk for congenital CMV infection. *Obstetrics and Gynecology* **82**, 481–6.

Dorfman, D. H. and Glaser, J. H. (1990). Congenital syphilis presenting in infants after the newborn period. *New England Journal of Medicine* **323**, 1299–302.

Dudgeon, J. A. (1976). Infective causes of human malformation. *British Medical Bulletin* **32**, 77–83.

Easmon, C. S. F., Hastings, M. J. G., Deeley, J., Bloxham, B., Rivers, R., and Marwood, R. (1983). The effect of intrapartum chemoprophylaxis on the vertical transmission of group B streptococci. *British Journal of Obstetrics and Gynaecology* **90**, 633–5.

Easmon, C. S. F., Hastings, M. J. G., Neill, J., Bloxham, B., and Rivers, R. P. A. (1985). Is group B streptococcal screening during pregnancy justified? *British Journal of Obstetrics and Gynaecology* **92**, 197–207.

Eder, S. E., Apuzzio, J. J., and Weiss, G. (1988). Varicella pneumonia during pregnancy. Treatment of two cases with acyclovir. *American Journal of Perinatology* **5**, 16–18.

Ehrnst, A., Lindgran, S., Dictor, M., Johansson, B., Sonarburg, A., Czajkowski, J., et al. (1991). HIV in pregnant women and their offspring: evidence for late transmission. *Lancet* **38**, 203–7.

Embril, J. A., Ozere, R. L., and Haldane, E. V. (1970). Congenital CMV infection to siblings from consecutive pregnancies. *Journal of Paediatrics* **77**, 417–21.

European Collaborative Study (1991). Children born to women with HIV-1 infection. *Lancet* **337**, 253–60.

European Collaborative Study (1992). Risk factors for mother-to-child transmission of HIV-1. *Lancet* **339**, 1007–12.

Ferenczy, A. (1984). Treating genital condyloma during pregnancy with the carbon dioxide lazer. *American Journal of Obstetrics and Gynecology* **148**, 9–12.

Ferrieri, P., Cleary, P. P., and Seeds, A. (1977). Epidemiology of group B streptococcal carriage in pregnant women and newborn infants. *Journal of Medical Microbiology* **10**, 103–14.

Fleming, D. W., Cochi, S. I., MacDonald, K. L., Brandum, J., Hayes, P. S., Plikaytis, B. D., et al. (1985). Pasteurized milk as a vehicle of infection in an outbreak of listeriosis. *New England Journal of Medicine* **312**, 404–7.

Forestier, F., Cox, W. L., Daffas, F., and Rainaut, M. (1988). The assessment of fetal blood samples. *American Journal of Obstetrics and Gynaecology* **158**, 1184–8.

Foulon, W., Naessens , A., Lauwers, S., De Meuter, F., and Amy, J. J. (1988). Impact of primary prevention on the incidence of toxoplasmosis during pregnancy. *Obstetrics and Gynecology* **72**, 363–6.

Foulon, W., Naessens, A., Mahler, T., De Waele, M., De Catte, L., and De Meuter, F. (1990). Prenatal diagnosis of congenital toxoplasmosis. *Obstetrics and Gynecology* **76**, 769–72.

Franciosi, R. A., Knostman, J. D., and Zimmerman, R. A. (1973). Group B streptococcal neonatal and infant infections. *Journal of Paediatrics* **82**, 707–18.

Frommell, G. T., Rothenberg, R., Wong, S., and McIntosh, K. (1979). Chlamydial infection of mothers and their infants. *Journal of Paediatrics* **95**, 28–32.

Gardner, S. E., Yo, W. M. D., Leeds, L. J., Thompson, P. K., Mason, E. D., and Clark, D. J. (1979). Failure of penicillin to eradicate group B streptococcal colonisation in the pregnant woman. *American Journal of Obstetrics and Gynecology* **135**, 1062–5.

Ghidini, A., Sepulveda, W., Lockwood, C. J., and Romero, R. (1993). Complications of fetal blood sampling. *American Journal of Obstetrics and Gynecology* **168**, 1339–44.

Gibbs, R. S., Amstey, M. S., Sweet, M. L., Mead, P. B., and Sever, J. L. (1988). Management of genital herpes infection in pregnancy. *Obstetrics and Gynecology* **71**, 779–80.

Gilbert, G. L. (1988). Congenital syphilis — should we worry? *Medical Journal of Australia* **148**, 162–3.

Gilbert, G. L. (1993). Chicken pox during pregnancy. *British Medical Journal* **306**, 1079–80.

Gordon, R. C., Barrett, F. F., and Clark, D. J. (1972). Influence of several antibiotics, singularly and in combination, on the growth of *Listeria monocytogenes. Journal of Paediatrics* **80**, 667–70.

Gray, O. P., Campbell, A. G. M., Kerr, M. M., Forfar, J. U., Keay, A. J., Uttley, S. S., *et al.* (1984). The newborn. In *Textbook of paediatrics* (ed. J. O. Forfar and G. C. Arneil), pp. 117–258, Churchill Livingstone, Edinburgh.

Greenspoon, J. S., Wilcox, J. G., and Kirschbaun, T. H. (1991). Group B streptococcus the effectiveness of screening and chemoprophylaxis. *Obstetrics and Gynecological Survey* **46**, 499–504.

Griffiths, P. D. and Baboonian, C. (1984). A prospective study of primary cytomegalovirus infection during pregnancy. *British Journal of Obstetrics and Gynaecology* **91**, 307–15.

Griffiths, P. D., Baboonian, C., Rotter, D., and Peckham, C. (1991). Congenital and maternal CMV infection in a London population. *British Journal of Obstetrics and Gynaecology* **98**, 135–40.

Grossman, J. H., Wallen, W. C., and Sever, J. L. (1981). Management of genital herpes simplex virus infection during pregnancy. *Obstetrics and Gynecology* **58**, 1–4.

Guinness, L. F., Sibandze, S., McGrath, E., and Cornelis, A. L. (1988). Influence of antenatal screening on perinatal mortality caused by syphilis. *Genitourinary Medicine* **64**, 294–7.

Haddad, G., Langer, B., Astruc, D., Messer, J., and Lokiec, F. (1993). Oral acyclovir doesn't prevent asymptomatic shedding of virus or prevent transmission to fetus. *Obstetrics and Gynecology* **81**, 750–2.

Halliday, H. L. and Hirata, T. (1979). Perinatal listeriosis — review of 12 patients. *American Journal of Obstetrics and Gynecology* **133**, 405–10.

Hammerschlag, M. R., Cummings, C., Roblin, P. M., Williams, T. H., and Delke, I. (1989). Efficacy of neonatal occular prophylaxis for the prevention of chlamydial and gynococcal conjunctivitis. *New England Journal of Medicine* **320**, 769–72.

Hankins, G. D., Gilstrap, L. C., and Patterson, A. R. (1987). Acyclovir treatment of varicella pneumonia in pregnancy. *Critical Care Medicine* **15**, 336–7.

Hanngren, K., Grandien, M., and Grandstrom, G. (1985). Effects of zoster immunoglobulin for varicella prophylaxis in the newborn. *Scandinavian Journal of Infectious Diseases* **17**, 343–7.

Hare, M. J. (1973). Serological tests for treponemal disease in pregnancy. *Journal of Obstetrics and Gynaecology of the British Commonwealth* **80**, 515–19.

Harris, R. E. and Rhoades, E. R. (1965). Varicella pneumonia complicating pregnancy. *Obstetrics and Gynecology* **25**, 734–40.

Harter, C. A. and Benisschke, K. (1976). Fetal syphilis in the first trimester. *American Journal of Obstetrics and Gynecology* **124**, 705–11.

Hermann, K. L. (1982). Congenital and perinatal varicella. *Clinical Obstetrics and Gynecology* **25**, 605–9.

Higa, K., Dan, K., and Manabe, H. (1987). Varicella–zoster infections in pregnancy: Hypothesis concerning the mechanisms of congenital malformations. *Obstetrics and Gynecology* **69**, 214–22.

Hobson, D., Rees, E., and Viswalingham, N. D. (1983). Chlamydial infection in neonates and older children. *British Medical Bulletin* **39**, 138–32.

Holliman, R. E., Johnson, J. D., Constantine, G., Bissenden, J. G., Nicolaides, K., and Savva, D. (1991). Difficulties in the diagnosis of congenital toxoplasmosis by cordocentesis. *British Journal of Obstetrics and Gynaecology* **98**, 832–4.

Horn, K. A., Zimmerman, R. A., Knotsman, J. D., and Meyer, W. T. (1974). Neurological sequelae of group B streptococcal neonatal infection. *Paediatrics* **53**, 501–4.

Hume, O. S. (1976). Maternal *Listeria monocytogenes* septicaemia with sparing of the fetus. *Obstetrics and Gynecology* **48**, 33s–44s.

Hurley, R. and De Louvois, J. (1979). Candida vaginitis. *Postgraduate Medical Journal* **55**, 645–7.

Hurley, R., Lesk, B. G. S., Faktor, J. A., and De Foneska, C. I. (1973). Incidence and distribution of yeast species and of *Trichomonalis vaginalis* in the vagina of pregnant women. *Journal of Obstetrics and Gynaecology of the British Commonwealth* **80**, 252–7.

Iams, J. D. and O'Shaughnessey, R. (1982). Antepartum versus intrapartum selection screening for maternal group B streptococcus colonization. *American Journal of Obstetrics and Gynecology* **143**, 153–6.

Ingraham, N. R. (1951). Syphilis in pregnancy and congenital syphilis. *Acta Dermatovenereologica* **Supp. 24**, 60–87.

Italian Multicentre Study (1988). Epidemiology, clinical features, and prognostic features of paediatric HIV infection. *Lancet* **ii**, 1043–5.

Jackson, F. R., Vanderstoep, E. M., Knox, J. M., Desmond, M. M., and Moore, M. B. (1962). Use of aqueous benzathine penicillin G in the treatment of syphilis in pregnant women. *American Journal of Obstetrics and Gynecology* **83**, 1389–92.

Jacobs, M. R., Stein, H., Buqwana, A., Dubb, A., Segal, F., Rabinowitz, L., *et al.* (1978). Epidemic listeriosis *South African Medical Journal* **54**, 389–92.

Jeannel, D., Niel, G., Costagliola, D., Danis, M., Traore, B. M., and Gentilini, M. (1988). Epidemiology of toxoplasma infection of pregnant women in the Paris area. *International Journal of Epidemiology* **17**, 595–602.

Jeannel, D., Costagliola, D., Niel, G., Hubert, B., and Danis, M. (1990). What is known about the prevention of congenital toxoplasmos? *Lancet* **336**, 359–61.

Johnson, D. E., Thompson, T. R., Green, T. P., and Ferrieri, P. (1984). Systemic candidiosis in very low birth-weight infants. *Pediatrics* **73**, 138–43.

Johnson, F. W. A., Matheson, B. A., Williams, H., Laing, A. G., Jandial, B., Davidson-Lamb, R., *et al.* (1985). Abortion due to infection with *Chlamydia psittaci* in a sheep farmer's wife. *British Medical Journal* **290**, 592–4.

Johnson, M. A. and Webster, A. (1989). Human immunodeficiency virus infection in women. *British Journal of Obstetrics and Gynaecology* **96**, 129–32.

Johnstone, F. D., MacCallum, L., Brettle, R., Inglis, J. M., and Peutherer, J. F. (1988). Does infection with HIV affect the outcome of pregnancy? *British Medical Journal* **296**, 467.

Johnstone, F. D., Willox, L., and Brettle, R. P. (1992). Survival time after AIDS in pregnancy. *British Journal of Obstetrics and Gynaecology* **99**, 633–6.

Joynson, D. H. M. and Payne, R. (1988). Screening for toxoplasmosis in pregnancy. *Lancet* **ii**, 795–6.

Kalstone, C. (1991). Successful antepartum treatment of listeriosis. *American Journal of Obstetrics and Gynecology* **164**, 57–8.

Kelly, J. (1988). Genital herpes during pregnancy. *British Medical Journal* **297**, 1146–7.

Kerr, K., Dealler, S. F., and Lacey, R. W. (1988). Listeria in cook–chill food. *Lancet* **ii**, 37–8.

Knott, P. D., Welpley, G. A. C., and Anderson, M. J. (1984). Serologically proven intra-uterine infection with parvovirus. *British Medical Journal* **289**, 6660.

Kovar, I. and Harvey, D. (1981). Current problems in TORCH and other viral perinatal infections. In *Progress in obstetrics and gynaecology*, Vol. 1, (ed J. Studd), pp. 39–50. Churchill Livingstone, Edinburgh.

Kozinn, P. J., Taschdjan, C. L., Dragutsky, D., and Minsky, A. (1957). Cutaneous candidiasis in early infancy and childhood. *Pediatrics* **20**, 827–30.

Krasinski, K., Burkowsky, W., Bebenroth, D., and Moore, T. (1988). Failure of voluntary testing for HIV to identify infected parturient women. *New England Journal of Medicine* **318**, 185.

Kumar, M. L., Nankervis, G. A., Cooper, A. R., and Gold, E. (1984a). Postnatally acquired CMV infection in infants of CMV-excreting mothers. *Journal of Paediatrics* **104**, 669–73.

Kumar, M. L., Nankervis, G. A., Jacobs, I. B., Ernhart, C. B., Glasson, C. E., McMillan, P. M., et al. (1984b). Congenital and postnatally acquired cytomegalovirus infections. *Journal of Paediatrics* **104**, 674–9.

Lancet (1989). Listeriosis. *Lancet* **i**, 83–4.

Lancet (1991). TORCH syndrome and TORCH screening. *Lancet* **335**, 1559–61.

Landesman, S., Minkoff, H., Holman, S., McCalla, S., and Sijin, O. (1987). Serosurvey of HIV infection in parturients. *Journal of the American Medical Association* **258**, 2701–3.

Landsberger, E. J., Hager, W. D., and Grossman, J. H. (1986). Successful management of varicella pneumonia complicating pregnancy. *Journal of Reproductive Medicine* **31**, 311–14.

Lay, K. M. and Russell, C. (1977). Candida species and yeasts in mouths of infants from a special care baby unit of a maternity hospital. *Archives of Diseases in Childhood* **52**, 794–804.

Leck, I. (1963). Incidence of malformation following influenza epidemics. *British Journal of Preventative and Social Medicine* **17**, 70–80.

Lewin, E. B. and Amstey, M. S. (1981). Natural history of group B streptococcus colonization during pregnancy. *American Journal of Obstetrics and Gynecology* **139**, 512–15.

Linnan, M. J., Mascola, L., Lou, X. D., Goulet, V., May, S., Salminen, C., et al. (1988). Epidemic listeriosis associated with Mexican-style cheese. *New England Journal of Medicine* **319**, 823–8.

Lissauer, T. and Jeffries, D. (1989). Preventing neonatal herpes infection. *British Journal of Obstetrics and Gynaecology* **96**, 1015–23.

Lundstrom, S. (1962). Rubella during pregnancy. *Acta Paediatrica Scandinavica* **Supp. 133**, 9–11.

MacDonald, M. G., Ginzburg, H. M., and Bolan, J. C. (1991). HIV infection in pregnancy. *Journal of the Acquired Immunodeficiency Syndrome* **4**, 100–8.

McGregor, J. A. and French, J. I. (1991). *Chlamydia trachomatus* infection during pregnancy. *American Journal of Obstetrics and Gynecology* **164**, 1782–9.

McLauchlin, J. (1992). Listeriosis. *British Medical Journal* **304**, 1583–4.

McLauchlin, J., Saunders, N., Ridley, A. M., and Taylor, A. G. (1988). Listeriosis and food-borne transmission. *Lancet* **i**, 177–8.

Macnaughton, M. C. (1962). *Listeria monocytogenes* in abortion. *Lancet* **ii**, 484.

Magat, A. H., Alger, L. S., Nagey, D. A., Hatch, V., and Lovchik, J. C. (1993). Double-blind randomized study comparing amoxycillin and erythromycin for the treatment of Chlamydia trachomatis in pregnancy. *Obstetrics and Gynecology* **81**, 745–9.

Manson, M. M., Logan, W. P. D., and Loy, R. M. (1960). Rubella and other infections during pregnancy. *Reports on Public Health and Medical Subjects* **101**, 33–48.

Marion, R. W., Wiznia, A. A., Huthceon, G., and Rubinstein, A. (1986). Human T-cell lymphotrophic virus type III embryopathy. *American Journal of Diseases of Children* **140**, 638–40.

Mascola, L., Pelosi, R., and Alexander, C. (1984). Inadequate treatment of syphilis in pregnancy. *American Journal of Obstetrics and Gynecology* **150**, 945–7.

Meyers, J. D. (1974). Congenital varicella in term infants: Risks considered. *Journal of Infectious Diseases* **129**, 215–17.

Miller, C. L., Miller, E., Sequerira, P. J. L., Crodock-Watson, J. E., Langson, M., and Wiseberg, E. (1985). Effect of selective vaccination on rubella susceptibility and infection in pregnancy. *British Medical Journal* **291**, 1398–401.

Miller, E., Crodock-Watson, J. E., and Pollock, T. M. (1982). Consequences of confirmed maternal rubella at successive stages of pregnancy. *Lancet* ii, 781–4.

Milsom, I. and Forssman, L. (1985). Repeated candidiosis – reinfection or recrudescent? *American Journal of Obstetrics and Gynecology* **152**, 956–9.

Montgomery, C. H., Knox, J. M., Sciple, G. W., and Stoep, E. M. V. (1961). *Archives of Internal Medicine* **107**, 732–5.

Morales, W. J., Lim, D., and Walsh, A. F. (1986). Prevention of neonatal group B streptococcal sepsis by the use of a rapid screening test and selective intrapartum chemoprophylaxis. *American Journal of Obstetrics and Gynecology* **155**, 979–83.

Morbidity and Mortality Weekly Report. (1986). Rubella vaccination during pregnancy. *Morbidity and Mortality Weekly Report* **35**, 275–85.

Mortimer, P. P., Cohen, B. J., Buckley, M. M., Crocock-Watson, J. E., Ridhalgh, M. K. S., Burkhardt, F., *et al.* (1985). Human Parvovirus in the fetus. *Lancet* ii, 1012.

Munday, P. E., Porter, R., Falder, P. S., Carder, J. F., Holliman, R., Lewis, B. V., *et al.* (1984). Spontaneous abortion – an infectious aetiology? *British Journal of Obstetrics and Gynaecology* **81**, 1177–80.

Music, S. I., Fine, E. M., and Togo, Y. (1971). Zoster-like disease in the newborn due to herpes simplex virus. *New England Journal of Medicine* **284**, 24–6.

Nagington, J., Wreghitt, T. G., Gandy, G., Robertson, N. R. C., and Berry, P. J. (1978). Fetal echovirus infections in outbreak in special care baby unit. *Lancet* ii, 725–8.

Nahmias, A. J., Josey, W. E., Naib, Z. M., Freeman, M. G., Fernandez, R. G., and Wheeler, J. M. (1971*a*). Perinatal risk associated with maternal genital herpes simplex virus. *American Journal of Obstetrics and Gynecology* **101**, 825–37.

Nahmias, A. J., Walls, K. W., Stewart, J. A., Herrman, K. L., and Flint, W. J. (1971*b*). The 'TORCH' complex. *Paediatric Research* **5**, 405–6.

Newell, M. L. and Peckham, C. S. (1994). Working towards a European strategy for intervention to reduce vertical transmission of HIV. *British Journal of Obstetrics and Gynaecology* **101**, 192–6.

Oriel, J. D. (1992). Sexually transmitted diseases in children: Human papillomavirus infection. *Genito-Urinary Medicine* **68**, 80–3.

O'Sullivan, M. J., Boyer, P. J., Scott, G. B., Parkes, W. P., Weller, S., Blum, M. R., *et al.* (1993). The pharmaco-kinetics and safety of zidovudine in the third trimester of pregnancy. *American Journal of Obstetrics and Gynecology* **168**, 1510–16.

Parker, M. T. (1977). Infection with group B streptococci. *Journal of Antimicrobiol Chemotherapy* **5**, Supp. A, 27–37.

Paryani, S. G. and Arvin, A. M. (1986). Intrauterine infection with varicella–zoster virus after maternal varicella. *New England Journal of Medicine* **314**, 1542–6.

Payne, R. A., Joynson, D. H. M., Balfour, A. H., Harford, J. P., Fleck, D. G.,

Mythen, M., *et al.* (1987). Public Health Laboratory Service. ELISA for detecting Toxoplasma specific IgM antibody. *Journal of Clinical Pathology* **40**, 276–81.

Pearl, K. N., Preece, P. M., Adez, A., and Peckham, C. S. (1986). Neurodevelopment assessment after congenital cytomegalovirus infection. *Archives of Diseases of Childhood* **61**, 323–6.

Pearson, H. E. (1964). Parturition varicella–zoster. *Obstetrics and Gynecology* **32**, 21–7.

Peckham, C. S., Chin, K. S., Coleman, J. C., Henderson, K., Hurley, R., and Preece, P. M. (1983). Cytomegalovirus infection in pregnancy. *Lancet* i, 1352–5.

Piper, J. M., Mitchell, E. F., and Ray, W. A. (1993). Pre-natal use of metronidazole and birth defects. *Obstetrics and Gynecology* **82**, 348–52.

Pizzo, P. A. and Butler, K. M. (1991). In the vertical transmission of HIV, timing may be everything. *New England Journal of Medicine* **325**, 652–4.

Prober, C. G., Sullender, W. A., Yasukawa, L. L., Au, D. S., Yeager, A. S., and Arvin, A. M. (1987). Low risk of herpes simplex virus infection, in neonates exposed to the virus at various times of vaginal delivery to mothers with recurrent congenital herpes simplex virus infection. *New England Journal of Medicine* **316**, 240–4.

Public Health Laboratory Service Communicable Disease Surveillance Centre (1989). Sexually transmitted disease in Britain: 1985–6. *Genitourinary Medicine* **69**, 117–21.

Quick, C. A., Watts, S., Krzyzek, L. A., and Faras, A. J. (1980). Relationship between condylomata and laryngeal papilloma. *Annals of Otology, Rhinology, and Laryngology* **89**, 467–71.

Rappaport, F., Rabinovitz, M., Toaff, R., and Crochi, K. (1960). Genital listeriosis as a cause of repeated abortion. *Lancet* i, 1273–5.

Readett, M. D. and McGibbon, C. (1961). Neonatal varicella. *Lancet* i, 644–5.

Rees, D. A. and Hamlett, J. D. (1972). Screening for gonorrhoea in pregnancy. *Journal of Obstetrics and Gynaecology of the British Commonwealth* **79**, 344–7.

Relier, J. P. (1975). Listeriosis. *Journal of Antimicrobial Chemotherapy* **5**, Supp. A51–7.

Revised Report of the RCOG Subcommittee on Problems Associated with AIDS in Relation to Obstetrics and Gynaecology (1990). *HIV Infection in Maternity Care and Gynaecology*, pp. 6–23. RCOG, London.

Ricci, J. M., Fojacor, M., and O'Sullivan, M. J. (1989). Congenital syphilis. *Obstetrics and Gynecology* **74**, 687–93.

Roos, T., Martius, J., Gross, V., and Schroo, L. (1993). Systemic serological screening for Toxoplasmosis in pregnancy. *Obstetrics and Gynecology* **81**, 243–50.

Rouss, C. F. and Bourne, G. L. (1972). Toxoplasmosis in pregnancy. *Journal of Obstetrics and Gynaecology of the British Commonwealth* **79**, 1115–18.

Ryan, G. M., Abdella, T. N., McNeeley, S. G., Basclski, V. S., and Drummond, D. E. (1990). *Chlamydia trachomatus* infection in pregnancy and effect of treatment on outcome. *Obstetrics and Gynecology* **162**, 34–9.

Saigal, S., Lunyk, O., Larke, R. P. B., and Chernesky, M. A. (1982). The outcome in children with congenital cytomegalovirus infection. *American Journal of Diseases of Children* **136**, 896–901.

St Geme, J. W., Noren, G. R., and Adams, P. (1966). Mumps and endocardial fibroelastosis. *New England Journal of Medicine* **275**, 339–47.

Samaranayake, L. P. and MacFarlane, T. W. (1982). The effect of dietary carbohydrates on the *in vitro* adhesion of *Candida albicans* to epithelial cells. *Journal of Medical Microbiology* **15**, 511–17.

Schachter, G., Grossman, M., Holt, J., Sweet, R., Goodner, E., and Mills, E. (1979). Prospective study of chlamydial infection in neonates. *Lancet* ii, 377–9.

Schachter, G., Sweet, R., Grossman, M., Landers, D., Robbie, M., and Bishop, E.,

(1986). Experience with the routine use of erythromycin for chlamydial infection in pregnancy. *New England Journal of Medicine* **314**, 276–9.

Schlech, W. F., Lavingne, P. M., Bortolucci, R. A., Allen, A. A., Haldane, E. V., Wort, A. J., *et al.* (1983). Epidemic listeriosis–evidence for transmission by food. *New England Journal of Medicine* **308**, 203–8.

Schofield, C. B. S. (1979). Congenital syphilis. In *Sexually transmitted diseases*, pp. 113–22. Churchill Livingstone, Edinburgh.

Schwartz, B., Liesielski, C. A., Broome, C. V., Gaventa, S., Brown, G. R., Gellin, B. G., *et al.* (1988). Association of sporadic listeriosis with consumption of uncooked hot dogs and undercooked chicken. *Lancet* **ii**, 779–82.

Schwartz, D. B., Greenberg, D., Daoud, Y., and Reid, R. (1988). Congenital condylomas in pregnancy: use of trichloractic acid and lazer therapy. *American Journal of Obstetrics and Gynecology* **158**, 1407–16.

Scott, G. B., Fischl, M. A., Klimnas, N., Fletcher, M. A., Dickinson, G. M., Levine, R. S., *et al.* (1985). Mothers of infants with AIDS. *Journal of the American Medical Association* **253**, 363–6.

Selwyn, P. A., Schoenbaum, E. E., Davenny, K., Robertson, V. J., Feingold, A. R., Schulman, J. F., *et al.* (1989). Prospective study of HIV infection and pregnancy outcome in intravenous drug users. *Journal of the American Medical Association* **261**, 1289–94.

Senturia, Y. D., Ades, A. E., and Peckham, C. S. (1987). Breast feeding and HIV infection. *Lancet* **ii**, 400–1.

Sever, J. and White, L. R. (1968). Intrauterine viral infections. *Annual Review of Medicine* **19**, 471–86.

Sizmmur, K. and Walker, C. W. (1988). Listeria in prepacked salads. *Lancet* **i**, 1167.

Slater, G. E., Rumack, R. H., and Peterson, R. G. (1978). Podophyllin poisoning. *Obstetrics and Gynecology* **52**, 94–6.

South, M. A., Short, D. H., and Know, J. M. (1964). Failure of erythromycin therapy in *in utero* syphilis. *Journal of the American Medical Association* **190**, 70–1.

Sparks, R. A., Williams, G. L., Boyce, J. M. H., Fitzgerald, T. L., and Shelley, G. (1975). Antenatal screening for candidiasis, toxoplasmosis and gonorrhoea. *British Journal of Venereal Diseases* **51**, 110–15.

Spencer, J. A. D. (1987). Perinatal listeriosis. *British Medical Journal* **295**, 349.

Sperling, R. S., Stratton, P., and the Gynecologic Working Group (1992). Treatment options for human immunodeficiency virus infected pregnant women. *Obstetrics and Gynecology* **79**, 443–4.

Srabstein, J. C., Morrin, N., and Larke, R. P. B. (1974). Is there a congenital varicella syndrome? *Journal of Pediatrics* **84**, 239–43.

Stagno, S., Pass, R. F., Dworsky, M. E., Henderson, R. E., Moore, E. G., Walton, P. D., *et al.* (1982). Congenital cytomegalovirus infection. *New England Journal of Medicine* **306**, 945–9.

Stehr-Green, P. A., Cochi, S., Preblud, S. R., and Orenstein, W. A. (1990). Evidence of increasing rubella seronegativity among adolescent girls. *American Journal of Public Health* **80**, 88.

Stern, H. and Tucker, S. M. (1973). Prospective study of cytomegalovirus infection in pregnancy. *British Medical Journal* **2**, 268–70.

Stratton, T., Matherson, L. N., and Willoughby, A. D. (1992). Human immunodeficiency virus infection in pregnant women. *Obstetrics and Gynecology* **79**, 364–8.

Stray-Pedersen, B. (1990). Acyclovir in late pregnancy to prevent neonatal herpes simplex. *Lancet* **336**, 756.

Tang, C. K., Shermeta, D. W., and Wood, D. (1978). Congenital condylomata acuminata. *American Journal of Obstetrics and Gynecology* 131, 912-13.

Thin, R. N. T. and Michael, A. M. (1970). Sexually transmitted diseases in antenatal patients. *British Journal of Venereal Diseases* 46, 126-8.

Tobin, J. O. H. (1970). Cytomegalovirus infection in the North West of England. *Archives of Diseases in Childhood* 45, 513-22.

Van De Perre, P., Simonana, A., Msellati, P., Hitimani, D. G., Vaira, D., Bazubagria, A., *et al.* (1991). Postnatal transmission of human immunodeficiency virus type I from mother to infant. *New England Journal of Medicine* 325, 593-8.

Vontner, L. A., Hickok, D. E., Brown, Z., Reid., L., and Corey, L. (1982). Recurrent genital herpes simplex virus infection in pregnancy. *American Journal of Obstetrics and Gynecology* 143, 75-84.

Webster, A. and Johnson, M. (1990). HIV infection. In *Progress in obstetrics and gynaecology*, Vol. 8 (ed. J. Studd), pp. 175-90. Churchill Livingstone, Edinburgh.

Weller, M. H. (1971a). The cytomegaloviruses. *New England Journal of Medicine* 285, 203-14.

Weller, M. H. (1971b). The cytomegaloviruses. *New England Journal of Medicine* 285, 267-74.

Weller, T. H. and Hanshaw, J. B. (1962). Virologic and clinical observations on cytomegalic inclusion disease. *New England Journal of Medicine* 266, 1233-44.

Whitley, R. J., Nahmias, A. J., Visintine, A. M., Fleming, C. L., and Alford, C. A. (1980). The natural history of herpes simplex virus infection of mothers and newborns. *Pediatrics* 66, 489-94.

Williams, K. (1985). Screening for syphilis in pregnancy. *Community Medicine* 7, 37-42.

Wilson, C. B., Remmington, J. S., Stagno, S., and Reynolds, D. W. (1980). Development of adverse sequelae in children born with subclinical congenital toxoplasmosis infections. *Pediatrics* 66, 767-74.

Wright, D. J. M. and Gerken, A. (1981). Antenatal screening for syphilis. *British Journal of Venereal Diseases* 57, 147-8.

Wright, E. P., Dyson, A. J., and Alaily, A. (1985). Infection with parvovirus during pregnancy. *British Medical Journal* 290, 241.

Yeager, A. S. and Arvin, A. M. (1984). Reasons for the absence of a history of recurrent congenital infections in mothers of neonates infected with herpes simplex virus. *Pediatrics* 73, 188-93.

Yow, M. D., Mason, E. O., Leeds, L. J., Thompson, P. R., Clark, D. J., and Garner, S. E. (1979). Ampicillin prevents intra-partum transmission of group B streptococci. *Journal of the American Medical Association* 781, 1245-7.

Ziegler, J. B. (1993). Breastfeeding and HIV. *Lancet* 342, 1437-8.

22 The management of preterm labour

The incidence of preterm delivery has remained static at 7–9 per cent of all births for many years (Creasy 1991). The importance of preterm birth in terms of the perinatal mortality rate has already been stressed (Chapter 15 – 'Antenatal care'), with premature delivery accounting for up to 25 per cent of perinatal deaths (Bucknell and Wood 1985; McIlwaine *et al.* 1979; Rush *et al.* 1978). The importance of the association between multiple pregnancy and prematurity can be exemplified by the work of Rayburn *et al.* (1986) who reported that 18 per cent of 239 women in preterm labour had a multiple pregnancy, whilst MacGillivray (1989) reported that 'approximately 30 per cent' of twin pregnancies are delivered prematurely.

Neonatal survival rates will depend upon both gestational age at delivery and birthweight, and figures need to be continued beyond the neonatal period for a more accurate prognosis to be given. Thus Yu *et al.* (1986) reported 108 deaths related to prematurity and demonstrated that 74 per cent of all deaths occurred within the first week of life – 23 per cent within one hour, 33 per cent within one day, and a further 18 per cent up to the end of the first week. However, some 26 per cent of deaths were later – 14 per cent during the late neonatal period and 12 per cent in the post-neonatal period. In the same series of 356 infants born between the 23rd and 28th weeks of gestation, boys had a lower survival rate than girls, 19 per cent of survivors had some degree of impairment of which 12 per cent was major, i.e. cerebral palsy or developmental delay.

In the days before neonatal intensive care units, Drillien (1961) reviewed 69 children whose birthweights were less than 1.36 kg (3 lb), of whom 50 were of school age. Only 24 per cent attended a normal school, 10 per cent being 'so grossly handicapped as to be ineducable'. Only 10 per cent of those children given an intelligence test had an IQ of 100 or over.

With the advent of neonatal intensive care units, we are able to reassess the survival rates based on gestational age and birthweight, whilst information is accumulating concerning the quality of survival and the occurrence of handicap in those survivals. Survival following delivery before the 23rd week of gestation is rare, and an analysis of survival rate and impairment by gestational age and birthweight has been assessed in a series of 1425 preterm infants weighing less than 2 kg (Powell *et al.* 1986). This analysis is summarized in Table 22.1 and demonstrates the relatively good survival with low incidences of handicap to be expected following delivery at the 31st week or later.

However, the incidence of survival with and without handicap, following delivery before the 31st week of gestation is more disappointing with evidence

Table 22.1 The results of preterm birth

Gestational age and birthweight	% Survival	% Survival with impairment
25–30 weeks		
(a) 501–1500 g	43	7
(b) 1501–2000 g	76	10.5
31–34 weeks		
(a) 501–1500 g	77	7
(b) 1501–2000 g	92	6
> 34 weeks		
(a) 501–1500 g	88	3
(b) 1501–2000 g	91	2

From Powell *et al.* 1986

to suggest an increased rate of handicap in the survivors. An accurate estimate of the morbidity in survivors born before the 25th week of gestation is yet to be adequately assessed (Hack and Fanaroff 1989; Powell *et al.* 1986) (please see Tables 22.1 and 22.2.). Despite the improvements in neonatal intensive care, survival of 500–750 g neonates is still relatively poor, with a 35 per cent overall survival rate and a 9 per cent incidence of severe handicap (Roussounis *et al.* 1993; Young and Stevenson 1990). Advances in neonatal intensive care together with a detailed assessment of a greater number of survivors will allow for a better assessment of prognosis in these infants.

The prevention of preterm labour

The prediction of women at increased risk of preterm labour would be valuable if prophylaxis could then be instituted successfully. Single women, women below the age of 25 years, and social class V women are all at increased risk of preterm labour, the relative risk for these factors ranging from 1.8–3.3 (Berkowitz 1981). Other risk factors include low maternal pre-pregnancy weight (relative risk of 2.34 women who weigh 60 kg or less), whilst the major single risk factor is the history of a previous preterm delivery, the relative risk of preterm labour ranging between 3 and 29.8 compared with women without such a history. The relative risk of preterm delivery after antepartum haemorrhage is 25.9, urinary tract infection 6.1, and a previous induced abortion 4.6 (Berkowitz 1981; Carr-Hill and Hall 1985; De Haas *et al.* 1991; Sanjose *et al.* 1991; Wen *et al.* 1990).

There are also some vaginal microorganisms the presence of which represents a risk for preterm labour, even when other factors have been taken into account

Table 22.2 The result of preterm birth

Gestational age (weeks)	% Survival
20	0
21	0
22	5
23	5
24	15
25	64
26	71
27	76

From Hack and Fanaroff (1989)

by regression analysis. It would appear that *Gardnerella vaginalis* is the most important of these (Hay *et al*. 1994; McDonald *et al*. 1991; Read and Klebanoff 1993). It is yet to be proven whether screening for this organism, and treatment should it be found, would reduce the incidence of preterm labour (Kirschbaum 1993; Romero *et al*. 1993).

The assessment of such risk factors may be used to quantify the risk of preterm delivery by the use of a formal scoring system. Several such systems have been devised, but the predictive value of such a score is relatively poor and may be unlikely to improve upon clinical judgement (Creasy *et al*. 1980; Main *et al*. 1987; Owen *et al*. 1990). Although repeated vaginal examination in order to predict changes in the cervix have traditionally been used to predict preterm labour, it is of poor sensitivity and specificity and adds little to the clinical assessment of risk (Blondel *et al*. 1990).

There has been much recent interest in the use of equipment for home monitoring of uterine contractions. Although this is a poor discriminator between Braxton–Hicks contractions and early labour, it may allow the opportunity for earlier intervention including the use of tocolysis (Morrison 1990; Rhoads *et al*. 1991). Two recent randomized trials of home monitoring of uterine activity have suggested that the technique is associated with a lower incidence of preterm delivery. In one trial, patients were randomly allocated to either home monitoring, in addition to regular antenatal assessments, or regular antenatal assessments alone. Some 42 per cent of 55 high-risk pregnancies resulted in delivery before the 32nd week of gestation in the home monitored group compared with 65 per cent of 43 non-monitored pregnancies (Hill *et al*. 1990). In a second similar randomized trial, 47 per cent of 33 home monitored high-risk pregnancies delivered before the 37th week of pregnancy compared with 84 per cent of 34 non-monitored pregnancies (Watson *et al*. 1990).

However, rather more trials exist which have failed to demonstrate any benefit from intensive antenatal regimes which include a combination of patient education, home daily uterine activity monitoring, intermittant cervical assessment, and daily contact and support by specialist nurses (Creasy and Merkatz 1990). Such randomized trials have been designed to allow for an earlier intervention in threatened premature labour in order that pregnancy may be prolonged. The results have tended to show no differences in the rates of preterm birth between the active and the control group despite the greater use of tocolytic agents in the active group (Grimes and Schultz 1992; Main *et al.* 1985; Mueller-Heubach *et al.* 1989). In the Alabama project, 1000 high-risk women were randomized into intervention or control groups, the intervention groups receiving tocolytic agents whenever the patient or the specialist nurses reported increased uterine activity. The intervention group also had regular support and contact from specialist medical and nursing staff. Although tocolytics were used widely in the intervention groups, there were no statistical significant differences between the groups for gestational age, birthweight, or neonatal morbidity (Goldenberg *et al.* 1990). Moreover, a prospective controled trial of social support in the UK showed little evidence for a reduction in preterm labour in high-risk patients, being 13 per cent in the social support group and 15 per cent in controls (Bryce *et al.* 1991).

It is going to take a large multicentre randomized trial of intervention if any statistically significant benefit is to be demonstrated, assuming it exists, from the vigorous use of tocolytic agents in high-risk patients in whom increased uterine activity or cervical changes are noted.

Several treatment modalities have been advocated in order to prevent preterm labour in women at increased risk without waiting for evidence of increased uterine activity. The major modalities which have been used include rest, cervical cerclage, and prophylactic drug therapy.

Bedrest, in order to prevent preterm labour in the presence of a multiple pregnancy, was advocated by Russell (1952) and became a traditional part of obstetric teaching. Powers and Miller (1979) stated 'Already in the reported English literature, a minimum of 88 women-years of bedrest has been expended on healthy mothers solely to prolong their twin pregnancies and, still, its efficacy is unproved.'

Persson *et al.* (1979) reported that when 86 women with twin pregnancies were admitted to hospital for bedrest between the 29th and 36th week of pregnancy, only 20 per cent had delivered before the 37th week, whereas a decade before this policy was introduced, 33 per cent would have delivered before the 37th week. Although the conclusions may be valid, the two series are not strictly comparable. Saunders *et al.* (1985) randomly allocated 212 women with twin pregnancies either to routine admission ($n = 105$) or to selective admission ($n = 107$). Some 30 per cent of those patients admitted for bedrest delivered before the 37th week of pregnancy, whereas only 19 per cent of the controls did so, suggesting that there was no benefit, and possible hazard, for those admitted for bedrest.

Crowther *et al.* (1989) randomized 139 women with twin pregnancies and a high risk of preterm labour, based on cervical reassessment, to receive either bedrest in hospital ($n = 70$) or no specific advice ($n = 69$) at a mean of 33.5

weeks' gestation. There were no differences in outcome between the two groups, the mean gestational age at delivery in both groups being 35.8 weeks and there being two perinatal deaths in each group. It would seem unlikely that bedrest is an effective prophylaxis against preterm labour.

Similarly, it seems unlikely that prophylactic cervical cerclage will prevent preterm labour in women with a past history of this complication, other than, perhaps, those with a classical history of cervical incompetence. Rush *et al.* (1984) admitted 194 women with singleton pregnancies considered to be at high risk of preterm labour, based on past history, into a randomly allocated trial of cervical cerclage ($n = 96$) against no suture ($n = 98$). Some 34 per cent of those patients with a cervical suture delivered before the 37th week of pregnancy compared with 32 per cent of those without, these results not reaching statistical significance. Weekes *et al.* (1977) reported three non-randomly allocated groups of patients with a twin pregnancy into bedrest in hospital between the 28th and 34th weeks of gestation ($n = 60$), cervical suture ($n = 37$), and no active treatment ($n = 36$). Delivery before the 36th week occurred in 23.3 per cent of patients in the first group, 27 per cent in the second, and 22 per cent in the third. The mean gestation age at delivery was 37 weeks in the first group, 36.9 weeks in the second, and 37.3 in the third. Although the allocation was not random, the results suggested that neither treatment modality prevented premature labour in this group of patients.

The beta-2 sympathomimetic agonists, have been used prophylactically, and Mathews *et al.* (1967) reported 64 patients with a singleton pregnancy who were considered to be at high risk of preterm delivery based on their history. Of 31 patients who received isoxsuprine two delivered before the 36th week of pregnancy as did two of 33 patients who received placebo. The trial was abandoned prematurely because of side-effects, 16 per cent of the patients taking the active agent complained of palpitations and there was an unwilling-ness on behalf of patients to take 12 tablets per day prophylactically. Walters and Wood (1977) reported 38 women considered at high risk of premature labour because of a dilated internal cervical os. Some 21 women received oral ritodrine and 17 placebo. The mean gestational age at delivery in the ritodrine group was 38.5 weeks and the placebo group 39.2 weeks. Gummerus and Halonen (1987) randomly allocated 200 patients with a multiple pregnancy to receive either salbutamol (20 mg per day) and to have bedrest from the 31st week of gestation ($n = 101$), or to receive bedrest from the 31st week of gestation alone ($n = 99$). The mean gestational age at delivery in both groups was 37.6 weeks.

Prophylactic therapy with progesterone has been more successful. Yemini *et al.* (1985) allocated 80 pregnant women at high risk of preterm labour, based on past history, into a double-blind study of 250 mg 17-alpha-hydroxyprogesterone caproate intramuscularly weekly or a placebo. Preterm labour occurred in 29 per cent of the treated group and 59 per cent of the control group. Preterm delivery occurred in 16 per cent of the treated group and 38 per cent of the control group. Keirse (1990) reported a meta-analysis of five published controlled trials involving approximately 450 patients with singleton pregnancies considered to be at risk of preterm labour. These patients had been randomly allocated to receive either 17-alpha-hydroxyprogesterone caproate or placebo. The progestogen therapy reduced the incidence of preterm labour by 50 per cent, compared with placebo, providing the therapy was commenced by the start of the third trimester.

It would seem that the most effective prophylactic agent against preterm labour, so far, would appear to be 17-hydroxyprogesterone therapy commenced before the start of the third trimester, although there is a limited evidence that a *combination* of prophylactic measures (bedrest, cervical circlage, and beta-2 agonist treatment) may be more helpful than any one agent alone (White *et al.* 1989).

The suppression of preterm labour

There are numerous problems in interpreting the data available from the literature on the use of drugs to suppress preterm labour. This is partly because of the large number of uncontrolled studies, partly because of a lack of a common end-point, and partly because of an absence of information on longer term infant survival. Moreover, there is a significant placebo rate, which in one study reached 73 per cent for the postponement of delivery for longer than seven days (Castren *et al.* 1975).

Beta-2 agonists

The use of beta-2 agonists in order to suppress preterm labour has resulted in a wide range of results, sometimes contradictory. Overall, ritodrine tocolysis has been reported as suppressing preterm labour in between 19–72 per cent of labours in which it has been used (Newton *et al.* 1991). In view of the high placebo rate recorded above, it seems inappropriate to include any studies which have not compared either ritodrine or terbutaline to a placebo. Moreover, the use of different end-points must also be noted. Most studies have demonstrated that the use of a beta-2 agonist is superior to placebo in delaying delivery for greater than 24 hours and perhaps even up to seven days, but it does not tend to alter either the percentage of patients who reach term or have an effect on overall perinatal outcome (Beall *et al.* 1985; Larsen *et al.* 1980, 1986; Spellacy *et al.* 1979). Overall, up to 39 per cent of women given a beta-2 agonist in order to suppress preterm labour may expect to be undelivered by the 35th week of gestation (Besinger *et al.* 1991; Hollander *et al.* 1987; Newton *et al.* 1991).

In a recent meta-analysis, based on data from 890 women in 16 randomized controlled trials, of a beta-2 agonist in the inhibition of active preterm labour, King *et al.* (1988) reported that these agents were superior to placebo in delaying delivery beyond 48 hours, but they only had a minimally superior effect in delaying delivery beyond the 37th week of pregnancy. Despite these modest delays, there were no reductions in the incidence of respiratory distress syndrome or in survival. The available evidence also suggests that terbutaline and ritodrine are equally effective in the suppression of preterm labour compared with a placebo (Beall *et al.* 1985; Caritis *et al.* 1984).

In clinical practice, the use of beta-2 agonists is often inhibited by the occurrence of maternal side effects, of which tachycardia with or without palpitations is the most common (Higby *et al.* 1993). There is evidence to suggest that this side effect is less common with terbutaline than with ritodrine; for instance, in one trial some 30 per cent of patients developed a tachycardia with terbutaline whilst 65 per cent developed one with ritodrine (Caritis *et al.* 1984). A more worrying side effect is pulmonary oedema (Katz *et al.* 1981; Lampert *et al.* 1993; Rayburn *et al.* 1986). The incidence of acute pulmonary oedema may be greater when a beta-2 agonist is combined with betamethasone or dexamethasone, an unfortunate result when one of the major reasons for attempting to suppress preterm labour in the short term is the use of corticosteroids in order to accelerate fetal lung maturity (Elliott *et al.* 1978).

There is not, as yet, sufficient information to be able to state whether or not there is any benefit from maintaining therapy with these agents after tocolysis. There is evidence from randomized controlled trials that women who receive oral terbutaline after tocolysis will remain undelivered longer than those who receive a placebo (Brown and Tejani 1981), whilst Ridgway *et al.* (1990) reported that 82 per cent of 27 women whose labour was arrested with a beta-2 agonist and who remained on a maintenance dose were still undelivered by the 36th week of pregnancy. The need for further information on this point is clear.

Inhibitors of prostaglandin synthesis

There is good evidence that antiprostaglandin agents are as effective as beta-2 agonists in the inhibition of preterm labour (Besinger *et al.* 1991; Niebyl *et al.* 1980). However, there is a significant risk that these agents will result in premature closure of the ductus arteriosus *in utero* with potentially lethal consequences (Wilkinson 1980).

Indomethacin is a potent agent for the closure of a persistent ductus arteriosus in the neonatal period (Gersony *et al.* 1983), and even the short-term use of indomethacin antenatally has resulted in ductal constricition in 50 per cent of fetuses studied by echocardiography (Eronen *et al.* 1991; Moise *et al.* 1988).

The Editor of *The Lancet* (1980) advised that 'during pregnancy and lactation, therefore, non-steroidal anti-inflammatory drugs should be prescribed with extreme caution, if at all'. It may be that this agent can be used before the 27th week of pregnancy since constriction of the ductus is unlikely at this gestation (Moise 1993; van den Veyver *et al.* 1993).

Alcohol

Intravenous ethanol is superior to placebo and almost as effective as beta-2 agonists in the short-term suppression of preterm labour (Fuchs 1976; Spearing 1979). The mechanism of action is presumed to be the inhibition of posterior pituitary secretion of oxytocin and the inhibition of oxytocic stimulation of the myometrium. However, the dangers of intravenous alcohol therapy are significant, and include nausea, vomiting, delayed gastric emptying, headaches, and inebriation (Zlatnik and Fuchs 1972). This agent is now rarely used in clinical practice because of these side effects.

Progesterone

The evidence for the benefit of progesterone therapy in the inhibition of preterm labour is contradictory. One placebo-controlled trial failed to show any benefit of intramuscular progesterone over intramuscular placebo (Fuchs and Stakemann 1960). Whilst a more recent trial (Erny *et al.* 1986) reported that progestogen therapy suppressed uterine activity in 76 per cent of patients compared with 43 per cent after placebo. Again, this is an area where further information is required.

Magnesium sulfate

It is well known that magnesium sulfate exerts an effect on skeletal muscle by decreasing the amplitude of the motor end-plate potential, reducing acetylcholine release and reducing the motor end-plate sensitivity, thus making muscular activity more difficult to initiate. However, such a mechanism cannot apply to the smooth muscle of the uterus and if magnesium sulfate has an effect, it must be by a direct action.

Magnesium sulfate is an active agent for the suppression of preterm labour. After administration of this agent up to 88 per cent of patients will be undelivered after 72 hours and 75 per cent undelivered after seven days (Hollander *et al.* 1987; Newton *et al.* 1991). However, magnesium sulfate had to be continued in 11 per cent of patients in one series because of toxicity, which included generalized muscle weakness and respiratory depression (Cox *et al.* 1990; Higby *et al.* 1993). It seems unlikely that this substance will receive widespread use for the suppression of preterm labour.

Other agents

There have been several recent suggestions of agents which may inhibit preterm labour but the clinical experience with these agents is, as yet, limited.

Hauksson *et al.* (1988) suggested that a synthetic antagonist against oxytocin might become useful in the prevention of preterm labour. The calcium channel blocking agent, nifedipine is also able to inhibit preterm labour (Glock and

Table 22.3 The value of corticosteroids

	Betamethasone	Control
No.	117	96
PMR (per 1000)	64	180
Early neonatal death rate	32	150
RDS (%)	9.0	25.8
Neonatal infection (%)	1.1	5.1

From Liggins and Howie (1972)

Morales 1993). In a randomized trial, it was as effective as ritodrine in delaying delivery for seven days in 70 per cent of patients and until the 36th week of gestation in 41 per cent. However, the role and safety of such therapy will require additional assessment (Ferguson *et al.* 1990).

It has been suggested that subclinical infection may be a factor in the failure of tocolytic agents to inhibit some preterm labours (Newton *et al.* 1989; Potkul *et al.* 1985). For this reason broad-spectrum antibiotics have been administered along with tocolytic agents in an attempt to increase the percentage of labours inhibited, but without any success (Newton *et al.* 1991; Romero *et al.* 1993).

The use of corticosteroids in preterm labour

Liggins (1969) reported that premature fetal lambs born after the induction of labour using an intravenous infusion of glucocorticoids resulted in the partial aeration of the lungs, possibly related to accelerated surfactant production. Liggins and Howie (1972) reported a trial on the use of betamethasone in 213 women with threatened and unplanned premature labour. The results are shown in Table 22.3. There was a significant reduction in the incidence of respiratory distress syndrome (RDS) in the fetuses of mothers who received betamethasone as opposed to those who received a weak steroid as a control. Caspi *et al.* (1981) suggested that there was a greater protective effect of dexamethasone against RDS before the 32nd week of pregnancy in the infants of mothers who had received dexamethasone, 4 mg intramuscularly eight-hourly for at least 24 hours. These results can be seen in Table 22.4.

The US Collaborative Study Group on Antenatal Steroids (1981) randomly allocated 696 women at risk of preterm labour to receive dexamethasone ($n = 349$) or placebo ($n = 347$). The overall incidence of RDS was 12.6 per cent in the treated patients and 18.0 per cent in the controls. As the effect of twin or triplet pregnancy was minimal, when the figures were corrected to take account of singleton pregnancies only, the incidence of RDS in the steroid group was 10.1 per cent and in controls 16.0 per cent. Virtually the whole effect was exclusive to females with no statistically significant benefit in male fetuses.

Table 22.4 The value of corticosteroids

Gestational age	Incidence RDS (%)	
	Dexamethasone (n = 200)	Control (n = 260)
28–32 weeks	23	60.8
33 weeks	0	17.9
34 weeks	2.4	18.2
35 weeks	0	3.6
Total	9.5	26.5

From Caspi *et al.* (1981)

There was no evidence of any increased infection in the steroid group. In the UK Collaborative Study (Gamsu *et al.* 1989) 139 women were randomly allocated to receive betamethasone, 4 mg eight-hourly in six doses, and 132 women to receive placebo. The incidence of RDS in the steroid group was 5.4 per cent whilst in the placebo group it was 12.1 per cent.

Crowley *et al.* (1990) reviewed 12 controlled clinical trials involving over 3000 patients in which there was an overall reduction of RDS in the region of 50 per cent in the fetuses of mothers who received steroids. The major benefit occurred within 24 hours of commencing the steroids and lasted for seven days. There was a real, but lesser, benefit thereafter. The effect was not gestational age dependent, but figures beyond the 34th week of pregnancy become small and perhaps difficult to interpret. Overall, the trials did not confirm a gender effect, and there was no evidence that steroids have a longterm adverse neurological effect.

There has been anxiety concerning the administration of steroids to women who were hypertensive during pregnancy. Liggins and Howie (1972) reported that there were no stillborn infants in their control group, but that there were five stillborn infants in the group receiving steroids and in whom there was maternal hypertension. However, this complication has not been confirmed following the accumulation of more data. Lamont *et al.* (1983), in a prospective, non-randomized trial, reported that 72 per cent of 32 infants who were delivered before the 34th week of pregnancy because of maternal hypertension and proteinuria, and whose mothers did not receive steroids, survived, whereas 88 per cent of 24 infants delivered before the 34th week of pregnancy because of maternal hypertension and proteinuria, but whose mothers did receive steroids, survived. Survival was related to a decrease in the incidences of both respiratory distress syndrome and intraventricular haemorrhage. The meta-analysis of 12 controlled trial by Crowley *et al.* (1990) substantiated the view that there is no increased fetal risk when steroids are administered in the presence of maternal hypertension.

It has already been stated that acute pulmonary oedema may occur when steroids are combined with a beta-sympathomimetic agent, thus patients need to be regularly assessed clinically for the possible development of this

Table 22.5 Some effects of preterm rupture of the membranes

State	No.	RDS (%)	Amnionitis (%)	Endometritis (%)
Premature rupture of membranes	151	4	8	7
Rupture for 0–23 h	79	4	4	4
Rupture for 24–47 h	41	6	4	10
Rupture for 48 + h	31	0	19	10

From Miller *et al.* (1978)

complication. There is some evidence that prenatal corticosteroids followed by postnatal surfactant will further reduce pulmonary complications and improve survival especially in infants born between the 28th and 32nd weeks of gestation (Jobe *et al.* 1990).

Preterm premature rupture of the membranes (PPROM)

Spontaneous rupture of the membranes occurs in the absence of uterine contractions in 1 per cent of pregnancies before the 37th week of gestation, and in 57 per cent of these pregnancies labour rapidly ensues (Gibbs and Blanco, 1982; White *et al.* 1986).

There are both benefits and complications from PPROM. There is evidence that prolonged rupture of the membranes has a sparing effect upon the development of respiratory distress syndrome, although this is not universally accepted and the benefits are probably only minimal (Eggers *et al.* 1979; Hallak and Bottoms 1993; Miller *et al.* 1978). This has to be balanced against the risk of chorioamniotis and post-partum endometritis, complications which increase in incidence the longer the membranes are ruptured prior to delivery (please see Table 22.5, Miller *et al.* 1978). If no attempt is made to expedite delivery because of extreme prematurity, the incidence of chorioamniotis reaches nearly 60 per cent and the incidence of post-partum endometritis 13 per cent (Bengston *et al.* 1989; Beydoun and Yasin 1986).

The following features are discussed below:

(1) vaginal examination;

(2) the use of C-reactive protein;

(3) the place of amniocentesis;

(4) the use of antibiotics;

(5) the use of oral tocolytics;

(6) the induction of labour;

(7) the use of corticosteroids;

(8) the route of delivery.

Vaginal examination

Although it is traditional to avoid vaginal examination in patients with PPROM in whom delivery is not to be expeditied, the evidence for this line of management is poor (Schutte *et al.* 1983). However, a sterile speculum examination is as useful as a vaginal examination if delivery is not to be expedited, and this does not seem to be associated with an increased risk of infection (Munson *et al.* 1985). If delivery is planned to take place within 24 hours, there is no reason to avoid vaginal examination (Schutte *et al.* 1983).

The use of C-reactive protein

There is an association between the levels of maternal circulating C-reactive protein (CRP) and intrauterine infection. Romen and Artal (1984) suggested that an increase in CRP in the presence of spontaneous rupture of the membranes more accurately heralded infection than did an increase in the white cell count, based upon the series of 25 patients tested daily and in whom 14 developed clinical chorioamnionitis. However, this association is neither specific nor sensitive for clinical or histological chorioamnitis (Cammu *et al.* 1989; Farb *et al.* 1983). The clinical use of this assay is, therefore, limited unless the level of CRP is greater than 40 mg/l, in which case there is 100 per cent positive predictive value for infection but a 53 per cent negative predictive value (Fisk *et al.* 1987).

The place of amniocentesis

In an attempt to diagnose subclinical infection and therefore expedite delivery of an infected baby, transabdominal amniocentesis has been performed with either a Gram stain or bacteriological culture performed on fluid obtained. Feinstein *et al.* (1986) attempted transabdominal amniocentesis in 73 patients with spontaneous rupture of the membranes who were not in labour and who had no evidence of infection. Fluid was obtained in 50 patients (68.5 per cent), and of the 50 samples 76 per cent were negative on Gram staining. Some 33 of these 38 infants were without any evidence of infection at delivery. Of 12 samples (24 per cent) with positive Gram staining, six infants showed evidence of infection at delivery. However, amniocentesis is not as sensitive or specific as the assay of CRP in maternal serum since there is only a 50 per cent positive predictive value for infection but an 87 per cent negative predictive value (Feinstein *et al.* 1986).

The use of antibiotics

The use of antibiotics in this situation may be indicated for two reasons. The first is the prevention of infection following PPROM but the second, and of more interest recently, is the possibility that infection was the cause of the PPROM.

Table 22.6 The use of prophylactic antibiotics

	Antibiotic	Placebo
No. of patients	81	85
% Chorioamnionitis	4	26
% Neonatal sepsis	5	10

From Morales *et al.* (1989)

Several recent randomized double-blind controlled trials have demonstrated that prophylactic antibiotics are associated with lower incidences of endometritis, chorioamnitis, and neonatal sepsis than is placebo therapy (Amon *et al.* 1988; Johnston *et al.* 1990; Krohn *et al.* 1991; Morales *et al.* 1989). The results from one such trial are shown in Table 22.6.

The use of antibiotics as a prophylaxis appears to be justified when PPROM occurs and, because of gestational age, delivery is not to be expedited. What is yet to be assessed is the size of any risk from a superimposed opportunistic organism, or whether the identification of a causative organism for preterm labour in general, or PPROM in particular, may be identified and appropriate antibiotic therapy commenced with an improvement in survival (Ernest and Givner 1994; Lockwood *et al.* 1993).

There is good evidence that certain microorganisms may be found more commonly in either the vagina or in the amniotic fluid in the presence of preterm labour or PPROM (Lamont *et al.* 1986; Wahbeh *et al.* 1984). Moreover, such microorganisms are more commonly found in the vaginae of women who will develop PPROM compared with controls (McDonald *et al.* 1991). The microorganisms which have been implicated in these situations include *Bacteroides* spp., group B streptococci, anaerobic organisms, ureaplasma, mycoplasma, and gardnerella (Lamont *et al.* 1986; McDonald *et al.* 1991; Mercer *et al.* 1992; Regan *et al.* 1981; Wahbeh *et al.* 1984).

It has been demonstrated that such microorganisms can migrate through the chorioamniotic membranes on to the fetal surface, and it is proposed that this results in either PPROM or preterm labour due to either the local inflammatory process or to the local release of prostaglandins (Bobitt *et al.* 1981; Galask *et al.* 1984; Wahbeh *et al.* 1984).

It has yet to be established whether the identification of such organisms, perhaps in the vagina during the second trimester, followed by the eradication using antimicrobial agents will result in a prevention of either PPROM or preterm labour.

The use of oral tocolytics

There is only limited evidence to suggest the efficacy or otherwise of oral tocolytic therapy in the prevention of preterm labour in patients with PPROM in whom there is a wish for labour to be delayed. In a randomized placebo-controlled trial, Levy and Warsof (1985) demonstrated a mean delay between spontaneous rupture of the membranes and delivery in patients who received ritodrine (33.5 days compared with 12.5 days). Further information is required upon this point.

The induction of labour

In view of the risk of infection related to conservative management, it would seem logical to induce labour should the risks of premature delivery be small. Although the period of gestation at which labour should be induced may vary from unit to unit, in most hospitals this will be between the 31st and 33rd week of pregnancy. However, there are suprisingly few randomized studies which show the benefits or otherwise of such management. Spinnato (1987) reported 47 patients whose membranes had ruptured between the 25th and 36th week of pregnancy but who had either 'a mature LS ratio' or a positive foam stability test. These patients were randomly assigned to either prompt delivery following oxytocin infusion ($n = 26$) or conservative management ($n = 21$). There were no failed inductions but no specific benefits either, in that the incidence of neonatal sepsis in the group following labour induction was 6 per cent whereas in the group allowed to labour spontaneously it was 3 per cent.

The use of corticosteroids

The place of corticosteroids in the prevention of RDS has already been discussed. However, the use of corticosteroids in the presence of ruptured membranes is complicated by the sparing effect of ruptured membranes on RDS itself and upon the theoretical possibility of increased maternal of fetal sepsis.

The only studies which have demonstrated an increased incidence in neonatal sepsis following beta-methasone administration in the presence of PPROM have been non-randomized ones (Simpson and Harbert 1985). Several randomized studies have failed to demonstrate any difference between the incidence of maternal infection and neonatal infection between patients in the control group and those who received a corticosteroid (Garite *et al.* 1981; Iams *et al.* 1985; Morales *et al.* 1986).

The evidence for a reduction in the incidence of respiratory distress syndrome following the administration of corticosteroids following PPROM is less strong than the evidence when the membranes are intact. Some studies have failed to demonstrate any reduction in the incidence of respiratory distress syndrome (Iams *et al.* 1985; Simpson and Harbert *et al.* 1985). Other studies have demonstrated a significant reduction in the incidence of respiratory distress syndrome in the corticosteroid treated group (17 per cent compared with 21 per cent (Garite *et al.* 1981), 25 per cent compared with 51 per cent (Morales *et al.* 1986).

On balance, evidence from current practice would suggest that if labour is not to be expedited immediately the use of corticosteroids does not involve a

Table 22.7 The route of delivery

Birthweight	Vaginal		Caesarean	
	No.	% Mortality	No.	% Mortality
750–999 g	132	55	9	56
1000–1249 g	165	28	24	46
1250–1499 g	145	17	16	19

From Main *et al.* (1983)

significant increase in the risk of sepsis but may well offer a significant decrease in the risk of respiratory distress syndrome.

The route of delivery

This section will debate the route of delivery of a preterm infant with a vertex presentation. The debate concerning the route of delivery of a preterm infant presenting by the breech was discussed in Chapter 20 (Breech presentation).

The use of forceps in order 'to protect' the head of a preterm baby delivering by the vertex has been assessed in a randomly allocated clinical trial of 46 infants delivering between the 28th and 35th weeks of pregnancy allocated to receive either a gentle forceps delivery ($n = 23$) or a spontaneous vertex delivery ($n = 23$) (Maltau *et al.* 1984). There were no differences between the two groups for any complication, including the incidence of retinal haemorrhage (6 per cent in both groups) this generally being considered to relate to fetal head compression and venous congestion. O'Driscoll *et al.* (1981), however, reported a series, coverina a 17-year period, of 27 babies with autopsy evidence of traumatic intracranial haemorrhage, all of whom had presented by the vertex. All 27 infants had been delivered by forceps, no other infant in the series of over 35 000 infants, excluding breech deliveries, had died from a traumatic intracranial haemorrhage.

Main *et al.* (1983) reported 491 babies with a cephalic presentation delivering at a birthweight of less than 1500 g. Some 442 babies delivered vaginally, with a mortality of 33 per cent, and 49 babies delivered abdominally, with a mortality of 39 per cent. As shown in Table 22.7, the route of delivery was not relevant in any of the three birthweight categories for cephalic presentation. Olshan *et al.* (1984) analysed 345 infants born between 700 and 1500 g birthweight, and found that delivery by Caesarean section or vaginally had no influence upon the survival statistics once these were corrected for presentation and divided into birthweight groups.

There is, therefore, no good evidence that preterm babies presenting by the head will have a lower mortality or morbidity if they are delivered abdominally rather than vaginally, and the use of forceps for these specific indication of preterm delivery is to be avoided.

Conclusions

Preterm delivery remains one of the major causes of perinatal mortality and infant handicap in the civilized world, yet we know very little about the aetiology of preterm labour or the most appropriate way to manage the condition. The major advances have probably come from improved neonatal care rather than obstetric intervention, whilst many trials of obstetric management have been too small to allow satisfactory conclusions to be drawn. This area is an example where meta-analysis may allow more satisfactory conclusions to be drawn.

The need for collaboration in management between obstetrician and neonatologist should be stressed (Liggins 1990). A future trend may be the identification of a chemical marker, such as fetal fibronectin, derived from trophoblast and found in cervical and vaginal secretions, which may predict preterm labour and allow for earlier intervention (Creasy 1991; Lockwood *et al.* 1991).

References

Amon, E. A., Lewis, S. V., Sibai, B. M., Villar, M. A., and Arheart, K. L. (1988). Ampicillin prophylaxis in pre-term premature rupture of the membranes. *American Journal of Obstetrics and Gynecology* **159**, 539–43.

Beall, M. H., Edgar, B. W., Paul, R. H., and Smith-Wallace, T. (1985). A comparison of ritodrine, terbutaline and magnesium sulphate for the suppression of pre-term labour. *American Journal of Obstetrics and Gynecology* **153**, 854–9.

Bengston, J. M., Van Marter, L. J., Barss, V. A., Green, M. F., Tulmala, R. E., and Epstein, M. F. (1989). Pregnancy outcome after premature rupture of the membranes at or before 26 weeks' gestation. *Obstetrics and Gynecology* **73**, 941–6.

Berkowitz, G. S. (1981). An epidemiologic study of preterm delivery. *American Journal of Epidemiology* **113**, 81–92.

Besinger, R. E., Niebyl, J. R., Keyes, W. G., and Johnson, T. R. B. (1991). Randomized comparative trial of indomethacin and ritodrine for the long-term treatment of preterm labour. *American Journal of Obstetrics and Gynecology* **164**, 981–8.

Beydoun, S. N. and Yasin, S. Y. (1986). Premature rupture of the membranes before 28 weeks. *American Journal of Obstetrics and Gynecology* **155**, 471–9.

Blondel, B., Le Coutour, X., Kaminski, M., Chavigny, C., Breart, G., and Sureau, C. (1990). Prediction of pre-term delivery: Is it substantially improved by routine vaginal examination? *American Journal of Obstetrics and Gynacology* **162**, 1042–8.

Bobitt, J. R., Hayslip, C. C., and Damato, J. D. (1981). Amniotic fluid infection as determined by transabdominal amniocentesis in patients with intact membranes in preterm labour. *American Journal of Obstetrics and Gynecology* **140**, 947–52.

Brown, S. M. and Tejani, N. A. (1981). Terbutaline sulphate in the prevention of recurrence of preterm labour. *Obstetrics and Gynecology* **57**, 22–5.

Bryce, R. L., Stanley, F. J., and Garner, J. B. (1991). Randomized control trial of antenatal social support to prevent preterm birth. *British Journal of Obstetrics and Gynaecology* **98**, 1001–8.

Bucknell, E. W. C. and Wood, B. S. B. (1985). The Wessex perinatal mortality survey. *British Journal of Obstetrics and Gynaecology* **92**, 550–8.

Cammu, H., Goossens, A., Derde, M. P., Tennerman, M., Foulon, W., and Amy, J. (1989). C-reactive protein in preterm labour. *British Journal of Obstetrics and Gynaecology* **96**, 314–19.

Caritis, S. N., Toig, G., Heddinjer, L. A., and Ashmead, G. (1984). A double-blind study comparing ritodrine and terbutaline in the treatment of pre-term labour. *American Journal of Obstetrics and Gynecology* **150**, 7–14.

Carr-Hill, R. A. and Hall, M. H. (1985). The repetition of spontaneous preterm labour. *British Journal of Obstetrics and Gynaecology* **92**, 921–8.

Caspi, E., Schreyer, P., Weinraub, Z., Lifshitz, Y., and Goldberg, M. (1981). Dexamethasone for prevention of respiratory distress syndrome. *Obstetrics and Gynecology* **57**, 41–7.

Castren, O., Gummerus, N., and Saarikoski, S. (1975). Treatment of imminent preterm labour. *Acta Obstetrica et Gynaecologica Scandinavica* **54**, 95–100.

Cox, S. M., Sherman, M. L., and Leveno, H. J. (1990). Randomized investigation of magnesium sulfate for prevention of prevention of preterm birth. *American Journal of Obstetrics and Gynecology* **163**, 767–73.

Creasy, R. K. (1991). Preventing preterm birth. *The Journal of Medicine* **325**, 727–8.

Creasy, R. K. and Merkatz, I. R. (1990). Preventing preterm birth: Clinical opinion. *Obstetrics and Gynecology* **76**, Supp. 2S–4S.

Creasy, R. K., Gummar, B. A., and Liggins, G. C. (1980). System for predicting spontaneous preterm birth. *Obstetrics and Gynecology* **55**, 692–5.

Crowley, P., Chalmers, I., and Keirse, M. J. N. C. (1990). The effects of cortiocosteroid administration before pre-term delivery: an overview. *British Journal of Obstetrics and Gynaecology* **97**, 11–25.

Crowther, C. A., Neilson, J. P., Verkuil, D. A. A., Bannerman, C., and Ashurst, H. M. (1989). Pre-term labour in twin pregnancy. *British Journal of Obstetrics and Gynaecology* **96**, 850–3.

De Haas, I., Harlow, B. L., Cramer, D. W., and Frigolett, F. D. (1991). Spontaneous preterm birth: a case controlled study. *American Journal of Obstetrics and Gynecology* **165**, 1290–6.

Drillien, C. M. (1961). The incidence of mental and physical handicaps in school-aged children of very low birthweight. *Paediatrics* **27**, 452–64.

Eggers, T. R., Doyle, L. W., and Pepperell, R. J. (1979). Premature rupture of the membranes. *Medical Journal of Australia* **1**, 209–13.

Elliott, H. R., Abdulla, S., and Hayes, P. J. (1978). Pulmonary oedema associated with ritodrine infusion and beta-methasone administration in premature labour. *British Medical Journal* **2**, 799–800.

Ernest, J. L. and Givner, L. B. (1994). A prospective randomized placebo-controlled trial of penicillin in pre-term premature rupture of the membranes. *American Journal of Obstetrics and Gynecology* **170**, 516–20.

Erny, R., Pigne, A., Prouvost, C., Gamerre, M., Malet, C., Serment, H., *et al.* (1986). The effects of oral administration of progesterone for premature labour. *American Journal of Obstetrics and Gynecology* **154**, 525–9.

Eronen, M., Pesonen, E., Kurki, T., Ylikorkala, O., and Hallman, M. (1991). The effects of indomethacin and beta-sympathomimetic agents on the fetal ductus arteriosus during treatment of preterm labour. *American Journal of Obstetrics and Gynecology* **164**, 141–6.

Farb, H. R., Amesen, M., Geistler, P., and Knox, G. E. (1983). C-reactive protein with premature rupture of membranes and premature labour. *Obstetrics and Gynecology* **62**, 49–51.

Feinstein, S. J., Vintzileos, A. M., Lodeiro, J. G., Campbell, W. A., Weinbaum, P. J., and Nochimson, D. J. (1986). Amniocentesis with premature rupture of the membranes. *Obstetrics and Gynecology* **68**, 147–52.

Ferguson, J. E., Dyson, D. C., Schutz, T., and Stevenson, D. K. (1990). A comparison of tocolysis with nifedipine or ritodrine. *American Journal of Obstetrics and Gynecology* **163**, 105–11.

Fisk, N. M., Fysh, J., Chitd, A. G., Gatenby, P. A., Jeffery, H., and Bradfield, A. H. (1987). Is C-reactive protein really useful in preterm premature rupture of the mebranes? *British Journal of Obstetrics and Gynaecology* **94**, 1159–64.

Fuchs, F. (1976). Prevention of post-maturity. *American Journal of Obstetrics and Gynecology* **126**, 809–20.

Fuchs, F. and Stakemann, G. (1960). Treatment of threatened premature labour with large doses of progesterone. *American Journal of Obstetrics and Gynecology* **79**, 172–6.

Galask, R. P., Varnar, M. W., Petzold, C. R., and Wilbur, S. L. (1984). Bacterial attachment to the chorioamniotic membrane. *American Journal of Obstetrics and Gynecology* **148**, 913–26.

Gamsu, H. R., Mullinger, B. M., Donnai, P., and Dash, C. H. (1989). Antenatal administration of betamethasone to prevent respiratory dexamethasone in preterm infants. *British Journal of Obstetrics and Gynaecology* **96**, 401–10.

Garite, T. J., Freeman, R. K., Linzey, M., Braly, P. S., and Dorchester, W. L. (1981). Prospective randomized study of corticosteroids in the management of premature rupture of the membranes. *American Journal of Obstetrics and Gynecology* **141**, 508–15.

Gersony, W. M., Peckham, G. J., Ellison, R. C., Meittinem, O. S., and Nadis, A. S. (1983). Effects of indomethacin in premature infants with patent ductus arteriosus. *Journal of Paediatrics* **102**, 895–906.

Gibbs, R. S. and Blanco, J. D. (1982). Premature rupture of the membranes. *Obstetrics and Gynecology* **60**, 671–9.

Glock, J. L. and Morales, W. J. (1993). Efficacy and safety of nifedipine versus magnesium sulphate in the management of pre-term labour. *American Journal of Obstetrics and Gynecology* **169**, 960–4.

Goldenberg, R. J., Davis, R. O., Copper, R. L., Corliss, D. K., Andrews, J. B., and Carpenter, A. H. (1990). The Alahbama preterm birth prevention project. *Obstetrics and Gynecology* **75**, 933–9.

Grimes, D. and Schultz, K. F. (1992). Randomized controlled trials of home uterine activity monitoring. *Obstetrics and Gynecology* **79**, 137–42.

Gummerus, M. and Halonen, O. (1987). Prophylactic long-term oral tocolysis of multiple pregnancy. *British Journal of Obstetrics and Gynaecology* **94**, 249–51.

Hack, M. and Fanaroff, A. A. (1989). Outcome of extremely low birthweight infants. *New England Journal of Medicine* **321**, 1642–7.

Hallak, M. and Bottoms, S. F. (1993). Accelerated pulmonary maturity for pre-term premature rupture of the membranes—a myth. *American Journal of Obstetrics and Gynecology* **169**, 1045–9.

Hauksson, A., Akerlund, M., and Melin, P. (1988). Uterine blood flow and myometrial activity at menstruation, and the action of vasopressin and a synthetic antagonist. *British Journal of Obstetrics and Gynaecology* **95**, 898–904.

Hay, P. E., Lamont, R. F., Taylor-Robinson, D., Morgan, D. J., Ison, C., and Pearson, J. (1994). Abnormal bacterial colonisation of the genital tract and subsequent pre-term delivery and late miscarriage. *British Medical Journal* **308**, 295–8.

Higby, K., Xanakis, E. M., and Paverstein, C. J. (1993). Do tocolytic agents stop preterm labour? *American Journal of Obstetrics and Gynecology* **168**, 1247–59.

Hill, W. C., Fleming, A. D., Martin, R. W., Hamer, C., Knuppel, R. A., Lake, M. F., *et al.* (1990). Home uterine activity monitoring is associated with a reduction in preterm birth. *Obstetrics and Gynecology* **76**, Supp. 135–185.

Hollander, D. I., Nagey, D. A., and Pupkin, M. J. (1987). Magnesium sulphate and ritodrine hydrochloride: a randomized comparison. *American Journal of Obstetrics and Gynecology* **156**, 631–7.

Iams, J. D., Talbert, M. L., Barrows, H., and Sachs, L. (1985). Management of preterm prematurely ruptured membranes. *American Journal of Obstetrics and Gynecology* **151**, 32–8.

Jobe, A. H., Mitchell, B. R., and Gunkel, J. H. (1993). Beneficial effects of continued use of pre-natal corticosteroids and post-natal surfactant. *American Journal of Obstetrics and Gynecology* **168**, 508–13.

Johnston, M. M., Sanchez-Ramos, L., Vaughan, A. J., Todd, M. W., and Benrobi, G. I. (1990). Antibiotic therapy in preterm premature rupture of the membranes: A randomized prospective double-blind trial. *American Journal of Obstetrics and Gynecology* **163**, 743–7.

Katz, M., Robertson, P. A., and Creasy, R. K. (1981). Cardiovascular complications associated with terbutaline treatment for pre-term labour. *American Journal of Obstetrics and Gynecology* **139**, 605–8.

Keirse, M. J. N. C. (1990). Progestogen administration in pregnancy may prevent pre-term delivery. *British Journal of Obstetrics and Gynaecology* **97**, 149–54.

King, J. F., Grant, A., Keirse, M. J. N. C., and Chalmers, I. (1988). Betamimetics in pre-term labour: an overview of the randomized controlled trials. *British Journal of Obstetrics and Gynaecology* **95**, 211–22.

Kirschenbaum, T. (1993). Antibiotics in the treatment of pre-term labour. *American Journal of Obstetrics and Gynecology* **168**, 1239–46.

Krohn, M. A., Hillier, S. L., Lee, M. L., Rabe, L. K., and Eschenbach, D. A. (1991). Vaginal *Bacteroides* species are associated with an increased rate of pre-term delivery among women in pre-term labour. *Journal of Infectious Diseases* **164**, 88–92.

Lamont, R. F., Dunlop, P. D. M., Levene, M. I., and Elder, M. G., (1983). Use of glucocorticoids in pregnancy complicated by severe hypertension and proteinuria. *British Journal of Obstetrics and Gynaecology* **90**, 199–202.

Lamont, R. F., Taylor-Robinson, D., Newman, M., Wigglesworth, J., and Elder, M. G. (1986). Spontaneous early pre-term labour associated with abnormal genital tract bacterial colonization. *British Journal of Obstetrics and Gynaecology* **93**, 804–10.

Lampert, M. B., Hibbard, J., Weiner, T. L., Briller, J., Lindheimer, M., and Lang, R. (1993). Peri-partum heart failure associated with prolonged tocolysis. *American Journal of Obstetrics and Gynecology* **168**, 291–3.

Lancet (1980). Prostaglandin synthetase inhibitors in Obstetrics and after. *Lancet* **ii**, 185–6.

Larsen, J. F., Hansen, M. K., Hesseldahl, H., Kristofferson, K., Larsen, P. K., Osler, M., *et al.* (1980). Ritrodrine in the treatment of preterm labour. *British Journal of Obstetrics and Gynaecology* **87**, 949–57.

Larsen, J. F., Oldon, K., Lange, A. P., Leegaard, M., Osler, M., Oslen, J. S., *et al.* (1986). Ritodrine in the treatment of preterm labour. *Obstetrics and Gynecology* **67**, 607–13.

Levy, D. L. and Warsof, S. L. (1985). Oral ritodrine and preterm premature rupture of the membranes. *Obstetrics and Gynecology* **66**, 621–3.

Liggins, G. C. (1969). Premature delivery of fetal lambs infused with glucocorticoids. *Journal of Endocrinology* **45**, 515-23.

Liggins, G. C. (1990). Obstetric and paediatric collaboration to reduce morbidity after pre-term birth. *British Journal of Obstetrics and Gynaecology* **97**, 1-3.

Liggins, G. C. and Howie, R. N. (1972). A controlled trial of antepartum glucocorticoids treatment for the prevention of respiratory distress syndrome in premature infants. *Pediatrics* **50**, 515-25.

Lockwood, C. J., Senyei, A. E., Gifche, M. R., Cafal, D., Shah, K. D., Thung, S. N., *et al.* (1991). Fetal fibronectin in cervical and vaginal secretions as a predictor of preterm delivery. *New England Journal of Medicine* **325**, 669-74.

Lockwood, C. J., Costigan, K., Ghidini, A., Wein, R., Chien, D., Brown, B. L., *et al.* (1993). Double-blind placebo controlled trial of piperacillin prophylaxis and pre-term membrane rupture. *American Journal of Obstetrics and Gynecology* **169**, 970-6.

McDonald, H. M., O'Loughlin, J. A., Jolley, P., Vigneswaran, R., and McDonald, P. J. (1991). Vaginal infection and preterm labour. *British Journal of Obstetrics and Gynaecology* **98**, 427-35.

MacGillivray, I. (1989). Multiple pregnancies. In *Obstetrics* (ed. A. Turnbull and G. Chamberlain), pp. 493-502. Churchill Livingstone, Edinburgh.

McIlwaine, G. M., Howat, R. C. L., Dunn, F., and MacNaughton, M. C. (1979). The Scottish perinatal mortality survey. *British Medical Journal* **2**, 1103-6.

Main, D. M., Main, E. K., and Maurer, M. M. (1983). Caesarean section versus vaginal delivery for the breech fetus weighing less than 1500 grams. *American Journal of Obstetrics and Gynecology* **146**, 580-4.

Main, D. M., Gabb, E. S. G., Richardson, D., and Strong, S. (1985). Can preterm delivery be prevented? *American Journal of Obstetrics and Gynecology* **151**, 892-8.

Main, D. M., Richardson, D., Gabb, E. S. G., Strong, S., and Weller, S. C. (1987). Prospective evaluation of a risk scoring system for predicting preterm delivery in black inner-city women. *Obstetrics and Gynecology* **69**, 61-6.

Maltau, J. M., Egge, E., and Moe, N. (1984). Retinal haemorrhages in the pre-term neonate. *Acta Obstetrica et Gynaecologica Scandinavica* **63**, 219-21.

Mathews, D. D., Friend, J. D., and Michael, C. A. (1967). A double-blind trial of oral isoxsuprine in the prevention of premature labour. *Journal of Obstetrics and Gynaecology of the British Commonwealth* **74**, 68-70.

Mercer, B. M., Moretti, M. L., Prevost, R. R., and Sibai, B. M. (1992). Erythromycin treatment in pre-term premature rupture of the membranes. *American Journal of Obstetrics and Gynecology* **166**, 794-802.

Miller, J. M., Pupkin, M. J., and Crenshaw, C. (1978). Premature labour and premature rupture of the membranes. *American Journal of Obstetrics and Gynecology* **132**, 1-6.

Moise, K. J. (1993). Effect of advancing gestational age and frequency of fetal ductal constriction in association with internal indomethacin use. *American Journal of Obstetrics and Gynecology* **168**, 1350-3.

Moise, K. J., Huhta, J. C., Sharif, D. S., Ou, C. N., Kirshon, B., Wasserstrum, N., *et al.* (1988). Indomethacin in the treatment of premature labour. *New England Journal of Medicine* **319**, 327-31.

Morales, W. J., Diebel, D., Lazar, A. J., and Zadrozny, D. (1986). The effects of antenatal dexamethasone administration on the prevention of respiratory distress syndrome in gestations with premature rupture of the membranes. *American Journal of Obstetrics and Gynecology* **154**, 591-5.

Morales, W. J., Angel, J., O'Brien, W., and Knuppel, R. (1989). Use of ampicillin and corticosteroids in premature rupture of the membranes. *Obstetrics and Gynecology* **73**, 721-6.

Morrison, J. C. (1990). Preterm birth: a puzzle worth solving. *Obstetrics and Gynecology* **76**, Supp. 5S–12S.

Mueller-Heubach, E., Reddick, D., Barrett, B., and Bente, R. (1989). Preterm birth prediction: evaluation of a prospective controlled randomized trial. *American Journal of Obstetrics and Gynecology* **160**, 1172–8.

Munson, L. A., Graham, A., Koos, B. J., and Valenzuela, G. J. (1985). Is there a need for digital examination in patients with spontaneous rupture of the membranes? *American Journal of obstetrics and Gynecology* **153**, 562–3.

Newton, E. R., Dinsmour, M. J., and Gibbs, R. S. (1989). A randomized blinded placebo controlled trial of antibiotics in idiopathic preterm labour. *Obstetrics and Gynecology* **74**, 562–6.

Newton, E. R., Shields, L., Ridgway, L. E., Berkus, M. D., and Elliott, B. D. (1991). Combined antibiotic and indomethacin in idiopathic preterm labour. *American Journal of Obstetrics and Gynecology* **165**, 1753–9.

Niebyl, L. J., Blake, D. A., White, R. D., Kumor, K. M., Dubin, N. H., Robinson, J. C., *et al.* (1980). The inhibition of premature labour with indomethacin. *American Journal of Obstetrics and Gynecology* **136**, 1014–19.

O'Driscoll, K., meagher, D., MacDonald, D., and Jeoghejan, F. (1981). Traumatic intracranial haemorrhage in firstborn infants and delivery with obstetric forceps. *British Journal of Obstetrics and Gynaecology* **88**, 577–81.

Olshan, A. F., Shy, K. K., Luthy, D. A., Hickok, D., Weiss, N. S., and Daling, J. R. (1984). Caesarean birth and neonatal mortality in very low birthweight infants. *Obstetrics and Gynecology* **64**, 267–70.

Owen, J. O., Goldenberg, R. L., Davis, R. O., Kirk, K. A., and Copper, R. L. (1990). Evaluation of a risk scoring system as a predictor of preterm birth in an indigent population. *American Journal of Obstetrics and Gynecology* **163**, 873–9.

Persson, P. H., Greenert, L., Gennser, G., and Kullander, S. (1979). On improved outcome of twin pregnancies. *Acta Obstetrica et Gynaecologica Scandinavica* **58**, 3–7.

Potkul, R. K., Moawad, A. H., and Ponto, K. L. (1985). The association of subclinical infection with preterm labour. *American Journal of Obstetrics and Gynecology* **153**, 642–5.

Powell, T. G., Pharoah, P. O. D., and Cooke, R. W. I. (1986). Survival and morbidity in a geographically defined population of low birthweight infants. *Lancet* **i**, 539–43.

Powers, W. F. and Miller, T. C. (1979). Bedrest in twin pregnancy. *American Journal of Obstetrics and Gynecology* **134**, 23–9.

Rayburn, W., Piehl, E., Schork, M. A., and Kierse, H. T. J. (1986). Intravenous ritodrine therapy: a comparison between twin and singleton gestation. *Obstetrics and Gynecology* **67**, 243–8.

Read, J. S. and Klebenoff, M.A. (1993). Sexual intercourse during pregnancy and preterm delivery. *American Journal of Obstetrics and Gynecology* **168**, 514–19.

Regan, J. A., Chao, S., and James, L. S. (1981). Premature rupture of the membranes, preterm delivery, and group B streptococcus. *American Journal of Obstetrics and Gynecology* **141**, 184–9.

Rhoads, G. G., McNellis, D. C., and Kessel, S. S. (1991). A home monitoring of uterine contractivity. *American Journal of Obstetrics and Gynecology* **165**, 2–6.

Ridgway, L. E., Muise, K., Wright, J. W., Patterson, R. M., and Newton, E. R. (1990). A prospective randomized comparison of oral terbutaline and magnesium oxide for the maintenance of tocolysis. *American Journal of Obstetrics and Gynecology* **163**, 879–82.

Romen, Y. and Artal, R. (1984). C-reactive protein as a predictor for chorioamnionitis

UNIVERSITY OF CHICAGO BOOKSTORE

894 CASH-1   6223 0491

978140284112 TRADE
College Madams May   MDS 1   9.
            DISCOUNT 75.0   7.
                SUBTOTAL   2.
        8.75% SALES TAX   :
                TOTAL   2.

Cash   5.
            CHANGE   2.
        DISCOUNT TOTAL   7.
last day spring qtr text returns:

                    5/13/05 3:1

in cases of premature rupture of the membranes. *American Journal of Obstetrics and Gynecology* **150**, 546–50.

Romero, R., Sibai, B., Caritis, S., Paul, R., Depp, R., Rosen, M., *et al.* (1993). Antibiotic treatment of pre-term labour with intact membranes. *American Journal of Obstetrics and Gynecology* **169**, 764–74.

Roussounis, S. H., Hubley, P. A., and Dear, P. R. F. (1993). Five-year follow-up of very low birthweight infants. *Childcare, Health and Development* **19**, 45–59.

Rush, R. W., Davey, D. A., and Segall, M. L (1978). The effect of premature delivery on perinatal mortality. *British Journal of Obstetrics and Gynaecology* **85**, 806–11.

Rush, R. W., Isaacs, S., McPherson, K., Jones, L., Chalmers, I., and Grant, A. (1984). A randomised controlled trial of cervical cerclage in women of high risk of spontaneous premature labour. *British Journal of Obstetrics and Gynaecology* **91**, 724–30.

Russell, J. K. (1952). Maternal and fetal hazards associated with twin pregnancy. *Journal of Obstetrics and Gynaecology of the British Commonwealth* **59**, 208–13.

Sanjose, S., Roman, E., and Beral, V. (1991). Low birthweight and preterm delivery, Scotland, 1981–4. *Lancet* **338**, 428–31.

Saunders, M. C., Dick, J. C., Brown, I. M., McPherson, K., and Chalmers, I. (1985). The effects of hospital admission for bedrest on the duration of twin pregnancy. *Lancet* **ii**, 793–5.

Schutte, M. F., Treffers, P. E., Kloosterman, G. J., and Saepatmi, S. (1983). Management of 'premature rupture of the membranes. *American Journal of Obstetrics and Gynecology* **146**, 395–400.

Simpson, G. F. and Harbert, G. M. (1985). Use of betamethasone in the management of preterm gestation with premature rupture of the membranes. *Obstetrics and Gynecology* **66**, 168–75.

Spearing, G. (1979). Alcohol, indomethacin and salbutamol. *Obstetrics and Gynecology* **53**, 171–4.

Spellacy, W. N., Cruz, A. C., Birk, S. A., and Buhi, W. C. (1979). Treatment of premature labour with ritodrine. *Obstetrics and Gynecology* **54**, 220–3.

Spinnato, J. A. (1987). Preterm premature rupture of the membranes with fetal maturity present. *Obstetrics and Gynecology* **69**, 196–201.

US Collaborative Study Group on Antenatal Steroids (1981). Effect of antenatal dexamethasone administration on the prevention of respiratory distress syndrome. *American Journal of Obstetrics and Gynecology* **141**, 276–87.

van den Veyver, I. B., Moise, K. J., Ou, C. N., and Carpenter, R. J. (1993). Effect of gestational age on the constriction of the fetal ductus arteriosis. *Obstetrics and Gynecology* **81**, 500–3.

Wahbeh, C. J., Hill, G. B., Eden, R. D., and Gall, S. A. (1984). Intra-amniotic bacterial colonization in premature labour. *American Journal of Obstetrics and Gynecology* **148**, 739–42.

Walters, W. A. W. and Wood, C. (1977). A trial of oral ritodine in the prevention of premature labour. *British Journal of Obstetrics and Gynaecology* **84**, 26–30.

Watson, D. L., Welch, R. A., Marion, F. G., Lake, M. F., Canuppel, R. A., Martin, R. W., *et al.* (1990). Management of preterm labour patients at home. *Obstetrics and Gynecology* **76**, Supp. 32S–5S.

Weekes, A. R. L., Menzies, D. N., and De Boer, C. H. (1977). The relative efficacy of bedrest, cervical suture and no treatment in the management of twin pregnancy. *British Journal of Obstetrics and Gynaecology* **84**, 161–4.

Wen, S. W., Goldenberg, R. L., Cutter, G. R., Hoffman, H. J., and Oliver, S. P. (1990). Intrauterine growth retardation and preterm delivery: prenatal risk factors. *American Journal of Obstetrics and Gynecology* **162**, 213–18.

White, B., Lamont, R. F., and Tetchorth, A. T. (1989). An approach to the problem of recurrent middle trimester abortion. *Journal of Obstetrics and Gynaecology* **10**, 8–9.

White, D. R., Hall, M. H., and Campbell, D. M. (1986). Aetiology of preterm labour. *British Journal of Obstetrics and Gynaecology* **93**, 733–8.

Wilkinson, A. R. (1980). Naproxen levels in preterm infants after maternal treatment. *Lancet* **ii**, 591–2.

Yemini, M., Borenstein, W., Dreaze, N. E., Applerman, Z., Mogilner, B. M., Kessler, I., *et al.* (1985). Prevention of premature labour by 17-alpha-hydroxyprogesterone caproate. *American Journal of Obstetrics and Gynecology* **151**, 574–7.

Young, E. W. D. and Stevenson, D. K. (1990). Limiting treatment for extremely premature, low birthweight infants. *American Journal of Diseases of Children* **144**, 549–52.

Yu, V. Y. H., Loke, H. L., Bajuk, B., Szymonowicz, W., Orgill, A. A., and Astbury, J. (1986). Prognosis for infants born 23 to 28 weeks' gestation. *British Medical Journal* **293**, 1200–3.

Zlatnik, F. J. and Fuchs, F. (1972). A controlled study of ethanol in threatened preterm labour. *American Journal of Obstetrics and Gynecology* **112**, 610–12.

23 Diabetes and pregnancy

This chapter is concerned with glucose tolerance and intolerance during pregnancy, the diagnosis of diabetes, and the implications of that diagnosis.

Diabetes is a relatively common disorder with insulin-dependent diabetes affecting 0.2 per cent of Caucasians below the age of 30 years with a peak age incidence of 11–14 years (Brudenell 1989).

Gestational diabetes is the condition in which a woman becomes diabetic during pregnancy, regardless of whether or not the condition continues after delivery. Although it may seem more sensible to distinguish between the gestational diabetic woman who reverts to normal after delivery and the gestational diabetic woman who is really only a newly diagnosed diabetic patient, this distinction does not specifically influence management during the pregnancy and indeed cannot. Traditionally, the perinatal risks to the fetus of a gestational diabetic mother are considered to be greater than those without diabetes, but are now less than those for established diabetes. The British Survey of Diabetic Pregnancies reported a perinatal mortality rate of 60.2 per 1000 for women with gestational diabetes (Beard and Lowy 1982). Maresh *et al.* (1989) quoted a perinatal mortality rate of 14 per 1000 for patients with gestational diabetes compared with 9.4 per 1000 for non-diabetic controls. However, some recent series have not confirmed an excess risk from gestational diabetes (Coustan 1991). For example, Brudenell and Doddridge (1989*a*) quoted a perinatal mortality rate of 12 per 1000 for established diabetes and zero for gestational diabetes. This current lack of excess risk is presumably due to care and intervention and should not be equated with a need for reduced vigilance in attempting to diagnose gestational diabetes, since diagnosed but untreated gestational diabetes does carry a significant risk (Pettitt *et al.* 1980).

Perinatal morbidity also occurs in gestational diabetes. Widness *et al.* (1985) reported a greater incidence of macrosomia, shoulder dystocia, birth trauma, hypoglycaemia, polycythaemia, hyperbilirubinaemia, and respiratory distress in the 62 infants of women with gestational diabetes compared with 62 controls. Moreover, the prophylactic use of insulin in women with gestational diabetes may reduce neonatal morbidity. Coustan and Imarah (1984) reported that macrosomia complicated 7 per cent of 115 insulin treated gestational diabetic pregnancies, 18.5 per cent of 184 dietary restricted gestational diabetic pregnancies and 17.8 per cent of 146 untreated gestational diabetic pregnancies. Similarly, the insulin treated group had a reduced incidence of operative delivery and birth trauma. Thompson *et al.* (1990) randomized 68 gestational diabetics to receive either insulin and dietary advice or dietary advice alone. Macrosomia occurred in 6 per cent of the diet and insulin treated group compared with 27 per cent of the diet alone group. Not all authors have demonstrated that insulin and diet are superior to diet alone when treating a gestational diabetic patient. Persson *et al.* (1985) randomly allocated 202 gestational diabetic women to receive either diet or diet and insulin. The incidence of macrosomia was similar in both groups, but it is possible that this was a reflection of dietary advice rather than a lack of effect of insulin. In this series, 14 per cent of patients allocated to diet alone required additional insulin during the pregnancy. Thus, gestational diabetes is a clinically important entity and may require as enthusiastic treatment as insulin-dependent diabetes prior to pregnancy.

The incidence of gestational diabetes appears to vary, according to the literature, from between 0.4 to 6 per cent of patients (Amankwah *et al.* 1977; Coustan *et al.* 1989; Gillmer *et al.* 1980; Maresh *et al.* 1989; Merkatz *et al.* 1980; Sepe *et al.* 1985).

Gestational diabetes does not invariably recur in subsequent pregnancies and hence the diagnosis should not be assumed but checked by means of a glucose tolerance test. The literature would suggest that gestational diabetes recurs in between 34–56 per cent of pregnancies (Grant *et al.* 1986; Philipson and Super 1989).

There are also longterm implications from gestational diabetes. Grant *et al.* (1986) retested 447 women who had gestational diabetes 1–12 years earlier. Of these, 11 per cent were diabetic and a further 8 per cent had impaired glucose tolerance. Mestman (1988) reported that 65 per cent of women with gestational diabetes ultimately became overtly diabetic. Other authors quote statistics in excess of 50 per cent (Dornhorst 1994).

Abnormal glucose tolerance during pregnancy

Pregnancy is diabetogenic. As the levels of maternal cortisol and placental lactogen increase, especially during the third trimester, relative insulin resistance occurs, for these substances are insulin antagonists. Maternal insulin production increases and a state of relative glucose intolerance develops. Glucose is able to cross the placenta and, in a state of maternal hyperglycaemia, fetal hyperinsulinaemia will occur (Kuhl 1991).

Since gestational diabetes is largely asymptomatic, screening is necessary in order to select those patients who need some formal test of their carbohydrate metabolism. The clinical criteria for performing a glucose tolerance test are well known and are shown in Table 23.1 Brudenell (1989) argued that such criteria will fail to detect 'most cases of impaired glucose tolerance' and 'some women' with gestational diabetes. These criteria will only identify approximately 60 per cent of the antenatal gestational diabetic population (Coustan 1991) and although they represent the major indications of *selective* diabetic screening during pregnancy, they are of limited value. These criteria will now be further discussed.

Genetic factors play a role in the development of diabetes. Up to 5 per cent of the offspring of a diabetic parent will ultimately become diabetic, whilst

Table 23.1 Criteria for glucose tolerance testing

(1) Potential diabetes (first-degree relative, previous baby weighing more than 4.5 kg);

(2) Obesity (over 20% of ideal weight for height);

(3) Glycosuria on two or more occasions (preferably fasting);

(4) Previous congenital abnormality, unexplained stillbirth or neonatal death;

(5) Hydramnios in current pregnancy;

(6) Previous gestational diabetes;

(7) Developing fetal macrosomia.

6 per cent of diabetics will have a diabetic parent compared with 3 per cent of the general population. Some 21 per cent of diabetics have a first degree relative with diabetes compared with 8 per cent amongst a control population (Pyke 1968; Tillil and Kobberling 1987).

The association between maternal diabetes and large babies has long been recognized. Thus Kriss and Futcher (1948) reported 100 diabetic women who had delivered 360 babies prior to the diagnosis of diabetes being made. Some 35 per cent of these women delivered a baby weighing more than 4.5 kg compared with 11 per cent of controls. O'Sullivan and Mahan (1980) reported that 13 per cent of infants born to mothers with gestational diabetes weighed in excess of 4 kg compared with 4 per cent of controls. There is evidence that the increased incidence of macrosomia in the offspring of gestational diabetic patients is a reflection of maternal obesity rather than the diabetes. Maresh *et al.* (1989) reported 213 women with abnormal glucose tolerance tests during pregnancy. The incidence of macrosomia in the offspring of non-obese diabetic women was 10 per cent but was 24 per cent in the offspring of obese gestational diabetic patients.

Although maternal obesity tends to be associated with maturity onset diabetes, there is only limited evidence for an excess of gestational diabetes in obese obstetric patients.

Random glycosuria, related to increased glomerular filtration and reduced tubular reabsorption of glucose, will occur in two-thirds of healthy pregnant women at some stage during their pregnancy (Lind and Hytten 1972). Sutherland *et al.* (1970) found glycosuria in a single random urine test in 11 per cent of 1418 pregnant women. Only 4 per cent of these women had gestational diabetes. However, 15 per cent of patients with glycosuria in their 'second fasting' sample had gestational diabetes making this a more logical urine screening test.

A past history of previous unexplained perinatal loss, or of a fetal abnormality, is a weak but important criterion for glucose tolerance testing. The past history of perinatal loss was assessed by Maresh *et al.* (1989) who reported such losses in 9 per cent of 213 gestational diabetics compared with 6 per cent of 213 matched controls.

Hydramnios has been reported in up to 31 per cent of established diabetic pregnancies. Kitzmiller *et al.* (1978) reported that it is least common in those diabetic patients with the lowest blood glucose concentrations. Brudenell and Doddridge (1989*b*) reported hydramnios in 25 per cent of pregnancies in established diabetes and 13 per cent in gestational diabetes. It is argued that fetal hyperglycaemia, related to poor maternal diabetic control, results in polyuria and hence hydramnios. As the diabetic control improves, the hydramnios decreases.

The relationship between gestational diabetes in a previous pregnancy and in the index pregnancy has already been discussed. The diagnosis of developing fetal macrosomia, based on ultrasound, is an indication for glucose tolerance testing.

The glucose tolerance test may be considered reliable and reproducible should it be clearly normal or clearly abnormal, but should only one blood glucose result be abnormal, the test should be repeated later in the pregnancy (Harlass *et al.* 1991).

The criteria for the diagnosis of gestational diabetes are based upon plasma glucose estimations in fasting venous blood or on the interpretation of a glucose tolerance test. It is now generally accepted that a fasting blood glucose concentration of 8 mmol/l, or more, is diagnostic for gestational diabetes, as is a concentration of 11 mmol/l or more after food. A fasting concentration of less than 6 mmol/l excludes diabetes, whilst a concentration of between 6 and 8 represents impaired glucose tolerance and is an indication for performing a glucose tolerance test (Keen *et al.* 1979; National Diabetes Data Group 1979; World Health Organization 1980). These authorities also recommend that a glucose tolerance test following an overnight fast is conducted using a 75 g oral glucose load in 250 ml water with blood taken at both one and two hours after drinking. A concentration equal to, or greater than, 11.0 mmol/l for both venous plasma glucose samples at one and two hours confirms the diagnosis, but the two-hour concentration alone may be accepted as diagnostic of diabetes if it is greater than 11.0 mmol/l should diabetic symptoms be present. Impaired glucose tolerance will be diagnosed when there is only one abnormal value for blood glucose concentration on the glucose tolerance test. This is generally the blood glucose concentration at one hour and is an indication for repeating the glucose tolerance test later in pregnancy (Harlass *et al.* 1991).

Testing for diabetes during pregnancy

Since the above clinical criteria are of limited value and since gestational diabetes is seen in the absence of glycosuria, interest has developed in antenatal screening, using single plasma glucose levels as an indicator for an oral glucose tolerance test. Lind and Anderson (1984) sampled venous blood from 2403 pregnant women attending an antenatal clinic between the 28th and 32nd weeks without a previous glucose load. They considered that a plasma glucose level of 6.1 mmol/l within two hours of a meal, or 5.6 mmol/l after two hours, were indications for a 75 g oral glucose tolerance test. Some 1.6 per cent of their population satisfied these criteria, 0.5 per cent of the population being diagnosed as having gestational diabetes. Similarly, a fasting blood glucose concentration of less than 4.1 mmol/l will exclude 92 per cent of pregnant diabetic women when used as a screening test (Jowett *et al.* 1987).

Screening may be refined by means of a previous glucose load. Gillmer *et al.* (1980) sampled venous plasma one hour after the ingestion of a 50 g glucose load in 948 antenatal patients selected randomly. An abnormal result (defined as equal to or greater than 7.7 mmol/l) was obtained in 7.8 per cent of the population who then underwent a glucose tolerance test. Some 1.5 per cent of the original population were diagnosed as having gestational diabetes.

Glycosylated haemoglobin measurements have also been used for screening. For instance, Cousins *et al.* (1984) reported that if an HbA_1 of 6.9 per cent was chosen, 40 per cent of normal subjects would require further evaluation but 60 per cent would have glucose intolerance, whilst Morris *et al.* (1986) reported that if an HbA_1 of 6.3 per cent was chosen as the threshold for further investigation, only 7 per cent of gestational diabetic patients would be missed, whilst only 14 per cent of normal women would be subjected to a glucose tolerance test.

Fasting blood glucose estimations have not been evaluated widely as a screening method, but a fasting cut-off of 4.1 mmol/l would detect approximately 90 per cent of diabetic patients but also 50 per cent of normal subjects.

It would, therefore, appear that specific screening tests in an antenatal population will detect a greater number of women with abnormal glucose tolerance over and above those detected using the classical indications shown in Table 23.1.

Perinatal mortality

As management has been improved and refined, the perinatal mortality rate associated with diabetes during pregnancy has steadily fallen. Table 23.2 is based on an analysis of 1451 babies born to diabetic mothers between 1951 and 1990. During this time the perinatal mortality rate fell from 225 to 18 per 1000, whilst the cause of that perinatal mortality also altered (Brudenell, personal communication). The major cause of perinatal mortality is now lethal fetal abnormality and this is discussed further in the next subsection. The significance of the timing of delivery and of obstetric complications in diabetic mothers is also discussed in a later subsection.

Congenital abnormalities of the fetus

There is no doubt that the fetus of a diabetic mother is more likely to be abnormal than the fetus of a non-diabetic mother. Thus Johnson *et al.* (1988)

Table 23.2 Perinatal mortality

Year	Perinatal deaths			Major causes of perinatal mortality				
	No. of patients	No. of deaths	%	Obstetric	Diabetic	Congenital abnormality	Respiratory distress	Unexplained
1951–60	319	72	22.5	26	5	6	17	18
1961–70	390	39	10.0	9	2	5	8	15
1971–80	352	13	3.7	3	1	6	1	2
1981–90	390	7	1.8	0	0	4	0	3

From Brudenell (personal communication)

reported an incidence of fetal abnormality of 3.3 per cent in 238 diabetic pregnancies compared with 1.5 per cent of the overall clinic population. The United Kingdom Survey reported a malformation rate of 5.7 per cent for established diabetes and 1.8 per cent for gestational diabetes (Beard and Lowy 1982), whilst Lemons *et al.* (1981) reported that the incidence of major fetal abnormalites in 225 infants of diabetic mothers was 4.6 per cent, with minor fetal abnormalities occurring in 3.2 per cent. The major abnormalities were mainly cardiac, neural tube, and skeletal, whilst the non-lethal defects included hypospadias, cleft palate, hairlip, talipes, and phocomelia. Rosenn *et al.* (1990) scrutinized the infants of 171 insulin-dependent diabetic mothers and identified a minor congenital malformation rate of 18.7 per cent.

There is evidence that the incidence of fetal abnormality in the infants of diabetic mothers is decreasing with time, and that, although it is still greater than the fetal abnormality rate for the overall population, factors over and above tight diabetic control may be involved. Damm and Molsted-Pedersen (1989) reported that, in an unselected population of diabetic pregnant women, the incidence of fetal abnormality fell from 7.4 per cent between 1977 and 1981 to 2.7 per cent between 1982 and 1986. Moreover, Mills *et al.* (1988*a*) were unable to find any relationship between the incidence of fetal abnormality and mean blood glucose concentration, swings in blood glucose concentration, episodes of hypoglycaemia, and glycosylated haemoglobin levels. They reported that the incidence of fetal abnormality was 2 per cent for 389 non-diabetic pregnant women, 5 per cent for 347 diabetic women who were assessed within 21 days of conception, and 9 per cent for 279 diabetic women assessed later than this.

It is not clear which, if any, of the haematological indices which can be measured in pregnant diabetic women during the first trimester will give the most accurate prediction for the risk of fetal abnormality (*Lancet* 1988; Mills *et al.* 1988*a*). Interest has focused upon glycosylated haemoglobin which is a normal variant of human haemoglobin HbA characterized by the presence of carbohydrate irreversibly bonded to a beta chain. Whilst HbA constitute over 90 per cent of the haemoglobin of adults, glycosylation occurs within the red cell to form HbA_1, such that some 4–8 per cent of HbA is glycosylated in the non-diabetic patient and rises inversely with the degree of diabetic control in diabetic patients (Leslie *et al.* 1978). Should diabetic control improve during pregnancy, the percentage of HbA_1 falls. Several studies have suggested that the HbA_1 concentrations during the first trimester were greater in pregnancies in diabetic women complicated by congenital abnormality compared with those diabetic pregnancies without this complication (Shields *et al.* 1993; Stubbs *et al.* 1987; Ylinen *et al.* 1984).

Since glycosylated haemoglobin will give a retrospective measurement of diabetic control, it might be anticipated that there should be an association between raised levels of HbA_1 and fetal abnormality. Although this is true in general terms, no threshold for the concentration for HbA_1 may be found below which fetal abnormality will not occur. This is, in fact, a more logical situation since diabetes is a pan-metabolic disease and it is likely that 'tight diabetic control' during early pregnancy is required rather than specific control of. any one measurable substance (*Lancet* 1988).

Since organogenesis occurs during the first eight weeks of intrauterine life, interest has focused upon diabetic care prior to conception. The concept of tight diabetic control initiated at a pregnancy clinic has arisen (Goldman *et al*. 1986; Steel *et al*. 1982). Fuhrman *et al*. (1983) reported a congenital abnormality rate of 7.5 per cent in 292 diabetic patients with strict control after the eighth week of pregnancy compared with 0.8 per cent in 128 diabetic women seen for strict control prior to a planned pregnancy. Steel *et al*. (1990) reported 143 insulin-diabetic women who attended a prepregnancy clinic. Two (1.4 per cent) of these patients delivered an infant with a major congenital malformation compared with 10 per cent of 96 insulin-diabetic women who did not attend. Whilst it is possible that those who attended were also better motivated towards their diabetic control, it nevertheless seems that tight prepregnancy control will significantly reduce the incidence of fetal malformation.

It is likely, therefore, that prepregnancy management which results in tight diabetic control will significantly reduce the incidence of major fetal abnormality.

Obstetric management

Peel (1972) advised that pregnant diabetic women were best managed in specialist units, in order that expertise may be concentrated and liaison between an obstetrician and diabetic physician take place. In his unit, these principles resulted in a perinatal mortality rate of 252 per 1000 for 141 diabetic pregnancies compared with a perinatal mortality rate of 401 per 1000 for 458 diabetic pregnancies occurring in a survey of the United Kingdom teaching hospitals.

The basic obstetric management of the pregnant diabetic patient does not differ greatly from other pregnant patients other than at the two extremes of pregnancy.

The benefit of prepregnancy management in the reduction of fetal abnormalities has been discussed above, and there is evidence that attendance at a prepregnancy clinic, in order to achieve tighter control of the diabetes, will result in an improved obstetric outcome over and above the malformation rate. Steel *et al*. (1982, 1990) reported that the diabetic control throughout pregnancy in insulin-dependent diabetic women who attended the prepregnancy clinic prior to a planned pregnancy was superior to that of women who did not attend, but this may reflect the motivation and attitude of the patient rather than any other feature.

The increased incidence of fetal abnormality should be an indication for mid-trimester ultrasound screening for fetal anomaly, and Milunsky *et al*. (1982) reported a 10-fold increase in the frequency of neural tube defects in the fetuses of insulin-dependent diabetic patients. However, alphafetoprotein screening is of limited value in diabetic patients. Wald *et al.* (1979) reported that the mean AFP level amongst singleton pregnancies in insulin-dependent diabetics was 60 per cent that of controls without diabetes, matched for gestational age.

The fetus of a mother whose pregnancy is complicated by diabetes needs to be monitored. Regular clinical assessments of fetal growth should commence at the 26th week of pregnancy and be supplemented by bi-weekly ultrasound measurement and liquor assessment (Lagrew *et al.* 1993). Bi-weekly cardiotocography is recommended after the 35th week of pregnancy or earlier if there is any departure from normal growth rate, either too much or too little, or if there is diabetic vascular disease (Teramo *et al.* 1983). Some authors also advocate the use of formal biophysical profiles (Johnson *et al.* 1988; Salvesen *et al.* 1993), whilst the use of Doppler studies have been shown to be of limited value unless intrauterine growth retardation co-exists (Dicker *et al.* 1990; Landon *et al.* 1989). Despite such monitoring, late intrauterine death may be unexpected and has been blamed upon fetal hypoglycaemia, fetal hypergylcaemia, and fetal hypoxia.

Pre-eclampsia is only minimally increased in diabetic pregnancies, occurring in 14 per cent of established diabetic pregnancies and 12 per cent of pregnancies in patients with gestational diabetes (Brudenell 1989). However, this author also reported that pre-eclampsia is becoming less common in association with diabetes and that there is no increase in perinatal mortality due to the pre-eclampsia in such patients. However, this lack of mortality is not universal. Garner *et al.* (1990) reported a prospective study in which pre-eclampsia was diagnosed in 10 per cent of 334 diabetic pregnancies compared with 4 per cent of 16 534 non-diabetic ones. Despite similar maternal age, parity, and blood glucose control, the perinatal mortality rate was 60 per 1000 in 33 pre-eclamptic diabetic pregnancies, some 18 times higher that the 3.3 per 1000 in 301 normotensive diabetic pregnancies, suggesting that pre-eclampsia is still a potential cause of mortality (and hence morbidity) in these patients. The incidence of pre-eclampsia during diabetic pregnancy may be reduced by improved diabetic control throughout the pregnancy (Saddiqi *et al.* 1991) and may represent underlying incipient diabetic nephropathy (Combs *et al.* 1993).

Fetal macrosomia, defined as the occurrence of birthweight above the 90th centile for gestational age, occurred in 29 per cent of pregnancies in established diabetics and in 26 per cent in gestational diabetics (Beard and Lowy 1982). This complication is associated with birth trauma, shoulder dystocia, and a 4 per cent incidence of serious fetal morbidity (Erb's palsy, fracture of the humerus, or fracture of the clavicle). Fetal macrosomia appears to be related to an increase in the adipose tissue and, although it is associated with maternal hyperglycaemia and fetal hyperinsulinaemia, it may also occur in well-controlled diabetic women (Brudenell and Carr 1984; Milner and Hill 1984; Willman *et al.* 1986). Willman *et al.* (1986) reported 95 infants of diabetic mothers of whom 24 were macrosomic. Macrosomia occurred in 65 per cent of women whose peak third trimester blood glucose levels were in excess of 7.2 mmol/l compared with 27 per cent of those whose peak level was below this. This evidence, therefore,

Table 23.3 Perinatal mortality

Year	Perinatal deaths	Deaths due to fetal abnormality	Unexplained late deaths
1972–8 (n = 35)	2	2	0
1979–84 (n = 45)	3	1	1

From Murphy *et al.* (1984)

suggests that the quality of diabetic control is a major factor in the occurrence of fetal macrosomia.

A major dilemma in obstetric management relates to the timing of delivery. One of the major factors in perinatal mortality used to be unexplained stillbirth during the latter part of the third trimester. Thus, Peel (1972) advocated that all such infants should be delivered by the 36th week of pregnancy in order to avoid this complication, whilst Drury *et al.* (1983) analysed 22 intrauterine deaths occurring in 600 pregnancies to diabetic mothers and found eight unexplained intrauterine deaths after the 37th week of pregnancy. The concept of premature delivery, in order to avoid late unexplained intrauterine death, is no longer universally accepted, and there is a tendency to allow the diabetic pregnancy to be prolonged towards term, thus avoiding the risk of respiratory distress syndrome which was itself a potent cause of perinatal wastage. Coustan *et al.* (1980) allowed 73 patients with established diabetes to go as close as possible to the 40th week of pregnancy but associated with tight control of blood glucose levels. Some 51 per cent of patients delivered at or beyond the 38th week with a perinatal mortality rate, corrected for fetal abnormality, of 14 per 1000. Similarly, Murphy *et al.* (1984) reported no significant deterioration in their perinatal mortality rate between the periods 1972–1978 when 35 patients were delivered by the 38th week of pregnancy compared with 1979–1984 when 45 women were delivered by the 40th week. These results are shown in Table 23.3.

In a recent review of the evidence for the timing of delivery, Hunter (1989) concluded that 'there would seem little reason to terminate an otherwise uncomplicated pregnancy in a diabetic woman before term', although if the fetus is considered to be large, delivery before the 38th week may be indicated to avoid the incidence of shoulder dystocia (Kjos *et al.* 1993).

The infants of diabetic mothers are particularly prone to respiratory problems. Roberts *et al.* (1976) reported perinatal data on 805 such infants compared with 10 152 infants of non-diabetic mothers. Respiratory distress syndrome occurred in 24 per cent of the diabetic infants compared with 1.3 per cent in the non-diabetic group, with an increased risk at all gestational ages up to the 39th week. Although the precise mechanism of this predisposition is not understood, it is apparent that fetal hyperinsulinaemia can limit the production of surfactant (Stubbs and Stubbs 1978). Other authors have reported increased incidences of RDS, but not as high as those reported by Roberts *et al.* (Piper and Langer 1993) Lemons *et al.* (1981) reported an incidence of respiratory distress syndrome of 2.8 per cent, whilst Brudenell *et al.* (1976) reported an incidence of 2.3 per cent. Whether there really is a major increase in the incidence of respiratory distress syndrome is confused by several factors, including the premature delivery of the infants of diabetic mothers, the increased incidence of Caesarean section with its increase in neonatal respiratory morbidity, and the increase in polyhydramnios with resultant retained lung liquid causing transient tachypnoea of the newborn.

Whilst the estimation of fetal lung maturity by the lecithin–sphingomyelin ratio may predict RDS or indicate the need for corticosteroids, this estimation is now rarely performed as it no longer has a significant influence upon management, partly as a result of improved neonatal care and partly because the lecithin–sphingomyelin ratio, suggesting mature lungs in the infant of a non-diabetic mother, may still be associated with an incidence of RDS in the infant of a diabetic one, a false-positive rate in the region of 3 per cent being quoted (Tchobroutsky *et al.* 1978; Kitzmiller *et al.* 1978).

The mode of delivery

There is general agreement that the Caesarean section rate in pregnant diabetic patients should exceed that in the general population. Drury *et al.* (1986) reported a Caesarean section rate of 26 per cent, whilst most other authors report a Caesarean section rate of 50 per cent (Brudenell 1989). The major indications for Caesarean section are fetal distress and cephalopelvic disproportion.

Over the last decade, there has been a trend towards a slight decrease in the incidence of Caesarean section and this relates primarily to a reduction in the incidence of elective procedures. Between 1971 and 1978, 34 per cent of patients underwent an elective Caesarean section, whereas between 1981 and 1985 this figure was 24 per cent (Brudenell 1989). Similarly, Murphy *et al.* (1984) reported that the overall Caesarean section rate between 1973 and 1978 was 35 per cent but between 1979 and 1982 it was 25 per cent.

In the absence of other obstetric complications, the main danger of vaginal delivery in these patients relates to birth trauma, particularly brachial plexus injury secondary to shoulder dystocia and macrosomia (Hunter 1989). The diagnosis of a macrosomic infant in a diabetic mother may, therefore, be an indication for Caesarean section.

Fetal distress is observed more commonly during labour in the presence of diabetes than would otherwise be expected. The incidence of fetal distress, based on either cardiotocography or a scalp pH of less than 7.26, was reported in 17 per cent of insulin-dependent diabetic labours compared with 11 per cent of matched controls. The same authors reported a Caesarean section rate for fetal distress of 13 per cent in the diabetic patients compared with zero in the controls, and an incidence of an Apgar score of less than seven at five minutes in 2 per cent of the infants of diabetic mothers compared with 0 per cent in the controls (Olofsson *et al.* 1986). Brudenell (1978) reported an overall incidence of fetal distress of 25 per cent for diabetic pregnancies or 33.3 per cent in all induced or spontaneous diabetic labours. Such labours should, therefore, involve continuous electronic fetal heart monitoring.

The infants of diabetic mothers

The major problems of fetal malformation, macrosomia, and respiratory distress syndrome have already been discussed. Hypoglycaemia as a result of fetal hyperinsulinaemia is well recognized in the early neonatal period. Lemons *et al.* (1981) reported that hypoglycaemia occurred in 47 per cent of macrosomic infants and in 21 per cent of normal birthweight infants of 225 diabetic mothers. Kitzmiller *et al.* (1978) found hypoglycaemia in 22 per cent of 147 infants of diabetic mothers. There is also an increased incidence of birth trauma, polycythaemia (probably related to fetal hyperinsulinaemia), and jaundice (related to neonatal polycythaemia).

There is an increased risk that such infants will themselves become diabetic. Thus Persson (1986) reported that 3 per cent of 73 such infants had been diagnosed as diabetic in the first ten years of life. Infants born to mothers with impaired glucose tolerance in gestational diabetes are also at greater risk of developing glucose intolerance, and there is some evidence to suggest that this may be associated with poor maternal diabetic control rather than genetic factors or the relationship with obesity (Pettitt *et al.* 1985).

Diabetes and spontaneous abortion

There is debate as to whether spontaneous abortion occurs more commonly in diabetic mothers. Miodovnik *et al.* (1984) reported a prospective study of spontaneous abortion in insulin-dependent diabetics evaluated prior to pregnancy. Spontaneous abortion occurred in 30 per cent of 132 pregnancies, 87 per cent of these occurring in the first trimester. The more severe the diabetes, the greater the risk of abortion. Wright *et al.* (1983) reported 58 consecutive pregnancies in insulin-dependent diabetic women in whom glycosylated haemoglobin levels were abnormally high in 78 per cent at the time of booking. The mean glycosylated haemoglobin level in the 15 patients who aborted were statistically significantly higher than the mean in 43 patients who did not.

However, Kalter (1987) reviewed some 58 studies from the literature, involving 8041 pregnancies, and concluded that the spontaneous abortion rate of 10 per cent was not different from the overall population, but rather that some studies with an excess abortion might have been methologically unsound since the quoted incidences of abortion range from 3.8 to 28 per cent. Mills *et al.* (1988*b*) recruited 386 insulin-dependent diabetic women and 432 women without diabetes within 21 days of conception and followed both groups. Spontaneous abortion occurred in 16.1 per cent of cases and 16.2 per cent of the controls, demonstrating that diabetic women as a group do not have an increased risk of abortion. However, in the subgroup of women with poorly controlled diabetes, as evidenced by a raised glycosylated haemoglobin level, the risk of spontaneous abortion rose in an approximately linear fashion with increasing levels of glycosylated haemoglobin.

It would seem that good prepregnancy and early pregnancy diabetic control reduces the likelihood of spontaneous abortion (Miodovnik *et al.* 1990).

The management of the diabetes

Perhaps the most important single principle in managing the diabetes of a pregnant diabetic patient is the close liaison between the obstetrician and the diabetic physician. Although some dietary advice with restriction on calorie intake is appropriate, it is only in a small minority of patients that diet alone will be sufficient to maintain blood glucose at the required concentrations. Moreover, poor dietary habits should be corrected (Vaughan 1987).

There is evidence that even patients with gestational diabetes may require insulin in addition to dietary restriction during pregnancy. Recent randomized trials have demonstrated that blood glucose concentrations were better controlled by insulin and diet than by diet alone, although the incidence of macrosomia was similar in both groups (Maresh *et al.* 1985; Persson *et al.* 1985).

Insulin is traditionally given to pregnant women on a minimum of two occasions per day, generally using a mixture of short- and medium-acting insulins. Insulin is administered some 30 minutes before the main morning and evening meal. There are recent trends towards the use of non-antigenic insulin preparations and towards the use of 'pen' regimes in which patients administer three doses of short-acting insulin immediately prior to meals and one dose of long-acting insulin, usually at night. Such a regime allows for greater flexibility with regard to diet.

The two major points of interest relate to the level of blood glucose which is required and the place where such monitoring should occur.

Many authors have advocated the principle of tight control of maternal diabetes, advocating that the fasting blood glucose should always be below 5.5 mmol/l whilst post-prandial blood glucose should remain below 6.6 mmol/l (Coustan *et al.* 1980; Karlsson and Kjellner 1972; Thompson *et al.* 1994). These latter authors demonstrated a close relationship between the mean blood glucose concentrations during the last two weeks prior to delivery in 179 diabetic pregnant women and the perinatal mortality rate, as shown in Table 23.4.

In practical terms, control is assessed by means of blood glucose profiles estimated either at regular intervals or before and after a standard meal (Hadden 1991). The benefit of this tight control has been demonstrated by Farrag (1987) who allocated (but not randomly) 60 insulin-dependent diabetic

Table 23.4 Tight blood glucose control

Mean blood sugar level (mmol/l)	Perinatal mortality rate (per 1000)
Greater than 8.3	236
5.5–8.3	153
Less than 5.5	38

From Karlsson and Kjellner (1972)

Table 23.5 Tight blood glucose control

	Blood glucose levels		
	less than 5.6 mmol/l	5.6–6.7 mmol/l	6.7–8.9 mmol/l
No.	16	29	15
Maternal hypoglycaemia	7	0	0
Maternal hypertension of any cause	1	1	6
RDS	1	2	6
Caesarean section	2	3	6
Mean birthweight (kg)	3.2	3.3	4.25
Macrosomia	0	0	13
Perinatal death	0	0	2

From Farrag (1987)

women to one of three regimens. As can be seen from Table 23.5, the tighter the blood glucose control, the lower the incidence of obstetric complications, although the higher the incidence of maternal hypoglycaemic episodes.

Third-trimester measurement of HbA_1c may also be used as a guide to tight diabetic control. Ylinen *et al.* (1981) reported 526 HbA_1c estimations in 112 insulin-dependent diabetics. In the six pregnancies which terminated in a perinatal death, the mean HbA_1c levels were significantly higher than the rest of the group, suggesting that metabolic derangement is associated with a poor outcome.

Such tight diabetic control is no longer considered to require universal in-patient management and many patients can achieve good control at home by repeated monitoring using a glucose meter.

Stubbs *et al.* (1980) allocated 13 insulin-dependent diabetic women to either home self-monitoring of capillary blood glucose, using a meter on seven occasions per day, twice per week ($n = 7$), whilst others ($n = 6$) tested urine four times every day and underwent random blood glucose checks at a weekly or fortnightly hospital clinic. Although all patients spent some time in hospital being monitored as an in-patient, there was no real difference between the quality of diabetic control achieved either at home or in hospital, or using a meter or not using a meter. Peacock *et al.* (1979) demonstrated that glucose control at home was superior to that in hospital in 25 diabetics (24 taking insulin) undergoing 4247 observations of their blood glucose levels based on the use of a glucose meter for capillary blood sampling. Other authors have demonstrated the safety of home monitoring (Goldberg *et al.* 1986). However, some patients, by virtue of their motivation, intellect, or difficulty in controlling their diabetes, will need admission to hospital (occasionally prolonged).

The management of the insulin-dependent diabetic woman during labour is best achieved using a continuous insulin infusion pump balanced by a continuous glucose intravenous infusion to maintain the blood glucose concentration at between 3.9 and 6.0 mmol/l (Hadden 1991; Jovanovic and Peterson 1983). These authors reported that insulin requirements varied throughout labour, being minimal during the active phase of labour and increasing during the late first stage and second stage. Immediately after delivery, the insulin requirement falls to prepregnancy levels.

The twin complications of diabetic retinopathy and diabetic nephropathy may worsen during pregnancy. Diabetic proliferative retinopathy is a progressive vascular lesion associated with blindness and generally related to the duration of the diabetes. Pregnancy is itself a risk factor for deteriorating diabetic retinopathy, the relative risk of this complication progressing being 2.3 times that of the non-pregnant woman (Klein *et al.* 1990). Moloney and Drury (1982) reported a prospective study involving repeated retinal examinations throughout pregnancy in 53 insulin-dependent diabetic women and 39 non-pregnant diabetic controls. Of the controls 46.2 per cent already had some degree of retinopathy but none progressed during the 15 months of the study. Of the 53 pregnant diabetics, 62 per cent had retinopathy at the first examination but a further 15 per cent developed this complication during the pregnancy. Over half of the pregnant diabetics showed some progression of their retinopathy during the pregnancy, although this regressed by six months after delivery. Progressive retinopathy may be treated with argon laser photocoagulation during pregnancy (Elman *et al.* 1990).

Diabetic nephropathy is a chronic condition which may deteriorate during pregnancy. Grenfell *et al.* (1986) reported 22 pregnancies in 20 insulin-dependent diabetic women with proteinuria noted in, or before, the first trimester, out of 396 diabetic pregnancies (5.6 per cent). The 20 women delivered 23 liveborn infants including one with a non-fatal congenital malformation. Four of these patients developed end-stage renal failure at a range of six months to ten years after the pregnancy, suggesting the need for counselling about parenthood in this group of patients.

Contraception

Whilst no method of contraception is absolutely contraindicated for the diabetic woman, certain reservations are appropriate concerning both IUCDs and oestrogen-containing oral contraception.

It had been suggested that there was a higher than expected pregnancy rate in diabetic women using an IUCD (Gosden *et al.* 1982). However, larger and more recent studies have demonstrated that the accidental pregnancy rate in diabetic women using a copper-containing IUCD was similar to that in non-diabetic controls (Mestman and Schmidt-Sarosi 1993; Skouby *et al.* 1984, 1991).

Both oral contraceptives and diabetes are risk factors for myocardial infarction and cerebral ischaemia in young women. Moreover, the pharmacological properties and the concentration of the hormonal constituents in combined oral contraceptives are of fundamental significance for the development of adverse metabolic effects. This has resulted in some caution in prescribing combined oral contraception to women with previous gestational diabetes or current insulin-dependent diabetes.

The newer low-dose oestrogen and progestogen pills have little or no effect on carbohydrate metabolism in healthy women (Mestman and Schmidt-Sarosi 1993; Van der Vange *et al.* 1987). Furthermore, Kjos *et al.* (1990) were unable to find any differences in glucose tolerance testing in 156 women with recent gestational diabetes regardless of their use of hormonal or non-hormonal contraception. It would seem that low-dose combined oral contraception may be administered without running the risk of inducing glucose intolerance, although the long-term effects in patients with a past history of gestational diabetes are not yet available (Skouby *et al.* 1991).

In insulin-dependent diabetic women, combined oral contraception may be administered in the short term, although 19 per cent of such patients have an increased insulin requirement (Steel and Duncan 1980). These authors advised the cessation of oral contraception as soon as the family was completed, presumably giving serious consideration to either female or male sterilization.

In well-motivated patients, barrier methods of contraception may prove both acceptable and reliable.

Conclusions

Huge improvements have been made in the third quarter of this century in the management of the pregnant diabetic patient. The major factors in the reduction of perinatal mortality relate to the joint management between obstetrician and diabetologist, tight control of diabetes, and prepregnancy counselling.

References

Amankwah, K. S., Prentice, R. L., and Fleury, F. J. (1977). The incidence of gestational diabetes. *Obstetrics and Gynecology* **49**, 7–8.

Beard, R. W. and Lowy, C. (1982). The British Survey of diabetic pregnancies. *British Journal of Obstetrics and Gynaecology* **89**, 783–6.

Brudenell, J. M. (1978). Delivering the baby of the diabetic mother. *Journal of the Royal Society of Medicine* **71**, 207–11.

Brudenell, J. M. (1989). Diabetic pregnancy. In *Obstetrics* (ed. A. Turnbull and G. Chamberlain), pp. 585–603. Churchill Livingstone, Edinburgh.

Brudenell, J. M. and Carr, J. (1984). Conservative management of pregnancy in diabetic women. *British Medical Journal* **288**, 195.

Brudenell, M. and Doddridge, M. C. (1989a). *Diabetic pregnancy*, p. 56. Churchill Livingstone, Edinburgh.

Brudenell, M. and Doddridge, M. C. (1986b). *Diabetic pregnancy*, pp. 90–8. Churchill Livingstone, Edinburgh.

Brudenell, J. M., Gamsu, H. R., and Roberts, A. B. (1976). Fetal lung maturity in diabetic pregnancy. *British Journal of Obstetrics and Gynaecology* **87**, 638–41.

Combs, C. A., Rosenn, B., Kitzmiller, J. L., Khoury, J. C., Wheeler, B. C., and Miodovnik, M. (1993). Early pregnancy proteinuria and diabetes related to pre-eclampsia. *Obstetrics and Gynecology* **82**, 802–7.

Cousins, L., Dattel, B. J., Hollingworth, D. R., and Zettner, A. (1984). Glycosylated haemoglobin as a screening test for carbohydrate intolerance in pregnancy. *American Journal of Obstetrics and Gynecology* **150**, 455–60.

Coustan, D. R. (1991). Screening and diagnosis. *Ballière's Clinical Obstetrics and Gynaecology* **5**, 293–313.

Coustan, D. R. and Imarah, J. (1984). Prophylactic insulin treatment of gestational diabetes reduces the incidence of macrosomia, operative delivery and birth trauma. *American Journal of Obstetrics and Gynecology* **150**, 836–42.

Coustan, D. R., Berkowitz, R. L., and Hobbins, J. C. (1980). Tight metabolic control of overt diabetes in pregnancy. *American Journal of Medicine* **68**, 845–52.

Coustan, D. R., Nelson, C., Carpenter, M. W., Carr, S. R., Rotondo, L., and Widness, J. (1989). Maternal age and screening for gestation diabetes. *Obstetrics and Gynecology* **73**, 557–61.

Damm, P. and Molsted-Pedersen, L. (1989). Significant decrease in congenital malformation in newborn infant of an unselected population of diabetic women. *American Journal of Obstetrics and Gynecology* **161**, 1163–7.

De Swiet, M. (1991). Blood pressure measurement in pregnancy. *British Journal of Obstetrics and Gynaecology* **98**, 239–40.

Dicker, D., Goldman, J. A., Yeshaya, A., and Peleg, D. (1990). Umbilical artery velocimetry in insulin dependent diabetes mellitus in pregnancies. *Journal of Reproductive Medicine* **18**, 391–5.

Dornhorst, A. (1994). Implications of gestational diabetes for the health of the mother. *British Journal of Obstetrics and Gynaecology* **101**, 286–90.

Drury, M. I. (1986). Management of the pregnant diabetic patient. *Diabetologia* **29**, 10–12.

Drury, M. I., Stronge, J. M., Foley, M. E., and MacDonald, D. W. (1983). Pregnancy in the diabetic patient: timing and mode of delivery. *Obstetrics and Gynecology* **62**, 279–82.

Elman, K. D., Welch, R. A., Franks, R. N., Goyert, G. L., and Sokol, R. J. (1990). Diabetic retinopathy in pregnancy. *Obstetrics and Gynecology* **75**, 119-27.

Farrag, O. A. M. (1987). Prospective study of three metabolic regimens in pregnant diabetics. *Australian and New Zealand Journal of Obstetrics and Gynaecology* **27**, 6-9.

Fuhrman, K., Reiher, Hl, Senner, K., Fischer, F., Fischer, M., and Glockner, E. (1983). Prevention of congenital malformation in infants of insulin-dependent diabetic mothers. *Diabetes Care* **6**, 219-23.

Garner, P. R., D'Alton, M. E., Dudley, D. K., Huard, P., and Hardie, N. (1990). Pre-eclampsia in diabetic pregnancy. *American Journal of Obstetrics and Gynecology* **163**, 505-8.

Gillmer, M. D. G., Oakley, N. W., Beard, W., Nithyananthan, R., and Cawston, M. (1980). Screening for diabetes during pregnancy, *British Journal of Obstetrics and Gynaecology* **87**, 377-82.

Goldberg, J. D., Franklin, B., Lasser, D., Jornsay, D. L., Hawsknecht, R. U., Ginsberg-Fellner, F., *et al.* (1986). Gestational diabetes: effect of home glucose monitoring on neonatal birthweight. *American Journal of Obstetrics and Gynecology* **154**, 546-50.

Goldman, J. A., Dicker, D., Feldberg, D., Yeshaya, A., Samuel, N., and Karp, M. (1986). Pregnancy outcome in patients with insulin-dependent diabetes with pre-conceptual diabetic control. *American Journal of Obstetrics and Gynecology* **155**, 293-7.

Gosden, C., Steel, J., Ross, R., and Springbett, A. (1982). Intrauterine contraceptive devices in diabetic women. *Lancet* **i**, 530-4.

Grant., P. T., Oates, J. N., and Beischer, N. A. (1986). The long-term follow-up of women with gestational diabetes. *Australian and New Zealand Journal of Obstetrics and Gynaecology* **26**, 17-22.

Grenfell, A., Brudenell, J. M., Doddridge, M. C., and Watkins, P. J. (1986). Pregnant diabetic women who have proteinuria. *Quarterly Journal of Medicine* **59**, 379-86.

Hadden, D. R. (1991). Medical management of diabetes in pregnancy. *Ballière's Clinical Obstetrics and Gynaecology* **5**, 369-94.

Harlass, R. E., Brady, A. K., and Read, J. A. (1991). Reproducibility of the oral glucose tolerance test in pregnancy. *American Journal of Obstetrics and Gynecology* **164**, 564-8.

Hunter, D. J. S. (1989). Diabetes in pregnancy. In *Effective care in pregnancy and childbirth* (ed I. Chalmers, M. Enkin, and M. J. C. Keirse), pp. 578-93. Oxford University Press, Oxford.

Johnson, J. M., Lange, I. R., Harman, C. R., Torchin, M. G., and Manning, F. A. (1988). Biophysical profile screening in the management of the diabetic pregnancy. *Obstetrics and Gynecology* **72**, 841-6.

Jovanovic, L. and Peterson, C. M. (1983). Insulin and glucose requirements during the first stage of labour in insulin-dependent diabetic women. *American Journal of Medicine* **75**, 607-12.

Jowett, N. I., Samanta, A. K., and Burden, A. C. (1987). Screening for diabetes in pregnancy. *Diabetic Medicine* **4**, 160-3.

Kalter, H. (1987). Diabetes and spontaneous abortion. *American Journal of Obstetrics and Gynecology* **156**, 1243-53.

Karlsson, K. and Kjellner, I. (1972). The outcome of diabetic pregnancies in relation to the mother's blood sugar level. *American Journal of Obstetrics and Gynecology* **111**, 213-20.

Keen, H., Jarrett, R. J., and Alberti, K. G. M. M. (1979). Diabetes mellitus: a new look at diagnostic criteria. *Diabetologica* **16**, 283-5.

Kitzmiller, J. L., Cloherty, J. P., Younger, M. D., Tabatabaii, A., Rothchild, S. B., Sosenko, I., *et al.* (1978). Diabetic pregnancy and perinatal mortality. *American Journal of Obstetrics and Gynecology* 131, 560–80.

Kjos, S. L., Shoupe, D., Douyan, S., Friedman, R. L., Bernstein, G. S., Mestman, J. H., *et al.* (1990). Effect of low-dose oral contraceptives on carbohydrate and lipid metabolism in women with recent gestational diabetes. *American Journal of Obstetrics and Gynecology* 163, 1822–7.

Kjos, S. L., Henry, O. A., Montero, M., Buchanan, T. A., and Mestman, J. H. (1993). Insulin-requiring diabetes in pregnancy. *American Journal of Obstetrics and Gynecology* 169, 611–15.

Klein, B. E. K., Moss, S. E., and Klein, R. (1990). Effect of pregnancy on progression of diabetic retinopathy. *Diabetes Care* 13, 34–40.

Kriss, J. P. and Futcher, P. H. (1948). The relationship between infant birthweight and subsequent development of maternal diabetes mellitus. *Journal of Clinical Endocrinology* 8, 380–9.

Kuhl, C. (1991). Aetiology of gestational diabetes. *Ballière's Clinical Obstetrics and Gynaecology* 5, 279–92.

Lagrew, D. C., Pircon, R. A., Towers, C. V., Dorchester, W., and Freeman, R. K. (1993). Ante-natal fetal surveillance in patients with diabetes. *American Journal of Obstetrics and Gynecology* 168, 1820–6.

Lancet (1988). Congenital abnormalities in infants of diabetic mothers. *Lancet* i, 1313–15.

Landon, M. B., Gabbe, S. G., Bruner, J. P., and Ludmir, J. (1989). Doppler umbilical artery velocimetry in pregnancy complicated by insulin dependent diabetes mellitus. *Obstetrics and Gynecology* 73, 961–5.

Lemons, J. A., Varga, P., and Delaney, J. J. (1981). Infant of the diabetic mother: a review of 225 cases. *Obstetrics and Gynecology* 57, 187–92.

Leslie, R. D. G., Pyke, D. A., John, P. N., and White, J. N. (1978). Haemoglobin A1 in diabetic pregnancy. *Lancet* ii, 958–9.

Lind, T. and Anderson, J. (1984). Does random blood glucose sampling outdate testing for glycosuria in the detection of diabetes during pregnancy? *British Medical Journal* 289, 1569–71.

Lind, T. and Hytten, S. E. (1972). The excretion of glucose during normal pregnancy. *Journal of Obstetrics and Gynaecology of the British Commonwealth* 79, 961–5.

Maresh, M., Gillmer, M. D. G., Beard, R. W., Alderson, G. S., Bloxham, B. A., and Elkeles, R. S. (1985). The effect of diet and insulin on metabolic profiles of women with gestational diabetes mellitus. *Diabetes* 34, Supp. 2. 88–93.

Maresh, N., Beard, R. W., Bray, C. S., Elkles, R. S., and Wadsworth, J. (1989). Factors predisposing to an outcome of gestational diabetes. *Obstetrics and Gynecology* 74, 342–6.

Merkatz, I. R., Duchon, N. A., Yamashita, J. S., and Hooser, H. B. (1980). A pilot community based screening programme for gestational diabetes. *Diabetic Care* 3, 453–7.

Mestman, J. H. (1988). Follow-up studies in women with gestational diabetes. In *Gestational diabetes* (ed. P. A. M. Weiss and D. R. Coustan), pp. 191–8. Springer, Vienna.

Mestman, J. H. and Schmidt-Sarosi, C. (1993). Diabetes mellitus and fertility control. *American Journal of Obstetrics and Gynecology* 168, 2012–20.

Mills, J. L. Knopp R. H., Simpson, J. L., Juvanovic-Peterson, L., Metzger, B. E., Holmesc, B., *et al.* (1988a). Lack of relation of increase malformation rate in infants of diabetic mothers to glycaemic control during organogenesis. *New England Journal of Medicine* 318, 671–6.

Mills, J. L., Simpson, J. L., Driscoll, S. G., Juvanovic-Peterson, L., Allen, M. V., Aarons, J., *et al.* (1988*b*). Incidence of spontaneous abortion among normal women and insulin-dependent diabetic women whose pregnancies were identified within 21 days of conception. *New England Journal of Medicine* **319**, 1617–23.

Milner, R. D. and Hill, D. J. (1984). Fetal growth control: the role of insulin and related peptides. *Clinical Endocrinology* **21**, 315–33.

Milunsky, A., Alpert, E., Kitzmiller, J. L., Younger, M. D., and Neff, R. K. (1982). Prenatal diagnosis of neural tube defects. *American Journal of Obstetrics and Gynecology* **142**, 1030–2.

Miodovnik, N., Lavin, J. P., Knowles, H. C., Holroyde, J., and Stys, S. J. (1984). Spontaneous abortion amongst insulin-dependent diabetic women. *American Journal of Obstetrics and Gynecology* **150**, 372–6.

Miodovnik, N., Mimouni, F., Saddiqi, T., Khoury, J., and Berk, M. A. (1990). Spontaneous abortion in repeat diabetic pregnancies. *Obstetrics and Gynecology* **75**, 75–8.

Moloney, J. B. M. and Drury, M. I. (1982). The effect of pregnancy on the natural outcome of diabetic retinopathy. *American Journal of Ophthalmology* **93**, 745–56.

Morris, M. A., Grandis, A. S., and Litton, J. (1986). Glycosylated haemoglobin. *Obstetrics and Gynecology* **68**, 357–61.

Murphy, J. A., Peters, J., Morris, P., Hayes, T. M., and Pearson, J. F. (1984). Conservative management of pregnant diabetic women. *British Medical Journal* **288**, 1203–5.

National Diabetes Data Group (1979). Classification and diagnosis of diabetes mellitus and other categories of glucose tolerance. *Diabetes* **28**, 1039–57.

Olofsson, P., Ingermarsson, I., and Solum, T. (1986). Fetal distress during labour in diabetic pregnancies. *British Journal of Obstetrics and Gynaecology* **93**, 1067–71.

O'Sullivan, J. B. and Mahan, C. (1980). Diabetes subsequent to the birth of a large baby. *Journal of Chronic Diseases* **33**, 37–45.

Peacock, I., Hunter, J. C., Walford, S., Allison, S. P., Davison, J., Clarke, P., *et al.* (1979). Self-monitoring of blood glucose in diabetic pregnancy. *British Medical Journal* **2**, 1333–6.

Peel, J. (1972). A historical review of diabetes and pregnancy. *Journal of Obstetrics and Gynaecology of the British Commonwealth* **79**, 385–95.

Persson, B. (1986). Long-term morbidity in the offspring of diabetic mothers. *Acta Endocrinologica* **Supp. 277**, 150–5.

Persson, B., Stangenberg, B., Hansson, B., and Nordlander, E. (1985). Gestational diabetes mellitus. *Diabetes* **34**, Supp. 2, 101–5.

Pettitt, D. J., Knowler, W. C., Baird, H. R., and Bennett, P. H. (1980). Gestational diabetes. *Diabetes Care* **3**, 458–64.

Pettitt, D. J., Bennett, P. H., Knowler, W. C., Baird, H. R., and Aleck, K. A. (1985). Gestational diabetes mellitus and impaired glucose tolerance during pregnancy. *Diabetes* **34**, Supp. 2, 119–22.

Philipson, E. H. and Super, D. M. (1989). Gestational diabetes mellitus: does it recur? *American Journal of Obstetrics and Gynecology* **160**, 1324–31.

Piper, J. M. and Langer, O. (1993). Does maternal diabetes delay fetal pulmonary maturity? *American Journal of Obstetrics and Gynecology* **168**, 783–6.

Pyke, D. A. (1968). Aetiological factors. In *Clinical diabetes* (ed. W. G. Oakley, D. A. Pyke, and K. W. Taylor), pp. 210–51. Blackwell Scientific Publications, Oxford.

Roberts, M. F., Neff, R. K., Hubbell, J. P., Taeusch, H. W., and Avery, M. E. (1976). Relationship between maternal diabetes and the respiratory distress syndrome in the newborn. *New England Journal of Medicine* **294**, 357–60.

Rosenn, B., Miodovnik, N., Dignan, P. S. J., Saddiqi, T., Khoury, J., and Mimouni, F. (1990). Minor congenital malformation in the infants of insulin-dependent diabetic women. *Obstetrics and Gynecology* **76**, 745-9.

Saddiqi, T., Rosenn, B., Mimouni, F., Khoury, J., and Miodovnik, N. (1991). Hypertension during pregnancy in insulin-dependent diabetic women. *Obstetrics and Gynecology* **77**, 514-19.

Salvesan, D. R., Freeman, J., Brudenell, J. M., and Nicolaides, K. H. (1993). Prediction of fetal acidaemia in pregnancies complicated by maternal diabetes mellitus. *British Journal of Obstetrics and Gynaecology* **100**, 227-33.

Sepe, S. J., Connell, F. A., Geiss, L. S., and Teutsch, S. M. (1985). Gestational diabetes. *Diabetes* **34**, Supp. 2, 13-16.

Shields, L. E., Gan, E. A., Murphy, H. F., Sahn, D. J., and Moore, T. R. (1993). The prognostic value of haemoglobin A_1C in predicting fetal heart disease in diabetic pregnancies. *Obstetrics and Gynecology* **81**, 954-7.

Skouby, S. O., Molsted-Pedersen, L., and Kosonen, A. (1984). Consequences of intrauterine contraception in diabetic women. *Fertility Sterility* **42**, 568-73.

Skouby, S. O., Molsted-Pedersen, L., and Petersen, K. R. (1991). Contraception for women with diabetes. *Clinical Obstetrics and Gynaecology* **5**, 493-503.

Steel, J. M. and Duncan, L. J. P. (1980). Contraception for the insulin-dependent diabetic women. *Diabetes Care* **3**, 557-60.

Steel, J. M., Johnstone, F. D., Smith, A. F., and Duncan, L. J. P. (1982). Five years' experience of a prepregnancy clinic for insulin-dependent diabetes. *British Medical Journal* **285**, 353-6.

Steel, J. M., Johnstone, F. D., Hepburn, D. A., and Smith, A. F. (1990). Can prepregnancy care of diabetic women reduce the risk of abnormal babies? *British Medical Journal* **301**, 1070-4.

Stubbs, W. A. and Stubbs, S. M. (1978). Hyperinsulinism, diabetes mellitus, and respiratory distress syndrome of the newborn: a common link? *Lancet* **i**, 308-9.

Stubbs, S. M., Brudenell, J. M., Pyke, D. A., Watkins, P. J., Stubbs, W. A., and Alberti, K. G. M. M. (1980). Management of the pregnant diabetic: home or hospital, with or without glucose meters? *Lancet* **ii**, 1122-4.

Stubbs, S. M., Doddridge, M. C., John, P. M., Steel, J. M., and Wright, A. D. (1987). Haemoglobin A_1c and congenital malformation. *Diabetic Medicine* **4**, 156-9.

Sutherland, H. W., Stowers, J. M., and McKenzie, C. (1970). Simplifying the clinical problem of glycosuria in pregnancy. *Lancet* **i**, 69-71.

Tchobroutsky, C., Amiel-Tison, C., Cedard, L., Eshwege, E., Rouvillois, J. L., and Tchobroutsky, G. (1978). The lecithin–sphingomyelin ratio in insulin-dependent pregnancy. *American Journal of Obstetrics and Gynecology* **130**, 754-60.

Teramo, K., Ammala, P., Ylinen, K., and Raivic, K. O. (1983). Pathologic fetal heart rate associated with poor metabolic control in diabetic pregnancy. *Obstetrics and Gynecology* **61**, 559-65.

Thompson, D. J., Porter, K. B., Gunnells, D. J., Wagner, P. C., and Spinnato, J. A. (1990). Prophylactic insulin in the management of gestational diabetes. *Obstetrics and Gynecology* **75**, 960-4.

Thompson, D. M., Dansereau, J., Creed, M., and Ridell, L. (1994). Tight glucose control results in normal peri-natal outcome. *Obstetrics and Gynecology* **83**, 362-6.

Tillil, H. and Kobberling, J. (1987). Age-correlated empirical genetic risk estimates for first degree relatives of insulin-dependent diabetic patients. *Diabetes* **36**, 93-9.

Van der Vange, N., Kloosterboer, H. J., and Haspels, A. (1987). Effect of seven low-dose combined oral contraceptive preparations on carbohydrate metabolism. *American Journal of Obstetrics and Gynecology* **156**, 918-22.

Vaughan, N. J. A. (1987). Treatment of diabetes in pregnancy. *British Medical Journal* **294**, 558-60.

Wald, N. J., Cuckle, H., Boreham, J., Stirrat, G. M., and Turnbull, A. C. (1979). Maternal serum alpha-fetoprotein and diabetes mellitus. *British Journal of Obstetrics and Gynaecology* **86**, 101-5.

Widness, J. A., Cowett, R. M., Coustan, D. R., Carpenter, M. W., and Oh, W. (1985). Neonatal morbidity in infants of mothers with glucose intolerance in pregnancy. *Diabetes* **34**, (Supp. 2), 61-5.

Willman, S. P., Leveno, K. J., Guzick, D. S., Williams, M. L., and Whalley, P. J. (1986). Glucose threshold for macrosomia in pregnancy complicated by diabetes. *American Journal of Obstetrics and Gynecology* **154**, 470-5.

World Health Organization (1980). Expert Committee on Diabetes Mellitus. Second report. *World Health Organization Technical Report Series* **646**, Geneva.

Wright, A. D., Nicholson, H. O., Pollock, A., Taylor, K. G., and Betts, S. (1983). Spontaneous abortion and diabetes mellitus. *Postgraduate Medical Journal* **59**, 295-8.

Ylinen, K., Raivio, K., and Teramo, K. (1981). Haemoglobin A_1c predicts the perinatal outcome in insulin-dependent diabetic pregnancy. *British Journal of Obstetrics and Gynaecology* **88**, 961-7.

Ylinen, K., Aula, P., Stenman, U. A., Kesaniemi-Kuokhanen, T., and Teramo, K. (1984). Risk of minor and major fetal malformation in diabetes with high haemoglobin A_1c values in early pregnancy. *British Medical Journal* **289**, 345-6.

24 Pre-eclampsia

This chapter deals with difficulties and dilemmas in the managements of hypertension during pregnancy, with special emphasis on hypertension commencing during, and not prior to, pregnancy. There is no single term which is used universally in the literature and many names for this disease process, therefore, exist, although they are not always entirely synonymous. Such terms include pre-eclampsia, pre-eclamptic toxaemia, pregnancy-related hypertension, pregnancy-induced hypertension, hypertensive disease of pregnancy, gestosis, and EPH gestosis (Oedema–Proteinuira–Hypertension). The one term which should probably be avoided is toxaemia, in that there is no convincing evidence for the existence of a circulating toxin. There have been several attempts made to define pre-eclampsia, largely in order that it may be distinguished from other causes of hypertension, of which mild chronic hypertension would be the commonest. There have been three definitions which are particularly worthy of note. Nelson (1955) divided hypertension diagnosed for the first time during pregnancy into mild pre-eclampsia and proteinuric hypertension (or severe pre-eclampsia). Davey and MacGillivray (1988) redefined pre-eclampsia as gestational proteinuric hypertension, whilst hypertension itself was defined as a diastolic blood pressure of equal to or greater than 90 mmHg on two or more occasions at least four hours apart, or a single measurement of a diastolic blood pressure equal to or greater than 110 mmHg. Redman and Jefferies (1988) defined pre-eclampsia as a first diastolic blood pressure of less than 90 mmHg, a subsequent rise of at least 25 mmHg, and a maximum reading of at least 90 mmHg, but proteinuria was not mandatory for the definition.

Of all these definitions, the one finding current favour is that of Davey and MacGillivray (1988), in that mild chronic hypertension would be excluded and special emphasis placed on proteinuric hypertension. Using such a definition, pre-eclampsia would be found in 4.8 per cent of all pregnancies, 6.1 per cent of first pregnancies, and 1.9 per cent of second pregnancies (Campbell et al. 1985).

The importance of pre-eclampsia is that it is a potentially lethal disease, both for the fetus and for the mother. The perinatal effects of pre-eclampsia will be discussed below, but hypertensive disorders during pregnancy consistently remain one of the three major causes of maternal mortality, the other two being thromboembolic disease and the complications of anaesthesia. During the 18-year period 1970–87, there were 192 deaths related to hypertensive disease during pregnancy in England and Wales, an average of 11 per year. Some 54 per cent of these deaths were associated with eclampsia whilst 46 per cent occurred in the absence of fitting. The commonest cause of death, whether or not fits occurred, was cerebral haemorrhage (Report on Confidential Enquiries into Maternal Deaths 1991).

Clinical and pathological features

Pre-eclampsia is a syndrome which involves some, but not all, of the clinical features and pathological processes discussed below:

(1) hypertension;

(2) proteinuria;

(3) oedema;

(4) placental pathology;

(5) clotting system;

(6) liver pathology;

(7) central nervous system;

(8) the fetus.

Hypertension

Hypertension is the main clinical feature of pre-eclampsia and is associated with a raised systemic vascular resistance and a reduced cardiac output antenatally but an increased cardiac output during labour (Wallenburg 1988). The level at which a pregnant woman's blood pressure is considered to be elevated is a matter for debate; the criteria for diagnosis, as laid down by Nelson (1955), Davey and MacGillivray (1988), and Redman and Jefferies (1988) have already been described. Whichever of these definitions is used, levels cited must have excluded the effect of anxiety and ideally should be observed on at least two consecutive occasions, four or more hours apart, after rest (World Health Organization 1987).

In order to be meaningful, the technique of blood pressure measurement should itself be consistent. Whilst the level of systolic blood pressure tends to be relatively consistently recorded, the level of diastolic is not. The World Health Organization recommend that the diastolic blood pressure should be recorded at the level of the fourth Korotkoff sound (muffling) and not the fifth (disappearance) (World Health Organization 1987). Yet, in a survey of 91 obstetricians and midwives in the UK, 53 per cent used the fifth sound (Perry *et al.* 1991). Furthermore, a variety of cuff sizes should be available in order that the length of the inflation bladder is at least 80 per cent of the circumference around the arm. Errors are generally greater when using too small a cuff rather than one which is too large (Petrie *et al.* 1986; De Swiet 1991). The blood pressure should be measured in the sitting or left lateral positions rather than supine because of the fall in blood pressure related to obstruction of the inferior vena cava (De Swiet 1991).

Proteinuria

Proteinuria is defined as the presence of urinary protein in concentrations of greater than 0.3 g/l in a 24-hour urine collection, or in a concentration of greater than 1 g/l in a random urine collection on two or more occasions at least four hours apart (Davey and MacGillivray 1988). The proteinuria is essentially albuminuria and reflects the severity of the disease in the absence of pre-existing renal pathology. The British Perinatal Mortality Survey (Butler and Bonham 1963) reported that the perinatal mortality rate in 10 966 normotensive patients was 76 per cent that of the population of 16 994 patients as a whole, but the perinatal mortality rate in 'moderate toxaemia' was 107 per cent, in 'severe' 147 per cent, and in proteinuric hypertension, 294 per cent. Naeye and Friedman (1979) reported that the perinatal mortality rate was 17.2 per 1000 for normotensive pregnancies and 37.9 per 1000 for pregnancies complicated by proteinuric hypertension. Some 70 per cent of these perinatal deaths were related to macroscopic placental infarction, severe IUGR, or placental abruption.

Although there is rarely, if ever, an indication for renal biopsy in pre-eclamptic patients, Spargo *et al.* (1959) reported the characteristic lesion on electron microscopy of glomerular capillary endothelial cell changes which he termed 'endotheliosis', and which involved a swelling of the cytoplasm. Fisher *et al.* (1969) reported this change together with mesangial thickening in the glomerula of patients with proteinuric hypertension and non-proteinuric hypertension during pregnancy. The occurrence and degree of hyperuricaemia may be an early indicator of renal involvement, preceding the proteinuria, whilst a rapid deterioration of renal function may occur, leading to renal failure (Redman 1989; Sagen *et al.* 1984).

The finding of proteinuria during pregnancy may be due to unsuspected renal disease and not due to pre-eclampsia. The commonest underlying renal disorders which may become apparent are chronic glomerulonephritis and polycystic kidneys. If renal impairment persists beyond pregnancy, renal biopsy may then be indicated. When pre-eclampsia is the cause of proteinuric hypertension with raised creatinine levels, no longterm detectable renal impairment seems to occur providing that no co-existing renal pathology is present, unless acute renal failure due to tubular necrosis has occurred (Chugh *et al.* 1976; Fisher *et al.* 1977; Seidman *et al.* 1991).

Oedema

Oedema is a common non-specific clinical sign during pregnancy. During normal pregnancy, the only reduction in serum albumin levels relates to haemodilution whilst the total circulating albumin levels remain unchanged. This, via Starling's law, will tend to increase tissue fluid and hence allow oedema to occur. The oedema of proteinuric hypertension, however, may relate to a true reduction in albumin levels. Thus, Studd *et al.* (1970) reported a mean reduction of 34 per cent in the circulating levels of albumin in 10 patients with severe pre-eclampsia or eclampsia when compared with non-pregnant levels.

In pre-eclampsia, the presence of oedema does not necessarily imply an increase in total body water but may in fact reflect a relative reduction in plasma volume. Thus MacGillivray (1967) showed that the mean plasma volume in normal pregnancy. was 4.04 litres compared with 3.44 litres in 'mild pre-eclampsia; and 3.32 litres in 'severe pre-eclampsia', even though the total body water was largely similar in the three groups. Similarly, Gallery *et al.* (1979) reported that whilst 189 normotensive pregnant women expanded their blood volume by the third trimester by 40 per cent, 84 women who became hypertensive during the third trimester only increased their blood volume by 22 per cent. Similar findings have been confirmed in more recent studies (Brown *et al.* 1992).

Placental pathology

The role of trophoblastic tissue in the aetiology of pre-eclampsia will be discussed in the section on aetiology below. Impaired trophoblastic infiltration of the uterine arterial walls during placentation is now considered to be pivotal to the onset of the syndrome (Redman 1989; Roberts *et al.* 1989). The conversion of spiral arteries into uteroplacental arteries appears to be dependent upon trophoblastic invasion of the vascular vessel walls and, should this process be impaired, the pathological process which follows may be pre-eclampsia, intrauterine growth retardation, or both (Pijnenborg *et al.* 1991; Shepherd and Bonnar 1981). These changes are, therefore, not characteristic of any one clinical entity. These changes, as seen on the histological examination of placental bed biopsies, may include fibrin deposition, arteriosclerosis, endothelial vacuolation, and thrombosis (Brosens 1964; Pijnenborg *et al.* 1991; Robertson *et al.* 1967).

Since these changes will have become apparent by the mid-trimester, it is possible that examination of the placental bed using Doppler ultrasound to assess the uterine (arcuate) vessels may predict those women who will develop the syndrome of pre-eclampsia before any of the clinical features become apparent (Campbell *et al.* 1986; Steel *et al.* 1990). Thus, Steel *et al.* (1990) reported the results of mid-trimester Doppler screening of the uteroplacental circulation in 1014 nulliparous women. Of the 118 women with persistently abnormal wave forms, 25 per cent developed hypertension later in pregnancy and 13 per cent delivered a growth retarded infant. Of 896 women with normal wave forms, only 5 per cent developed hypertension and none delivered a growth retarded infant. This may represent a valid early screening test.

Clotting system

The changes within the clotting system during early pregnancy are well documented. Bonnar *et al.* (1969) reported that the haemostatic mechanism appeared to be altered towards an enhanced capacity to form fibrin and a diminished ability to lyse it, as demonstrated by a 200 per cent increase in plasminogen and fibrinogen levels, allowing for plasma volume expansion, during pregnancy. The platelet count remained relatively stable during the pregnancy, but rose by some 30 per cent during the first week of the puerperium.

The clotting defects in pre-eclampsia are also well known. Redman *et al.* (1978*b*) reported early platelet consumption in pre-eclampsia with decreases of between 20–30 per cent occurring in the platelet count before the hypertension became evident. Other authors have detected alterations in platelet function as early as in the first trimester in patients destined to become pre-eclamptic (Redman 1990; Zemel *et al.* 1990). Overt intravascular coagulopathy may occur in severe pre-eclampsia or eclampsia. Thus the Birmingham Eclampsia Study Group (1971) demonstrated thrombocytopenia, hypofibrinogenaemia, and hypoplasminogenaemia, a fall in the platelet count, an increase in fibrinogen degradation products, or a combination of some of these in 10 of 19 patients with severe pre-eclampsia (a blood pressure of 160/100 mmHg and proteinuria) and six out of eight eclamptic patients. No patient will develop evidence of coagulopathy in the presence of a normal platelet count (Leduc *et al.* 1992).

It is not clear why these changes occur, but Pritchard *et al.* (1976) believe that they relate to platelet adherence at sites of vascular endothelial damage as a consequence of vasospasm rather than by thromboplastin release from the placenta, whilst Redman (1989) suggests that they may be related either to disorders of prostanoid metabolism or liver pathology. However, there is no good evidence which explains these changes.

Haemolysis (microangiopathic haemolytic anaemia) may also occur in pre-eclampsia, and the syndrome of Haemolysis, Elevated Liver enzymes, and Low Platelet count (HELLP syndrome) is now well recognized, but rare, and presents with right upper quadrant pain, jaundice, and nausea, mimicking cholecystitis (Duffy and Watson 1988; Sibai 1990*a*; Weinstein 1982). It is considered to be an indication for delivery (Sibai 1990*a*).

Liver pathology

Jaundice may occur, especially in relation to eclampsia, due to either acute fatty liver, intravesicle coagulopathy, Gram-negative septicaemia, or coincidental viral hepatitis (Duffy and Watson 1988; Sibai 1990*a*; Studd 1977). The characteristic hepatic lesion in pre-eclampsia is haemorrhage and ischaemia around both the portal tract and under the liver capsule, perhaps related to the fibrin deposits in the liver vasculature (Studd 1977).

Central nervous system

The incidence of eclampsia would appear to lie between 1 in 1390 pregnancies and 1 in 4250 pregnancies (Redman 1989; Svensson *et al.* 1984; Wightman *et al.* 1978). The perinatal mortality rate in eclampsia seems to lie between

Table 24.1 Consequences of pre-eclampsia

Condition	No.	Number of perinatal deaths	Perinatal morbidity rate (per 1000)
Total	14 686	294	20.0
Normotensive	10 787	207	19.2
Pre-eclampsia			
—mild	2459	48	19.5
—moderate	610	11	18.0
—severe	830	28	33.7

From Chamberlain et al. (1978)

86 and 213 per 1000 (Sibai et al. 1981). There is also an appreciable maternal mortality. This has been reported to be in the region of 2 per cent (Lopez-Llera et al. 1976), (Chesley 1984; Pritchard et al. 1984; Sibai et al. 1981).

It is important to observe that not all eclampsia occurs before delivery. Some 46 per cent of patients had their first convulsion antenatally, 17 per cent during labour, and 37 per cent postnatally (Sibai et al. 1981).

Eclampsia has been likened to a hypertensive encephalopathy (Redman 1989) but with superimposed features, such as cerebral oedema, haemorrhage, and infarction. The cause of the cerebral dysfunction is unclear, but it is associated with intense vasoconstriction which some believe to be a cause (Sheehan and Lynch 1973) and others believe to be a protective mechanism against haemorrhage (Redman 1989).

Traditionally, the eye is considered to be part of the central nervous system and ocular complications of eclampsia do occur. Narrowing of the retinal arterioles due to vasoconstriction occurs in some degree in up to 70 per cent of hypertensive pregnant women, and this vasoconstriction reverses when the blood pressure subsides (Seidman et al. 1991). However, 'cotton-wool' exudates and retinal oedema may occur in up to 1 per cent of women with pre-eclampsia and 10 per cent of those with eclampsia, and rarely these may lead to retinal detachment in 1 in 700 such women (Dornan et al. 1982; Seidman et al. 1991). Spontaneous retinal re-attachment follows, but some degree of visual impairment may persist (Dornan et al. 1982). Transient cortical blindness has also been reported in up to 5 per cent of women who have had eclamptic fits (Sibai et al. 1981).

The fetus

The fetus can be affected by acute and/or chronic changes in the uteroplacental circulation. The increased perinatal mortality associated with severe pre-eclampsia, but not with mild or moderate pre-eclampsia, is shown in Table 24.1 (Chamberlain et al. 1978). This increased perinatal mortality rate with eclampsia and severe pre-eclampsia has been referred to in the above section,

Table 24.2 Consequences of pre-eclampsia

	Pre-eclampsia	Normotensive
No.	271	2850
Birthweight % < 5 lb (2.3 kg)	32.1	12.8
Birthweight % 5–7 lb	55.3	68.4
Birthweight % > 7 lb (3.2 kg)	12.6	18.8

From MacGilliray (1967)

the commonest cause of perinatal death being abruptio placentae (Sibai *et al.* 1981, 1984). That pre-eclampsia is associated with a reduction in birthweight has been well demonstrated, as illustrated in Table 24.2 (MacGillivray 1967). Moore and Redman (1983) matched 24 women with pre-eclampsia, including proteinuria, with 48 randomly selected controls matched for age and parity. Some 8 per cent of controls delivered a baby whose birthweight was below the 10th centile compared with 82 per cent of the patients with pre-eclampsia. Sibai *et al.* (1984) reported 91 patients with severe pre-eclampsia superimposed upon chronic hypertension and 212 patients with pre-eclampsia alone. Intrauterine growth retardation occurred in 14 per cent of the fetuses born to mothers with pre-eclampsia but occurred in 33 per cent of the fetuses born to mothers with pre-eclampsia superimposed upon chronic hypertension. Other authors confirm this association (Eskenazi *et al.* 1993).

Predisposing factors to pre-eclampsia

The following factors would appear to affect the likelihood of pre-eclampsia developing in a given pregnancy:

(1) nulliparity;

(2) previous pre-eclampsia or eclampsia;

(3) maternal age;

(4) family history;

(5) maternal weight;

(6) associated obstetric conditions.

Nulliparity

The predilection of both mild pre-eclampsia and severe pre-eclampsia for a first pregnancy as compared with subsequent pregnancies has long been recognized (MacGillivray 1961). The incidences of proteinuric hypertension and mild pre-eclampsia was seen to fall in higher parity groups (please see Table 24.3, Campbell *et al.* 1985). Should the first pregnancy have ended in spontaneous

Table 24.3 The influence of parity

Pregnancy	No. of pregnancies	% With proteinuric hypertension	% With mild pre-eclampsia
First	11 534	6.1	27.5
Second	9730	1.9	17.7
Third	5002	1.2	15.7
Fourth	2155	0.6	15.9
5–15	1430	1.1	18.0

From Campbell *et al.* (1985)

abortion, the incidence of proteinuric hypertension (4.8 per cent) was more similar to that in a first pregnancy (6.1 per cent) than a second pregnancy (1.9 per cent) (Campbell *et al.* 1985).

Previous pre-eclampsia

It has been stated that the incidence of proteinuric hypertension is 1.9 per cent in a second pregnancy. However, should proteinuric hypertension have occurred during the first pregnancy, then there is an incidence of 7.5 per cent in a subsequent pregnancy (Campbell *et al.* 1985).

Maternal age

A graph of the incidence of pre-eclampsia against maternal age is generally considered to be a J-shaped curve. It is uncertain whether or not the incidence of pre-eclampsia is increased in the very young (MacGillivray 1983). Osbourne *et al.* (1981) were unable, in a retrospective case record analysis, to find any difference between the incidence of severe pre-eclampsia between teenage pregnancies and other primigravidae. The World Health Organization Study Group (1987) suggested that the apparent increased incidence in teenage girls may relate to the increased incidence of concealed pregnancies in this group. However, a recent survey of over one and a half million pregnancies in the USA did confirm the traditional J-shaped curve, with a relative risk of 1.9 for the development of pre-eclampsia in women aged 17 years or less compared with those aged 20–24 years (Saftlas *et al.* 1990).

The effect of increasing maternal age may be complicated by an increase in the incidence of essential hypertension, but the evidence for an increased incidence of both mild pre-eclampsia and severe pre-eclampsia is more convincing in this age group. The British Perinatal Mortality Survey (Butler and Alberman 1969) demonstrated a significant increase in the incidence of severe pre-eclampsia in women over the age of 35 years, applicable both to primigravidae and multigravidae (please see Table 24.4).

Table 24.4 The influence of maternal age

Parity	Maternal age	Singleton pregnancies			
		Number of deliveries	Mild pre-eclampsia (%)	Moderate pre-eclampsia (%)	Severe pre-eclampsia (%)
All	All	16 981	17.4	4.0	6.1
Primigravidae	<25	3619	18.4	4.4	8.5
	25–34	2412	21.4	5.2	7.9
	>35	249	30.9	6.8	15.3
Multigravidae	<25	2288	12.4	2.0	3.5
	25–34	6459	15.9	3.7	3.7
	>35	1954	19.4	4.7	6.5

From The British Perinated Mortality Survey (Butler and Alberman 1969)

Family history

There would appear to be an increased incidence of both mild pre-eclampsia and severe pre-eclampsia in the female relatives of patients who have themselves had this disease, and this may be of importance when aetiology is considered. Chesley and Cooper (1986) reported that of women who had pre-eclampsia during the first viable pregnancy, 25 per cent of their daughters had pre-eclampsia, as did 20 per cent of their granddaughters, but only 6 per cent of daughters-in-law. Sutherland *et al.* (1981) analysed the first pregnancies of 158 mothers and 160 mothers-in-law of pre-eclamptic women and of matched controls. Some 14 per cent of mothers of pre-eclamptic women had severe pre-eclampsia compared with 3 per cent of controls and 4 per cent of mothers-in-law.

Similarly Arngrimsson *et al.* (1990) reported families descended from women who had either eclampsia or pre-eclampsia; some 23 per cent of daughters, but only 10 per cent of daughters-in-law, had either eclampsia or pre-eclampsia.

These observations suggest a maternal genotype susceptibility to pre-eclampsia which would be compatible with either a Mendelian recessive condition or a dominant gene with incomplete penetrance (Arngrimsson *et al.* 1990; Cooper and Liston 1979).

If this genetic aetiology is correct, then a significant incidence of proteinuric pre-eclampsia should be found in identical twins during their first pregnancies, even if the gene was recessive and of limited penetrance. However, Thornton and Onwude (1991) analysed the first pregnancies of 108 pairs of adult identical twins and could not identify a single pregnancy in which both women were affected with proteinuric pre-eclampsia. This study does not rule out a single gene hypothesis for pre-eclampsia, but does make it more difficult to accept. It may be that the maternal genetic susceptibility may be influenced by antigen sharing between the maternal and fetal genotype (Cooper *et al.* 1988; Liston and Kilpatrick 1991).

Maternal weight

There is conflicting evidence concerning the influence of maternal obesity upon the incidence of pre-eclampsia. Edwards *et al.* (1978) reported that 23 per cent of obese women had some form of hypertensive disorder during pregnancy compared with 10 per cent non-obese controls matched for age and parity. However, Chesley (1984) reported 242 women with eclampsia and found that the condition 'has a slight predilection for underweight women', but was unable to find any association between eclampsia and obesity. However, such studies should always use the appropriate size of cuff for the patient's arm (see also p. 618).

One of the reasons put forward for the routine weighing of patients during pregnancy was the belief that excessive weight gain may identify those patients who are at increased risk of pre-eclampsia. However, such weight gain is of little value for predicting pre-eclampsia in that it has both a low specificity and sensitivity, demonstrated as long ago as 1942. Waters (1942) reported the weight gain during pregnancy in 3230 women and found that a maternal weight gain of 21–45 lb was associated with an incidence of pre-eclampsia of 3.5 per cent, a weight gain of 26–30 lb with an incidence of pre-eclampsia of 5.5 per cent, and 31–35 lb with an incidence of pre-eclampsia of 11.8 per cent, whilst the mean weight gain for the group (23.2 lb) was associated with an overall incidence of pre-eclampsia of 6.1 per cent. In this series, therefore, almost 90 per cent of those who gained weight 'excessively' did not develop pre-eclampsia.

Associated obstetric conditions

There is an association between the presence of a hydatidiform mole and pre-eclampsia. Curry *et al.* (1975) reported 347 pregnancies complicated by hydatidiform moles and found an overall incidence of 12 per cent for pre-eclampsia in this population. Since the excess of hydatidiform moles in primigravidae compared with multigravidae is only 5 per cent, this would seem to represent a true relationship. Eclampsia may also occur (Newman and Eddy 1988).

There is an association between pre-eclampsia and diabetic pregnancies. Brudenell (1989), reporting the United Kingdom Diabetic Pregnancy Survey, found that the overall incidence of pre-eclampsia in established diabetics was 14.4 per cent.

It is difficult to quote an exact incidence for pre-eclampsia superimposed upon pre-existing hypertension, renal disease, or both, partly because of a blurring of terminology, but there would seem to be an incidence of acute exacerbations of proteinuric hypertension during the second half of some of these pregnancies (Redman 1989).

Twinning is associated with a greater incidence of pre-eclampsia. The incidence of severe pre-eclampsia in primigravid twin pregnancy is 29 per cent compared with 5.5 per cent in singleton primigravidae (MacGillivray 1983). This

Table 24.5 Pre-eclampsia and twin pregnancy

Group	No.	Incidence of pre-eclampsia (%)
All twins	1858	26.2
Twins, same sex	1156	24.1
Twins, opposite sex	702	29.6
Twins, presumed monozygous	454	15.6
Twins, presumed dizygous	1404	29.6

From Stevenson *et al.* (1976)

increase cannot be explained by age alone since severe pre-eclampsia only occurs in 15 per cent of primigravidae over the age of 35 years with a twin pregnancy (Butler and Alberman 1969). Stevenson *et al.* (1976) combined the data from five studies on the relationship between pre-eclampsia and twinning. The overall incidence of pre-eclampsia in 1858 twins was 26 per cent (please see Table 24.5). It can also be seen that the incidence of pre-eclampsia was higher in the presence of twins of the opposite sex than the same sex, and higher in twin pregnancies which were presumed to be dizygous (29.6 per cent) compared with those that were presumed to be monoyzgous (15.6 per cent). These data are used to lend support to the hypothesis that pre-eclampsia may depend upon a maternofetal incompatibility (as discussed in the section below on aetiology).

The aetiology of pre-eclampsia

There is no universally accepted theory for the aetiology of pre-eclampsia. The conditions which any theory would have to satisfy were enumerated by Browne (1946), later augmented by MacGillivray (1983), and are shown below.

1. This is a disease of pregnancy occcurring mainly within the second half of pregnancy. The disease occasionally becomes worse or may even arise for the first time shortly after delivery.
2. It occurs preferentially during first pregnancies.
3. It requires the presence of placental tissue but not of the fetus.
4. There are extrauterine diseases associated with pre-eclampsia, such as renal and hepatic disease.
5. It is more likely to occur in the presence of twin pregnancies, diabetes, and maternal obesity.
6. There is a family tendency, and a change of partner alters the incidence.

There are numerous theories concerning the aetiology of pre-eclampsia which are now largely of historical interest, including the presence of a circulating toxin, placental infarcts, uterine over-distension, a uterorenal reflex, dietary deficiencies, salt excess, water intoxication, enzyme deficiencies, and an increase in the circulating level of oestrogen, adrenaline, noradrenaline, and antidiuretic hormone. What must be stressed, however, is that the hypertension which is so characteristic of pre-eclampsia is an effect of the disease and not an aetiological factor since other features of pre-eclampsia, such as the reduced platelet count and the alteration in uteroplacental circulation, may be seen before the onset of the hypertension.

The theories which have to be considered at the current time involve:

(1) renin–angiotensin–aldosterone system;

(2) immunological factors;

(3) disseminated intravascular coagulopathy;

(4) prostacyclin and thromboxane;

(5) maternal endothelial damage.

Renin–angiotensin–aldosterone system

Renin is an enzyme which acts upon renin substrate to form angiotensin I. Angiotensin I is then converted to angiotensin II by angiotensin-converting enzyme. Angiotensin II is an extremely potent circulating vasoconstrictor which also stimulates the synthesis of aldosterone (Symonds 1988). It is also synthesized locally in some vascular beds. These characteristics link it closely to arterial blood pressure control and thence to pregnancy-induced hypertension.

The changes in the renin–angiotensin–aldosterone system in pre-eclampsia remain both controversial and contradictory. There is general agreement that plasma renin activity and plasma renin concentrations are lower in pre-eclamptic patients than in non-hypertensive pregnant patients (Carr and Gant 1983; Weir *et al*. 1973). The main disagreement concerns the circulating levels of angiotensin II. Some authors report that angiotensin II levels are lower in pre-eclamptic than in non-hypertensive pregnant patients (Hanssens *et al*. 1991; Weir *et al*. 1973), some report that there are no significant differences in the levels (Massani 1967), whilst others report that the circulating levels are raised (Symonds *et al*. 1975; Symonds and Broughton-Pipkin 1978).

It may be that sensitivity to angiotensin II is of more importance than the actual circulating level, and there is evidence that patients with pregnancy-related hypertension or patients who are destined to develop pregnancy-related hypertension are more sensitive to the pressor effect of angiotensin II than are non-hypertensive pregnant patients (Baker *et al*. 1991; Gant *et al*. 1977; Symonds 1988).

It is difficult, however, with our current state of knowledge to explain how alterations in the renin–angiotensin–aldosterone system can act as the primary aetiological event in pre-eclampsia.

Immunological factors

There is evidence that pre-eclampsia is associated with an immunological reaction, either as a primary aetiological feature or as a factor which determines susceptibility to the development of pre-eclampsia.

Most of the immunological evidence supports the view that those patients who are free from pre-eclampsia either do not have the gene that predisposes to it, or the immunological reaction is not sufficiently strong to cause a clinically recognizable effect, or it is efficiently blocked by an immunological reaction which overcomes the immunological reaction due to maternal–fetal dissimilarity. The observation that pre-eclampsia is commoner in primigravidae and has an increased incidence in multigravidae following a change of male partner could be explained upon the basis that pre-eclampsia associated with an immunological reaction is either less vigorous or blocked upon subsequent exposure to an antigen (Alderman *et al.* 1986; Feeney *et al.* 1977; Ikedife 1980).

The above observations suggest that a greater antigenic dissimilarity between fetus and mother increased the likelihood of pre-eclampsia. This hypothesis is supported by the previous observations on twinning, where there is some evidence that the incidence of pre-eclampsia is greater when twins are of the opposite sex than of the same sex or when they are dizygous rather than monozygous (Table 24.5) (Stevenson *et al.* 1976).

However, other workers have produced evidence which suggests that it is a reduced maternal immunological response perhaps related to greater fetomaternal histocompatibility that is an aetiological factor in pre-eclampsia. (Jenkins *et al.* 1978; Redman *et al.* 1978a).

The balance of evidence would appear to be compatible with the view that the immune system may modify the patient's susceptibility to pre-eclampsia, but it is unlikely to be a primary aetiological factor.

Disseminated intravascular coagulopathy

The association between the clotting system and pre-eclampsia is well recognized and has been described earlier in this chapter. However, there is very little evidence to suggest that the changes in the coagulation-fibrinolytic system may precede the clinical finds of pre-eclampsia. They are more likely to be the result of this condition (Roberts *et al.* 1989). The one abnormality of clotting which does seem to precede the onset of hypertenison, however, is a fall in the platelet count (Zemel *et al.* 1990).

Prostacyclin and thromboxane

There is evidence for a role for the more recently described eicosanoid, prostacyclin, which is a potent vasodilator and an inhibitor of platelet aggregation, and the prostaglandin, thromboxane, which is a potent vaso-constrictor and a platelet aggregation (McParland and Pearce 1991). In a normal pregnancy, synthesis of prostacyclin is increased so that the prostacyclin: thromboxane ratio is tipped heavily towards vasodilatation and anti-aggregation. However, in women who will become hypertensive during pregnancy, there is inadequate prostacyclin synthesis in both maternal and fetoplacental tissues. The result is that the prostacyclin: thromboxane ratio is tipped towards vasoconstriction and a tendency to platelet aggregation. The diminution in prostacyclin synthesis is present from early in the first trimester and may thus be one of the primary aetiological factors in the condition (Fitzgerald *et al.* 1987; Friedman 1988). This would result in an increased sensitivity to angiotensin II, elevated blood pressure, and an activation of intravascular coagulation.

There is experimental evidence to support this concept. Demers and Gabbe (1976) assayed prostaglandin levels in placental tissue from 22 patients with hypertension developing during pregnancy and 20 following a normotensive pregnancy. In those with hypertension, the levels of PGE (a vasoconstrictor) were significantly elevated compared with the results from the placentae of the normotensive patients. Walsh *et al.* (1985) performed a similar study assaying prostacyclin production in the placentae after delivery of 12 normotensive women and 12 women with severe pre-eclampsia. The ability of the placentae from the pre-eclamptic women to produce prostacyclin was less than that produced by the placentae of the normotensive women.

Broughton-Pipkin *et al.* (1982) studied 22 normotensive women during the second trimester and 10 non-pregnant controls during the infusion of angiotensin II without and with a simultaneous infusion of prostaglandin E_2. As expected, the pressor response to angiotensin II alone was less in the pregnant than the non-pregnant woman. Furthermore, the simultaneous administration of prostaglandin E_2 had a greater blunting effect on the pressor response to angiotensin II in pregnant than in non-pregnant women. In a subsequent study they showed prostacyclin to have a similar effect (Broughton-Pipkin *et al.* 1989). Thus the increased synthesis of E-series prostaglandins and prostacyclin may be partly responsible for blunting the pressor response to angiotensin II in a normal pregnancy. By extrapolation, the lesser synthesis of prostacyclin may account for the enhanced pressor responsiveness to angiotensin II in pre-eclampsia. A greater pressor responsiveness to noradrenaline and possibly vasopressin has also been reported in hypertensive women (Talledo *et al.* 1968). It also appears that the intracellular smooth muscle calcium concentration may be increased in women with pre-eclampsia, and this would contribute to an enhanced pressor sensitivity to a variety of agents (Baker *et al.* 1992; Kilby *et al.* 1990).

Maternal endothelial damage

It has been suggested recently that the abnormalities of pre-eclampsia can be explained by the dysfunction of vascular endothelial cells (Roberts *et al.* 1989). The most consistent morphological abnormality in pre-eclampsia is the renal lesion which has been termed 'glomerular endotheliosis', in which the glomerular capillary endothelial cells are engorged with intracellular inclusions (Roberts *et al.* 1989). The same authors draw attention to the observation that when the endothelium becomes damaged, less prostacyclin is produced and platelets become activated, subsequently releasing thromboxane.

The cause of the endothelial cell disorder is not clear, but Roberts *et al.* (1989) have suggested that the reduced trophoblastic perfusion associated with pre-eclampsia may be an earlier aetiological factor than the endothelial cell disorder, and that this reduced perfusion releases a circulating factor or factors injurious to vascular endothelium. It is suggested that endothelin, a peptide synthesized in endothelial cells and with potent vasoconstrictor and platelet-aggregating properties, may be an aetiological agent (Ferris 1991).

The treatment of pre-eclampsia

Whilst the most effective treatment of pre-eclampsia at the current time is, ultimately, delivery, there will be situations – related to prevention, gestational age, or an acute clinical or laboratory observation – which require treatment without termination of the pregnancy. Such treatment may involve the reduction of maternal hypertension, the prevention of convulsions, the protection from hepatic or renal failure, the management of a coagulopathy, and the prevention of harm to the fetus either by disease or by treatment. Such lines of management are now discussed.

Prevention and treatment—historical aspects

Hamlin (1952) suggested that good obstetric care with patient education and regular blood pressure checks will reduce the incidence of pre-eclampsia. So convinced was he as to the value of regular antenatal checks that he advocated both domiciliary visits for chronic non-attenders and further encouragement by a visit from the local police to inform them that an immediate visit to the hospital 'was expected'! The strict control of weight gain by diet was also encouraged. Baird *et al.* (1962) were unable to show any reduction in the incidence of pre-eclampsia in women given strict dietary advice.

The other aspect of dietary advice which is no longer followed relates to salt restriction. A prospective randomly allocated trial failed to demonstrate a lower incidence of pre-eclampsia in women who were asked to reduce their salt intake in both cooking and eating (Robinson 1958).

The effect of bedrest on hypertension outside pregnancy is well documented, but this cannot necessarily be extrapolated to pre-eclampsia. Mathews (1977) recruited 135 patients with a singleton pregnancy and a diastolic blood pressure of 90–109 mmHg without proteinuria after the 28th week of pregnancy, and randomly allocated them to bedrest in hospital, with or without sedation (using barbiturates) or to normal activity at home (with or without the same sedation).

Table 24.6 The effect of bedrest

	Bedrest in hospital		Normal activity at home	
	Sedation	No sedation	Sedation	No sedation
No.	36	35	36	28
Diastolic BP > 109 mmHg	8	7	5	1
Albuminuria	1	4	1	2
Eclampsia	1	0	0	0
Fetal death	1	0	1	0
Apgar < 7 at 5 minutes	2	0	1	0
Mean birthweight (g)	3229	3087	3110	3249
IUGR	5	9	6	4

From Mathews (1977)

These results, shown in Table 24.6, suggest that bedrest and/or sedation are of no direct benefit either to the patient or to the fetus. Mathews *et al.* (1982) randomly allocated 40 women with severe pre-eclampsia to either complete bedrest in hospital or to free activity within the hospital wards. The ambulatory group showed no significant increase in the levels of either blood pressure or proteinuria but did have some worsening of biochemical placental function testing, an excess of stillbirth due to intrauterine growth retardation (15 per cent compared with 3 per cent), whilst the resting group were more likely to complain of the premonitory symptoms of eclampsia and to be delivered. Sibai *et al.* (1987) randomly allocated 200 primigravid women with mild pre-eclampsia to receive bedrest in hospital alone or bedrest and antihypertensive agents. There were no significant differences between the two groups in the occurrence of superimposed severe pre-eclampsia, the need for delivery, the birthweights of the babies, the occurrence of fetal distress, or any other measured parameter of neonatal morbidity.

There is no good evidence, therefore, for the use of either bedrest or sedation in the prevention or treatment of pre-eclampsia.

The use of diuretic therapy in hypertensive women who are not pregnant is well documented. However, there is little if any place in modern practice for the use of diuretic therapy in the treatment of pre-eclampsia.

Collins *et al.* (1985) reported an overview of nine randomized trials, involving nearly 7000 patients, designed to assess the prevention of pre-eclampsia using diuretics. Mild pre-eclampsia could be prevented, occurring in 8 per cent of the treated patients and 11 per cent of controls, but there was no statistical difference between the occurrence of severe pre-eclampsia in controls and treated patients. The use of diuretics is now rarely practised since there are more effective ways to reduce blood pressure, and since diuretics could further deplete the relative hypovolaemia associated with pre-eclampsia and thus precipitate renal failure (Redman 1989).

When to admit?

There is accumulating evidence that patients whose blood pressure does not exceed 100 mmHg, and in whom there is no proteinuria, could be managed at home with frequent blood pressure checks by either a midwife or general practitioner (Redman 1989). Such patients could even be taught to check their own urine for protein. Mathews *et al.* (1971) kept 128 such patient at home performing their own urine testing for albuminuria daily. Compared to the two-year period when 105 such patients were admitted to hospital, there was a small reduction in perinatal mortality and none of the 128 patients became eclamptic. However, there was one maternal death, but this was related to cardiomyopathy following a Caesarean section for antepartum haemorrhage in a patient in the domiciliary group. Feeney (1984) reported a series of pregnant women with a diastolic blood pressure of between 90 and 100 mmHg, without albuminuria, who were visited at home two or three times per week by a community midwife and who were only admitted to hospital if the diastolic blood pressure exceeded 100 mmHg or if albuminuria occurred. Some 38 patients were so managed, 19 requiring admission without any apparent detriment.

The emergence of the fetal surveillance unit in obstetric practice may enable patients, including those with mild hypertension, to undergo tests of fetal well-being together with blood pressure and urine checks on an out-patient basis in situations where they would previously have been admitted to hospital. The effect of such units is to reduce the antenatal bed occupancy rate by some 22 per cent without detriment to patient care (Soothill *et al.* 1991; Tuffnell *et al.* 1992).

The indications for admission to hospital then become either a diastolic blood pressure of 100 mmHg or greater, the presence of proteinuria in association with a diastolic blood pressure of 90 mmHg, the prodromal signs of eclampsia, or anxiety concerning fetal well-being.

Current aspects of treatment

The following five aspects of current management should be addressed:

(1) drugs and hypertension;

(2) drugs and convulsions;

(3) the use of plasma volume expansion;

(4) the use of aspirin as a prophylactic agent;

(5) delivery.

Drugs and hypertension

In general terms, there are three situations in which drug treatment may be indicated in order to reduce the level of blood pressure in hypertensive pregnant women. The first situation is in patients without proteinuria, especially before

Table 24.7 The use of methyldopa

	Early		Late	
	Control	Treated	Control	Treated
No.	107	101	18	16
Livebirths	101	100	15	16
Mid-trimester abortions	4	0	0	0
Stillbirths	1	1	2	0
Neonatal deaths	1	0	1	0
Proteinuric hypertension	5	6	—	—
Mean birthweight (g)	3130	3090	2690	3090

From Redman *et al.* (1976)

the third trimester, in the hope that later complications of pregnancy, including the onset of proteinuria (? superimposed pre-eclampsia) may be prevented. The second situation arises when pre-eclampsia has developed and antihypertensive therapy might be expected to prevent deterioration or allow the fetus a few days, or possibly weeks, more intrauterine development. The third situation is the management of an acute hypertensive crisis.

The most common drugs used in the first two situations are either methyldopa or a beta-blocking agent. Methyldopa is one of the best known drugs for the treatment of essential hypertension and its efficacy and safety during pregnancy is well known. It has the disadvantage that it takes approximately four hours to become effective after administration. Beta-blocking agents became popular more recently than methyldopa and are suitable alternatives.

The progression from hypertension, during early pregnancy, to proteinuric hypertension or severe pre-eclampsia is well documented (Mabie *et al.* 1978). It would seem that either with or without antihypertensive drug therapy, between 32 and 38 per cent of patients with mild chronic hypertension will develop worsening hypertension or proteinuria during the pregnancy (Blake and MacDonald 1991; Mabie *et al.* 1978). There would, however, appear to be some small advantage from the treatment of such patients.

Redman *et al.* (1976) reported 242 women who developed a blood pressure of 140/90 mmHg, substratified into early onset (before the 28th week of pregnancy) or late onset (after 28th week of pregnancy). The women were randomly allocated to receive either methyldopa or no specific treatment. The groups were well matched as regards age, gestation at entry to the trial, socio-economic class, and parity. The results are shown in Table 24.7. Although there were nine pregnancy losses in the control group compared with only one in the treatment group, the major benefit appeared to be the reduction in mid-trimester abortion in the early treated group. Superficially, it would appear that the mean birthweight was higher in the late treated than in the late control group, but once these figures were corrected for gestational age there was no longer a statistically significant difference. Sibai *et al.* (1990) randomly allocated 263 pregnant women with mild chronic hypertension to receive either methyldopa ($n = 87$), labetalol ($n = 86$), or placebo ($n = 90$). Although those patients treated with either antihypertensive agent had a similar reduction in blood pressure which was itself superior to the placebo, there were no differences between the three groups as regards the incidences of either super-imposed pre-eclampsia, abruptio placentae, preterm delivery, gestational age at birth, or the incidence of IUGR. Blake and MacDonald (1991) randomly allocated 36 women who were hypertensive during pregnancy to receive either treatment (methyldopa or atenolol) or no specific treatment (unless there was substantial clinical concern). Proteinuric hypertension developed in 32 per cent of the untreated group and in 6 per cent of the treated group. Whilst such treatment may reduce the frequency of acute hypertensive episodes during pregnancy, and may even reduce the incidence of Caesarean section, it does not seem to have a beneficial (or adverse) effect on either gestational age at birth or birthweight (Plouin *et al.* 1990). Other studies have also failed to demonstrate an improved outcome from antihypertensive treatment compared with placebo (Butters *et al.* 1990; Pickles *et al.* 1992).

Once pre-eclampsia is established, there is also little, if any, benefit from the institution of antihypertensive therapy outside an acute hypertensive episode. Thus, Pickles *et al.* (1989) compared labetalol to placebo in a randomized double-blind trial of 144 women with mild pre-eclampsia. Although there was some fall in the blood pressure in the placebo group on rest, the fall was statistically greater in the treated group. The mean birthweight for babies in both groups was statistically similar. Fidler *et al.* (1983) compared the use of methyldopa with that of oxprenolol in 100 women with mild pre-eclampsia in a randomized trial. There was no significant difference in the degree of maternal blood pressure control, but methyldopa controlled the blood pressure sooner than did oxprenolol. There was no difference in neonatal outcome as judged by birthweight, placental weight, Apgar scores, or head circumferences. Gallery *et al.* (1985) reported a randomized trial of methyldopa ($n = 87$) with oxprenolol ($n = 96$) in patients with pre-eclampsia. The control of hypertension was equivalent in both groups, but they did find a statistically significant increase in the birthweight in the oxprenolol group (mean 3122 g) compared with the methyldopa group (mean 2981 g) even allowing for parity and fetal gender.

Since these drugs, if they are to be given in the antenatal period, may have to be given for several weeks, an examination of their safety from the fetal viewpoint is required. Ounsted *et al.* (1980) reviewed, at four years of age, 86 children whose mothers had received methyldopa antenatally and compared them with 82 children whose mothers were hypertensive during pregnancy but did not receive antihypertensive drug therapy, and 107 random controls. Although there were no gross differences, the children in the control group were more advanced on a global score of development than were those in the treated group, the boys in the treated hypertension group having smaller head circumferences than the other groups, suggesting that the treatment of maternal hypertension with methyldopa may be associated with some developmental delay. However, Cockburn *et al.* (1982) reviewed 195 of the children born to women in the above trial when they were aged seven years or older. There were no significant differences between the children in the treated group or in the untreated group in 14 tests of ability, suggesting that methyldopa is a safe drug during pregnancy.

Beta-blocking agents are able to cross the placenta, and MacPherson *et al.* (1986) reported a 'mild reduction' in the blood pressure of 11 neonates born to mothers who took labetalol compared with 11 controls. This reduction, from a mean systolic blood pressure of 63.3 mmHg to 58.8 mmHg, was only observed for the first 24 hours of life. Although this gives rise to concern about possible neonatal side-effects, these appear to be very low, and De Swiet (1985) advises that 'the short-term safety of beta-blockade has been proven'. Reynolds *et al.* (1984) assessed, at the age of one year, 110 children whose mothers had received atenolol for pregnancy-related hypertension. All children were developing normally and no short-or medium-term complication relating to the use of beta-blockers was identified.

There would appear to be no advantage in favouring either methyldopa or a beta-blocking agent should the clinician wish to treat hypertension in either of the above two situations. The choice of drug will probably depend upon the clinician's familiarity with these agents and the patient's side-effects rather than any therapeutic efficacy.

The angiotensin-converting enzyme inhibitors are being used increasingly in the treatment of hypertension in the non-pregnant patient, but these agents (ACE inhibitors) are contraindicated during pregnancy since there is evidence for teratogenicity, a possible excess of fetal death, and neonatal oliguria and even renal failure (*Lancet* 1989; Thorpe-Beeston *et al.* 1993).

When antihypertensive treatment is required in the acute situation, especially for women with prodromal signs of eclampsia, methyldopa is generally considered to be too slow, although some of the faster-acting beta-blocking agents may be used (for example, labetalol).

However, other agents are available for use in this situation. Hydralazine is a vasodilator which inhibits the contractile activity of smooth muscle and increases the cardiac output, but it may be associated with a marked maternal tachycardia which limits its use. Mabie *et al.* (1978) reported, in a randomized trial, the use of intravenous injections of either labetalol ($n = 40$) or hydralazine ($n = 20$) in patient with a diastolic blood pressure of 110 mmHg or higher. Labetalol successfully lowered the blood pressure in 90 per cent of patients, whilst hydralazine was effective in 100 per cent. Since the rapid reduction of maternal blood pressure may precipitate fetal heart rate abnormalities suggestive of fetal distress, fetal monitoring is required (Vink *et al.* 1980).

Diazoxide is a rapid and powerful vasodilator and, hence, a useful hypotensive agent (Michael 1986). However, the fall in blood pressure with a diazoxide may be too rapid and too severe, and, hence, it is rarely used in obstetric practice.

Nifedipine is a calcium-channel blocking agent that reduces blood pressure and increases renal blood flow. As a sublingual agent, in an initial dose of 10–30 mg followed by 40–120 mg per day, it rapidly reduces blood pressure (3–15 minutes) without any apparent reduction in uteroplacental blood flow and without causing fetal heart rate abnormalities (Fenakel *et al.* 1991). Some 13 per cent of patients will experience vasodilator side-effects, such as headache, flushing, and palpatations (Opie and Jennings 1985). Sublingual nifedipine is rapidly becoming the agent of choice in acute hypertensive crises (Chua and Redman 1991; *Lancet* 1991). There is also increasing experience in the use of sublingual nifedipine as an antihypertensive agent in the less acute situation during pregnancy (Impey 1993; Lowe and Rubin 1992).

Drugs and convulsions

It is accepted wisdom that the patient with prodromal signs of eclampsia requires protection from convulsions over and above the treatment of hypertension, and this requires the use of anticonvulsant agents, which should not be confused with sedation. There are, however, two areas of significant debate within this area, the first concerns the choice of available agents whilst the second, and perhaps more important, relates to whether a prophylactic anticonvulsant is required at all.

Diazepam is the treatment of choice for stopping fits, but not necessarily the treatment of choice to prevent them, either primarily, or after the cessation of fitting (Moodley 1990; Redman 1989). In a combined assessment of the data from four trials involving 136 eclamptic patients, Wood (1982) reported that an initial intravenous bolus injection of up to 40 mg of diazepam abolished fits in 88 per cent of the cases. However, its effect is only shortlived and the drug may cause respiratory depression of the mother and sedate the fetus.

Once the initial fitting has been abolished, there is a choice of agents which can be used in an attempt to prevent further fits. In the United States, intravenous magnesium sulfate is the most commonly used drug, and this has the advantage of being able to stop the initial fits as well as having a use in prophylaxis. In a series of 245 eclamptic patients, fits were controlled in 96 per cent but 5 per cent had further convulsions despite magnesium sulfate prophylaxis (Pritchard *et al.* 1984). In another series of 262 women with eclampsia, 14 per cent had an additional convulsion despite treatment with magnesium sulfate (Sibai 1990*b*). Magnesium sulfate has generally been avoided in the United Kingdom because of the risks of respiratory depression and cardiac arrest. In the series from Pritchard *et al.* (1984) two patients developed respiratory depression and a further two respiratory arrest, one patient dying. This represents a serious complication in 1.6 per cent of patients. The mechanism of action of magnesium sulfate is not known, but it does not cross the blood–brain barrier. The first sign of magnesium sulfate toxicity is said to be the loss of patellar reflexes (Sibai 1990*b*). In a small randomized trial of magnesium sulfate with diazepam in 51 eclamptic women, there were no statistically significant differences in the ability of either agent to stop convulsions, prevent their recurrence, or result in side-effects (Crowther 1990).

There is some popularity for the use of chlormethiazole in a continuous infusion of 0.8 per cent. This is an effective anticonvulsant and although having a minimal effect upon the fetus, it may suppress the maternal cough reflex (Duffus 1968; Wood 1982).

Phenytoin is little used by obstetricians yet it has a long half-life making it, theoretically, a good drug for preventing the recurrence of fits once under control (Robson *et al.* 1993). Slater *et al.* (1989) reported that none of 70 patients with severe pre-eclampsia or eclampsia had a fit after the commencement of a phenytoin infusion. However, other reports have been less enthusiastic. Tuffnell *et al.* (1989*a*) reported that 17 per cent of 18 eclamptic patients treated with phenytoin had further convulsions, whilst Dommisse (1990) found that phenytoin was less effective than magnesium sulfate in the prevention of further convulsions in eclamptic patients. Should phenytoin be used, cardiac dysrhythmias may occur and electrocardiograph monitoring is desirable.

Some authors question whether anticonvulsant therapy is needed at all in severe pre-eclampsia providing that the blood pressure is controlled pharmacologically. Thus, Chua and Redman (1991) treated 78 women with severe pre-eclampsia with nifedipine and methyldopa but without an anticonvulsant; one patient developed eclampsia. They questioned whether anticonvulsants should be given to 78 women to prevent fits in one (1.3 per cent), a result better than that quoted for the recurrence of convulsions in most drug trials. However, in order to have an 80 per cent chance of demonstrating, at the 5 per cent significance level, that a drug has a 50 per cent chance of reducing eclampsia, it has been estimated that a population of 200 000 pregnant women would be required (Tuffnell *et al.* 1989*b*). It seems unlikely that, even on a multicentre basis, such a trial will ever occur and the question may never be answered.

The use of plasma volume expansion

The concept of plasma volume expansion in order to combat the relative hypovolaemia of pre-eclampsia has been advocated, especially when a vasodilatory antihypertensive agent is also used (Goodlin *et al.* 1978). Such management should probably only be given under strict central venous pressure control and urine output monitoring (Morris and O'Grady 1979). More recently, experience has accumulated to suggest that plasma volume expansion under either central venous pressure or pulmonary capillary wedge pressure measurement is of therapeutic benefit in the severely hypertensive patient with a low cardiac index (Belfort *et al.* 1989).

The use of aspirin as a prophylactic agent

Low-dose aspirin has a series of actions which may explain why it has been tried as a preventative agent in pre-eclampsia. It inhibits platelet thromboxane synthesis yet leaves endothelial prostacyclin synthesis intact (Benigni *et al.*

Table 24.8 The prevention of pre-eclampsia

	Antiplatelet therapy	Control
No.	48	45
Normal pregnancy	29	12
Hypertension alone	19	22
Proteinuric hypertension	0	6
Perinatal death	0	5
IUGR (<10th centile and alive)	0	4

From Beaufils *et al.* (1985)

1989). It also inhibits both platelet adhesion to collagen and platelet aggregation (McParland and Pearce 1991).

Although the use of aspirin in the prevention of pre-eclampsia must still be considered experimental, there is increasing clinical evidence which suggests that low-dose aspirin may be of value (McParland *et al.* 1990).

Beaufils *et al.* (1985) randomly allocated 102 patients at high risk of pre-eclampsia or IUGR, based on previous obstetric history, to receive either 300 mg dipyridamole and 150 mg aspirin daily from the 12th week of pregnancy or no specific treatment. The outcomes, as shown in Table 24.8, suggest that the treatment is effective and without serious side-effects. Wallenburg *et al.* (1986) admitted 46 normotensive women at the 28th week of pregnancy to a placebo-controlled double-blind trial based on their increased sensitivity to an angiotensin II infusion. Of the 23 women who received 60 mg aspirin daily, two developed mild pre-eclampsia but none developed severe pre-eclampsia, whereas four of the 23 women who received placebo developed mild pre-eclampsia and a further seven severe pre-eclampsia, while one patient became eclamptic. Schiff *et al.* (1989) reported the use of aspirin in a prospective randomized double-blind placebo-controlled trial of patients believed to be at risk of developing pre-eclampsia. Some 791 pregnant women with risk factors for pre-eclampsia underwent a 'roll-over' test. Of 69 women with a positive roll-over test, 65 were recruited to receive either aspirin, 100 mg per day, ($n = 34$) or placebo ($n = 31$), from the 28th week of pregnancy. As can be seen from Table 24.9, aspirin was more effective than placebo in the prevention of either mild pre-eclampsia or severe pre-eclampsia, and had a significant effect on the metabolism of thromboxane and prostacyclin. There were no serious side-effects in either mothers or babies.

A recent meta-analysis of low-dose aspirin for the prevention of pregnancy-induced hypertensive disease among 394 subjects in six trials has shown that the relative risk of pregnancy-induced hypertension amongst women who took low-dose aspirin was 0.35, whilst the risk of severe intrauterine growth retardation in their infant was 0.56 (Imperiale and Petrulis 1991). The multi-centre collaborative trial on the use of low-dose aspirin as a prophylaxis for

Table 24.9 The prevention of pre-eclampsia

	Aspirin	Placebo
No.	34	31
Mild pre-eclampsia (%)	11.8	35.5
Severe pre-eclampsia (%)	2.9	22.6
Mean ratio thromboxane to prostacyclin	34.7	51.2

From Schiff *et al.* (1989)

pregnancy-induced hypertension and pre-eclampsia (The CLASP Study) has now reported on almost 7000 patients entered as a prophylaxis against pre-eclampsia and over 1000 for the treatment of pre-eclampsia. Low dose aspirin was not statistically significant to placebo in either the prevention of pre-eclampsia and the results do not support widespread routine use of this drug (CLASP 1994). Similar results were found in the Italian Study (1993).

Caution is required since aspirin can cross the placenta and its effects upon either the fetus or upon complications of pregnancy have not yet been fully studied. From a review of the literature, aspirin in low dose is not considered to be teratogenic, to cause premature closure of the ductus arteriosus, or to be secreted in breast milk (De Swiet and Fryers 1990). Anxiety does exist because the haemostatic changes associated with aspirin could theoretically potentiate a placental abruption, but the evidence from large clinical trials will be required in order that this risk be assessed. Once pre-eclampsia has arisen, aspirin will not arrest the course of the disease (Schiff *et al.* 1990).

Delivery

The timing and mode of delivery is a multifactorial decision taking into account gestational age, maternal condition, and fetal well-being, but it is unlikely that an eclamptic woman beyong the 34th week of pregnancy will be left undelivered or that a woman with persistent proteinuric hypertension will be left undelivered beyond the 36th week.

The use of epidural analgesia is generally recommended, but not universally so, providing that disseminated intravascular coagulopathy has been excluded. Willcocks and Moir (1968) pointed out the ability of epidural analgesia to reduce maternal blood pressure, by a mean of 36 mmHg systolic and 27 mmHg diastolic, in 20 patients in labour with pre-eclampsia. Although hypotension may result in fetal heart rate changes, Moore *et al.* (1985) found such changes in 20 per cent of 116 pre-eclamptic women with epidural analgesia during labour and 20 per cent of 69 normotensive women with an epidural *in situ* during labour. Lindheimer and Katz (1985) recommended the avoidance of an epidural during labour since the risk of hypotension in the presence of a relatively hypovolaemic circulation may result in vascular collapse. This complication should be avoidable by the judicious use of intravenous fluids.

The use of epidural anaesthesia, rather than general anaesthesia, avoids the risk of failure to intubate due to pharyngolaryngeal oedema (Heller *et al*. 1983).

Patients with pre-eclampsia are not at greater risk for primary post-partum haemorrhage than other patients, but they may be able to cope less well with circulatory compromise. However, ergometrine should be avoided for patients with pre-eclampsia since it may elevate blood pressure further. Baillie (1963) reported that intravenous ergometrine elevated the systolic blood pressure in 17 per cent of normotensive women and 86 per cent of hypertensive women when used after delivery. Therefore, syntocinon is the agent of choice for the management of the third stage in patients with pre-eclampsia (Redman 1989).

The longterm effects of eclampsia

Patients who survive an eclamptic fit and have no other complication may be reassured. Sibai *et al*. (1985) assessed 65 women, some six months after one or more eclamptic fits. No patient had any neurological deficit.

It has already been stated that a patient with severe pre-eclampsia in her first pregnancy has an approximately 4 per cent chance of a recurrence in a subsequent pregnancy, whilst a patient with eclampsia has a 1.9 per cent chance of a recurrence (Chesley *et al*. 1962). These authors reported 466 pregnancies in 189 women who had an eclamptic fit in a previous pregnancy. Of the women who had an elamptic fit in their first pregnancy, 25 per cent had mild pre-eclampsia in a subsequent pregnancy, 10 per cent had severe pre-eclampsia, and 1.9 per cent had a recurrence of eclampsia. Of 31 women who had an eclamptic fit in a pregnancy other than their first some 50 per cent subsequently had pre-eclampsia, although the incidence of severe pre-eclampsia was not specifically stated and one patient had recurrent eclampsia.

The risk of hypertension in later life relates primarily to the patient who develops eclampsia in a pregnancy other than her first. Chesley *et al*. (1962) reported a group of 270 women who survived eclampsia and who were reassessed some 9–28 years later. There was no increase in the observed over the expected incidence of hypertension in women who had eclampsia during their first pregnancy (13 per cent of women), but the incidence of observed hypertension in women who had eclampsia when multiparous was 60 per cent compared with an expected incidence of 21 per cent based on age. In a longer follow-up study at between 23 and 43 years, the incidence of hypertension in the primiparous eclamptic group was still that expected from an age-matched population (22 per cent), wheeas it was again increased from the multiparous group to 51 per cent as opposed to the age-expected incidence of 33 per cent, perhaps suggesting that chronic hypertension was an aetiological factor in eclampsia in multiparous patients (Chesley *et al*. 1976).

It has been suggested (Chesley *et al*. 1962) that diabetes was seven times more common in women after eclampsia than would have been expected, but this was later retracted in the longer term study on the same patients by the same authors (Chesley *et al.* 1976) and by Singh *et al.* (1973). However, Singh (1976) did show that women with severe pre-eclampsia during pregnancy have some degree of glucose intolerance based on the use of an intravenous glucose tolerance test.

Conclusions

There is much confusion in the literature relating to this condition. To some degree this confusion could be reduced by the adoption of agreed terms and definitions.

Until the aetiology of pre-eclampsia is discovered, treatment will remain empirical. However, the ideal would be that the condition may be prevented. Although it cannot be recommended for routine clinical practice at the current time, the use of low-dose aspirin may represent a major step towards this. There is also a renewal in interest in the possible prevention of pre-eclampsia by fish-oil supplementation in pregnancy (Secher and Olsen 1990). Such supplementation increases the availability of the precursors from which predominantly vasodilator prostanoids synthesize (*Lancet* 1992).

In the patient with prodromal signs of eclampsia, or one who has become eclamptic, there is an indication for intensive care management in the labour ward should the baby not yet be delivered or perhaps in the intensive care unit after delivery. The close liaison between obstetrican, anaesthetist, and physician may serve to refine management and reduce morbidity and mortality.

References

Alderman, B. W., Sperling, R. S., and Darling, J. R. (1986). An epidemiological study of the immunogenic aetiology of pre-eclampsia. *British Medical Journal* **292**, 372–4.

Arngrimsson, R., Bjornsson, S., Geirsson, R. T., Bjornsson, H., Walker, J. J., and Snaedal, G. (1990). Genetic and familial predisposition to eclampsia and pre-eclampsia in a defined population. *British Journal of Obstetrics and Gynaecology* **97**, 762–9.

Baillie, G. W. (1963). Vasopressor activity of ergometrine maleate in anaesthetised parturient women. *British Medical Journal* **1**, 585–8.

Baird, D., Thompson, A. M., and Hytten, F. E. (1962). Weight gain in pre-eclampsia. *Lancet* **1**, 1297–8.

Baker, P. N., Broughton-Pipkin, F., and Symonds, E. M. (1991). Platelet angiotensin 2 binding sites in normotensive and hypertensive women. *British Journal of Obstetrics and Gynaecology* **98**, 436–48.

Baker, P. N., Kilby, M. D., and Broughton-Pipkin, F. (1992). The effect of angiotensin 2 on platelet intracellular free calcium concentration in human pregnancy. *Journal of Hypertension* **10**, 55–60.

Beaufils, M., Uzan., S., Donismone, R., and Colau, J. C. (1985). Prevention of pre-eclampsia by antiplatelet therapy. *Lancet* **i**, 840–2.

Belfort, M., Uys, P., Dommisse, J., and Davey, D. A. (1989). Haemodynamic changes in gestationl proteinuric hypertension. *British Journal of Obstetrics and Gynaecology* **96**, 634–41.

Benigni, A., Gregorini, G., Frusca, T., Chiabrando, C., Ballerina, S., Valcamonicho, A., *et al.* (1989). Effects of low-dose aspirin on fetal and maternal generation of thromboxane by platelets in women at risk for pregnancy-induced hypertension. *New England Journal of Medicine* **321**, 357–62.

Birmingham Eclampsia Study Group (1971). Intravascular coagulation and abnormal lung scans in pre-eclampsia and eclampsia. *Lancet* **ii**, 889–91.

Blake, S. and MacDonald, D. (1991). The prevention of maternal manifestations of pre-eclampsia by intensive anti-hypertensive therapy. *British Journal of Obstetrics and Gynaecology* **98**, 244–8.

Bonnar, J., McNicol, G. P., and Douglas, A. S. (1969). Fibrinolytic enzyme systems and pregnancy. *British Medical Journal* **3**, 387–9.

Brosens, I. (1964). A study of the spiral arteries in the decidua basalis in normotensive and hypertensive pregnancies. *Journal of Obstetrics and Gynaecology of the British Commonwealth* **71**, 222–30.

Broughton-Pipkin, F., Hunter, J. C., Turner, S. R., and O'Brien, P. M. S. (1982). Prostaglandin E$_2$ attenuates the pressor response to angiotensin II in pregnant subjects but not in non-pregnant subjects. *American Journal of Obstetrics and Gynecology* **142**, 168–76.

Broughton-Pipkin, F., Morrison, R., and O'Brien, P. M. S. (1989). Prostacyclin attenuates both the pressor and adrenocortical response to angiotensin 2 in human pregnancy. *Clinical Science* **76**, 529–34.

Brown, M. A., Zammit, V. C., and Micar, D. M. (1992). Extracellular fluid volumes in pregnancy-induced hypertension. *Journal of Hypertension* **10**, 61–8.

Browne, F. J. (1946). The significance of signs and symptoms of toxaemia of pregnancy. *Edinburgh Medical Journal* **51**, 449–53.

Brudenell, M. (1989). Diabetic pregnancy. In *Obstetrics* (ed. A. C. Turnbull and G. Chamberlain), pp. 596. Churchill Livingstone, Edinburgh.

Butler, N. R. and Alberman, E. D. (1969). High risk predictors at booking and in pregnancy. In *Perinatal problems*, pp. 36–9. Churchill Livingstone, London.

Butler, N. R. and Bonham, D. G. (1963). *The First Report of the 1958 British Perinatal Mortality Survey*, pp. 86–100. Churchill Livingstone, London.

Butters, L., Kennedy, S., and Rubin, P. C. (1990). Atenolol in essential hypertension during pregnancy. *British Medical Journal* **301**, 587–9.

Campbell, D., MacGillivray, I., and Carr-Hill, R. (1985). Pre-eclampsia in second pregnancies. *British Journal of Obstetrics and Gynaecology* **92**, 131–40.

Campbell, S., Pearce, J. M. F., Hackett, G., Cohen-Overbeek, J., and Hernandez, C. (1986). Qualitative assessment of uteroplacental blood flow. *Obstetrics and Gynecology* **68**, 649–53.

Carr, B. R. and Gant, N. F. (1983). The endocrinology of pregnancy-induced hypertension. *Clinics in Perinatology* **10**, 737–61.

Chamberlain, G. V. P., Philip, E., Howlett, B., and Masters, K. (1978). *British births, 1970*, pp. 80–107. Heinemann, London.

Chesley, L. (1984). Habitus and eclampsia. *Obstetrics and Gynecology* **64**, 315–18.

Chesley, L. C. and Cooper, D. W. (1986). Genetics of hypertension in pregnancy. *British Journal of Obstetrics and Gynaecology* **93**, 898–908.

Chesley, L. C., Cosgrove, R. A., and Annitto, J. E. (1962). A follow-up study of eclamptic women. *American Journal of Obstetrics and Gynaecology* **83**, 1360–72.

Chesley, L. C., Annitto, J. E., and Cosgrove, R. A. (1976). The remote prognosis of eclamptic women. *American Journal of Obstetrics and Gynaecology* **124**, 446–59.

Chua, S. and Redman, C. W. G. (1991). Are prophylactic anti-convulsants required in severe pre-eclampsia? *Lancet* **337**, 250-1.

Chugh, K. S., Singhal, P. C., Sharma, B. K., Pal, Y., Mathew, M. T., Dhall, K., *et al.* (1976). Acute renal failure of obstetric origin. *Obstetrics and Gynecology* **48**, 642-6.

CLASP (1994). A randomized trial of low dose aspirin for the prevention and treatment of pre-eclampsia amongst pregnant women. *Lancet* **434**, 619-29.

Cockburn, J., Moar, V. A., Ounsted, M., and Redman, C. W. G. (1982). Final report on study of hypertension during pregnancy. *Lancet* **i**, 647-9.

Collins, R., Yusuf, S., and Peto, R. (1985). Overview of randomized trials of diuretics in pregnancy. *British Medical Journal* **290**, 17-23.

Cooper, D. W. and Liston, W. A. (1979). Genetic control of severe pre-eclampsia. *Journal of Medical Genetics* **16**, 409-16.

Cooper, D. W., Hill, J. A., Chesley, L. C., and Bryans, C. I. (1988). Genetic control of susceptibility to eclampsia and miscarriage. *British Journal of Obstetrics and Gynaecology* **95**, 644-53.

Crowther, C. (1990). Magnesium sulphate versus diazepam in the management of eclampsia. *British Journal of Obstetrics and Gynaecology* **97**, 110-17.

Curry, S. L., Hammond, C. B., Tyree, L., Creasman, W. T., and Parker, R. (1975). Hydatidiform mole: diagnosis, managment and longterm follow-up of 347 patients. *Obstetrics and Gynecology* **45**, 1-12.

Davey, D. A. and MacGillivray, I. (1988). The classification and definition of hypertensive disorders of pregnancy. *American Journal of Obstetrics and Gynecology* **158**, 892-8.

De Swiet, M. (1985). Hypertensive drugs in pregnancy. *British Medical Journal* **291**, 365-6.

De Swiet, M. (1991). Blood pressure measurement in pregnancy. *British Journal of Obstetrics and Gynaecology* **98**, 239-40.

De Swiet, M. and Fryers, G. (1990). The use of aspirin in pregnancy. *Journal of Obstetrics and Gynaecology* **10**, 467-82.

Demers, L. M. and Gabbe, S. G. (1976). Placental prostaglandin levels in pre-eclampsia. *American Journal of Obstetrics and Gynecology* **126**, 137-9.

Dommisse, J. (1990). Phenytoin sodium and magnesium sulphate in the management of eclampsia. *British Journal of Obstetrics and Gynaecology* **97**, 104-9.

Dornan, K. J., Mallek, D. R., and Wittmann, B. K. (1982). The sequelae of serous retinal detachment in pre-eclampsia. *Obstetrics and Gynecology* **60**, 653-63.

Duffus, G. M., Turnstall, M. E., and MacGillivray, I. (1968). Intravenous chlormethiazole in pre-eclamptic toxaemia in labour. *Lancet* **i**, 335-7.

Duffy, B. L. and Watson, R. I. (1988). The HELLP syndrome mimicks cholecystitis. *Medical Journal of Australia* **148**, 473-6.

Edwards, L. E., Dickes, W. F., Alton, I. R., and Hakanson, E. Y. (1978). Pregnancy in the massively obese. *American Journal of Obstetrics and Gynecology* **131**, 479-83.

Eskenazi, B., Fenster, L., Sidney, S., and Elkin, E. P. (1993). Fetal growth retardation in infants of multiparous and nulliparous women with pre-eclampsia. *American Journal of Obstetrics and Gynecology* **169**, 1112-18.

Feeney, J. G. (1984). Hypertension in pregnancy managed at home by community midwives. *British Medical Journal* **288**, 1046-7.

Feeney, J. G., Tovey, L. A. D., and Scott, J. S. (1977). Influences of previous blood transfusion on the incidence of pre-eclampsia. *Lancet* **i**, 874-5.

Fenakel, K., Fenakel, G., Appleman, Z., Lurie, S., Katz, Z., and Schwartz, Z. (1991). Nifedipine in the treatment of severe pre-eclampsia. *Obstetrics and Gynecology* **77**, 331-7.

Ferris, T. F. (1991). Pregnancy, pre-eclampsia, and the endothelial cell. *New England Journal of Medicine* **325**, 1439–40.

Fidler, J., Smith, V., Fayres, P., and De Swiet, M. (1983). Randomised controlled comparative study of methyldopa and oxprenolol in treatment of hypertension in pregnancy. *British Medical Journal* **286**, 1927–30.

Fisher, E. R., Pardo, V., Paul, R., and Hayashi, T. T. (1969). Ultrastructural studies in hypertension. *American Journal of Pathology* **55**, 109–31.

Fisher, K. A., Ahuja, S., Luger, A., Spargo, B. H., and Lindheimer, M. D. (1977). Nephrotic proteinuria with pre-eclampsia. *American Journal of Obstetrics and Gynecology* **129**, 643–6.

Fitzgerald, D. J., Emptman, S. S., Mulloy, K., and Fitzgerald, G. A. (1987). Decreased prostacyclin biosynthesis preceeding the clinical manifestations of pregnancy-induced hypertension. *Circulation* **75**, 956–63.

Friedman, S. A. (1988). Pre-eclampsia: a review of the role of prostaglandins. *Obstetrics and Gynecology* **71**, 122–37.

Gallery, E. D. M., Hynyor, S. N., and Gyory, A. Z. (1979). Plasma volume contraction. *Quarterly Journal of Medicine* **48**, 593–602.

Gallery, E. D. M., Ross, M. R., and Gyory, A. Z. (1985). Antihypertensive treatment in pregnancy. *British Medical Journal* **291**, 563–6.

Gant, N. F., Jimenez, J. N., Whalley, P. J., Chand, S., and MacDonald, P. C. (1977). A prospective study of angiotensin II pressor responsiveness in pregnancies complicated by chronic essential hypertension. *American Journal of Obstetrics and Gynecology* **127**, 369–75.

Goodlin, R. C., Cotton, D. B., and Haesslein, H. C. (1978). Severe edemaproteinuria, hypertension gestosis. *American Journal of Obstetrics and Gynecology* **132**, 595–8.

Hamlin, R. H. J. (1952). The prevention of eclampsia and pre-eclampsia. *Lancet* i, 64–8.

Hanssens, M., Keirse, M. J. N. C., Spitz, B., and von Assche, F. A. (1991). Angiotensin II levels in hypertensive and normotensive pregnancies. *British Journal of Obstetrics and Gynaecology* **98**, 155–61.

Heller, P. H., Scheider, E. P., and Marx, G. F. (1983). Pharyngolaryngeal oedema as a presenting sign in pre-eclampsia. *Obstetrics and Gynecology* **62**, 533–5.

Ikedife, D. (1980). Eclampsia in multipara. *British Medical Journal* **280**, 985–6.

Imperiale, T. F. and Petrulis, A. S. (1991). A meta-analysis of low-dose aspirin for the prevention of pregnancy-induceed hypertensive disease. *Journal of the American Medical Association* **266**, 261–5.

Impey, L. (1993). Severe hypotension and fetal distress following sublingual administration of nifedipine. *British Journal of Obstetrics and Gynaecology* **100**, 959–51.

Italian Study of Aspirin in Pregnancy (1993). Low dose aspirin in the prevention and treatment of intra-uterine growth retardation and pregnancy-induced hypertension. *Lancet* **341**, 396–400.

Jenkins, D. M., Need, J. A., Scott, H. S., Morris, H., and Pepper, M. (1978). Human leucocyte antigens and mixed lymphocyte reaction in severe pre-eclampsia. *British Medical Journal* **1**, 542–4.

Kilby, M. D., Broughton-Pipkin, F., Cockbill, S., Heptinstall, S., and Symonds, E. M. (1990). A cross-sectional study of platelet intracellular free calcium in normotensive and hypertensive pregnancy. *Clinical Science* **78**, 75–80.

Lancet (1989). Are ACE inhibitors safe in pregnancy? *Lancet* ii, 482–3.

Lancet (1991). Hypertensive emergencies. *Lancet* **338**, 220–1.

Lancet (1992). Fish oils in pregnancy. *Lancet* **339**, 127–8.

Leduc, L., Wheeler, J. M., Kirshon, B., Mitchell, P., and Cotton, D. B. (1992). Coagulation profile in severe pre-eclampsia. *Obstetrics and Gynecology* **79**, 14–18.

Lindheimer, M. D. and Katz, A. I. (1985). Hypertension in pregnancy. *New England Journal of Medicine* **313**, 675–80.

Liston, W. A. and Kilpatrick, D. C. (1991). Is genetic susceptibility to pre-eclampsia conferred by homozygocity for the same recessive gene in mother and fetus? *British Journal of Obstetrics and Gynaecology* **98**, 1079–86.

Lopez-Llera, M., Linares, G. R., and Horta, J. L. H. (1976). Maternal mortality rates in eclampsia. *American Journal of Obstetrics and Gynecology* **124**, 149–55.

Lowe, S. A. and Rubin, P. B. (1992). The pharmacological management of hypertension in pregnancy. *Journal of Hypertension* **10**, 201–7.

Mabie, W. C., Gonzalez, A. R., Sabai, B. M., and Amon, E. (1978). A comparative trial of labetalol and hydralazine in the acute management of severe hypertension complicating pregnancy. *Obstetrics and Gynecology* **70**, 328–33.

MacGillivray, I. (1961). Hypertension in pregnancy and its consequences. *Journal of Obstetrics and Gynecology* **68**, 557–69.

MacGillivray, I. (1967). The significance of blood pressure and bodywater changes in pregnancy. *Scottish Medical Journal* **12**, 237–45.

MacGillivray, I. (1983). *Pre-eclampsia*, pp. 1–12; p. 310. W. B. Saunders, London.

McParland, P. and Pearce, J. M. (1991). Prostaglandins, aspirin, and pre-eclampsia. In *Progress in obstetrics and gynaecology*, Vol. 9 (ed. J. Studd), pp. 55–81. Churchill Livingstone, Edinburgh.

McParland, P., Pearce, J. M., and Chamberlain, G. V. P. (1990). Doppler ultrasound and aspirin in recognition and prevention of pregnancy-induced hypertension. *Lancet* **335**, 1552–5.

MacPherson, M., Broughton-Pipkin, F., and Rutter, N. (1986). The effect of maternal labetalol on the newborn infant. *British Journal of Obstetrics and Gynaecology* **93**, 539–42.

Massani, Z. M., Sanguinetti, R., Gallegos, R., and Raimondi, D. (1967). Angiotensin blood levels in normal and toxaemic patients. *American Journal of Obstetrics and Gynecology* **99**, 313–17.

Mathews, D. D. (1977). A randomised controlled trial of bedrest and sedation or normal activity and non-sedation in the management of non-proteinuric hypertension in later pregnancy. *British Journal of Obstetrics and Gynaecology* **84**, 108–14.

Mathews, D. D., Patel, I. R., and Sengupta, M. (1971). Outpatient management of toxaemia. *Journal of Obstetrics and Gynaecology of the British Commonwealth* **78**, 610–19.

Mathews, D. D., Agarwai, V., and Shuttleworth, T. P. (1982). A randomised controlled trial of complete bedrest versus ambulation in the management of proteinuric hypertension during pregnancy. *British Journal of Obstetrics and Gynaecology* **89**, 128–31.

Michael, C. A. (1986). Intravenous labetalol and intravenous diazoxide in severe hypertension complicating pregnancy. *Australia and New Zealand Journal of Obstetrics and Gynaecology* **26**, 26–9.

Moodley, J. (1990). Treatment of eclampsia. *British Journal of Obstetrics and Gynaecology* **97**, 99–101.

Moore, M. A. and Redman, C. W. G. (1983). Case-controlled study of severe pre-eclampsia of early onset. *British Medical Journal* **287**, 580–3.

Moore, T. R., Key, T. C., Reisner, L. S., and Resnick, R. (1985). Evaluation of the use of continuous lumbar epidural anaesthesia for hypertensive women in labour. *American Journal of Obstetrics and Gynecology* **152**, 404–12.

Morris, J. A. and O'Grady, J. P. (1979). Volume expansion in severe EPH gestosis. *American Journal of Obstetrics and Gynecology* **135**, 276.

Naeye, R. L. and Friedman, E. A. (1979). Causes of perinatal death associated with gestational hypertension and proteinuria. *American Journal of Obstetrics and Gynecology* **133**, 8-10.

Nelson, T. R. (1955). A clinical study of pre-eclampsia. *Journal of Obstetrics and Gynaecology of the British Commonwealth* **62**, 47-8.

Newman, R. B. and Eddy, G. L. (1988). Association of eclampsia and hydatidiform mole. *Obstetric and Gynecological Survey* **43**, 185-90.

Opie, L. H. and Jennings, A. (1985). Sublingual captopril versus nifedipine in hypertensive crises. *Lancet* **ii**, 555.

Osbourne, G. K., Howat, R. C. L., and Jordan, M. N. (1981). The obstetric outcome of teenage pregnancies. *British Journal of Obstetrics and Gynaecology* **88**, 215-31.

Ounsted, M. K., Moar, V. A., Good, F. J., and Redman, C. W. G. (1980). Hypertension during pregnancy with or without specific treatment; the development of children at the age of four years. *British Journal of Obstetrics and Gynaecology* **88**, 19-24.

Perry, I. J., Wilkinson, L. S., Shinton, R. A., and Beavers, D. G. (1991). Conflicting views on the measurement of blood pressure in pregnancy. *British Journal of Obstetrics and Gynaecology* **98**, 241-3.

Petrie, J. C., O'Brien, E. T., Littler, W. A., and De Swiet, M. (1986). Recommendations on blood pressure measurement. *British Medical Journal* **293**, 611-15.

Pickles, C. J. Symonds, E. M., and Broughton-Pipkin, F. (1989). Fetal outcome in a randomised double blind controlled trial of labetalol versus placebo in pregnancy-induced hypertension. *British Journal of Obstetrics and Gynaecology* **96**, 38-43.

Pickles, C. J., Broughton-Pipkin, F., and Symonds, E. M. (1992). A randomized placebo-controlled trial of labetalol in the treatment of mild-to-moderate pregnancy-induced hypertension. *British Journal of Obstetrics and Gynaecology* **99**, 964-8.

Pijnenborg, R., Anthony, J., Davey, D. A., Rees, A., Tiltman, A., Vercruysse, L., *et al.* (1991). Placental bed spiral arteries in the hypertensive disorders of pregnancy. *British Journal of Obstetrics and Gynaecology* **98**, 648-55.

Plouin, P. F., Breart, G., Llado, J., Dalle, M., Keller, M. E., Goujon, H., *et al.* (1990). A randomised comparison of early with conservative use of antihypertensive drugs in the management of pregnancy-induced hypertension. *British Journal of Obstetrics and Gynaecology* **97**, 134-41.

Pritchard, J. A., Cunningham, F. G., and Mason, R. A. (1976). Coagulation changes in eclampsia. *American Journal of Obstetrics and Gynecology* **124**, 855-64.

Pritchard, J. A., Cunningham, F. G., and Pritchards, S. A. (1984). The Parkland Memorial Hospital protocol for the treatment of eclampsia. *American Journal of Obstetrics and Gynecology* **148**, 951-63.

Redman, C. W. G. (1989). Hypertension in pregnancy. In *Obstetrics*, (ed. A. C. Turnbull and G. Chamberlain), pp. 515-54. Churchill Livingstone, Edinburgh.

Redman, C. W. G. (1990). Platelets and the beginnings of pre-eclampsia. *New England Journal of Medicine* **323**, 478-80.

Redman, C. W. G. and Jefferies, M. (1988). Revised definition of pre-eclampsia. *Lancet* **i**, 809-12.

Redman, C. W. G., Beilin, L. J., Bonnar, J., and Ounsted, M. K. (1976). Fetal outcome in trial of antihypertensive treatment in pregnancy. *Lancet* **ii**, 753-6.

Redman, C. W. G., Bodmer, J. G., Bodmer, W. F., Beilin, L. J., and Bonnar, J. (1978*a*). HLA antigens in severe pre-eclampsia. *Lancet* **ii**, 397-9.

Redman, C. W. G., Bonnar, J., and Beilin, L. J. (1978*b*). Early platelet consumption in pre-eclampsia. *British Medical Journal* **1**, 467-9.

Report on Confidential Enquiries into Maternal Deaths in England and Wales 1985-7 (1991). pp. 18-27. Her Majesty's Stationery Office, London.

Reynolds, B., Butters, L., Evans, J., Adams, T., and Rubin, P. C. (1984). First year of life after the use of atenolol in pregnancy-associated hypertension. *Archives of Diseases in Childhood* **59**, 1061–3.

Roberts, J. M., Taylor, R. M., Musci, T. J. Rodgers, G. M., Hubel, C. A., and McLaughlin, M. K. (1989). Pre-eclampsia and endothelial cell disorder. *American Journal of Obstetrics and Gynecology* **161**, 1200–4.

Robertson, W. B., Brosens, I., and Dixon, H. G. (1967). The pathological response of the vessels of the placental bed to hypertensive pregnancies. *Journal of Pathology and Bacteriology* **93**, 581–92.

Robinson, M. (1958). Salt in pregnancy. *Lancet* i, 178–81.

Robson, S. J., Redfern, N., Seviour, J., Campbell, M., Walkinshaw, S., Rodeck, C., *et al.* (1993). Phenytoin prophylaxis in severe pre-eclampsia and eclampsia. *British Journal of Obstetrics and Gynaecology* **100**, 623–8.

Saftlas, A. F., Olson, D. R., Franks, A. L., Atrash, H. K., and Pokras, R. (1990). Epidemiology of pre-eclampsia and eclampsia in the US, 1979–86. *American Journal of Obstetrics and Gynecology* **163**, 460–5.

Sagen, N., Haram, K., and Nilsen, S. T. (1984). Serum urates as a predictor of fetal outcome in severe pre-eclampsia. *Acta Obstetrica et Gynaecologica Scandinavica* **63**, 71–5.

Schiff, E., Peleg, E., Goldenberg, M., Rosenthal, T., Ruppin, E., Tamarkin, T., *et al.* (1989). The use of aspirin to prevent pregnancy-induced hypertension and lower the ratio of thromboxane to prostacyclin in relatively high risk pregnancies. *New England Journal of Medicine* **321**, 351–6.

Schiff, E., Barkai, G., Ben-Barush, G., and Mashiach, S. (1990). Low-dose aspirin does not influence the clinical course of women with mild pregnancy-induced hypertension. *Obstetrics and Gynecology* **76**, 742–4.

Secher, N. J. and Olsen, S. F. (1990). Fish-oil and pre-eclampsia. *British Journal of Obstetrics and Gynaecology* **97**, 1077–9.

Seidman, D. S., Seer, D. M., and Ben-Rafael, Z. (1991). Renal and ocular manifestations of hypertensive diseases of pregnancy. *Obstetrics and Gynaecological Survey* **46**, 71–6.

Sheehan, H. L. and Lynch, J. B. (1973). *Pathology of toxaemia in pregnancy*, pp. 524–53. Churchill Livingstone, Edinburgh.

Shepherd, B. and Bonnar, J. (1981). An ultrastructural study of utero-placental spiral arteries in hypertensive and normotensive pregnancies and fetal growth retardation. *British Journal of Obstetrics and Gynaecology* **88**, 695–705.

Sibai, B. M. (1990*a*). The HELLP syndrome: much ado about nothing? *American Journal of Obstetrics and Gynecology* **162**, 311–16.

Sibai, B. M. (1990*b*). Magnesium sulphate is the ideal anticonvulsant in pre-eclampsia–eclampsia. *American Journal of Obstetrics and Gynecology* **162**, 1141–5.

Sibai, B. M., McCubbin, J. H., Anderson, G. D., Lipshitz, J., and Dilts, P. V. (1981). Eclampsia. *Obstetrics and Gynecology* **58**, 609–13.

Sibai, B. M., Spinnato, J. A., Watson, D. L., Hill, G. A., and Anderson, G. D. (1984). Pregnancy outcome in 303 cases with severe pre-eclampsia. *Obstetrics and Gynecology* **64**, 319–25.

Sibai, B. M., Spinnato, J. A., Watson, D. L., Lewis, J. A., and Anderson, G. D. (1985). Eclampsia: neurological findings and future outcome. *American Journal of Obstetrics and Gynecology* **152**, 184–92.

Sibai, B. M., Gonzales, A. R., Mabie, W. C., and Moretti, M. (1987). A comparison of labetolol plus hospitalisation versus hospitalisation alone in the management of pre-eclampsia remote from term. *Obstetrics and Gynecology* **70**, 323–7.

Sibai, B. M., Mabie, W. C., Shamsa, F., Villar, M. A., and Anderson, G. D. (1990). A comparison of no medication versus methyldopa or labetalol in chronic hypertension during pregnancy. *American Journal of Obstetrics and Gynecology* **162**, 960–7.

Singh, M. M. (1976). Carbohydrate metabolism in pre-eclampsia. *British Journal of Obstetrics and Gynaecology* **83**, 124–31.

Singh, M. M., MacGillivray, I., and Sutherland, H. W. (1973). A late follow-up study of glucose tolerance after pre-eclampsia. *Journal of Obstetrics and Gynaecology of the British Commonwealth* **80**, 708–11.

Slater, R. M., Wilcox, F. L., Smith, W. D., and Maresh, M. J. A. (1989). Phenytoin in pre-eclampsia. *Lancet* **ii**, 1224.

Soothill, P. W., Ajayi, R., Campbell, S., Gibbs, J., Chandran, R., Gibb, D., *et al.* (1991). Effect of a fetal surveillance unit on admission of antenatal patients to hospital. *British Medical Journal* **303**, 269–71.

Spargo, B. McCartney, C. P., and Winemiller, R. (1959). Glomerular capillary epitheliosis in toxaemia of pregnancy. *Archives of Pathology* **68**, 593–9.

Steel, S. A., Pearce, J. M., McParland, P., and Chamberlain, G. V. P. (1990). Early Doppler ultrasound screen in the prediction of hypertensive disorders of pregnancy. *Lancet* **335**, 1548–51.

Stevenson, A. C., Say, B., Ustaoglu, S., and Dermus, Z. (1976). Aspects of pre-eclamptic toxaemia of pregnancy, consanguinity and twinning in Ankara. *Journal of Medical Genetics* **13**, 1–8.

Studd, J. (1977). Pre-eclampsia. *British Journal of Hospital Medicine* **18**, 52–62.

Studd, J. W. W., Blainey, J. D., and Bailey, D. E. (1970). Serum protein changes in the pre-eclampsia–eclampsia syndrome. *Journal of Obstetrics and Gynaecology of the British Commonwealth* **77**, 796–801.

Sutherland, A., Cooper, H., Howie, W., Liston, W. A., and MacGillivray, I. (1981). The incidence of severe pre-eclampsia amongst mothers and mothers-in-law of pre-eclamptic and controls. *British Journal of Obstetrics and Gynaecology* **88**, 785–91.

Svensson, A., Andersch, B., and Hannsson, L. (1984). Hypertension in pregnancy. *Acta Medica Scandinavica* **Supp. 693**, 33–9.

Symonds, E. M. (1988). Renin and reproduction. *American Journal of Obstetrics and Gynecology* **158**, 754–61.

Symonds, E. M. and Broughton-Pipkin, F. (1978). Pregnancy hypertension, parity, and the renin–angiotensin system. *American Journal of Obstetrics and Gynecology* **132**, 473–9.

Symonds, E. M., Broughton-Pipkin, F., and Craven, D. J. (1975). Changes in the renin–angiotensin system in primigravidae with hypertensive disease of pregnancy. *British Journal of Obstetrics and Gynaecology* **82**, 643–50.

Talledo, O. E., Chesley, L. C., and Zuspan, F. P. (1968). Renin–angiotensin system in normal and toxaemic pregnancies. *American Journal of Obstetrics and Gynecology* **100**, 218–21.

Thornton, J. and Onwude, J. L. (1991). Pre-eclampsia: discordance among twin pregnancies. *British Medical Journal* **303**, 1241–2.

Thorpe-Beeston, J. G., Armar, N. A., Dancy, M., Cochrane, G. W., Ryan, G., and Rodeck, C. H. (1993). Pregnancy and ACE inhibitors. *British Journal of Obstetrics and Gynaecology* **100**, 692–3.

Tuffnell, D. J., O'Donovan, P., Lilford, R. J., Prys-Davies, A., and Thornton, J. (1989*a*). Phenytoin in severe pre-eclampsia. *Lancet* **ii**, 273–4.

Tuffnell, D. J., O'Donovan, P., Lilford, R. J., Prys-Davies, A., and Thornton, J. G. (1989*b*). Phenytoin in pre-eclampsia. *Lancet* **ii**, 1224–5.

Tuffnell, D. J., Lilford, R. J., Buchan, P. C., Prendiville, V. M., Tuffnell, A. J., Holgate, M. P., *et al.* (1992). Randomised controlled trial of day care for hypertension in pregnancy. *Lancet* **339**, 224–7.

Vink, G. J., Moodley, J., and Philpott, R. H. (1980). Effect of dihydralazine on the fetus in the treatment of maternal hypertension. *Obstetrics and Gynecology* **55**, 519–22.

Wallenburg, H. C. S. (1988). Haemodynamics in hypertensive pregnancy. In *Handbook of hypertension, Vol. 10: Hypertension in pregnancy* (ed P. C. Rubin), pp. 66–101. Elsevier Scientific Publishers, Amsterdam.

Wallenburg, H. C. S., Decker, G. A., Makovitz, J. W., and Rotmans, P. (1986). Low-dose aspirin prevents pregnancy-induced hypertension and pre-eclampsia in angiotensin-sensitive primigravidae. *Lancet* **i**, 1–3.

Walsh, S. W., Behr, M. J., and Allen, N. H. (1985). Placental prostacyclin production in normal and toxaemia pregnancies. *American Journal of Obstetrics and Gynecology* **151**, 110–15.

Waters, E. G. (1942). Weight studies in pregnancy. *American Journal of Obstetrics and Gynecology* **43**, 826–32.

Weinstein, L. (1982). Syndrome of haemolysis, elevated liver enzymes, and low platelet count. *American Journal of Obstetrics and Gynecology* **149**, 159–67.

Weir, R. J., Brown, J. J., Fraser, R., Kraszewski, A., Lever, A. F., McIlwaine, G. M., *et al.* (1973). Plasma renin, renin substrate, angiotensin II and aldosterone in hypertensive disease of pregnancy. *Lancet* **i**, 291–4.

Wightman, H., Hibbard, B. M., and Rosen, M. (1978). Perinatal mortality and morbidity associated with eclampsia. *British Medical Journal* **2**, 235–7.

Willcocks, J. and Moir, D. M. (1968). Epidural analgesia in the management of hypertension in labour. *Journal of Obstetrics and Gynaecology of the British Commonwealth* **75**, 225–8.

Wood, S. M. (1982). Drugs in the treatment of hypertension in pregnancy. In *Progress in obstetrics and gynaecology*, Vol. 2 (ed. J. Studd), pp. 97–107. Churchill Livingstone, Edinburgh.

World Health Organization (1987). The hypertensive disorders of pregnancy. *World Health Organization Technical Report Series*, 758.

Zemel, M. B., Zemel, P. C., Berry, S., Norman, G., Kowalczyk, C., Sokol, R. J., *et al.* (1990). Altered platelet calcium metabolism as an early predictor of increased peripheral vascular resistance and pre-eclampsia in urban black women. *New England Journal of Medicine* **323**, 434–8.

25 The management of red cell alloimmunization

The reduction in intrauterine and neonatal death rates due to rhesus allo-immunization must be classed as one of the major achievements in contemporary obstetrics and neonatal care. In the 1950s, haemolytic disease of the newborn contributed 1.5 per 1000 to the perinatal mortality rate, equivalent to more than 1000 deaths per year in England and Wales. By 1969, there were 708 such deaths (Urbaniak 1985), and by 1989, there were between approximately 100 pregnancies lost from haemolytic disease in England and Wales (MacKenzie et al. 1992). The commonest reason for the onset of rhesus-D sensitization ultimately resulting in fetal or neonatal death is failure to administer immuno-globulin prophylaxis when generally considered appropriate; Clarke et al. (1987) reported that among 58 deaths due to rhesus-D alloimmunization, prophylaxis had been omitted in 48 per cent. There is, therefore, still considerable room for improvement in clinical practice if these potentially avoidable losses are to be avoided.

Even when anti-D is administered appropriately, sensitization may still occur. It has been demonstrated that anti-D immunoglobulin administered within 72 hours of delivery prevents 90 per cent of the sensitizations that would otherwise have occurred (Selinger 1991). However, unprovoked transplacental micro-haemorrhages from the fetal to maternal circulation must occur, since 16 per cent of patients who are sensitized by the end of pregnancy have developed antibodies during the antenatal period without any evidence of a traumatic event; the idea of routine antenatal prophylaxis has thus been promoted (Clarke et al. 1987; Tovey 1986).

The prevention of rhesus alloimmunization

An immunological mechanism for the development of rhesus disease was first recognized from the observation of Levine (1958) who reported that maternofetal ABO incompatibility was relatively protective against rhesus alloimmunization. The administration of anti-D immunoglobulin (Clarke et al. 1963) is designed to mop-up Rh(D)-positive fetal red cells following transplacental haemorrhage into the maternal circulation of a Rh(D)-negative mother and prevent the maternal antibody response. Transplacental haemorrhage may occur during threatened, inevitable, and therapeutic abortions, ectopic pregnancy, amniocentesis, antepartum haemorrhage, external version, in association with pre-eclampsia, and during delivery (Tabor et al. 1986; Tovey 1986).

Table 25.1 The use of anti-D

	Controls		Anti-D	
	No.	%	No.	%
Total	78	100	78	100
Immunized	19	24.4	3	3.8
Not immunized	59	75.6	75	96.2

From The Combined Study in England and Baltimore (1966)

Prophylaxis should, therefore, be given soon after each of these events, ideally within 72 hours (Dayton *et al.* 1990; Everett 1988; Tovey 1988).

The Combined Study in England and Baltimore (1966) reported the results of a controlled trial examining the value of intramuscular anti-D immuno-globulin at delivery in rhesus-negative primigravidae with fetal red cells in the maternal circulation. The results, illustrated in Table 25.1, demonstrate the significant reduction in the incidence in sensitization six months after delivery in those patients who received anti-D compared with controls. Similar results were reported by Freda *et al.* (1966) with none of the 48 patients who received prophylaxis becoming sensitized compared with 12 per cent of 59 controls.

Failed prophylaxis

The administration of anti-D is not wholly effective in the prevention of sensitization, and failure of antibody suppression following appropriate prophylaxis accounts for 46 per cent of all new cases of rhesus alloimmunization and 27 per cent of all rhesus deaths (Clarke *et al.* 1987; Hughes *et al.* 1994; Tovey 1986).

It is possible that a factor in failed prophylaxis is that an adequate dose of anti-D immunoglobulin had not been given. It has long been known that the efficacy of anti-D is dose-dependent (Clarke *et al.* 1963). When anti-D is required, the UK practice is to give 250 IU (50 μg) anti-D immunoglobulin before 20 weeks' gestation and 500 IU (100 μg) after that gestation; in North America, the usual practice is to administer 750 IU (150 μg) after 20 weeks. In the UK, the size of the transplacental haemorrhage following delivery (and at other times) is estimated from the fetal red cell population in samples of maternal peripheral blood, using the Kleihauer test and giving an additional 100 IU (20 μg) for every 1 ml fetal haemorrhage estimated over 4 ml (Urbaniak 1985).

There is no good evidence upon which to compare the relative merits of the UK and North American policies, but it is possible that even larger doses of anti-D may reduce prophylaxis failure (Stangenberg *et al.* 1991).

The use of prophylaxis

Analysis of the circumstances surrounding sensitization have shown that 15–20 per cent of patients are sensitized during the antenatal period without any traumatic episode being identified. Thus 1 per cent of Rh(D)-negative women produce antibodies by the end of their first pregnancy, while a further 3–5 per cent have detectable antibody six months after delivery (Selinger 1991; Tovey *et al.* 1978). Clinical trials have, therefore, taken place to assess whether the administration of anti-D antenatally to rhesus-negative women without antibodies may reduce further the incidence of new cases of rhesus alloimmunization.

Bowman and Pollock (1978) gave 300 µg anti-D immunoglobulin at the 28th week of pregnancy and again after delivery to 1086 rhesus-negative primigravidae who delivered rhesus (D) babies: only two women (0.18 per cent) subsequently developed anti-D antibodies compared with the anticipated 14 had prophylaxis not been administered. It would seem that a single injection of anti-D immunoglobulin given at the 28th week of pregnancy will prevent approximately 86 per cent of cases of rhesus alloimmunization.

Tovey *et al.* (1983) gave 100 µg anti-D immunoglobulin at 28 and again at 34 weeks' gestation to 2069 non-sensitized rhesus-negative primigravidae. Those women who subsequently delivered a rhesus-positive baby received a third injection following delivery, whilst a non-randomized control group of 2000 rhesus-negative women delivering a rhesus-positive infant did not receive the two antenatal injections but did receive the same post-partum prophylaxis. Immunization during the first pregnancy occurred in 1 per cent of patients in the control group compared with 0.6 per cent of at-risk patients in the treated group. The benefits also seem to extend into a future pregnancy. Some 528 women in the control group had a second rhesus-positive baby, 11 (2 per cent) developing antibodies for the first time during their second pregnancy. Of 325 women in the treated group who delivered a second rhesus-positive baby only two (0.6 per cent) developed antibodies for the first time during the second pregnancy. Thornton *et al.* (1989) reported a longer follow-up on these patients and reached the same conclusion, namely that antenatal prophylaxis not only reduced the incidence of antibody formation during the index pregnancy but also reduced the incidence of rhesus alloimmunization in a subsequent pregnancy.

The sensitized pregnancy

Several features have played a role in the improved survival of babies affected by red cell alloimmunization, including maternal surveillance, intrauterine fetal transfusion, and neonatal care.

Maternal serological screening

There is clearly an association between the maternal serum concentration of antibodies and the effect upon the fetus (Economides *et al.* 1993). This, however, is relatively imprecise when involving a high concentration of antibody. With the introduction of automated quantitation of Rh(D) antibodies, much more precise and reproducible levels can be reported compared with the lack of precision provided by titres. At present automated quantitation has not been adopted for other red cell antibodies.

Using automated anti-D quantitation, Bowell *et al.* (1982) reported the results for 260 sensitized patients (Table 25.2) demonstrating the direct relationship between maternal anti-D concentrations and cord haemoglobin levels and bilirubin concentrations; there was also a direct association with the need for neonatal exchange transfusion. Importantly, no baby had a cord haemoglobin of less than 10 g/dl if the maximum maternal anti-D concentration was 4 IU/ml or less. Caution in interpretation was expressed for antibody levels of 4–8 IU/ml when further investigations such as amniocentesis or delivery should be considered, and this was positively advised when the level was 8 IU/ml or greater, a situation that occurs in less than 35 per cent of sensitized cases (MacKenzie *et al.* 1991). Similar observations had been reported by Tovey and Haggas (1971).

Failure to detect antibodies in maternal serum in an initial sample during pregnancy does not provide reassurance about rhesus sensitization, since antibodies may appear at any stage during pregnancy. Bowell *et al.* (1986) reported that 30 per cent of 726 women with rhesus antibodies did not have antibodies at their first antenatal testing, while Stangenberg *et al.* (1991) estimated that 50 per cent of women sensitized with rhesus antibodies had none at their first screen. There should be repeat serological assessment of all initially antibody-negative rhesus-negative women at 28 and 34 weeks' gestation. Moreover, maternal antibody levels may rise, fall, or stay the same, irrespective of the antigen status of the fetus (Bowell *et al.* 1982).

When antibody concentrations are higher, in the range when further investigation needs to be considered (> 4 IU/ml), paternal rhesus typing and antigen testing should be performed to confirm that the fetus could be antigen positive.

Biophysical assessment

Over and above a more precise assessment of gestational age (which is clearly a major factor in the management of rhesus alloimmunization) and in helping to localize structures for a more invasive assessment, ultrasound has been used to give some guide to the severity of fetal compromise (Saltzman *et al.* 1989). Although cardiotocography will identify the seriously anaemic fetus, significant changes appear as late indicators and the fetal heart pattern is not sufficiently sensitive to predict mild or moderate disease; there is recent evidence that heart-rate variability, analysed by computer, correlates very strongly with fetal

Table 25.2 Maternal serological studies

Maternal anti-D concentration (IU/ml)	No.	Mean cord haemoglobin (g/dl)	% With cord haemoglobin (<10 g/dl)	% With cord bilirubin (>80 Umol/l}	% Given exchange transfusion
0–2	52	16.2	0	0	2
2–4	26	16.8	0	9	7.7
4–8	29	15.3	37	26.9	55.2
8–16	34	13.7	57.9	55.6	70.8
16–13	38	12.0	74	64	82.1
>32	25	11.0	82.6	66.7	92

From Bowell *et al.* (1982)

haematocrit values and this could have a dramatic impact on antenatal assessment (Economides *et al.* 1992). The detection of signs of severe disease, such as those associated with hydrops, can be reliably made with real-time ultrasound, but this is not helpful in identifying early stage disease. Similarly, observation of fetal movements is insufficiently sensitive for any worthwhile management. Doppler studies on fetal blood flow unfortunately do not correlate well with the degree of fetal anaemia.

Amniocentesis

Once antibody concentrations are sufficiently high and delivery is not an option, an assessment of the effects upon the fetus should be made. Fetal haemolysis will result from the transplacental passage of antibodies; spectrophotometric analysis of bilirubinoid concentration at an optical density of 453 nm on samples of amniotic fluid obtained at amniocentesis will provide an indirect measurement of haemolysis. Bevis (1953) reported that bilirubin and non-haematin iron concentrations in liquor closely reflected the degree of fetal anaemia based on 205 specimens from 98 patients. Liley (1961) demonstrated, in a study of 101 affected fetuses, that the peak of the spectral absorption curve of liquor at 453 nm denoted the severity of the fetal anaemia and described zones of predictive risk. Whitfield (1970) described the use of an 'action line' superimposed upon Liley's data in order to determine the timing of delivery or intrauterine transfusion in 510 affected pregnancies. If the liquor bilirubin peak reached the 'action line' before the 33rd week of pregnancy, intrauterine transfusion was performed whilst after this gestation, delivery was advised.

The prediction of fetal anaemia based on optical density measurement may sometimes be misleading, either giving an overestimate or an underestimate of fetal compromise. Thus, MacKenzie *et al.* (1988) reported that the optical density gave a misleading prediction in 21 per cent of 63 estimates, thus they advocated direct fetal blood sampling as a more accurate alternative.

Fetal blood sampling

In those pregnancies where maternal antibody levels are high enough to warrant intervention and the father of the fetus is heterozygous for the offending antigen, fetal blood sampling to determine the fetal blood group and rhesus type can significantly influence subsequent management (MacKenzie *et al.* 1983). For antigen-positive fetuses, the estimation of fetal haematocrit on samples of fetal blood obtained under ultrasound guidance is the only direct method of assessing the effect of the disease on the fetus, since OD_{453} values on amniotic fluid can be misleading (Forestier *et al.* 1988; MacKenzie *et al.* 1988; Nicolaides *et al.* 1986). A recent study has suggested that fetal blood sampling from an umbilical cord vessel should be considered when maternal anti-D antibody concentration is greater than 15 IU/ml, since at or above this level the fetus could be severely anaemic whereas below this level, anaemia was, at most, mild (Nicolaides and Rodeck 1992).

The risks associated with fetal blood sampling include a fetal loss rate of 2–3 per cent (Daffos *et al.* 1985; MacKenzie *et al.* 1991) and preterm membrane rupture and delivery in 5 per cent (Daffos *et al.* 1985). In addition, further antibody production is stimulated in 28 per cent (Bowell *et al.* 1988; Pratt *et al.* 1989); this latter complication appears to be much more probable if the sampling needle passes transplacentally.

Plasmapheresis

Plasmapheresis, designed to reduce the amount of antibody in rhesus allo-immunized women, may be undertaken, removing plasma with or without reconstituted freeze-dried plasma or plasma protein fraction replacement. The technique has been advocated for the patient who has high antibody levels and the fetus is too immature for intrauterine transfusion (Clarke *et al.* 1970; Graham-Pole *et al.* 1977). The technique generally commences at the start of the second trimester, involves a mean total cumulative plasma exchange of 124 litres, with two or three litres being removed on up to three occasions per week; a mean fall in circulating antibody concentration of around 50 per cent can be achieved.

Robinson and Tovey (1980) reported 14 high-risk cases of rhesus alloimmuni-zation treated by repeated intensive plasma exchange. Although the fetal out-come looked encouraging, complications occurred in 16 per cent of 261 procedures, of which fainting, allergic reactions to the plasma, mild citrate toxicity, or mechanical difficulties were the commonest. Further studies are needed to prove the benefit of this technique.

Immunoglobulin therapy

It has been suggested that the augmentation of plasmapheresis by intravenous high-dose immunoglobulin may help to inhibit maternal antibody synthesis, block antibody transport across the placenta, and hence reduce both the maternal antibody levels and their effect (Berlin *et al.* 1985). As with plasma-pheresis, there is, as yet, no objective assessment to indicate that such an approach offers benefit.

Intrauterine fetal transfusion

If a severely affected fetus is mature enough to deliver, this is the treatment of choice, and even a mildly affected fetus is probably best delivered by 38 weeks' gestation (Stangenberg *et al.* 1991). Liley (1963) reported that selected induction in the presence of rhesus alloimmunization reduced the perinatal mortality rate from 22 to 9 per cent. However, in the most severe cases, some fetuses will be too immature to deliver and intrauterine transfusion will be required to preserve the fetus, this may be performed as early as 18 weeks' gestation (Reece *et al.* 1988).

The technique of fetal intraperitoneal transfusion using fresh group O rhesus-negative blood compatible with the mother was introduced by Liley (1961) and had a dramatic impact upon the management of severely affected cases. Queenan (1969) reported a series of 1097 intraperitoneal transfusions performed on 607 sensitized fetuses with an overall survival rate of 34 per cent. Whitfield *et al.* (1972) reported a series of 252 intraperitoneal transfusions on 166 affected fetuses and described an overall survival rate of 47 per cent with an immediate fetal mortality rate of 12 per cent following the procedure. Death was usually thought to be associated with overtransfusion, fetal damage, anaemia, or preterm labour. Ideally, intrauterine transfusions should occur before the fetus has become hydropic; Frigoletto *et al.* (1981) reported that following the introduction of transfusion under ultrasound control, the survival rate increased to 53 per cent of affected fetuses without hydrops, but only 7 per cent of fetuses with hydrops. Scott *et al.* (1984) reported that intrauterine transfusion under direct ultrasound control increased their salvage rate from 56 per cent of 34 pregnancies to 84 per cent of 37 pregnancies, with a mortality rate of 2.3 per cent per transfusion. Bowman and Manning (1983) demonstrated an overall survival rate of 58 per cent for 257 fetuses managed by 611 intraperitoneal transfusions.

During the past decade, intrauterine transfusion has been performed directly into the fetal circulation, initially using fetoscopy and more recently using ultrasound needle guidance. Rodeck *et al.* (1984) reported an 84 per cent survival in 25 affected fetuses (15 with hydrops) who underwent 77 intravascular transfusions. De Crespigny *et al.* (1985) and Berkowitz *et al.* (1986) reported similar results when transfusing blood into an umbilical vessel, whereas Westgren *et al.* (1988) advocated transfusion directly into the heart. Harman *et al.* (1990) gave the results of 173 transfusions on 44 fetuses using the intravascular approach; the procedure was technically successful in 52 per cent of cases but carried a mortality rate of 2.3 per cent.

The relative merits of the two methods of intrauterine transfusion are being debated, with considerable enthusiasm being expressed for the intravascular method. With the introduction of fetal haematocrit measurement prior to transfusion, the need for treatment can now be confirmed and the appropriate amount of blood to be transfused calculated. The volume of blood required depends upon the fetal haematocrit, the haematocrit of the donor blood, and ultrasound estimate of fetal weight, with the aim of elevating the recipient haematocrit to approximately 45 per cent. Transfusions should not be necessary unless the fetal haematocrit is below 25 per cent before 25 weeks' gestation and 30 per cent beyond that stage (MacKenzie *et al.* 1991).

The outcome of the two approaches has been compared with differing results, as shown in Tables 25.3 and 25.4. The study reported in Table 25.3 (MacKenzie *et al.* 1991) would suggest that with modern ultrasound equipment, the intraperitoneal route is safer, with fewer cases of transfusion-induced

Table 25.3 Intrauterine transfusion

	Intraperitoneal transfusion	Intravascular transfusion
No. of fetuses	14	12
No. of transfusions	38	32
Acute fetal distress with transfusion (%)	0	28
Emergency Caesarean section (%)	0	33
Survival (%)	79	67

From MacKenzie *et al.* (1991)

Table 25.4 Intrauterine transfusion

	Intraperitoneal transfusion	Intravascular transfusion
No. of fetuses	44	44
No. of transfusions	104	174
Failed attempts (%)	11.5	8.1
Procedural complications (%)	37.5	9.8
Traumatic deaths (%)	18.2	2.3
Gestational age at delivery (mean No. of weeks)	30.7	34.1
Mean No. of exchange transfusions	1.8	0.8
Survival (%)	66	91

From Harman *et al.* (1990)

fetal distress than are encountered using the intravascular route. There was a significant increase in the incidence of emergency Caesarean section for fetal distress following direct intravascular transfusion and with a higher survival following intraperitoneal transfusion. The second study, illustrated in Table 25.4 (Harman *et al.* 1990), also non-randomized, suggested that complications including traumatic deaths were greater following intraperitoneal transfusion than intravascular transfusion, with a greater survival after intravascular transfusion. It would seem that different workers are reporting a different experience with these two routes of transfusion and further information will be required in order that a firm conclusion may be reached. It must, however, be remembered that mothers of fetuses transfused *in utero* are very good antibody producers, and will readily develop increased and additional antibodies (Bowell *et al.* 1988; Pratt *et al.* 1989). It is evident that *in utero* transfusions should only be given when there is convincing evidence of impending serious fetal compromise.

Other red cell antibodies

While rhesus alloimmunization is the major cause of haemolytic disease of the newborn, other red cell antibodies are capable of producing the disease. Death from haemolytic disease related to other antigens is relatively rare. Thus, in 1985 in England and Wales, there were only four deaths due to antibodies other than anti-D (anti-E, anti-C, and anti-Kell), while there were 33 deaths due to anti-D alloimmunization (Clarke *et al*. 1987). With such low frequencies of the other alloimmunized cases, complacency and ignorance result about a disease which can be as lethal as that due to anti-D. Similar vigilance is thus required during pregnancy with recourse to amniocentesis or more appropriately, fetal blood sampling (amniotic fluid OD_{453} can be very misleading in Kell sensitization). Such investigations are not often required before 28 weeks' gestation and only when the antibody titration value is 1/64 or greater (MacKenzie *et al*. 1991).

Anti-A and anti-B antibodies may be seen when the mother is group O, and while mild neonatal jaundice occurs in 3 per cent of such situations, an exchange transfusion will only be needed in 0.003 per cent of cases. Intrauterine death due to ABO incompatibility has not been described. Amniocentesis or fetal blood sampling are thus not indicated.

Conclusions

The development of techniques to investigate the fetus directly *in utero* has been a major advance allowing more precise and appropriate management to be given. These investigative methods may well have applications for the management of more unusual causes of fetal anaemia due to circulating antibodies. In view of the significant reduction in the incidence of severe rhesus alloimmunization, the experience of individual obstetric units is so small that there is a strong case for directing referral of such patients to specialist units. Additionally, a continuing awareness of the risks to the small number of cases complicated by other antibodies that can cause severe fetal haemolysis during the antenatal period must be maintained (*Lancet* 1991).

While the perinatal mortality rate due to rhesus alloimmunization has fallen by approximately 96 per cent over the last 40 years, new cases still occur due either to a failure to administer any anti-D at the appropriate time, a failure to give an adequate dose, or to an unprovoked unrecognized sensitization during the antenatal period. Greater discipline in prophylactic administration of anti-D is still required. The routine antenatal administration of prophylaxis at 28 and 34 weeks' gestation should also help to reduce the incidence further. However, at present there are not limitless supplies of anti-D gammaglobulin and it is hoped that a synthetic form may become available in the near future.

References

Berkowitz, R. L., Chitkara, V., Goldberg, J. K., Wilkins, I., Chervenak, F. A., and Lynch, L. (1986). Intrauterine intravascular transfusion for severe red blood cell isoimmunisation. *American Journal of Obstetrics and Gynecology* 155, 574–81.

Berlin, G., Selbing, A., and Ryden, G. (1985). Rhesus haemolytic disease treated with high-dose intravenous immunoglobulin. *Lancet* i, 1153.

Bevis, D. C. A. (1953). The composition of liquor amnii in haemolytic disease of the newborn. *Journal of Obstetrics and Gynaecology of the British Empire* 60, 244–51.

Bowell, P., Wainscoat, J. S., Peto, T. E. A., and Gunson, H. H. (1982). Maternal anti-D concentrations and outcome in rhesus haemolytic disease of the newborn. *British Medical Journal* 285, 323–9.

Bowell, P. J., Allen, D. L., and Entwistle, C. C. (1986). Blood group antibody screening test during pregnancy. *British Journal of Obstetrics and Gynaecology* 93, 1038–43.

Bowell, P. J., Selinger, M., Ferguson, J., Giles, J., and MacKenzie, I. Z. (1988). Antenatal fetal blood sampling for the management of alloimmunized pregnancies. *British Journal of Obstetrics and Gynaecology* 95, 759–64.,

Bowman, J. M. and Manning, F. A. (1983). Intra-uterine transfusions: Winnipeg 1982. *Obstetrics and Gynecology* 61, 203–9.

Bowman, J. M. and Pollock, J. M. (1978). Antenatal prophylaxis of rhesus isoimmunisation. *Canadian Medical Association Journal* 118, 627–30.

Clarke, C. A., Donohoe, W. T. A., McConnell, R. B., Woodrow, J. C., Finn, R., Krevans, J. R., *et al.* (1963). Further experimental studies on the prevention of rhesus haemolytic disease. *British Medical Journal* 1, 979–84.

Clarke, C. A., Elson, C. J., Bradley, J., Donohoe, T. A., and Lehane, D. (1970). Intensive plasmapheresis as a therapeutic measure in rhesus immunised women. *Lancet* i, 793–8.

Clarke, C. A., Whitfield, A. G. W., and Mollison, P. L. (1987) Death from rhesus haemolytic disease in England and Wales in 1984 and 1985. *British Medical Journal* 294, 1001.

Combined Study in England and Baltimore (1966). Prevention of rhesus haemolytic disease. *British Medical Journal* 2, 907–14.

Daffos, F., Capella-Pavlovsky, M., and Forestier, F. (1985), Fetal blood sampling during pregnancy with the use of a needle guided by ultrasound. *American Journal of Obstetrics and Gynecology* 153, 655–60.

Dayton, V. D., Anderson, D. S., Crosson, J. T., and Cruikshank, S. H. (1990). A case of rhesus isoimmunization. *American Journal of Obstetrics and Gynecology* 163, 63–4.

De Crespigny, L., Robinson, H. P., Quinn, M., Doyle, L., Ross, A., and Cauchi, M. (1985). Ultrasound-guided fetal blood transfusion for severe isoimmunization. *Obstetrics and Gynecology* 66, 529–32.

Economides, D. L., Selinger, M., Ferguson, J., Bowell, P., Dawes, G., and MacKenzie, T. Z. (1992). Computerized measurement of heart rate variation in fetal anaemia secondary to rhesus alloimmunization. *American Journal of Obstetrics and Gynecology* 167, 689–93.

Economides, D. L., Bowell, P. J., Selinger, M., Pratt, G. A., Ferguson, J., and MacKenzie, I. Z. (1993). Anti-D concentrations in fetal and maternal serum and amniotic fluid and rhesus allo-immunized pregnancies. *British Journal of Obstetrics and Gynaecology* 100, 923–6.

Everett, C. B. (1988). Is anti-D immunoglobulin unnecessary in the domiciliary treatment of miscarriages? *British Medical Journal* **297**, 732–3.

Forestier, F., Cox, W. L., Daffos, F., and Rainaut, M. (1988). The assessment of fetal blood samples. *American Journal of Obstetrics and Gynecology* **158**, 1184–8.

Freda, V. J., Gorman, J. G., and Pollack, W. (1966). Rhesus factor: prevention of isoimmunization and clinical trials on mothers. *Science* **151**, 828–9.

Frigoletto, F. D., Umansky, I., Birnholz, J., Acker, D., Easterday, C. L., Harris, G. B. I., *et al.* (1981). Intra-uterine fetal transfusion in 365 fetuses during 15 years. *American Journal of Obstetrics and Gynecology* **139**, 781–90.

Graham-Pole, J., Barr, W., and Willoughby, M. L. M. (1977). Continuous-flow plasmapheresis in management of severe rhesus disease. *British Medical Journal* **1**, 1185–8.

Harman, C. R., Bowman, J. M., Manning, F. A., and Menticoglou, S. M. (1990). Intra-uterine transfusion — intraperitoneal versus intravascular approach: a case controlled study. *American Journal of Obstetrics and Gynecology* **162**, 1053–9.

Hughes, R. G., Craig, J. I. O., Murphy, W. G., and Greer, I. A. (1994). Causes and clinical consequences of Rhesus (D) haemolytic disease of the newborn. *British Journal of Obstetrics and Gynaecology* **101**, 297–300.

Lancet (1991). Dangers of anti-Kell in pregnancy. *Lancet* **337**, 1319–20.

Levine, P. (1958). The influence of the ABO system on rhesus haemolytic disease. *Human Biology* **30**, 14–15.

Liley, A. W. (1961). Liquor amnii analysis in the management of the pregnancy complication by rhesus isoimmunization. *American Journal of Obstetrics and Gynecology* **82**, 1359–70.

Liley, A. W. (1963). Intra-uterine transfusion of fetus in haemolytic disease. *British Medical Journal* **2**, 1107–9.

MacKenzie, I. Z., Guest, C. M., and Bowell, P. J. (1983). Fetal blood group studies during mid-trimester pregnancy and the management of severe isoimmunization. *Prenatul Diagnosis* **3**, 41–6.

MacKenzie, I. Z., Bowell, P. J., Castle, B. M., Selinger, M., and Ferguson, J. F. (1988). Serial fetal blood sampling for the management of pregnancy complicated by severe rhesus isoimmunization. *British Journal of Obstetrics and Gynaecology* **95**, 753–8.

MacKenzie, I. Z., Selinger, M., and Bowell, P. J. (1991). The management of red cell isoimmunization in the 1990s. In *Progress in obstetrics and gynaecology* Vol. 9 (ed. J. Studd), pp. 31–53. Churchill Livingstone, Edinburgh.

MacKenzie, I. Z., Bowell, P. J., and Selinger, M. (1992). Deaths from haemolytic disease of the newborn. *British Medical Journal* **304**, 1175–6.

Nicolaides, K. H. and Rodeck, C. H. (1992). Maternal serum anti-D antibody concentration and assessment of rhesus isoimmunization. *British Medical Journal* **304**, 1155–6.

Nicolaides, K. H., Rodeck, C. H., Mibashan, R. S., and Kemp, J. R. (1986). Have Liley charts outlived their usefulness? *American Journal of Obstetrics and Gynecology* **155**, 90–4.

Pratt, G. A., Bowell, P. J., MacKenzie, I. Z., Ferguson, J., and Selinger, M. (1989). Production of additional atypical alloantibodies in RhD-sensitized pregnancies managed by intra-uterine investigation methods. *Clinical Laboratory Haematology* **11**, 241–8.

Queenan, J. T. (1969). Intra-uterine transfusion. *American Journal of Obstetrics and Gynecology* **104**, 397–405.

Reece, E. A., Copel, J. L., Scioscia, L. A., Grannum, P. A. T., De Gennaro, N., and Hobbins, J. C. (1988). Diagnostic fetal umbilical blood sampling in the management of isoimmunization. *American Journal of Obstetrics and Gynecology* **159**, 1057–62.

Robinson, E. A. E. and Tovey, L. A. D. (1980). Intensive plasma exchange in the management of severe rhesus disease. *British Journal of Haematology* 45, 621–31.

Rodeck, C. H., Nicolaides, K. H., Warsof, S. L., Fysh, W. J., Gamsu, H. R., and Kept, J. R. (1984). The management of severe rhesus isoimmunisation by fetoscopic intravascular transfusions. *American Journal of Obstetrics and Gynecology* 150, 769–74.

Saltzman, D. H., Frigoletto, F. D., Harlow, B. L., Bass, V. A., and Benacerraf, B. R. (1989). Sonographic evaluation of hydrops fetalis. *Obstetrics and Gynecology* 74, 106–11.

Scott, J. R., Kochenour, N. K., Larkin, R. M., and Scott, M. J. (1984). Changes in the management of severely rhesus immunised patients. *American Journal of Obstetrics and Gynecology* 149, 336–41.

Selinger, M. (1991). Immunoprophylaxis for rhesus disease—expensive but worth it? *British Journal of Obstetrics and Gynaecology* 98, 509–12.

Stangenberg, G. M., Selbing, A., Lineman, G., and Westgren, M. (1991). Rhesus isoimmunisation. *Obstetric and Gynecological Survey* 46, 189–95.

Tabor, A., Jerne, D., and Bock, J. E. (1986). Incidence of rhesus immunisation after genetic amniocentesis. *British Medical Journal* 293, 533–6.

Thornton, J. G., Page, C., Foot, G., Arthur, G. R., Tovey, L. A. D., and Scott, J. S. (1989). Efficacy and long-term effects of antenatal prophylaxis with anti-D immunoglobulin. *British Medical Journal* 298, 1671–3.

Tovey, L. A. D. (1986). Haemolytic disease of the newborn—the changing scene. *British Journal of Obstetrics and Gynaecology* 93, 960–6.

Tovey, L. A. D. (1988). Anti-D and miscarriages. *British Medical Journal* 297, 977–8.

Tovey, L. A. D. and Haggas, W. K. (1971). Prediction of the severity of rhesus haemolytic disease by means of antibody titrations. *British Journal of Haematology* 20, 25–33.

Tovey, L. A. D., Murray, J., Stevenson, B. J., and Taverner, J. M. (1978). Prevention of rhesus haemolytic disease. *British Medical Journal* 2, 106–8.

Tovey, L. A. D., Townley, A., Stevenson, B. J., and Taverner, J. M. (1983). The Yorkshire antenatal anti-D immunoglobulin trial in primigravidae. *Lancet* ii, 224–6.

Urbaniak, S. J. (1985). Rhesus haemolytic disease of the newborn. *British Medical Journal* 291, 4–6.

Westgren, M., Selbing, A., and Strangenberg, M. (1988). Fetal intra-cardiac transfusion in patients with severe rhesus isoimmunization. *American Journal of Obstetrics and Gynecology* 108, 1239–44.

Whitfield, C. R. (1970). A three-year assessment of an 'action line' method of timing intervention in rhesus isoimmunization. *British Medical Journal* 296, 885–6.

Whitfield, C. R., Thompson, W., Armstrong, M. J., and Reed, M. M. (1972). Intra-uterine fetal transfusion for severe rhesus haemolytic disease. *Journal of Obstetrics and Gynaecology of the British Commonwealth* 79, 931–40.

26   Natural childbirth and intervention

There is no real definition of 'natural childbirth'. This blanket term tends to mean different things to different people. However, for the purpose of this chapter, the authors have chosen a selection of topics which represent situations where either the view of the obstetrician and the views of some of his or her patients have not always concurred, or situations where points of practice have become accepted without as full a scientific assessment as might be ideal.

The topics which will be discussed in this chapter are:

(1) antenatal preparation;

(2) supportive companionship during labour;

(3) routine procedures;

(4) analgesia — alternatives;

(5) the augmentation of labour;

(6) posture during labour and delivery;

(7) instrumental delivery;

(8) episiotomy;

(9) the third stage — active management;

(10) breast is best;

(11) the place of birth;

(12) the use of vitamin K.

Antenatal preparation

Numerous antenatal patients attend numerous antenatal classes given by numerous health-care professionals throughout the world, yet hard scientific evidence for the value of these classes is limited. Most of the trials involving antenatal classes or companionship during labour are uncontrolled (other than Hofmeyr *et al.* 1991 and Huttel *et al.* 1972). The uncontrolled evidence is more likely to describe the type of patient who attends antenatal classes or who has supportive companionship rather than provide information about the effect of these interventions. For instance, Cave (1978) reported 2302 patients of whom 678 had planned 'natural childbirth'. Those women who wished for natural childbirth were, when compared to a control group, slightly older (mean of two years), better educated, of higher socio-ecomonic status, more likely to be

Table 26.1 The value of antenatal classes

	Antenatal classes	No classes
No. of patients	123	66
% 1st stage less than 12 hours	41	26
% 1st stage less than 24 hours	80	56
% Forceps delivery	7	27
% Caesarean section	0	1

From Brant *et al.* (1962)

Jewish, and less likely to be Catholic. Leonard (1973) also reported the characteristics of 26 women who selected antenatal classes with 16 who did not; this author found that those who selected classes were more likely to be older, better educated, of higher socio-economic status, more likely to breast-feed, and more likely to have a planned pregnancy than those who did not select antenatal classes.

Brant (1962) compared the obstetric outcome of 123 primigravidae chosen for intense individual antenatal education by a childbirth educator who then accompanied the woman in labour with that of 66 primigravidae who received a less individualized form of antenatal education. Although this is an old study, it was an important one in that it demonstrated shorter labours with less operative delivery (see Table 26.1) in the women who received the more intensive education and support. However, as it was not a randomized trial the results may be subject to some of the biases already mentioned. In another unrandomized comparison, Davis and Morrone (1962) compared the labours of 355 primigravid patients who elected to attend antenatal classes with 108 who elected not to attend such classes. There were no differences in the duration of labour, amount of analgesia required, or the type of delivery between the two groups. A recent review of the evidence has concluded that antenatal classes themselves have little to do with obstetric outcomes (Simkin and Enkin 1989).

There is, however, reasonably good quality evidence to suggest that women who attend antenatal classes have a lesser requirement for analgesia during labour than women who do not attend such classes. Beck *et al.* (1980) used a multiple regression analysis for 67 patients who attended antenatal classes and 35 who did not. Those who attended were less anxious about their pain during labour than were those who did not attend, although the overall need for analgesia was similar in both groups. Melzack *et al.* (1981) measured pain during labour using the McGill Pain Questionnaire in 87 primigravidae and 54 multigravidae during labour. There was no difference in pain appreciation between those multigravidae who had attended classes and those who had not, but there was a decrease in pain appreciation in those primigravidae who had attended classes compared with those who did not. There was also a reduced need for analgesia in primigravidae who had attended classes. The use of 'coping techniques' for pain (such as breathing, relaxation, distraction, and yoga) may also delay the need for analgesia during labour in primigravidae (Copstick *et al.* 1986).

On a superficial basis, one may draw the conclusion from the above soft evidence that antenatal preparation, especially in primgravid patients, is associated with the need for less analgesia. Only if that analgesia should be a regional block is there then a significant difference in the mode of operative delivery.

The potential for antenatal classes to do harm has also been considered, but the evidence for this is flimsy. There have been some anecdotal reports concerning the feelings of failure which may occur in patients who elect to have natural childbirth but in whom a complication arises and intervention occurs. Stewart (1982) reported that each partner may blame themselves, or each other, and attributed the need for psychiatric help in five women and four men to be due to events which occurred during labour or delivery. The author concluded that 'flexibility' by both patients and staff, was the most appropriate attitude towards labour and delivery. The place of antenatal classes in the reduction of labour complications, as opposed to the education of the recipients, remains to be proven.

Supportive companionship during labour

Three randomized controlled trials have assessed the effect of a supportive companion in labour on obstetric outcome and the need for analgesia (Hofmeyr *et al.* 1991; Klaus *et al.* 1986; Sosa *et al.* 1980). In the two Guatemalan trials, the presence of a supportive labour companion was associated with a reduction in the duration of labour, the incidence of meconium-stained liquor, and of instrumental delivery. Although no such effects were seen in the Hofmeyr trial, social support was still beneficial in improving the maternal perception of coping well during labour, decreasing the perception of pain, and reducing the need for repeated analgesia (Hofmeyr *et al.* 1991). Such companionship may also reduce the risk of post-partum depression in randomized trials (Wolman *et al.* 1993).

Routine procedures

Recent years have resulted in a questioning of many routine procedures. These include shaving, the use of enemas, the use of masks, and the antenatal case record.

The shaving or clipping of pubic hair has been a traditional part of the preparation for childbirth (Johnston and Sidall 1922). Kantor *et al.* (1965) cultured the pubic skin at delivery in 50 women who were shaved during early labour and 50 who were not shaved. There was no significant difference in the percentage in whom microorganisms were grown. The authors concluded that merely clipping long hairs in order to avoid inclusion in obstetric forceps or in an episiotomy was all that was necessary. There was no post-partum advantage from shaving. Other non-randomized trials have come to similar conclusions (Romney 1980).

Traditional teaching has stated that the lack of an enema may delay descent of the presenting part, lead to unacceptable faecal contamination, and embarass the mother by the involuntary passing of faeces during the second stage of labour. Romney and Gordon (1981) reported a non-randomized trial in which 124 patients had an enema in early labour and 100 patients did not. Faecal contamination occurred during the second stage of labour in 35 per cent of patients who had an enema compared with 39 per cent of patients who did not. The authors then commenced a randomly allocated trial which had to be abandoned because 'the midwives were drawing their own conclusions and it was becoming difficult to adhere to the agreed protocol'. Drayton and Rees (1984) reported a randomly allocated trial of enemas in 222 women during labour. The mean duration of labour was the same in those primigravidae who had an enema compared with those multigravidae who did not. Faecal contamination during the second stage of labour occurred in 22 per cent of 109 women in the enema group but in 44 per cent of 113 women in the control group. Although there was statistically more faecal contamination in the control group, this was generally 'minimal faecal soiling' and 'unlikely to cause embarassment to the patient'. Perhaps, therefore, patients should be given the choice.

The use of face masks is becoming less common on our labour wards. Turner *et al.* (1984) reported that the incidence of puerperal infection in a controlled series of 1750 consecutive mothers when face masks were used routinely in the delivery room was statistically similar to the incidence of infection in a second series of 1750 consecutive mothers after the use of face masks had been abandoned other than at Caesarean section.

The available evidence still suggests that face masks should be used at Caesarean section. Orr (1981) reported a four-year period during which the incidence of wound infection was 4 per cent in 1634 general surgical wounds when masks were worn in the operating theatre, whereas in a six-month period over which time no masks were worn, the wound infection rate fell to 1.8 per cent of 432 wounds. However, Chamberlain and Houang (1984) randomly allocated the wearing of face masks by the team of surgeons and nurses in 41 gynaecological operations. Although there was no infection associated with unmasked vaginal surgery or minor abdominal surgery, there was an increased incidence of wound infection in the unmasked group compared with the masked group for patients undergoing major gynaecological surgery. The trial was abandoned following three wound infections in five patients undergoing major abdominal surgery without the use of masks compared with none when masks were worn. It will be well known to many readers of this book that Professor Chamberlain has a beard, and such studies may need to substratify for this feature. Substratification should also occur for 'mask wiggling' related to facial movements, including talking (Chamberlain and Houang 1984; Schweizer 1976). The type of mask worn will also influence the surgical infection rate;

synthetic material, in general, resulting in less infection than do paper masks (Rogers 1980).

It may, therefore, be reasonable to abandon the use of masks for vaginal procedures and delivery, but to continue their use at Caesarean section.

There is a recent vogue for patients to carry their own case records rather than a 'shared-care' card. Over and above any discussion on patients' rights, this is something which occurs not uncommonly in general practice (Bird and Walji 1986). Clearly, some patients may be upset by alarming apparently insulting, or sensitive information within the records, and communication between doctors concerning the patient may be inhibited (Sergeant 1986). Some authors have suggested that patients could be made more responsible for their own health by better education (including during consultations) rather than having access to their records (Sergeant 1986; Short 1986). There are two particular advantages when patients carry their own case records. There is evidence that patient compliance with therapy is enhanced (McLaren 1991) and that communication between doctors is improved (Bull 1983; Zander *et al*. 1978).

Not all patients wish to carry their own records. Draper *et al*. (1986) reported a study of 96 women of whom 74 per cent liked to carry their own notes, 86 per cent thought that there was some advantage to this system, 44 per cent considered that it gave them a more responsible attitude towards their pregnancy, but 46 per cent found the notes difficult to carry, 11 per cent forgot to bring them to a clinic visit, and 3 per cent were worried that there might be some information in the notes which they would rather not know.

There has been a randomized trial of 251 women allocated to carry either their own full obstetric case notes or a shared-care card (Elbourne *et al*. 1987). Some 36 per cent of the 132 women who held their own notes felt able to talk to doctors or midwives 'more easily' compared with 21 per cent of 119 women who held a shared-care card. The only other concrete advantage was a decreased work load for clerical staff. Notes were unavailable on 4 per cent of all occasions in both groups, either 'forgotten' by patients or 'lost' by the medical records department.

Whether or not this practice increases in relation to obstetric case records depends upon its perceived purpose. If it is perceived that greater patient involvement will be encouraged, or greater patient responsibility will result, it is likely to continue. If it is perceived that better communication between the providers of obstetric care will occur, then perhaps it should be superseded by the use of information technology. Finally, as of November 1991, patients in the UK have a right of access to their *written* medical records.

Analgesia—alternatives

The traditional analgesia for patients during labour consists of intramuscular pethidine and 'gas and oxygen'. Regional blockage, generally in the form of epidural anaesthesia, is now widely used during labour.

Table 26.2 The effects of analgesia

	Epidural group	Conventional analgesia group
No. of patients	100	102
% Second stage < 30 minutes	36	66.7
% Forceps delivery	30	5.9
% Apgar < 7 at 5 minutes	1	4.9
% Umbilical artery pH < 7.20	1	7.8
% Late decelerations on CTG	6	8.8

From Noble *et al.* (1971)

Table 26.3 The effects of analgesia

	Primigravid patients		Multigravid patients	
	Epidural	Pethidine	Epidural	Pthidine
No. of patients	28	30	17	18
% Forceps delivery	51	27	30	6

From Robinson *et al.* (1980)

There have been nine randomized controlled trials (of variable quality) comparing epidural analgesia with narcotic analgesia. Data from these trials have been analysed by Howell (1992). The available evidence confirms the obvious superiority of the pain relief provided by epidural analgesia. The effect of epidural analgesia on the first stage of labour is unclear, but there may be a tendency for women using epidural analgesia to have a longer first stage of labour and to require oxytocin augmentation more frequently. The effect on the second stage is more marked, with a three to four-fold increase in the instrumental vaginal delivery rate. The mean length of the second stage of labour is increased in nulliparous patients from 58 minutes to 97 minutes, whilst the mean length of the second stage of labour is increased in multiparous patients from 19 minutes to 54 minutes in the presence of an epidural (Paterson *et al.* 1992) but with delayed pushing, epidural analgesia need not be associated with an increased operative delivery rate (Reynolds 1993). No clear picture emerges from the randomized trials of the effect on the newborn. There may be a small benefit in that fewer babies in the epidural group have a low Apgar score.

A large observational study has raised the question of adverse maternal side-effects of epidural anaesthesia persisting up to a year after delivery. Women who had used epidural analgesia had a substantially increased incidence of backache, headache, tingling, and numbness compared with women who had not availed of epidural analgesia (MacArthur *et al.* 1990). Unfortunately, none of the investigators who carried out randomized trials had built in longterm follow-up into their study designs. It seems inevitable that great uncertainty about the longterm effects is going to remain until the hypothesis raised by MacArthur *et al.* (1990) has been tested in a randomized trial. For the woman aspiring towards 'natural childbirth' the chief disadvantages of epidural analgesia are the risk of assisted vaginal delivery and the impossibility of ambulation during labour.

There has been increased recent interest in non-pharmacological techniques of analgesia, including TENS (transcutaneous electrical nerve stimulation), hypnosis, and acupuncture.

The analgesic effects of transcutaneous electrical nerve stimulation may occur via the release of endorphins. Sjolund *et al.* (1977) reported a significant increase in cerebrospinal fluid endorphin levels following acupuncture or TENS in 67 per cent of nine patients who underwent repeated lumbar puncture. However, a similar percentage of control patients who underwent repeated lumbar puncture without TENS increased their cerebrospinal fluid endorphin levels. The available evidence suggests that TENS is a safe form of treatment, that it does not interfere with fetal heart monitoring, and that it has no demonstrable effect upon the fetus (Bunsden and Ericson 1982; Harrison *et al.* 1986).

Only uncontrolled trials have demonstrated a benefit as regards pain relief during labour. Augustinsson *et al.* (1977) reported 147 women who used TENS for analgesia during labour; 44 per cent considered their pain relief to be 'good' or 'very good', 44 per cent 'moderate', and 12 per cent 'without effect'. Harrison *et al.* (1986) randomly allocated 100 primigravid and 50 multigravid patients to receive either TENS or TENS-placebo machine during labour. There were no significant differences between the TENS and the TENS-placebo users in terms of their concept of pain, or the midwives' assessment of pain relief, or the need for additional analgesia. Neshein (1981) randomized 70 women in labour to receive TENS or a placebo apparatus. There were no differences in the degree of pain relief between the two groups. Some 14 per cent of both groups reported 'good pain relief', whilst opiate analgesia was required by 74 per cent of the women in the TENS group and 77 per cent of those in the control group.

It would, therefore, seem that the use of transcutaneous electrical nerve stimulation during labour for analgesia is a placebo effect.

The value of hypnosis has been assessed during labour. Freeman *et al.* (1986) randomly allocated 65 primigravidae, all of whom had attended antenatal preparation classes, to a trail of self-hypnosis. There were no differences in the need for conventional analgesia or in operative delivery rates between the 29 patients having self-hypnosis and the 36 controls.

Acupuncture has been evaluated during labour for both efficacy and safety. Wallis *et al.* (1974) administered acupuncture to 21 women during labour, either by manual manipulation of the needles or by battery-operated electro-acupuncture. Some 91 per cent of the patients considered their analgesia to have been 'inadequate', some 76 per cent of the patients requested additional analgesia, and the authors considered that no patient had adequate analgesia. There were no maternal or fetal complications from acupuncture. Abouleish and Depp (1975) reported the use of electro-acupuncture in 12 women during labour. Some 60 per cent of the patients felt that their pain had been reduced, but 83 per cent of the women ultimately requested regional analgesia. The authors concluded that the technique was time consuming, of limited value, and interfered with the electronic monitoring of the fetus.

All that can really be said about the non-pharmacological methods of pain relief during labour is that they are liked by some patients and that they seem to help some patients, but there is no evidence from more scientific studies that they offer any particular benefit other than the avoidance of the side-effects of those alternative methods in use.

The augmentation of labour

The place of augmentation during labour has been discussed in Chapter 18 (The management of labour). Readers should, therefore, consult that chapter for the information which assesses the efficacy and safety of the augmentation of labour.

Posture during labour and delivery

The effects of different postures upon the first and second stages of labour have been widely studied. Changes in posture are associated with certain physiological changes, especially in uterine blood flow, uterine activity, and in pelvic dimensions.

The posture of the patient may, during the first stage of labour, affect uterine blood flow, and, hence, potentially, placental function, uterine contraction, and the efficacy of those contractions. Veland and Hansen (1969), using catheter studies, demonstrated in 23 patients during early labour that a change from the supine to the lateral position produced an increase in cardiac output of 22 per cent, a decrease in heart rate of 6 per cent, and an increase in stroke volume of 27 per cent. The position of the patient is, hence, of some importance to maternal haemodynamics and may be particulary important in patients with compromised cardiac status. The haemodynamic changes associated with aortocaval compression have been confirmed by several authors (Eckstein and Marx 1974). The effect of these haemodyamic changes upon the fetal heart rate is well recognized. Abitbol (1985) described a cohort of 902 patients in labour of whom 14 per cent demonstrated late deceleratons of the fetal heart rate in the supine position, whereas only 11 per cent demonstrated such changes in the left lateral position.

Uterine activity will also vary with maternal position. The classical study of Caldeyro-Barcia *et al.* (1960) measured uterine activity by recording amniotic fluid pressure in 84 patients. They demonstrated that the mean intensity of contractions was 7.6 mmHg greater in the lateral than in the supine position, whilst the mean frequency of contractions was reduced by 0.7 contractions per 10 minutes in the lateral compared with the supine position. Not all publications have confirmed these findings. Chen *et al.* (1987) studied intrauterine pressure in 116 patients during labour and demonstrated that, whilst the resting pressure within the uterus was greater when sitting than when supine, the contraction pressure did not differ between these positions.

There is also some evidence that pelvic dimensions vary with the position of the patient. Lilford *et al.* (1989) performed X-ray pelvimetry on 43 women in the squatting and erect positions. The act of squatting increased the transverse and anteroposterior pelvic dimensions by 1 per cent.

There have been several trials which have made use of these concepts and these will now be discussed.

Posture and the first stage of labour

There is debate concerning the posture which patients should be encouraged to adopt during the first stage of labour. Flynn *et al.* (1978) randomized 68 women to be either ambulant or recumbent during labour. The mean length of the first stage of labour was 4 hours in the ambulant group compared with 6.7 hours in the recumbent group. All the patients in the recumbent group required analgesia, whereas only 41 per cent of the ambulant patients did so. There were no particular disadvantages in monitoring the ambulant patients who underwent fetal heart monitoring using telemetry. This study suggested that there were demonstrable advantages of ambulation during labour. Conversely, there have been more studies which have failed to demonstrate these results. Williams *et al.* (1980) reported a larger study with random allocation between ambulance and recumbency during labour. There were no differences between the two groups for the lengths of the first stage of labour. Other studies reached the same conclusion (McManus and Calder 1978). Similarly, other studies have failed to demonstrate any reduction in the need for analgesia in ambulant patients (Calvert *et al.* 1982; McManus and Calder 1978). It would seem unlikely, therefore, that maternal position during the first stage of labour has any significant effect upon the length of that stage or upon the need for analgesia.

There has been interest in the need for oxytocin in ambulant patients during labour. Read *et al.* (1981) reported 14 patients who had inadequate contractions during the first stage of labour; six patients were randomized to receive oxytocin and eight to be ambulatory. Both techniques appeared to stimulate uterine contractions to a similar degree. Similarly, Flynn *et al.* (1978) reported that 18 per cent of 34 ambulatory women required augmentation of labour compared with 35 per cent of 34 recumbent patients. Williams *et al.* (1980) found no difference in the incidence of augmentation between ambulatory and recumbent patients. Again, no consistent reduction in the need for oxytocin can be found in randomized trials.

There is no doubt, however, that some patients prefer to be ambulant. McManus and Calder (1978) reported that 60 per cent of ten multiparous patients allocated to be ambulant were keen to stay ambulant as were 30 per cent of ten primigravidae. Williams *et al.* (1980) were able to recruit 103 patients to their trial of ambulation, but a further 30 patients refused recruitment either because they wished for epidural analgesia or because they were too distressed and wished to lie down. Calvert *et al.* (1982) reported that of 100 women monitored by telemetry, 44 per cent elected to get out of bed and then 'often only for short periods'. Stewart and Calder (1984) reported 269 women who were asked to choose between remaining in bed or being ambulant during labour. Ambulation was chosen by 57 per cent of the patients in general, by 71 per cent of 139 women in induced labour, and by 41 per cent of 130 women in spontaneous labour, by 41 per cent of 68 primigravidae, and by 62 per cent of 201 multigravidae. When the ambulant group were considered as a whole, there were no differences in the length of labour, analgesic requirements, the need for oxytocic augmentation, or the mode of delivery as compared with the recumbent group as a whole, although the subgroup of ambulant multigravidae required less analgesia than any other subgroup and the subgroup of ambulant primigravidae had shorter first stages than recumbent primigravidae. This study, therefore, failed to show any consistent benefits, or harm, from ambulation even in women who actively chose ambulation during labour. It would seem that patients with an uncomplicated labour should be allowed to adopt the posture they prefer.

Posture and the second stage of labour

There is abundant but conflicting evidence concerning the relationship between ambulation during the first stage of labour, maternal position during the second stage, and the mode of delivery. The increased use of epidural analgesia by women allocated to recumbent positions in the first stage might be expected to increase the likelihood of instrumental delivery in that group. However, the majority of randomized studies demonstrated no differences in the modes of delivery (Calvert *et al.* 1982; McManus and Calder 1978; Stewart and Calder 1984).

Other studies have considered the effect of different positions during the second stage of labour upon its duration and outcome. The two major areas of evaluation relate to the use of a birth chair and squatting. The birth chair has ancient origins, referred to in the the Bible and in ancient Egyptian papyrus.

Several randomized studies have compared delivery in the conventional dorsal position with the use of a birth chair (Crowley *et al.* 1991; Hemminki *et al.* 1986; Stewart *et al.* 1983; Turner *et al.* 1986). In a recent overview of eight such randomized trials, there were no differences between delivery in the chair or in bed for the length of the second stage of labour, the length of time spent bearing down, or in the incidence of operative vaginal delivery. Some studies have failed to show any difference in the incidence of episiotomy between delivery in chair or bed (Turner *et al.* 1986), whilst other studies have suggested that episiotomy occurs less frequently in patients using the birth chair because of the increased difficulty in performing the procedure (Stewart *et al*. 1983). Similarly, some studies have suggested no difference in the incidence of perineal tears between the two groups (Crowley *et al*. 1991; Stewart *et al*. 1983), whilst other studies have found an increase in the incidence of perineal tears in patients delivering in the chair (Turner *et al*. 1986). Overall, it is unlikely that the incidence of perineal trauma will be significantly influenced one way or the other.

However, the one unexpected complication related to posture in the second stage of delivery has only emerged because of the use of these randomized trials. There is a significant increase in the risk of primary post-partum haemorrhage in women who deliver in the chair rather than in bed. For instance, Stewart *et al*. (1983) reported a primary post-partum haemorrhage in 13 per cent of women delivering in the chair and in 4 per cent of women delivering in bed. In the overview of eight such trials, the relative risk of primary post-partum haemorrhage following delivery in a birth chair was 1.4 that of delivery in bed. Presumably when an episiotomy or tear did bleed in patients in a birth chair, it was able to bleed more profusely in that there was increased perineal venous pressure, this being the most dependent area of the maternal trunk in a birth chair. Similarly, severe vulval oedema has been described in women who pushed for more than two hours in a birth chair (Goodlin and Frederick 1983).

Some interesting statistics have also emerged concerning the opinion of patients in these trials. Some 7 per cent of women allocated to the chair ultimately refused to delivery in it, whilst 85 per cent of those women who did deliver in the chair wished to use it for a subsequent delivery, as did 46 per cent of those who delivered in bed (Hemminki *et al*. 1986).

There would appear to be no proven benefit from the use of a birth chair, but there may well be a specific disadvantage namely, the risk of primary post-partum haemorrhage.

Squatting during delivery is also not new, being depicted in ancient vase paintings and sculptures. It has gained some recent popularity with patients in that the parturient may sink in to a birth cushion for a supported squat, Gardosi *et al*. (1989*a*) reported a randomized trial of 427 nulliparous women allocated to squatting ($n = 218$) or conventional delivery ($n = 209$). Spontaneous vaginal delivery occurred in 91 per cent of the squatting group as compared with 83 per cent of the recumbent group. The mean length of the second stage of labour was 39 minutes in the squatting group and 50 minutes in the recumbent group. Some 46 per cent of the mothers in the squatting group had an intact perineum compared with 32 per cent in the recumbent group. The incidence of primary post-partum haemorrhage was similar in both groups. Some 95 per cent of 140 women in the squatting group questioned two months after delivery wished to squat again in a subsequent delivery. Gardosi *et al*. (1989*b*) reported a randomized trial of 151 nulliparous patients allocated to conventional delivery or encouraged to assume any relatively upright posture of their choice, for example squatting, kneeling, sitting, or standing. The results, shown in Table 26.4, demonstrated that a more upright posture reduced the incidence of

Table 26.4 The effects of posture

	Recumbent posture	Upright posture
No. of patients	78	73
Mean duration of pushing (minutes)	47.1	48.8
% Spontaneous vaginal delivery	85	90
% Forceps delivery	15	10
Mean blood loss (ml)	223	201
% Intact perineum	26	37
Mean umbilical artery pH	7.24	7.26
% with Apgar score > 7 at 1 minute	87.2	98.6

From Gardosi *et al.* (1989 *b*)

operative delivery and increased the incidence of intact perineums without any detriment to the mother or baby.

An analysis of the adoption of alternative positions during labour would appear to result in a mixed conclusion. The use of a birth chair would not seem appropriate, but there would seem to be no reason to discourage any patient from adopting an upright posture should she so wish it. Upright positions in general appear to have a beneficial effect on the fetus, with a trend towards fewer fetal heart rate abnormalities in the fetus and more favourable Apgar scores and umbilical artery pH levels in those randomized to adopt more upright positions (Spiby 1992).

Finally, it has often been claimed that the use of a dorsal position during labour is artificial, being a device to make care easier for the modern obstetrician or midwife. This is not true. Chamberlain and Stewart (1987) reported that this position was discussed in the writings of William Smellie (circa 1718) and that 'traditional birth attendants in primitive tribes have for centuries nursed women horizontally'.

Instrumental delivery

The incidence of operative vaginal delivery varies greatly from country to country, as shown in Table 26.5 (Lomas and Enkin 1989). These figures almost certainly now represent an underestimate. When instrumental vaginal delivery is indicated, there has been debate between the use of forceps and vacuum extraction.

Forceps or vacuum extraction?

Seven randomized controlled trials have addressed the relative benefits and hazards of these instruments (Dell *et al.* 1985; Ehlers *et al.* 1974; Fall *et al.* 1986;

Table 26.5 Operative delivery rates

	Any operative delivery (%)	Forceps delivery (%)	Vacuum delivery (%)	Caesarean section (%)
Canada	34.4	17.8	0.5	16.1
USA	35.4	18.4	0.5	16.5
England and Wales	21.3	12.5	minimal	8.8
Scotland	24.0	13.0	0.3	10.7
Sweden	19.1	0.3	6.8	12.0
Norway	14.9	3.2	3.4	8.3

From Lomas and Enkin (1989)

Table 26.6 Forceps or vacuum?

	Forceps	Vacuum extraction
No. of patients	152	152
% Caesarean section	9.2	4.6
% Third degree tear	15.8	5.9
% Cephalhaematoma	5.3	9.2
% Endotracheal intubation	18.4	19.0
% Neonatal jaundice	19.1	30.3

Vacca *et al.* (1983)

Johanson *et al.* 1989; Lasbrey *et al.* 1964; Vacca *et al.* 1983; Williams *et al.* 1991). On the whole these trials are of good methodological quality and have been comprehensively reviewed by Johanson (1992). There is considerable consistency between the trials with respect to the more important outcomes. From the mother's point of view there is strong evidence that the vacuum extractor is the superior instrument with much less severe perineal and vaginal injury at delivery than is sustained with forceps. There is less need for regional or general analgesia for delivery by vacuum extraction. Attempts at delivery are much more likely to fail with vacuum extraction, but the benefits in terms of reduced maternal trauma persist in spite of this excess of failed procedures.

An increased risk of cephalhaematoma is the main disadvantage of vacuum extraction from the baby's point of view. Other injuries to the face and scalp are more common in those delivered by forceps, but not significantly so. One trial is inconsistent with the rest in showing an increase in retinal haemorrhage in babies delivered by vacuum extraction. (Ehlers *et al.* 1974). Further studies are needed to prove that there are no serious risks to the fetus or neonate that were too rare to be exposed by the moderately large sized trials that have been conducted to date. Meanwhile, the available evidence has placed many obstetricians in the uncomfortable position of having to

Table 26.7 Forceps or vacuum?

	Forceps	Vacuum extraction
No. of patients	45	73
% Failure	6.7	19.2
% Third degree tear	22.2	21.9
% Vaginal lacerations	37.8	6.8
% Cervical lacerations	15.6	11.0
% Cephalhaematoma	2.2	15.1

From Oell *et al.* (1985)

Table 26.8 Epidural analgesia and delivery

	Primigravidae		Multigravidae	
	No epidural	Epidural	No epidural	Epidural
No. of patients	503	80	899	46
% Spontaneous delivery	79.0	34.0	94.0	67.0
% Rotational delivery	0.8	20.0	0.2	4.3

From Studd *et al.* (1980)

recognize that the instrument with which they are more skilled may be the more harmful one for the mother (Johanson *et al.* 1993).

Kielland's forceps or Caesarean section?

A failure of rotation prior to delivery is not an uncommon problem. It is increased in the presence of epidural analgesia, probably due to reduced tone in the pelvic musculature.

Three randomized trials of epidural versus non-epidural analgesia in labour showed that epidural analgesia increased the incidence of malrotation of the fetal head in the second stage (Noble *et al.* 1971; Philipsen and Jensen 1989; Thalme *et al.* 1974). Hoult *et al.* (1977) reported that rotational delivery was performed in 3 per cent of patients without an epidural block and in 20 per cent of patients with an epidural block. As this is an observational study it is prone to the obvious bias that the women who had elected to have epidural analgesia were those who had more difficult labours to begin with. The same bias applies to the report of Studd *et al.* (1980) on the outcome of 1955 spontaneous labours where the incidence of rotational delivery was increased by over 20-fold in the presence of an epidural block (Table 26.8).

Maresh *et al.* (1983) have suggested that the use of rotational forceps would be decreased by an altered managment of the second stage of labour in the presence of an epidural block, demonstrating the benefit of delayed pushing in

Table 26.9 The value of delayed pushing

	Early pushing	Late pushing
No. of patients	40	36
Mean duration of waiting before pushing (minutes)	27	123
Range	0–95	15–220
% Spontaneous delivery	35	50
% Low forceps	35	33
% Rotational forceps	27	11
% Caesarean section	3	6
Mean umbilical artery pH	7.26	7.25
Mean umbilical vein pH	7.35	7.35

From Maresh *et al.* (1983)

women with an epidural block. They randomly allocated 76 primigravidae with epidural analgesia to one of two groups for the management of the second stage. The conventional groups were allowed to push as soon as they so desired after full dilatation, whilst the late pushing group continued to lie on their side and did not commence pushing until the head was visible on parting the labia. The results, shown in Table 26.9, demonstrated a more satisfactory outcome in the delayed pushing group without any detriment to the neonates.

When Kielland's forceps are then used, there would appear to be a significant association with neonatal trauma. It is possible that some degree of borderline cephalopelvic disproportion, especially in those patients with mid-cavity arrest in the absence of an epidural block, may explain some of these complications, but Chiswick and James (1979) argued that the trauma was inherent in the use of the instrument. They compared the outcomes in 86 consecutive liveborn singleton babies delivered by Kielland's forceps (or Caesarean section after attempted Kielland's forceps) with 86 babies born by spontaneous vertex vaginal delivery and matched for maternal age, parity, social class, gestational age, and whether labour was spontaneous or induced. These results, shown in Table 26.10, demonstrated that neonatal death in the study group was related to traumatic delivery (torn tentorium), and that the incidence of abnormal neurological behaviour was increased 10-fold in the Kielland's group compared with the control group. There were no differences between those infants who did or did not develop neonatal complications when compared for mean birthweight, maternal height, or occipitofrontal circumference. However, it seems scientifically unreasonable to compare babies delivered vaginally after rotation with Kielland's forceps with those delivered after spontaneous vaginal delivery. It would seem more appropriate to compare those babies delivered after a Kielland's rotation and forceps with either those babies delivered by

Table 26.10 Complications

	Kielland's forceps	Spontaneous delivery
No. of patients	86	86
% Neonatal deaths	4.7	0
% Delayed onset of respiration	17.4	3.5
% Birth trauma	15.1	3.5
% Abnormal neurological behaviour	23.3	2.3

From Chiswick and James (1979)

Table 26.11 Complications

	Kielland's forceps	Other rotational forceps	Manual rotation
No. of patients	552	95	160
% Neonatal death	1.27	1.05	0
% Vaginal or cervical lacerations	15	18	19
% Birth asphyxia	9	5	8
% Cephalhaematoma	7	6	3
% Neonatal seizures	3	2	0
% Facial nerve palsies	1	2	2

From Healey *et al.* (1982)

either manual rotation and forceps, by vacuum extraction, or with those babies delivered abdominally, since those are the alternatives.

Healey *et al.* (1982) undertook a retrospective survey of 552 deliveries by Kielland's rotation and delivery, 95 deliveries using other forceps for rotation and delivery, and 160 deliveries following manual rotation and low-cavity forceps. There were no differences in maternal or fetal morbidity between the groups (see Table 26.11), but there was an inverse association between the seniority of the operator and the incidence of maternal soft tissue damage, but not of neonatal morbidity. None of the eight neonatal deaths in the series were due to trauma.

The large difference in the incidence of maternal soft tissue trauma associated with vacuum extraction compared with forceps deliveries of all types indicates that some of the problems associated with Kielland's delivery may be inherent in the instrument itself, although the seniority of the operator and the indication for delivery may also be factors (Hutchon and McFa-dyen 1979; MacDonald and Scott 1979). What is perhaps needed is a skilled assessment before delivery is attempted (Drife 1983) and an increased use of 'trial of instrumental delivery' in an operating theatre available for immediate abdominal delivery if the outcome is in any doubt (MacDonald and Scott 1979). A large randomized trial of Kielland's forceps versus vacuum extraction versus Caesarean section is necessary to address the uncertainties that continue to exist (*British Medical Journal* 1979).

Episiotomy

Episiotomy is a widely used procedure and a source of much criticism from some quarters. Thorp and Bowes (1989) reported that 63 per cent of all vaginal deliveries in the USA were associated with an episiotomy, and that this figure rose to 80 per cent in nulliparous women. Sleep *et al.* (1984) reported a wide range in the incidence of episiotomy use between different hospitals in the UK, from 16 to 71 per cent of multiparous patients and from 14 to 96 per cent of nulliparous ones.

The disadvantages of episiotomy include excessive blood loss, trauma to the anal sphincter with subsequent risk of a rectovaginal fistula, perineal pain, and dyspareunia, all of which may also complicate perineal lacerations. The mean blood loss at delivery in women without an episiotomy or laceration was 207 ml compared with a mean of 245 ml in women with a laceration, and 360 ml in women with an episiotomy (Newton *et al.* 1961).

The advantages of an episiotomy are said to be an overall reduction in perineal trauma, especially third degree tears, prevention of trauma to the fetus, and the prevention of subsequent urinary incontinence. The evidence for these advantages will now be examined.

When considering the effect upon the incidence of third degree tears, one should distinguish between a midline episiotomy and a mediolateral episiotomy. The use of a midline episiotomy is not popular in current practice because of its association with anal sphincter damage. Thorp *et al.* (1987) reported a prospective non-randomized trial of midline episiotomy with unrestricted use of the episiotomy in 265 women and used only for fetal distress or operative delivery in 113 women. Damage to the anal sphincter and/or anal canal occurred in 1.8 per cent of patients with selected use and 13.2 per cent with unrestricted use, suggesting that damage may be less likely to occur following a tear than a midline episiotomy.

The advantages and disadvantages of mediolateral episiotomy have been well described in the Berkshire Episiotomy Trial, in which 1000 women were randomly allocated to undergo either a policy of liberal mediolateral episiotomy use or restricted use for fetal indication only (Sleep *et al.* 1984). These results have been summarized in Table 26.12. They demonstrated that the restricted use of episiotomy increases the percentage of patients with an intact perineum by 9 per cent. A similar but smaller trial suggested that this figure may be as high as 21 per cent (Harrison *et al.* 1984). However, the only third degree damage occurred in the restricted group. There is no evidence from randomized trials that patients with an intact perineum require less analgesia in the

Table 26.12 The place of episiotomy

	Liberal episiotomy use	Restricted episiotomy use
No. of patients	502	498
% Episiotomy alone	45.2	9.0
% Episiotomy with extension	6.0	1.2
% Perineal tear	24.5	55.8
% Labial tear	17.3	26.3
% Required no sutures	22	31
% Third degree tear	0	0.4
% Resumed coitus within one month	27	37
% Of above with dyspareunia within one month	51	52
% Persistent dyspareunia	18	22
% Involuntary urine loss at three months	19	19

From Sleep *et al.* (1984), Berkshire Episiotomy Trial

post-partum period than do patients with either an episiotomy or a tear (Coats *et al.* 1980; Harrison *et al.* 1984). The only evidence for increased pain from an episiotomy during the puerperium comes from uncontrolled studies (Reading *et al.* 1982) and, therefore, must carry less weight.

In a randomized trial which compared the use of midline with mediolateral episiotomies in 407 patients, patients resumed coitus earlier after a midline episiotomy, but there was no statistical difference with regard to the incidence of coitus by two months after delivery (Coats *et al.* 1980). However, the incidence of third degree tears was 5.5 per cent after midline episiotomy but only 0.4 per cent after mediolateral episiotomy.

There is no evidence that the restricted use of an episiotomy prejudices fetal outcome at delivery (Harrison *et al.* 1984; Sleep *et al.* 1984).

The above studies would seem to suggest that the restricted use of an episiotomy results in a smaller number of women requiring perineal sutures, but without any detriment to fetal condition or alteration in the need for post-partum analgesia. The frequently quoted view that 'a clean surgical incision into the perineum, correctly timed and repaired, is more likely that a ragged, bruised tear to heal by first intention' (Russell 1982) can no longer be substantiated.

One also needs to examine the view that the liberal use of episiotomy would prevent subsequent pelvic floor weakness (Aldridge and Watson 1935; Gainey 1955). Gordon and Logue (1985) assessed the ability to squeeze perineal musculature using a perineometer in 84 women one year after delivery. The ability to squeeze the pelvic floor bore no relationship to the type of delivery or the state of the perineum at delivery, but rather to the taking of exercise in general and pelvic exercise in particular. Sleep and Grant (1987) interviewed 674 of the 1000 patients in the Berkshire Episiotomy Trial some three years later. There were no differences between the liberal and restricted groups for the incidences of urinary incontinence (4 per cent) or dyspareunia (14 per cent). There is, therefore, little evidence to support the view that perineal trauma will be reduced by the use of an episiotomy.

The technique of perineal repair

There is now abundant evidence available to advise the obstetrician and midwife as to the technique of perineal repair and the choice of suture material. It is appropriate that the evidence concerning the perineal skin is considered separately from the evidence concerning vaginal skin and perineal musculature.

Perineal skin

There have been several studies which have compared the use of interrupted and subcuticular sutures for perineal skin repair. Isager-Sally *et al.* (1986) reported 802 women following an episiotomy repair and found that closure of the perineal skin was more comfortable after the use of subcuticular polyglycolic acid ($n = 267$) than after the use of interrupted polyglycolic acid ($n = 268$) or interrupted polyglycolic acid ($n = 267$). Pain was present within the first five days after delivery in 49 per cent of the group who had subcuticular sutures compared with 59 per cent of the group who had interrupted sutures. Tenderness in the episiotomy scar was present in 19 per cent of the patients who had subcuticular sutures and 25 per cent of those with interrupted sutures some three months after delivery. Buchan and Nicholls (1980) compared the use of subcuticular polyglycolic acid and interrupted silk sutures in 140 women; they found a significantly lower need for analgesia in the early puerperium in those sutured with polyglycolic acid. Mahomed *et al.* (1989), however, could find no difference in post-partum pain or dyspareunia in 1574 women whose perineal skin had been sutured with subcuticular or interrupted sutures, whatever the material used. Grant (1989) reviewed 14 controlled trials involving 5136 patients and concluded that subcuticular polyglycolic acid was the technique and suture material of choice for perineal skin.

Not all patients do, in fact, require *any* sutures in their perineal skin. Some authors have found that a tissue adhesive applied to the skin allowed for satisfactory healing and with less pain than did sutures (Adoni and Anteby 1991).

Vaginal skin and perineal muscle repair

Isager-Sally *et al.* (1986) compared the use of plain catgut in the vagina and perineal muscles ($n = 272$) with polyglycolic acid ($n = 530$) and found no significant difference in pain during the first five days of the puerperium or longterm. It was the technique and type of perineal skin suture which influenced their results. Spencer *et al.* (1986) randomly allocated 737 women with perineal tears to a repair using either glycerol-impregnanted chromic catgut or untreated chormic catgut for all layers. At ten days post-partum, the prevalence of 'severe' pain was greater in the treated catgut than the untreated catgut group (1.5 per cent compared with 0 per cent) as was the incidence of dyspareunia persisting beyond three months (26.0 per cent compared with 19.5 per cent), hence these problems would seem to preclude the use of treated catgut for perineal repair.

Beard *et al.* (1974) compared 100 patients whose perinea had been repaired throughout with polyglycolic acid with 100 repaired throughout with chromic catgut. There were no differences in the degree of perineal breakdown (12 per cent in both groups), but there was a lesser need for analgesia by the patients in the polyglycolic acid group. Mahomed *et al.* (1989) found the analgesic need to be reduced in those patients sutured with polyglycolic acid compared with chromic catgut, although more patients with polyglycolic acid needed removal of suture material than did those with catgut (25 per cent versus 21 per cent), whilst the need for resuture was similar in both groups (1 per cent) as was dyspareunia (23 per cent). Grant (1989), in the overview of 14 trials, found that the analgesia requirement was reduced by up to 40 per cent in patients sutured with polyglycolic acid as compared with chromic catgut. Thus, polyglycolic acid would appear to be the current choice of suture material for all layers.

The benefits of polyglycolic acid may relate to its lesser tissue reaction than catgut, dissolving by hydrolysis, whereas catgut dissolves by phagocytosis (Craig *et al.* 1975; Lawrie *et al.* 1959).

Additional techniques have been proposed in order to ease perineal discomfort after repair. Khan and Lilford (1987) reported that local infiltration of the perineal tissues with 15 ml of normal saline reduced post-operative pain significantly in a randomized trial of 150 patients sutured by a common technique. The authors postulated that the preliminary infiltration allowed the inflammatory oedema to be accommodated within the tissues under less pressure, and, hence, reduce pain. Grant *et al.* (1989), in a randomized trial, tested the use of ultrasound and pulsed electromagnetic energy in 414 women with moderate or severe perineal trauma compared with placebo machines. Over 90 per cent of the patients in both groups found the treatment to be comforting, no statistical difference being seen between the active and placebo treatment.

Ice, tap-water, and witch hazel have all been shown to be beneficial in the short-term relief of perineal pain. Local anaesthetic sprays and gels give more longterm relief. There is no good evidence to support the use of expensive aerosol foams containing hydrocortisone. Oral analgesia with paracetamol supplements local measures (Grant and Sleep 1989).

The third stage—active management

Blood loss at delivery is frequently underestimated. Pritchard *et al.* (1962) measured maternal blood loss at delivery using blood volume estimations from radiochromium red cell labelling techniques. The average blood loss in women who delivered normally was 505 ml whilst it was 930 ml following Caesarean section. Newton *et al.* (1961) reported that the mean blood loss in 41 women without an episiotomy or laceration was 270 ml at vaginal delivery, compared with a mean of 245 ml for 12 women with a laceration and 360 ml for 15 women with an episiotomy. These authors also reported that the estimated blood loss ranged from an underestimate of 82 per cent to an overestimate of 34 per cent.

The incidence of primary post-partum haemorrhage was 2 per cent of 605 120 deliveries (Hospital In-patient Enquiry 1988), but this was almost certainly an underestimate related to under-reporting. Hall *et al.* (1985) reported that primary post-partum haemorrhage complicated 4 per cent of 36 312 deliveries, but complicated 21 per cent of 812 deliveries in which a retained placenta occurred. Gilbert *et al.* (1987) recorded an incidence of 11 per cent of vaginal deliveries complicated by primary post-partum haemorrhage. The Report on the Confidential Enquiries into Maternal Deaths in England and Wales (1989) reported that 2.2 per cent of the 138 direct maternal deaths were due to primary post-partum haemorrhage, representing a mortality of 1.6 per 1 000 000 maternities.

The use of pharmacological agents to promote uterine contraction with a view to reducing the incidence of primary post-partum haemorrhage is well known. Martin and Dumoulin (1953) reported that the primary post-partum haemorrhage rate of 13.1 per cent for the 1000 deliveries prior to the introduction of intravenous ergometrine administration fell to 1.2 per cent for the first 1000 deliveries after the introduction of routine ergometrine administration. Embrey (1961) reported that intramuscular oxytocin alone or intramuscular oxytocin and ergometrine (syntometrine) took 2.5 minutes to exert an oxytocic effect, whereas intravenous ergometrine took 41 seconds, and intramuscular ergometrine alone took 7 minutes.

The use of intravenous oxytocin (5 units) has been preferred to the use of intravenous ergometrine because of a reduction in the complications of nausea, vomiting, and hypertension, without any detriment in the ability to prevent blood loss (McDonald *et al.* 1993; Moir and Amoa 1979; Moodie and Moir 1976). None of the patients who received oxytocin vomited but 13 per cent of the patients who received ergometrine did so, whilst 46 per cent of those patients who received ergometrine experienced nausea, wretching, or vomiting.

The hypertensive effect of ergometrine, which possesses both α-and β-adrenergic properties and hence causes vasoconstriction, has also been studied (Johnstone 1972). Vaughan-Williams *et al.* (1974) reported a significant elevation in central venous pressure following the administration of ergometrine or syntometrine (range 1.7–5.0 cm), but no elevation with oxytocin during the third state of labour. Baillie (1963) reported that women who were hypertensive, for whatever reason, before the third stage of labour had a greater pressor effect than did those who were not. Following the intravenous administration of 0.5 mg of ergometrine 14 per cent of 173 previously normotensive women showed an elevation of diastolic blood pressure of at least 10 mmHg, whilst

Table 26.13 The management of the third stage

	Physiological management	Active management
No. of patients	849	846
% Primary post-partum haemorrhage	17.9	5.9
% Haemorrhage > 1000 ml	3.1	0.8
% Post-partum haemoglobin $\leqslant$ 9 g/ml	6.0	3.2
% Transfused	5.7	2.1
% Retained placenta	2.6	1.9
Mean length of third stage (minutes)	15	5
% Given additional oxytocic therapy	29.7	6.4
% Babies with jaundice	6.4	4.6
% Babies with packed cell volume > 0.65	7.5	1.8

From Prendiville *et al.* (1988*a*), Bristol Third Stage Third

66 per cent of 59 women with a preinjection diastolic blood pressure of greater than 90 mmHg showed a rise of at least 10 mmHg, generally within three minutes of administration. Post-partum eclampsia has been described (Dua 1994).

The direct intrauterine injection of prostaglandin $F_{2\alpha}$ (0.25 mg) has been used to induce uterine contraction in the presence of post-partum haemorrhage and uterine hypotonus, but not in routine practice, without side-effects (Bruce *et al.* 1982; Toppozada *et al.* 1981).

There have been several recent randomized studies which have compared the active management of the third stage of labour, using an oxytocic agent, with the physiological management of the third stage of labour. In the Bristol Third Stage Trial (Prendiville *et al.* 1988*a*), patients were randomly allocated to physiological ($n = 849$) or active ($n = 846$) management, the latter involving the use of intramuscular syntometrine (or intramuscular oxytocin in hypertensive women), early cord clamping, and controlled cord traction, whilst the former received no oxytocic agents, leaving the baby attached to the cord until after delivery of the placenta, and delivering the placenta by maternal effort alone. These results, shown in Table 26.13, demonstrated a significant decrease in the blood loss related to active management and its associated reduction in neonatal packed cell volume and jaundice. Similar results have been reported from Dublin and the Netherlands demonstrating that the active management of labour reduces the incidence of post-partum haemorrhage by one-third (Begley 1990; Elbourne and Harding 1991; Poeschmann *et al.* 1991).

There are disadvantages to this line of management. There is an increase in the incidence of vomiting in patients who undergo active management, this risk being increased by 11 per cent in the Bristol trial but by 64 per cent in the Dublin trial. Significant hypertension (diastolic blood pressure greater than 100 mmHg) was also increased following active management, occurring in up to 1.3 per cent of patients in the active group but in none in the physiological group. These trials gave conflicting evidence on the incidence of manual removal of the placenta, there being no increase in the Bristol trial but a six-fold relative increase in the Dublin trial.

Prendiville *et al.* (1988*b*) analysed the data obtained from nine other controlled trials which compared an oxytocic drug (*n* = 2895 patients) with either a placebo or no prophylaxis (*n* = 1599). The use of any oxytocic agent reduced the incidence of primary post-partum haemorrhage by 40 per cent, preventing a post-partum haemorrhage in one in every 22 women given such an agent. Elbourne *et al.* (1988) analysed 27 trials from the literature, involving 11 281 patients. These results showed that both oxytocin and syntometrine are effective at preventing post-partum haemorrhage. Obviously if oxytocin can be shown to be as effective in preventing post-partum haemorrhage without the adverse effects of hypertension and nausea, it will become the drug of choice.

It would seem that the active management of the third stage carries advantages which significantly outweigh the disadvantages, and there can no longer be any scientific basis upon which to hold the view that physiological management of the third stage should occur. The prevention of post-partum haemorrhage is desirable in all circumstances but is vital when birth is occurring at home, where the consequences of post-partum haemorrhage are potentially more hazardous than in the hospital setting.

Breast is best

It is generally considered that breastfeeding has advantages over formula products, but it is not absolutely clear, in the First or Second World, how important these benefits currently are. 'Daddy' (1976), in an open letter to any 'son', recorded the usual reasons why 'breast is best': it is natural, the immunological properties of colostrum protect against infection, the infant is less likely to develop hypernatraemia or hypocalcaemia, there is less infant obesity, less cot deaths, less atopic disorders, and it increases maternal bonding.

Inch (1989) reported that the majority of women who decide to breastfeed had already made this decision prior to, or in very early pregnancy, and that once a woman had decided how she would feed her baby, no amount of persuasion or dissipation of knowledge was likely to change her mind.

Howie *et al.* (1990) demonstrated that breastfeeding still protected infants against gastrointestinal infection, but not against other infections. They reported 618 pairs of infants, one of each pair having a mother who elected to breastfeed whilst the other had a mother who elected to bottlefeed. If the infant was weaned before the 13th week of pregnancy, there was no protection against gastrointestinal infection but if breastfeeding continued beyond the 13th week, there was. There was a minimal benefit for protection against respiratory illnesses but no protection against others.

It has also been proposed that nutrition in early life has a longterm influence on neurodevelopment. Lucas *et al.* (1990, 1992) reported that the IQ of 210 children born preterm and fed mother's milk by tube was eight points higher at 7.5–8 years than was the IQ of 90 babies fed with artificial feeds, this difference being statistically significant even when adjusted for differences in maternal education and social class. The IQ of children whose mother chose to provide breastmilk but failed to do so was similar to the IQ in children whose mothers elected not to provide breastmilk, suggesting that this is a real observation not an effect of bias. If the significance of these findings is to be accepted, the results would need to be confirmed by a separate and larger study. The crucial group, namely the children whose mothers chose to provide breastmilk but were unable so to do, is the group which needs to be large enough to allow a regression analysis to take place.

In First and Second World countries, the use of breastmilk rather than artificial feeds is not a factor in infant survival, and whilst we may continue to encourage breast feeding this policy must be 'tempered with realism' (Jason 1991).

Perhaps the most compelling reason to encourage women to breastfeed is the negative association between breastfeeding and the risk of breast cancer. In a case controlled study, the risk of breast cancer in women below the age of 36 fell with the increasing duration of breastfeeding, but breastfeeding each baby for longer than three months conferred no additional benefit (United Kingdom National Case Controlled Study Group 1993).

The place of birth

There are a small, but significant, number of home confinements taking place and, no doubt, a significant number requested but refused. In England and Wales, 1.1 per cent of all deliveries take place at home and a further 6 per cent of all deliveries are under general practitioner care in hospital, 27 per cent of these deliveries occurring in general practitioner units and the rest in integrated units (Jewell 1985; Smith and Jewell 1991). This section will examine the role of consultant units, general practitioner units, and home deliveries in current obstetric practice.

A comparison of outcome between these three major options for delivery is difficult for numerous reasons. The cases are not comparable, since only carefully selected, low-risk patients should be delivered at home or in a general practioner unit; patients in whom complications do occur may then be transferred to the consultant units and will then appear in that unit's statistics; babies with serious congenital abnormalities will now be delivered almost exclusively in consultant units and should, therefore, be excluded from the statistics, as should preterm deliveries and multiple pregnancies. For these reasons, the crude statistics will rarely indicate a true assessment. However, the available evidence suggests that in carefully selected low-risk patients, the additional risk from delivery at home should be low, whilst satisfaction of that delivery should be high (Alberman 1986).

In a recent review of home births, 82 per cent of such planned deliveries took place at home, 9 per cent being transferred to a consultant unit antenatally, and 9 per cent being transferred during labour. Of those transferred during labour, 12 per cent (1 per cent of the total population) required the use of a Flying Squad. No baby delivered at home required intubation, but 2 per cent required oxygen via a face mask. There were no intrapartum or neonatal deaths (Ford *et al*. 1991). It would seem that in selected cases the risks of home confinement are small. It has been estimated that the perinatal mortality rate for patients booked and delivered at home is 4.1 per 1000 (Campbell *et al*. 1984).

There are two specific anxieties concerning home confinement. The first concerns the use of either an Obstetric or Paediatric Flying Squad which, when required, will deplete the hospital unit staff. Secondly, several series have suggested that up to 9 per cent of patients who plan to deliver at home will require transfer into hospital during labour (Ford *et al*. 1991; Hudson 1968; Scherjon 1986; Shearer 1985). This transfer during labour from home to hospital takes place against the background of an acute problem and is associated with an increased perinatal mortality rate (9.5 per 1000, Murphy *et al*. 1984). It should, therefore, be stressed to patients requesting a home confinement that this, in the absence of known obstetric problems, is low-risk but not no-risk.

The general practitioner unit offers the 'half-way house' of care by midwife and general practitioner, preferably within a hospital unit, and allows relatively easy transfer to a consultant unit should it be required, as it is in 11 per cent of cases (Roseveare and Bull 1982).

It would seem appropriate that the general practitioner unit should be integrated within the consultant unit and not isolated from it. Sangala *et al*. (1990) suggested that, whilst the integrated general practioner unit is as safe as the consultant unit for low-risk patients, the same is not true of the isolated general practioner unit. They analysed 14 415 deliveries, the results of which are shown in Table 26.14. It may be seen that whilst there were no perinatal deaths in the integrated general practitioner unit, there was an excess of deaths in the isolated general practioner unit, and 1.5 per 1000 of these deaths were due to asphyxia at birth. This complication accounted for 0.6 per 1000 deaths in the consultant unit and none in the integrated general practioner unit. Several other authors have reported favourable statistics from the delivery of selected low-risk patients in an integrated general practioner unit (Klein *et al*. 1983; Lowe *et al*. 1987; Marsh and Channing 1989; Taylor *et al*. 1980).

However, not all comparisons have found such favourable statistics, suggesting that low-risk deliveries are safe in the presence of enthusiastic general practitioners and midwives, and perhaps it is only such enthusiasts who report their results. The standard of care which would be expected from general practitioners using a general practitioner unit is not always met. Bryce *et al*. (1990) reported that of 1289 deliveries booked into a general practioner unit in a specific year, 29 per cent were transferred to a consultant unit antenatally and 20 per cent were transferred during labour. Only 14.3 per cent of those patients

Table 26.14 The place of birth

	No. of deliveries	Perinatal mortality rate per 1000
All		
Consultant unit	7950	2.8
Integrated general practitioner unit	1228	0
Isolated general practitioner unit	5237	4.8
Nulliparous		
Consultant unit	3740	3.2
Integrated general practitioner unit	502	0
Isolated general practitioner unit	1928	5.7
Multiparous		
Consultant unit	4210	2.4
Integrated general practitioner unit	726	0
Isolated general practitioner unit	3309	4.2

From Sangala *et al.* (1990)

Table 26.15 The place of birth

	Stillbirth rate per 1000	Perinatal mortality rate per 1000
All deliveries	9.0	13.8
Patients transferred antenatally	8.0	10.6
Patients transferred during labour	27.0	34.7

From Bryce *et al.* (1990)

transferred during labour were seen by any doctor before transfer; and 44.9 per cent of those patients who were transferred either antenatally or during labour either had at booking, or developed during pregnancy, complications which had been previously accepted as contraindications to booking in to the general practioner unit. As can be seen from Table 26.15, the perinatal mortality rate was significantly greater in those women transferred during labour than those transferred either antenatally, or for the unit as a whole.

It may be that such results represent either a poor quality of general practitioner care or poor communication between general practitioners and consultants in the management of some general practitioner units, a situation which cannot benefit patients (Campbell *et al.* 1991). Yet at least some patients want the choice and, if the risks are small, the patient may wish to make her own valued judgement and accept this risk. What is important is that these statistics are not used to mislead, but to provide information (Campbell *et al.* 1991; Charney 1990; Jenkinson 1990). It is possible that a consultant-led simulated home delivery in hospital may appeal to a considerable number of patients (MacVicar *et al.* 1993).

The use of vitamin K

Vitamin K is traditionally given to neonates as a prophylaxis against haemorrhagic disease of the newborn. This practice was called into question by a small retrospective case-controlled study on infants developing childhood malignancies (Golding *et al.* 1990). This study compared 33 children developing cancer with 99 controls matched for maternal age, parity, and social class. It suggested that the administration of vitamin K carried a relative risk of 1.8 for the development of childhood cancer compared with non-administration of vitamin K. Since this study is small and retrospective, and since the finding is unexpected and fitted no prior hypothesis, this possible association requires a superior methodological study in order to confirm or refute the findings. Recent studies from both Sweden and Denmark have failed to confirm this association (Ekelund *et al.* 1993; Olsen *et al.* 1994).

Against this possible, but unlikely, risk must be balanced the proven problem of haemorrhagic disease of the newborn. In a recent prospective study, haemorrhagic disease of the newborn occurred in 27 infants out of 1 671 000 livebirths, an incidence of 1.6 per 100 000 births or 1 in 62 500 births. Of these 27 infants, 10 developed an intracranial haemorrhage and two died. Of these 27 infants, 20 had received no vitamin K prophylaxis, seven had received oral prophylaxis, but none had received intramuscular vitamin K (McNinch and Tripp 1991). It has been estimated that, without intramuscular vitamin K prophylaxis, 40 infants would have an intracranial haemorrhage in the UK each year and eight would die, hence prophylactic intramuscular vitamin K would seem to be a safe option (von Kries 1991) and should be encouraged (Croucher and Azzopardi 1994).

Conclusions

As might be expected, there are some things which happen as a routine in many units, for example shaving and enemas, which cannot be justified scientifically, yet may assume great importance and inhibit the relationship between patients and obstetrician. Conversely, there are other tried and tested procedures, such as the active managment of the third stage of labour, which have clearly proven benefits. There are then a third group of practices, such as ambulation during labour, where flexibility is appropriate. This chapter also demonstrates the principle that all innovations should be tested before becoming part of established practice. Only when this happens, can unforeseen problems (such as the association of a birth chair with post-partum haemorrhage) become apparent.

Over the next few years, there are likely to be increasing numbers of patients requesting home confinement. Recently, a committee of the House of Commons received evidence upon the place of birth and concluded that home confinement was a relatively safe procedure and should be made more available to low-risk patients. Whether or not one approves of this conclusion, a satisfactory knowledge of the scientific literature is required if these patients are to be counselled appropriately.

References

Abitbol, M. M. (1985). Supine position in labour and associated fetal heart rate changes. *Obstetrics and Gynecology* **65**, 481-6.

Abouleish, E. and Depp, R. (1975). Acupuncture in obstetrics. *Anesthesia and Analgesia* **54**, 83-8.

Adoni, A. and Anteby, E. (1991). The use of Histoacryl for episiotomy repair. *British Journal of Obstetrics and Gynaecology* **98**, 476-8.

Alberman, E. (1986). The place of birth. *British Journal of Obstetrics and Gynaecology* **93**, 657-8.

Aldridge, A. H. and Watson, P. (1935). Analysis of end-results of labour in primiparas after spontaneous versus prophylactic methods of delivery. *American Journal of Obstetrics and Gynecology* **30**, 554-65.

Augustinsson, I. E., Bohlin, P., Bunsden, P., Carlsson, C. A., Forssman, L., Sjoberg, P., *et al.* (1977). Pain relief during delivery by TENS. *Pain* **4**, 59-65.

Baillie, T. W. (1963). Vasopressor activity of ergometrine maleate in anaesthetised parturient women. *British Medical Journal* **1**, 585-8.

Beard, R., Boyd, I., and Simms, C. (1974). A trial of polyglycolic acid and chromic catgut sutures in episiotomy repair. *British Journal of Clinical Practice* **28**, 409-10.

Beck, N. C., Siegel, L. J., Davidson, N. P., Kormeier, S., Breitenstien, A., and Hall, D. G. (1980). The prediction of pregnancy outcome. *Journal of Psychosomatic Research* **24**, 343-52.

Begley, C. (1990). A comparison of active and physiological management of the third stage of labour. *Midwifery* **6**, 3-17.

Bird, A. P. and Walji, M. T. I. (1986). Our patients have access to their medical records. *British Medical Journal* **292**, 595-6.

Brant, H. A. (1962). Childbirth, preparation, and support in labour. *New Zealand Medical Journal* **61**, 211-19.

British Medical Journal (1979). Keilland's forceps. *British Medical Journal* **1**, 362-3.

Bruce, S. I., Paul, R. H., and Van Dorsten, J. P. (1982). Control of post-partum uterine atony of intramyometrial prostaglandin. *Obstetrics and Gynecology* **59**, 47s-50s.

Bryce, F. C., Clayton, J. K., and Rand, R. J., Beck, I., Farquharson, D. I. M., and Jones, S. E. (1990). General practitioner obstetrics in Bradford. *British Medical Journal* **300**, 725-7.

Buchan, P. C. and Nicholls, J. A. J. (1980). Pain after episiotomy—a comparison of two methods of repair. *Journal of the Royal College of General Practitioners* **30**, 297-300.

Bull, M. H. V. (1983). The general practitioner and the specialist: obstetrics. *British Medical Journal* **286**, 141.

Bunsden, P. and Ericson, K. (1982). Pain relief in labour by transcutaneous electrical nerve stimulation. *Acta Obstetrica et Gynaecologica Scandinavica* **61**, 1-5.

Caldeyro-Barcia, R., Noriega-Guerra, L., Sibels, L. A., Alvarez, H., Poseiro, J. J., Pose, S. V., *et al.* (1960). Effect of position changes on the intensity and frequency of uterine contractions during labour. *American Journal of Obstetrics and Gynecology* **80**, 284–90.

Calvert, J. P., Newcombe, R. G., and Hibbard, B. M. (1982). An assessment of radiotelemetry in the monitoring of labour. *British Journal of Obstetrics and Gynaecology* **89**, 285–91.

Campbell, R., Davies, I. M., Macfarlane, A., and Beral, V. (1984). Home births in England and Wales, 1979. *British Medical Journal* **289**, 721–4.

Campbell, R., MacFarlane, A., and Cavenagh, S. (1992). Choice and chance in low risk maternity care. *British Medical Journal* **303**, 1487–8.

Cave, C. (1978). Social characteristics of natural childbirth users and non-users. *American Journal of Public Health* **68**, 898–900.

Chamberlain, G. V. P. and Houang, E. (1984). Trial of the use of masks in the gynaecological operating theatre. *Annals of the Royal College of Surgeons of England* **66**, 432–3.

Chamberlain, G. V. P. and Stewart, M. (1987). Walking through labour. *British Medical Journal* **295**, 902.

Charney, M. (1990). General practitioner maternity units. *British Medical Journal* **301**, 665–6.

Chen, S. Z., Aisaka, K., Mori, H., and Kigawa, T. (1987). Effects of sitting position on uterine activity during labour. *Obstetrics and Gynecology* **69**, 67–73.

Chiswick, M. and James, D. K. (1979). Kielland's forceps: association with neonatal morbidity and mortality. *British Medical Journal* **1**, 7–9.

Coats, P. M., Chan, A. K., Wilkins, M., and Beard, R. J. (1980). A comparison between midline and medio-lateral episiotomy. *British Journal of Obstetrics and Gynaecology* **87**, 408–12.

Copstick, S. M., Taylor, K. E., Hayes, R., and Morris, N. (1986). Parental support and the use of coping techniques in labour. *Journal of Psychosomatic Research* **30**, 497–503.

Craig, P. H., Williams, J. A., Davis, K. W., Magoun, A. D., Levy, A. J., Bogdansky, S., *et al.* (1975). A biologic comparison of polyglactin and polyglycolic acid synthetic absorbable sutures. *Surgery, Gynecology, and Obstetrics* **141**, 1–10.

Croucher, C. and Azzopardi, D. (1994). Compliance with giving vitamin K to newborn infants. *British Medical Journal* **308**, 894–5.

Crowley, P., Elbourne, D., Ashurst, H., Garcia, J., Murphy, D., and Duignan, N. (1991). Delivery in an obstetric birth chair: a randomized controlled trial. *British Journal of Obstetrics and Gynaecology* **98**, 667–74.

'Daddy' (1976). Breast is best. *Lancet* **ii**, 412–13.

Davis, C. D. and Morrone, F. A. (1962). An objective evaluation of a prepared childbirth program. *American Journal of Obstetrics and Gynecology* **84**, 1196–206.

Dell, D. C., Sightler, S. E., and Plauche, W. C. (1985). Soft cup vacuum extraction: a comparison of outlet delivery. *Obstetrics and Gynecology* **66**, 624–8.

Draper, J., Field, S., Thomas, H., and Mare, M. J. (1986). Should women carry their antenatal records? *British Medical Journal* **292**, 603.

Drayton, S. and Rees, C. (1984). They know what they're doing. *Nursing Mirror* **159**, (5), IV–VIII.

Drife, J. O. (1983). Kielland or Caesar? *British Medical Journal* **287**, 309–10.

Dua, J. A. (1994). Post-partum eclampsia associated with ergometrine administration. *British Journal of Obstetrics and Gynaecology* **101**, 72–3.

Eckstein, K. L. and Marx, G. F. (1974). Aortocaval compression and uterine displacement. *Anesthesiology* **40**, 92–6.

Ehlers, N., Krarup-Jensen, I. B., Brogard-Hansen, K. (1974). Retinal haemorrhage in the newborn. Comparison of delivery by forceps and by vacuum extractor. *Acta Opthalmologica* **52**, 73–82.

Ekelund, H., Finnstrom, O., Gunnarskog, J., Kallen, B., and Larsson, Y. (1993). Administration of vitamin K to newborn infants and childhood cancer. *British Medical Journal* **307**, 89–91.

Elbourne, D. and Harding, J. (1991). Routine management for the third stage of labour: evidence from two random controlled trials. *Journal of Obstetrics and Gynaecology* **11**, Supp 1. 523–7.

Elbourne, D., Richardson, M., Chalmers, I., Waterhouse, I., and Holt, E. (1987). The Newbury Maternity Care Study: a randomized controlled trial to assess a policy of women holding their own obstetric record. *British Journal of Obstetrics and Gynaecology* **94**, 612–19.

Elbourne, D., Prendiville, W., and Chalmers, I. (1988). Choice of oxytocic preparation for routine use in the management of the third stage of labour: an overview of the evidence from controlled trials. *British Journal of Obstetrics and Gynaecology* **95**, 17–30.

Embrey, M. P. (1961). Simultaneous intramuscular injection of oxytocin and ergometrine. *British Medical Journal* **1**, 1737–8.

Fall, O., Finnstrom, K., Finnstrom, O., and Leijon, I. (1986). Forceps delivery or vacuum extraction? *Acta Obstetrica et Gynaecologica Scandinavica* **65**, 75–80.

Flynn, A. M., Kelly, J., Hollins, G., and Lynch, P. F. (1978). Ambulation in labour. *British Medical Journal* **2**, 291–3.

Ford, C., Iliffe, S., and Franklin, O. (1991). Outcome of planned home births in an inner city practice. *British Medical Journal* **303**, 1517–19.

Freeman, R. M., Macauley, A. J., Eve, L., Chamberlain, G. V. P., and Bhat, A. V. (1986). Randomized trial of self-hypnosis for analgesia in labour. *British Medical Journal* **292**, 697–8.

Gainey, H. L. (1955). Postpartum observation of pelvic tissue damage. *American Journal of Obstetrics and Gynecology* **70**, 800–7.

Gardosi, J., Hutson, N., and Lynch, C. B. (1989*a*). Randomized controlled trial of squatting in the second stage of labour. *Lancet* **ii**, 74–7.

Gardosi, J., Sylvester, S., and Lynch, C. B. (1989*b*). Alternative positions in the second stage of labour. *British Journal of Obstetrics and Gynaecology* **96**, 1290–6.

Gilbert, L., Porter, W., and Brown, V. A. (1987). Post-partum haemorrhage—a continuing problem. *British Journal of Obstetrics and Gynaecology* **94**, 67–71.

Golding, J., Paterson, M., and Kinlen, L. J. (1990). Factors associated with childhood cancer in a national cohort study. *British Journal of Cancer* **62**, 304–8.

Goodlin, R. C. and Frederick, I. B. (1983). Postpartum vulval oedema associated with the birthing chair. *American Journal of Obstetrics and Gynecology* **146**, 334.

Gordon, H. and Logue, M. (1985). Perineal muscle function after childbirth. *Lancet* **ii**, 123–5.

Grant, A. (1989). The choice of suture materials and techniques for repair of perineal trauma: an overview of the evidence from controlled trials. *British Journal of Obstetrics and Gynaecology* **96**, 1281–9.

Grant, A. and Sleep, J. (1989). Relief of perineal pain and discomfort after childbirth. In *Effective care in pregnancy and childbirth* (ed. I. Chalmers, M. Enkin, and M. J. N. C. Keirse), pp. 1347–58. Oxford University Press, Oxford.

Grant, A., Sleep, J., McIntosh, J., and Ashurst, H. (1989). Ultrasound and pulsed electromagnetic energy treatment for perineal trauma. A randomized placebo-controlled trial. *British Journal of Obstetrics and Gynaecology* **96**, 434–9.

Hall, M. H., Halliwell, R., and Carr-Hill, R. (1985). Concomitant and repeated happenings of complications of the third stage of labour. *British Journal of Obstetrics and Gynaecology* **92**, 732-8.

Harrison, R. F., Brennan, M., North, P. M., Reed, J. V., and Wickham, E. A. (1984). Is routine episiotomy necessary? *British Medical Journal* **288**, 1971-5.

Harrison, R. F., Woods, T., Shore, M., Mathews, G., and Unwin, A. (1986). Pain relief in labour using transcutaneous electrical nerve stimulation. *British Journal of Obstetrics and Gynaecology* **93**, 739-46.

Healey, D. L., Quinn, M. A., and Pepperell, R. J. (1982). Rotation of the fetus: Kielland's forceps and two other methods compared. *British Journal of Obstetrics and Gynaecology* **89**, 501-6.

Hemminki, E., Virkkunen, A., Makela, A., Hanikainen, J., Pulkkis, E., Moilanen, K., *et al.* (1986). A trial of delivery in a birth chair. *Journal of Obstetrics and Gynaecology* **6**, 162-5.

Hofmeyr, G. J., Nikodem, V. J., Nikodem, V. C., Wolman, W. L., Chalmers, B. E., and Cramer, T. (1991). Companionship to modify the clinical birth environment: effect on progress and perceptions of labour, and breast feeding. *British Journal of Obstetrics and Gynaecology* **98**, 756-64.

Hospital In-patient Enquiry. (1988). *Maternity tables*, pp. 37-50. Her Majesty's Stationery Office, London.

Hoult, I. J., MacLennan, A. H., and Carrie, L. E. S. (1977). Lumbar epidural analgesia in labour: relation of fetal malposition and instrumental delivery. *British Medical Journal* **1**, 14-16.

Howell, C. J. (1992). Epidural versus non-epidural analgesia in labour. In *Oxford database of perinatal trials* (ed. I. Chalmers.), Version 1.3, Disk issue 7, Record 3399. Oxford University Press.

Howie, P. W., Forsyth, J. S., Ogston, S. A., Clark, A., and Florey, C. D. V. (1990). Protective effect of breastfeeding against infection. *British Medical Journal* **300**, 11-16.

Hudson, C. K. (1968). Domiciliary obstetrics in a group practice. *Practitioner* **201**, 816-22.

Hutchon, D. J. R. and McFadyen, Y. (1979). Kielland's forceps. *British Medical Journal* **1**, 408.

Huttel, F. A., Mitchell, I., Fischer, W. M., and Meyer, A. E. (1972). A quantitative evaluation of psychoprophylaxis in childbirth. *Journal of Psychosomatic Research* **16**, 81-92.

Inch, S. (1989). Antenatal preparation for breastfeeding. In *Effective care in pregnancy and childbirth* (ed. I. Chalmers, M. Enkin, and M. J. N. C. Keirse), pp. 335-42. Oxford University Press, Oxford.

Isager-Sally, L., Legarth, J., Jacobsen, B., and Bostof, T. E. (1986). Episiotomy repair—immediate and longterm sequelae. *British Journal of Obstetrics and Gynaecology* **93**, 420-5.

Jason, J. (1991). Breastfeeding in 1991. *New England Journal of Medicine* **325**, 1036-7.

Jenkinson, S. (1990). General practitioner maternity units. *British Medical Journal* **301**, 664.

Jewell, D. (1985). GP obstetrics: safe but endangered. *British Medical Journal* **291**, 711-12.

Johanson, R. (1992). Vacuum extractor versus forceps for delivery. In *Oxford database of perinatal trials*. (ed. I. Chalmers), Version 1.3. Disk issue 7, Record 3256. Oxford University Press.

Johanson, R, Pusey, J., Livera, N., and Jones, P. (1989). North Staffordshire/Wigan assisted delivery trial. *British Journal of Obstetrics and Gynaecology* **96**, 537-44.

Johanson, R. B., Rice, C., Doyle, M., Arthur, J., Anyanwu, L., Ibrahim, J., *et al.* (1993). A randomized prospective study comparing the new vacuum extractor policy with forceps delivery. *British Journal of Obstetrics and Gynaecology* **100**, 524–30.

Johnston, R. A. and Sidall, R. S. (1922). Preparation for delivery. *American Journal of Obstetrics and Gynecology* **4**, 645–50.

Johnstone, M. (1972). The cardiovascular effects of oxytocic drugs. *British Journal of Anaesthesia* **44**, 826–34.

Kantor, H. I., Rember, R., Tabio, P., and Buchanan, R. (1965). Value of shaving the pudendal–perineal area in delivery preparation. *Obstetrics and Gynecology* **25**, 509–12.

Khan, G. Q. and Lilford, R. J. (1987). Wound pain may be reduced by prior infiltration of the episiotomy site after delivery under epidural analgesia. *British Journal of Obstetrics and Gynaecology* **94**, 341–4.

Klaus, M. H., Kennell, J. H., Robertson, S. S., and Sosa, R. (1986). Effects of social support during parturition on maternal and infant morbidity. *British Medical Journal* **393**, 585–7.

Klein, M., Lloyd, I., Redman, C., Bull, M., and Turnbull, A. C. (1983). A comparison of low-risk pregnant women booked for delivery in two systems of care: shared care and integrated general practitioner unit. No. 1. Obstetric procedures and neonatal outcome. *British Journal of Obstetrics and Gynaecology* **90**, 118–22.

Lasbrey, A. H., Orchard, C. D., and Crichton, D. (1964). A study of the relative merits and scope of vacuum extraction as opposed to forceps delivery. *South African Journal of Obstetrics and Gynaecology* **1**, 2, 1–3.

Lawrie, P., Angus, G. E., and Reese, A. J. M. (1959). The absorption of surgical catgut. *British Journal of Surgery* **59**, 638–42.

Leonard, R. F. (1973). Evaluation of selection tendencies of patients preferring prepared childbirth. *Obstetrics and Gynecology* **42**, 371–7.

Lilford, R. J., Glanville, J. N., Gupta, J. K., Shrestha, R., and Johnson, N. (1989). The action of squatting in the early postnatal period marginally increases pelvic dimensions. *British Journal of Obstetrics and Gynaecology* **96**, 964–6.

Lomas, J. and Enkin, M. (1989). Variations in operative delivery rates. In *Effective care in pregnancy and childbirth* (ed. I. Chalmers, M. Enkin, and M. J. N. C. Keirse), pp. 1182–95. Oxford University Press, Oxford.

Lowe, S. W., House, W., and Garrett, T. (1987). Comparison of outcome of low-risk labour in an isolated general practitioner maternity unit and a specialised maternity hospital. *Journal of the Royal College of General Practitioners* **37**, 484–7.

Lucas, A., Gore, S. M., Cole, T. J., Gore, S. M., Lucas, P. J., Crowle, P., *et al.* (1990). Early diet in preterm babies and developmental status at 18 months. *Lancet* **335**, 1477–81.

Lucas, A., Morley, R., Cole, T. J., Lister, G., and Leeson-Payne, C. (1992). Breast milk and subsequent intelligence quotient in children born preterm. *Lancet* **339**, 261–4.

MacArthur, C. J., Lewis, M., Know, E. G., and Crawford, J. S. (1990). Epidural anaesthesia and long-term backache after childbirth. *British Medical Journal* **301**, 9–12.

MacDonald, R. R. and Scott, J. S. (1979). Kielland's forceps. *British Medical Journal* **1**, 408–9.

McDonald, S. J., Prendiville, W. J., and Blair, E. (1993). Randomized controlled trial of oxytocin alone versus oxytocin and ergometrine in active management of the third stage of labour. *British Medical Journal* **307**, 1167–71.

McLaren, P. (1991). The right to know. *British Medical Journal* **303**, 937–8.

McManus, T. J. and Calder, A. A. (1978). Upright posture for the efficiency of labour. *Lancet* **i**, 72–4.

McNinch, A. W. and Tripp, J. H. (1991). Haemorrhagic disease of the newborn in the British Isles. *British Medical Journal* **303**, 1105–9.

MacVicar, J., Dobbie, G., Owen-Johnstone, L., Jagger, C., Hopkins, M., and Kennedy, J. (1993). Simulated home delivery in hospital. *British Journal of Obstetrics and Gynaecology* **100**, 316–23.

Mahomed, K., Grant, A., Ashurst., H., and James, D. (1989). The Southmead Perineal Suture Study. A randomized comparison of suture materials and suturing techniques for repair of perineal trauma. *British Journal of Obstetrics and Gynaecology* **96**, 1272–80.

Maresh, M., Choong, K. H., and Beard, R. W. (1983). Delayed pushing with lumbar analgesia in labour. *British Journal of Obstetrics and Gynaecology* **90**, 623–7.

Marsh, G. N. and Channing, D. M. (1989). Audit of 26 years of obstetrics in general practice. *British Medical Journal* **298**, 1077–8.

Martin, J. D. and Dumoulin, G. G. (1953). Use of intravenous ergometrine to prevent postpartum haemorrhage. *British Medical Journal* **1**, 643–6.

Melzack, R., Taenzer, P., Feldman, P., and Kinch, R. A. (1981). Labour is still painful after prepared childbirth. *Canadian Medical Association Journal* **125**, 357–63.

Moir, D. D. and Amoa, A. B. (1979). Ergometrine or oxytocin? *British Journal of Anaesthesia* **51**, 113–17.

Moodie, J. E. and Moir, D. D. (1976). Ergometrine, oxytocin, and extradural analgesia. *British Journal of Anaesthesia* **48**, 571–4.

Murphy, J. F., Dauncey, M., Gray, O. P., and Chalmers, I. (1984). Planned and unplanned delivery at home. *British Medical Journal* **288**, 1429–32.

Neshein, B. I. (1981). The use of transcutaneous nerve stimulation for pain relief during labour. *Acta Obstetrica et Gynaecologica Scandinavica* **60**, 13–16.

Newton, M., Mosey, L. M., Egli, G. E., Gifford, W. B., and Hull, C. T. (1961). Blood loss during and immediately after delivery. *Obstetrics and Gynecology* **17**, 9–18.

Noble, A. D., Craft, I. L., Bootes, J. A. H., Edwards, P. A., Thomas, D. J., and Mills, K. L. M. (1971). Continuous lumbar epidural analgesia using bupivicaine. *Journal of Obstetrics and Gynaecology of the British Commonwealth* **78**, 559–63.

Olsen, J. H., Hertz, H., Blinkenberg, K., and Verder, H. (1994). Vitamin K regimens and incidence of childhood cancer in Denmark. *British Medical Journal* **308**, 895–6.

Orr, N. W. M. (1981). Is a mask necessary in the operating theatre? *Annals of the Royal College of Surgeons of England* **63**, 390–2.

Paterson, C. M., Saunders, N. S. G., and Wadsworth, J. (1992). The characteristics of the second stage of labour in 25 069 singleton deliveries in the North West Thames Health Region, 1992. *British Journal of Obstetrics and Gynaecology* **99**, 377–80.

Philipsen, T. and Jensen, N. H. (1989). Epidural block or parenteral pethidine as analgesic in labour, a randomized study concerning progress in labour and instrumental deliveries. *European Journal of Obstetrics, Gynaecology, and Reproductive Biology* **30**, 27–33.

Poeschmann, R. P., Doesburg, W. H., and Eskes, T. K. A. B. (1991). A randomized comparison of oxytocin, sulprostone and placebo in the management of the third stage of labour. *British Journal of Obstetrics and Gynaecology* **98**, 528–30.

Prendiville, W. J., Harding, J. E., Elbourne, D. R., and Stirrat, G. M. (1988a). The Bristol Third Stage Trial. *British Medical Journal* **297**, 1295–1300.

Prendiville, W. J., Elbourne, D., and Chalmers, I. (1988b). The effects of routine oxytocin administration in the management of the third stage of labour: an overview of the evidence from controlled trials. *British Journal of Obstetrics and Gynaecology* **95**, 3–16.

Pritchard, J. A., Baldwin, R. M., Dickey, J. C., Wiggins, K. M., Reed, G. P., and Bruce, D. M. (1962). Blood volume changes in pregnancy and puerperium. *American Journal of Obstetrics and Gynecology* **84**, 1271–82.

Read, J. A., Miller, F. C., and Paul, R. H. (1981). Randomized trial of ambulation versus oxytocin for labour enhancement. *American Journal of Obstetrics and Gynecology* **139**, 669–72.

Reading, A. E., Sledmore, C. M., Cox, D. N., and Campbell, A. L. (1982). How women view post-episiotomy pain. *British Medical Journal* **284**, 243–6.

Report on the Confidential Enquiries into Maternal Deaths in England and Wales, 1982–4, (1989). pp. 20–8. Her Majesty's Stationery Office, London.

Reynolds, F. (1993). Pain relief in labour. *British Journal of Obstetrics and Gynaecology* **100**, 979–83.

Rogers, K. B. (1980). An investigation into the efficacy of disposable face masks. *Journal of Clinical Pathology* **33**, 1086–91.

Romney, M. L. (1980). Pre-delivery shaving: an unjustified assault. *Journal of Obstetrics and Gynaecology* **1**, 33–5.

Romney, M. L. and Gordon, H. (1981). Is your enema really necessary? *British Medical Journal* **282**, 1296–71.

Roseveare, M. P. and Bull, M. J. V. (1982). General practitioner obstetrics: two styles of care. *British Medical Journal* **284**, 958–60.

Russell, J. K. (1982). Episiotomy. *British Medical Journal* **284**, 220.

Sangala, V., Dunster, G., Bohin, S., Osborne, J. P. (1990). Perinatal mortality rates in isolated general practitioner maternity units. *British Medical Journal* **301**, 418–20.

Scherjon, S. (1986). A comparison between the organisation of obstetrics in Denmark and The Netherlands. *British Journal of Obstetrics and Gynaecology* **93**, 694–9.

Schweizer, R. T. (1976). Mask wiggling as a potential cause of wound contamination. *Lancet* **ii**, 1129–30.

Sergeant, H. (1986). Should psychiatric patients be granted access to their hospital records? *Lancet* **ii**, 1322–4.

Shearer, J. M. L. (1985). Five-year prospective survey of risk of booking for a home birth in Essex. *British Medical Journal* **291**, 1478–80.

Short, D. (1986). Some consequences of granting patients access to consultants' records. *Lancet* **i**, 1316–18.

Simkin, P. and Enkin, M. (1989). Antenatal classes. In *Effective care in pregnancy and childbirth* (ed. I. Chalmers, M. Enkin, and M. J. N. C. Keirse), pp. 318–34. Oxford University Press, Oxford.

Sjolund, B., Terenius, L., and Eriksson, M. (1977). Increased cerebrospinal fluid levels of endorphins after electro-acupuncture. *Acta Physiologica Scandinavica* **100**, 382–4.

Sleep, J. and Grant, A. (1987). West Berkshire Perineal Management Trial: Three-year follow-up. *British Medical Journal* **295**, 749–51.

Sleep, J., Grant., A., Garcia, J., Elbourne, D., Spencer, J., and Chalmers, I. (1984). West Berkshire Perineal Management Trial. *British Medical Journal* **289**, 587–90.

Smith, L. F. P. and Jewell, D. (1991). Contribution of general practitioners to hospital intra-partum care in maternity units in England and Wales in 1988. *British Medical Journal* **302**, 13–16.

Sosa, R., Kennell, J. H., Klaus, M., Robertson, S., and Urrutia, J. (1980). The effect of a supportive companion on perinatal problems. Length of labour, and mother–infant interaction. *New England Journal of Medicine* **303**, 597–600.

Spencer, J. A. D., Grant, A., Elbourne, D., Garcia, J., and Sleep, J. (1986). A randomized comparison of glycerol-impregnanted chromic catgut with untreated chromic catgut for the repair of perineal trauma. *British Medical Journal of Obstetrics and Gynaecology* **93**, 426–30.

Spiby, H. (1992). Upright versus recumbent position during second stage of labour. In *Oxford database of perinatal trials* (ed. I. Chalmers), Version 1.3, Disk issue 7, Record 3335, Oxford University Press.

Stewart, D. E. (1982). Psychological symptoms following attempted natural childbirth. *Canadian Medical Association Journal* **127**, 713–16.

Stewart, P. and Calder, A. A. (1984). Posture in labour: patients' choice and its effects on performance. *British Journal of Obstetrics and Gynaecology* **91**, 1091–5.

Stewart, P., Hillam, E., and Calder, A. A. (1983). A randomized trial to evaluate the use of a birth chair for delivery. *Lancet* **i**, 1296–8.

Studd, J. W. W., Crawford, J. S., Duignan, N. M., Rowbottom, C. J. F., and Hughes, A. O. (1980). The effect of lumbar epidural analgesia on the rate of cervical dilatation and the outcome of labour of spontaneous onset. *British Journal of Obstetrics and Gynaecology* **87**, 1015–21.

Taylor, G. W., Edgar, W., Taylor, B. A., and Neal, D. G. (1980). How safe is general practitioner obstetrics? *Lancet* **ii**, 1287–9.

Thalme, B., Belfrage, P., Raabe, N. (1974). Lumbar epidural in labour. I. Acid–base balance and clinical condition of mother, fetus and newborn child. *Acta Obstetrica et Gynaecologica Scandinavika* **53**, 27–35.

Thorp, J. M. and Bowes, W. A., (1989). Episiotomy: can its routine use be defended? *American Journal of Obstetrics and Gynecology* **160**, 1027–30.

Thorp, J. M., Bowes, W. A., Brame, R. G., and Cefalo, R. (1987). Selected use of midline episiotomy. *Obstetrics and Gynecology* **70**, 260–2.

Toppozada, N., El-Bossaty, M., El-Rahman, H. A., and El-Din, A. H. S. (1981). Control of intractable atonic post-partum haemorrhage by 15-methyl PgF_{2A}. *Obstetrics and Gynecology* **58**, 327–30.

Turner, M. J., Crowley, P., and MacDonald, D. (1984). The unmasking of delivery room routine. *Journal of Obstetrics and Gynecology* **4**, 188–90.

Turner, M. J., Romney, M. L., Webb, J. B., and Gordon, H. (1986). The birthing chair; and obstetric hazard? *Journal of Obstetrics and Gynecology* **6**, 732–5.

United Kingdom National Case Controlled Study Group (1993). Breastfeeding and risk of breast cancer in young women. *British Medical Journal* **307**, 17–20.

Vacca, A., Grant, A., Wyatt, G., and Chalmers, I. (1983). Portsmouth operative delivery trial: a comparison of vacuum extraction and forceps delivery. *British Journal of Obstetrics and Gynaecology* **90**, 1107–12.

Vaughan-Williams, K., Johnson, A., and Ledward, G. (1974). A comparison of central venous pressure changes in the third stage of labour following oxytocic drugs and diazepam. *Journal of Obstetrics and Gynaecology of the British Commonwealth* **81**, 596–9.

Veland, K. and Hansen, J. M. (1969). Maternal cardiovascual haemodynamics. *American Journal of Obstetrics and Gynecology* **103**, 1–7.

von Kries, R. (1991). Neonatal vitamin K. *British Medical Journal* **303**, 1084–3.

Wallis, L., Shnider, S. M., Palahniuk, R. J., and Spivey, H. G. (1974). An evaluation of acupuncture analgesia in obstetrics. *Anesthesiology* **41**, 596–601.

Williams, M. C., Knuppel, R. A., Weiss, A., Kanarak, N., and O'Brien, W. F. (1991). A prospective randomized comparison of forceps and vacuum assisted delivery. *American Journal of Obstetrics and Gynecology* **164**, 323.

Williams, R. N., Thom, M. H., and Studd, J. W. W. (1980). A study of the benefits and acceptibility of ambulation in spontaneous labour. *British Journal of Obstetrics and Gynaecology* **87**, 122–6.

Wolman, W. L., Chalmers, L., Hofmeyr, G. J., and Nikodem, V. C. (1993). Post-partum depression and companionship in the clinical birth environment. *American Journal of Obstetrics and Gynecology* **168**, 1388–93.

Zander, L. I., Watson, M., Taylor, R. W., and Morrell, D. C. (1978). Integration of general practitioner and specialist antenatal care. *Journal of the Royal College of General Practitioners* **28**, 455–8.

Index